Intangible Spirits and Graven Images:
The Iconography of Deities in the Pre-Islamic Iranian World

Magical and Religious Literature of Late Antiquity

Series Editors

Shaul Shaked
Siam Bhayro

VOLUME 4

The titles published in this series are listed at brill.com/mrla

Intangible Spirits and Graven Images: The Iconography of Deities in the Pre-Islamic Iranian World

By

Michael Shenkar

BRILL

LEIDEN · BOSTON

This paperback was originally published in hardback as Volume 4 in the series *Magical and Religious Literature of Late Antiquity*.

Cover illustration: Investiture relief of Ardašīr I at Naqš-e Rağab (drawing E. Smekens © BAMI).

Library of Congress Cataloging-in-Publication Data

Shenkar, Michael.
Intangible spirits and graven images : the iconography of deities in the pre-Islamic Iranian world / by Michael Shenkar.
pages cm. – (Magical and religious literature of late antiquity ; VOLUME 4)
Revision of the author's thesis–Hebrew University of Jerusalem, 2013.
Includes bibliographical references and index.
ISBN 978-90-04-28148-6 (hardback : alk. paper) – ISBN 978-90-04-28149-3 (e-book)
1. Gods in art. 2. Art, Ancient–Iran. 3. Art and religion–Iran–History–To 1500. 4. Iran–Antiquities. 5. Iran–Civilization–To 640. I. Title.

N8191.I7S54 2014
704.9'4895–dc23

2014025537

Typeface for the Latin, Greek, and Cyrillic scripts: "Brill". See and download: brill.com/brill-typeface.

ISBN 978-90-04-36234-5 (paperback, 2018)
ISBN 978-90-04-28148-6 (hardback, 2014)
ISBN 978-90-04-28149-3 (e-book, 2014)

This book is printed on acid-free paper and produced in a sustainable manner.

CONTENTS

LIST OF FIGURES

LIST OF COLOR PLATES

LIST OF ABBREVIATIONS

1. *Texts*[1]

Ag.	Agat'angełos, *History of the Armenians* (Thomson 1976)
AWN	*Ardā Wīrāz Nāmag* (Vahman 1986)
BK	Theodore Bar Koni, *Scholia* (Hespel and Draguet 1982)
Bal'amī	*Mohammad b. Jarir Ṭabari, La chronique sur la version persane d'Abou-'Ali Mohammad Bel'ami* (Zotenberg 1867/1874)
Balādhurī	Al-Balādhurī, *The Origins of the Islamic State* (Murgotten 1924)
Bīrūnī	Al-Bīrūnī, *al-Āṯār al-bāqiya* (Sal'e 1957)
Dd	*Dādestān ī Dēnīg* (Jaafari-Dehaghi 1998)
Dk (M)	*Dēnkard* (Madan)
DMX	*Dādestān ī Mēnōg ī Xrad* (Chunakova 1997)
EK	Eznik Koghbac'i, *Refutation of the Sects* (Arevshatyan 2008)
GBd	*Greater or Iranian Bundahišn*
HN	*Hadōxt Nask*
IBd	*Indian Bundahišn*
Ibn Ḥauqal	Ibn Ḥauqal. *Configuration de la terre* (*Kitab surat al-ard*) (Kramers and Wiet 1964)
KAP	*Kār-nāmag ī Ardašīr ī Pābagān* (Grenet 2003b)
Kandia	*The Small Kandia* (Vyatkin 1905)
KC LK	*The Life of K'art'li* (*K'artlis C'xovreba*), *Life of the Kings* (Thomson 1996)
KC LN	*The Life of K'art'li* (*K'artlis C'xovreba*), *Life of St. Nino* (Thomson 1996)
Mart.Susan.	Iakob C'urtaveli, *Martyrdom of Saint Susan* (*Martwlobay Šušanikisi*)
Mas'ūdī	Al-Mas'ūdī, *Les prairies d'or* (Pellat 1965)
MHD	*Mādayān ī Hāzar Dādestān* (Perikhanian 1997)
MK LN	*The Conversion of K'art'li* (*Mok'c'evay K'art'lisay*) (*The Life of St. Nino*) (Lerner 2004)
MX	Moses Khorenats'i. *History of the Armenians* (Thomson 1976)
Narshakhī	Narshakhī. *The History of Bukhara* (Frye 1954)
PB	*The Epic Histories Attributed to P'awstos Buzand* (Garsoïan 1989)
PhlRDd	*The Pahlavi Rivāyat Accompanying the Dādestān ī Dēnīg* (Williams 1990)
WZ	*Wizīdagīhā ī Zādspram* (Gignoux and Tafazzoli 1993)
SE	*Šahrestānīhā ī Ērānšahr* (Daryaee 2002)
Shahrastānī	Al-Shahrastānī, *Livre des religions et des sects* (Jolivet and Monnot 1993)
Shāh-nāma	Firdausī, *Shāh-nāma* (Khaleghi-Motlagh 1988/2008)
ŠGW	Škand Gumānīg Wizār
ŠnŠ	*Šāyast nē Šāyast* (Kotwal 1969)
Sr	Sīh-rōzag (Raffaelli 2014)
ŠW	*Šā-Wahrām* (Jamasp-Asana 1992)
Ṭabarī	*The History of al-Ṭabarī*, 40 Vols. (Yarshater 1989–2007)
TS	*Tārīkh-i Sīstān* (Smirnova 1974)
Vd.	*Vīdēvdāt*
Y.	*Yasna*
Yt.	*Yašt*
ZWY	*Zand ī Wahman Yasn* (Cereti 1995)

[1] The abbreviations of the Greek and Latin texts usually follow those of *The Oxford Classical Dictionary*.

2. *Books, Series and Journals*

AA	*Acta Antiqua.*
AAASHB	*Acta Antiqua Academiae Scientiarum Hungaricae Budapest.*
ACSS	*Ancient Civilizations from Scythia to Siberia.*
AEPHE	*Annuaire de l'École pratique des hautes études, section des sciences religieuses.*
AI	*Acta Iranica.*
AIUO	*Annali del Istituto Universitario Orientale.*
AJA	*American Journal of Archaeology.*
AJN	*American Journal of Numismatics.*
AGE	*Arheologicheskiy sbornik Gosudarstvennogo Ermitazha* [*Archaeological Bulletin of the State Hermitage*].
AMI	*Archäologische Mitteilungen aus Iran und Turan.*
ANES	*Ancient Near Eastern Studies.*
ART	*Arkheologicheskie Raboty v Tadzhikistane* [*Archaeological Research in Tajikistan*].
BAI	*Bulletin of the Asia Institute.*
BAIPAA	*Bulletin of the American Institute for Persian Art and Archeology*
BAOM	*Bulletin of the Ancient Orient Museum.*
BAR	*Biblical Archaeology Review.*
BJRULM	*Bulletin of the John Rylands University Library of Manchester.*
BMM	*Bulletin of Miho Museum.*
BSOAS	*Bulletin of the School of Oriental and African Studies, University of London.*
CRAI	*Comptes rendus de l'Académie des Inscriptions et Belles-lettres*
DB	*Drevnyaya Baktriya* [*Ancient Bactria*].
EI2	*The Encyclopaedia of Islam 2nd Edition.*
EIr	*Encyclopedia Iranica.*
EV	*Epigrafika Vostoka*
EW	*East and West.*
IA	*Iranica Antiqua.*
IANT	*Izvestiya Akademii Nauk Turkmenskoy SSR* [*Proceedings of the Academy of Sciences of the Soviet Republic of Turkmenistan*].
IJ	*Irano-Judaica.*
IJAH	*Iranian Journal of Archaeology and History.*
IFZh	*Istoriko–filologicheskiy zhurnal* [*Historical–Philological Journal*].
IMKU	*Istoriya material'noy kul'tury Uzbekistana* [*History of the Material Culture of Uzbekistan*].
IANTSSR	*Izvestiya otdeleniya obshchestvennykh nauk Akademii nauk Tadzhikskoy SSR* [*Bulletin of the Section of Social Studies of Tajik SSR Academy of Science*].
JA	*Journal Asiatique.*
JAOS	*Journal of the American Oriental Society.*
JDAI	*Jahrbuch des Deutschen Archäologischen Instituts.*
JIAAA	*Journal of Inner Asian Art and Archaeology.*
JJS	*Journal of Jewish Studies.*
JMEOS	*Journal of the Manchester Egyptian and Oriental Society.*
JNES	*Journal of Near Eastern Studies.*
JNSL	*Journal of Northwest Semitic Languages.*
JONS	*Journal of the Oriental Numismatic Society.*
JPS	*Journal of Persianate Studies.*
JRAS	*Journal of the Royal Asiatic Society.*
JSAI	*Jerusalem Studies in Arabic and Islam.*
KSIIMK	*Kratkie soobshcheniya Instituta istorii material'noy kul'tury* [*Brief Notes of the Institute of History of Material Culture*].
LCL	*Loeb Classical Library.*
MMJ	*Metropolitan Museum Journal.*
MDAFA	*Mémoires de la Délégation Archéologique Française en Afghanistan.*
MDOG	*Mitteilungen der Deutschen Orient-Gesellschaft zu Berlin.*
MPAE	*Materialy Pendzhikentskoy arkheologicheskoy ekspeditsii* [*Proceedings of the Panjikent Archaeological Expedition*]

NIB	*Nāme-ye Irān-e Bāstān.*
NTA	*Numismatika Tsentral'noy Azii* [*The Numismatics of Central Asia*].
PBA	*Proceedings of the British Academy.*
PIFK	*Problemy istorii, filologii i kul'tury* [*Journal of Historical, Philological and Cultural Studies*].
PTKLA	*Protokoly Turkestanskogo kruzhka lyubiteley arkheologii* [*The Protocols of the Turkestan Archaeology Circle*].
RA	*Revue archéologique.*
RHR	*Revue de l'Histoire des Religions*
RIA	*Reallexikon der Assyriologie und Vorderasiatischen Archäologie.*
RSO	*Rivista degli Studi Orientali.*
SA	*Sovetskaya archeologiya* [*The Archaeology of the USSR*].
SI	*Studia Iranica.*
SGE	*Soobshcheniya Gosudarstvennogo Ermitazha* [*Bulletin of the State Hermitage Museum*].
SRAA	*Silk Road Art and Archaeology.*
TGE	*Trudy Gosudarstvennogo Ermitazha* [*Transactions of the State Hermitage Museum*].
Topoi	*Topoi Orient–Occident.*
TOVGE	*Trudy Otdela vostoka Gosudarstvennogo Ermitazha* [*Bulletin of the Oriental Section of the State Hermitage Museum*].
TSUS	*Tbilisis Saxelmtsipo Universitetis Shromebi* [*Proceedings of Tbilisi State University*].
TUTAKE	*Trudy Yuzhnoturkmenskoy arheologicheskoy kompleksnoy ekspeditsii* [*Proceedings of the South-Turkmenian Archaeological Complex Expedition*].
VDI	*Vestnik drevney istorii* [*Journal of Ancient History*].
VPSTBI	*Vestnik Pravoslavnogo Svyato-Tikhonovskogo Bogoslovskogo Instituta* [*Journal of Orthodox Svyato-Tikhonov Theological Institute*].
WZKM	*Wiener Zeitschrift für die Kunde des Morgenlandes.*
ZDMG	*Zeitschrift der Deutschen Morgenländischen Gesellschaft.*

ACKNOWLEDGEMENTS

This book is a revised version of my doctoral dissertation submitted to the Hebrew University of Jerusalem in 2013. It is a pleasure to express my gratitude and appreciation to my research supervisors, Joseph Patrich and Shaul Shaked. It was the suggestion and the instigation of Joseph Patrich that initially introduced me to the civilization of pre-Islamic Iran, eventually leading me to the fascinating area of ancient Iranian studies. Shaul Shaked guided me on this long path and was exceptionally generous in sharing with me his immense knowledge and deep understanding of everything Iranian, as well as the books from the unrivalled "Shaked's library".

This study has benefited from the advice, help and expertise of a great number of scholars, colleagues and friends. I would like to extend my special thanks to Domenico Agostini, Samra Azarnouche, Robert Bracey, Osmund Bopearachchi, Matteo Compareti, Joe Cribb, Vesta S. Curtis, Avner Ecker, Mark Garrison, Alexey Gorin, Mariam Gvelesiani, Rika Gyselen, Wouter Henkelman, Geoffrey Herman, Georgina Herrmann, Reuven Kiperwasser, Gunvor Lindström, Pavel Lurje, Sergey Minov, Tigran Mkrtychev, François Ory, Bruno Overlaet, Céline Redard, Edward Rtveladze, Julia Rubanovich, Véronique Schiltz, Yana Tchekhanovets, Nikolaus Schindel, François Thierry and Jörg Wagner. The comments made on the text of my dissertation by Pierfrancesco Callieri were priceless and helped me to avoid many mistakes. I am particularly grateful to Jean Kellens for generously hosting me at the Collège de France in 2011. The time that I was able to spend in Paris was invaluable for the progress of my research. I am indebted to Siam Bhayro for revising the manuscript and helping me to express my ideas in a more clear and readable way.

However, much more than can be acknowledged, this work owes a debt of gratitude to the intellectual and practical support, generous help, and constant encouragement, which I received from Frantz Grenet. He has shown limitless enthusiasm for my research and his groundbreaking and fundamental studies on ancient Iranian iconography have always been a source of inspiration for me.

This research was carried out with generous financial support from the Hebrew University of Jerusalem and the National Council for Higher Education in Israel. My research at the State Hermitage Museum in Saint Petersburg was made possible by a Mandel Travel Grant from the Faculty of Humanities of the Hebrew University of Jerusalem.

Finally, I would like to thank Shahar Shirtz. When I was just beginning to think about a subject for a dissertation, he told me that he would like to read a book on the iconography of Iranian deities.

PREFACE

The primary concern of this book is to investigate how the ancient Iranians perceived their deities, how they represented them and what was the place of these representations in the Iranian cults. Starting from the first millennium BCE, the ancient Near East was dominated by two ethno-linguistic groups, the Semites and the Iranians. While the religious world, temple architecture and the pantheon of the former have received much attention and are relatively well known, we are still far away from achieving the same degree of understanding of the latter. In sharp contrast with Mesopotamian, Syrian, Nabatean, Egyptian, Hittite and especially Canaanite and Israelite religious iconography, which have been extensively studied,[1] the iconographic repertoire of Iranian deities has not been subjected to systematic research.

The Iranian world occupied a unique position as the cultural crossroads of Eurasia. Iranian religious iconography was an important and integral component of ancient Near Eastern culture, and was formed in constant dialogue with both the Mespotamian and Graeco-Roman civilizations. However, it also played an important role in the formation of Hindu and Buddhist cultic imagery and in the later period came into contact with Chinese art.

This study is based on the analysis of pictorial depictions of Iranian deities on a variety of monuments and objects, which serves as a fundamental basis for the discussion of their meaning in relation to the historical evidence. During decades of exploration and excavations in Iran and Central Asia, a considerable body of religious iconographic data has accumulated. However, these monuments have never been studied as a group and they are assembled and systematically examined here for the first time. I have made every effort to collect all known representations of Iranian gods, although I am fully aware of the fact that some were inevitably overlooked and left out. Future discoveries will also undoubtedly add new exciting images and allow identifications of more deities.

In addition to the examination of the origins, development and significance of the iconography of each deity, this study explores the perception of anthropomorphism and aniconism in the religious imagery of the ancient Iranian world through the material evidence and the written sources. Despite a preference towards aniconic representations of deities, especially in Western Iran, I have attempted to show that the perception of the divine in ancient Iran was anthropomorphic from the very beginning.

The Iranian iconographic pantheon is arranged in alphabetical order and the developments in the iconography of each deity are treated separately for Western and for Eastern Iran, reflecting their cultural and historical disparity. Since the literature on certain objects discussed in this study is immense, no attempt has been made to provide an exhaustive bibliography. References are given only to the most important, comprehensive and recent discussions. The "pre-iconographical description" of the objects is kept to a necessary minimum. In fact, some monuments, like the Behestūn relief of Darius I have been so often discussed and reproduced that only a cursory description is necessary.

The Iranian names and toponyms used throughout the work usually conform to the form given in the *Encyclopædia Iranica*. Generally, Avestan forms of the divine names have been used for clarity and uniformity. However, in some cases, the forms other than Avestan that have become familiar in the scholarly literature have been preferred (e.g. MP. *Šahrewar* instead of Av. *xšaϑra vairiia*).

This study does not take upon itself the all-inclusive examination of the origin and historical development of the cults of Iranian gods; a task that will hopefully be undertaken by an interdisciplinary team

---

[1] For instance, see Patrich 1990; Dietrich and Loretz 1992; Green 1995; Mettinger 1995; Keel and Uehlinger 1998; Ornan 2005a.

of philologists, historians, archaeologists and historians of religion. My foremost goal was to create a reliable work of reference for anyone interested in Iranian religious iconography. It is my hope that it succeeds in also providing new insights into the religious and cultural situation in the Iranian world before its transformation following the Islamic conquest.

CHAPTER 1

INTRODUCTION

Unlike the Mesopotamian, Egyptian and Greek religions, for which there is a relative abundance of primary literary sources at our disposal, contemporary texts referring to Iranian religions and cults are extremely sparse and fragmentary. Art is the most important "text" of illiterate and oral societies. Ancient Iranians certainly belong to this category since, from the dawn of their history, they preferred to transmit their literary and religious compositions orally, while choosing to write down mainly administrative and economic texts. Therefore, iconography is of tremendous importance for the study of Zoroastrianism, and indeed for the entire religious and cultural history of the pre-Islamic Iranian world.

Iconography can be described as the study of the meaning of pictorial expression through the examination of its content, symbolism and context. One of the most prominent art historians of the twentieth century, Erwin Panofsky, proposed to distinguish between three layers in the analyses of iconography: (1) the "pre-iconographical description", which refers to the "primary or natural subject matter—(a) factual, (b) expressional, constituting the world of artistic motifs"; (2) "iconographical analyses", which is a "secondary or conventional subject matter, constituting the world of images, stories and allegories" and (3) "iconographical interpretation", which is an "intristic meaning or content, constituting the world of 'symbolical' values".[1]

One of the important preliminary questions that every scholar of religious iconography has to confront is defining the divine. In other words, how and according to which criteria does one distinguish between the representation of a mortal and of a deity? Broadly speaking, the Iranian tradition of pictorial expression followed the ancient Near Eastern one, which, as distinct from the artistic representations of ancient Egypt and Greece, was usually not provided with an accompanying text explaining and supplementing the picture. Fortunately for modern scholars, the Kushan kings labeled the deities of their extraordinary Numismatic Pantheon, probably following the example of contemporary Roman coinage.[2] Had the Kushans not adopted this practice, it undoubtedly would have been impossible to identify many of their gods by comparing their attributes and iconography with the data of extant Zoroastrian texts. This is, for example, one of the problems posed by Sogdian iconography that regrettably does not follow the Kushan tradition. Without the corresponding labels on the Kushan coins, nobody would ever imagine that the god whose iconography is that of the Indian Śiva could be in fact connected to the Iranian Vayu,[3] the odd four-armed deity with Hindu attributes wearing a Greek helmet could be identified with Vohu Manah,[4] and the male god standing before the horse is the same as Avestan goddess Drvāspā.[5] This should make us especially cautious when trying to recognize unlabeled Iranian divine images based upon the Zoroastrian written sources.[6]

Iranian art, with few exceptions, did not tend to depict mortals with superhuman attributes. Therefore, when a character has some supernatural trait or characteristic (such as standing on a beast, having

---

1 Panofsky 1962: 14–15.
2 Alram 2004: 55–56; Cribb 2007: 367.
3 See p. 154 ff.
4 See p. 163 ff.
5 See p. 96 ff.
6 For a detailed discussion, see below p. 6 ff.

wings or four arms or flames rising from its shoulders, or being accompanied by worshippers), we can be relatively confident that a deity is depicted. However, none of these attributes is obligatory. For instance, in Sogdian art, there are definite divine images that are of ordinary size, without nimbus or flames, and not enthroned,[7] as there are also royal representations of superior size, nimbate and with flames. Furthermore, some of these attributes, like burning shoulders, were also occasionally employed for royal representations. Numerous and nuanced interconnections and interrelations existed between divine and royal iconography and it is often not easy to distinguish between the two, especially if the context is lacking.

However, once the image has been successfully classified (with various degrees of certainty) as divine, another important question arises—how do we decide whether it is in fact "Iranian"? Can we define an "Iranian religious iconography", a collection of specific traits, characteristics and style that can be identified as peculiar to Iranian art? In the course of history, many foreign deities of various origins were venerated in the Iranian world. Some were incorporated into local Iranian pantheons,[8] while the adoration of others was limited, short-lived and supposedly left no iconographic traces.[9] This comes as no surprise, taking into account cultural contacts, conquests and population movements, which inevitably had a profound effect on cultural and religious patterns in Iran. In some cases, the interaction of the Iranian tradition with foreign ones resulted in a well-known phenomenon of religious and artistic syncretism; an Iranian deity was identified with a foreign one. This tendency is especially noteworthy during the Hellenistic and Kushan periods. Therefore, it is a natural desire among scholars to identify any statue of a Greek deity found in Iran as representing an Iranian divinity with similar characteristics and attributes.

However, in most cases, when there are no further indications, it is perhaps best to avoid such identifications. Without additional, preferably epigraphic evidence,[10] we simply do not know whether Iranians considered this Greek imagery to represent their own gods. Given the paucity of textual evidence, it is also problematic to draw firm conclusions from iconography about the name and spheres of responsibility of a given deity. Usually one has to rely exclusively on iconographical features and their analogies. Using the terminology of Panofsky, our ignorance of themes and concepts often does not allow us to confidently proceed beyond the "pre-iconographical description".

For our purpose, a divine image can be considered "Iranian" if it can be shown to depict a deity that specifically belongs to the Iranian religious tradition or those gods, like Nana, who have entered the Iranian pantheon(s) at a very early date and were certainly no longer understood by ancient Iranians themselves as "foreign" deities. Since our aim is to collect and discuss the representations of Iranian deities only, it is assumed, *a priori*, that all examples of foreign religious art not accompanied by an inscription, or any other markers that would allow its "Iranian" identification, represent foreign deities and not Iranian ones. Therefore, distinctive Mesopotamian, Greek, Hindu and Buddhist religious iconography from the Iranian world is excluded, as are mass-produced objects such as terracotta.[11] Only pictorial expressions of the divine from the Iranian world itself are incorporated in the discussion of the Iconographic Pantheon (with very few significant exceptions). Examples of Iranian iconography originating from regions beyond the borders of the Iranian world, like the reliefs of Commagene or Sino-Sogdian funeral art, are consistently referred to, but are not included among the representations of gods.

---

7 Marshak 1989: 118.

8 Like the goddesses Nana, see p. 116 ff.

9 For example, the enigmatic deity *ssn* who was worshipped in Parthiena during the Parthian period; see Schwartz 1996; Schwartz 1998; Gignoux 1998. According to Livshits 2008: 109, he was a Parthian god whose cult spread from Parthiena to Pars and whose name became popular as a personal name in early Sasanian Iran.

10 The statuette of Silenus-Marsyas playing the flute from Takht-i Sangin (p. 128) and the statue of Heracles from Mesene (p. 11) are exceptional instances.

11 See the study of Central Asian terracottas by Dvurechenskaya 2005.

I have made frequent use of data from the theophoric components of Iranian personal names as an indication of the existence of a cult of a certain deity in the region and period where this name is attested. However, one must note that it is by no means clear to what extent the prevalence such theophoric components reflect the deity's status. According to the important methodological observation made by Rüdiger Schmitt, only the newly created theophoric compounds, attested for the first time in a certain era, can provide a reliable indication of the popularity of those deities.[12]

Ancient Iranian art has been the subject of a number of general surveys, although all of them were composed several decades ago;[13] and there is little discussion devoted to Iranian religious iconography in general, most of which is quite limited in scope and/or outdated.[14] Scholars usually tended to limit their discussion to a certain deity, period or culture. Students of Iranian iconography have always been few in number. The studies of such scholars as Roman Ghirshman, Galina Pugachenkova, Boris Marshak, Martha Carter, Guitty Azarpay, Katsumi Tanabe, Markus Mode, Matteo Compareti and especially Frantz Grenet, have laid the foundations for any inquiry into the field of ancient Iranian art and it will be apparent from the following pages how much this book owes to their scholarship. However, an investigation, which covers the entire pre-Islamic Iranian world both chronologically and geographically, has not been yet attempted.

The modern study of Iranian religious anthropomorphism and cultic statuary has a longer history, going back to the entry in the *The Encyclopaedia of Religion and Ethics* published ninety-eight years ago by the noted American Iranist Abraham V.W. Jackson, which opens with the following statement:

> From the earliest antiquity the Persians had no idols in the sense of a representation of the godhead set up as an object of worship. Such allusions to the practice as are found are always in the way of condemning it as an abhorrent custom employed by foreigners and unbelievers. Zoroaster, the Prophet of Ancient Irān, makes no reference to idol-worship, even though his vision saw graphic pictures of the hosts of heaven. These vivid images, however, which might easily have been given a plastic form, remained, with the seer and with his people, simply a visualization of the ideal. Throughout the history of the religion of Irān, idolatry played no part.[15]

The only other systematic analysis of Iranian idolatry, which was undertaken by Mary Boyce in 1975,[16] is limited to Western Iran and I have critically revised it elsewhere.[17] The whole subject of idolatry and idol-worship in Iran has been so far insufficiently investigated. It is instructive that the articles "idol", "idol-worship" or "idol-temple" are missing in *EIr*, which is probably the most important scholarly enterprise ever undertaken in the area of Iranian studies.

About three decades ago the prominent Belgian archaeologist, Louis Vanden Berghe, reviewing the state of research into pre-Islamic Iranian art, noted that, contrary to the art of other peoples in the Near East, the Iranians were deprived of religious iconography.[18] And just seven years ago, the Italian specialist of Sogdian art, Matteo Compareti, remarked that, "... it is not possible to say much about Persian divinities during the Pre-Islamic period".[19] It is hoped that this book will demonstrate that pre-Islamic Iranians in fact possessed a rich, eclectic, complex and fascinating religious iconography about which much can be said.

---

12 See Schmitt 1991; Schmitt 1998.
13 The most notable are Pope and Ackerman 1964–1981; Ghirshman 1962; Ghirshman 1964; Godard 1965; Porada 1965; Lukonin 1977; Staviskiy 1974.
14 For instance, see Duchesne-Guillemin 1972; Basirov 2001.
15 Jackson 1915: 151.
16 Boyce 1975a.
17 Shenkar forthcoming a. See also p. 183.
18 Vanden Berghe 1985: 51.
19 Compareti 2006a: 163.

1. *The Iranian World*

1. *Geography*

The terms "Iran" and "Iranian world", as used in this study, refer to the region from the Hindu-Kush mountains in the East to the Zagros ridge in the West, and from the steppe zone of Southern Russia, Ukraine and Kazakhstan in the North to the Persian Gulf in the South, which in the first millennium BCE and the first millennium CE was dominated by Iranian-speaking people who shared a common cultural and religious background and ancestry (pl. 1). Historically, and in many senses also culturally, the Iranian world can be divided into two parts, Eastern and Western, with the great deserts of Dasht-i Lut and Dasht-i Kavir dividing them. However, despite considerable spatial and chronological diversity and many local variations, it is possible to speak of an Iranian unity sharing a number of common historical, cultural, linguistic and religious characteristics that could and should be studied as a unified phenomenon.

The Achaemenians, Parthians and Sasanians ruled empires that consisted of many different regions with heterogeneous populations. Historically and economically, the most significant region was undoubtedly Mesopotamia, which was an important province for all the western Iranian dynasties, serving as the royal seat of the Parthian and the Sasanian kings. However, Mesopotamia is excluded from this study because, although ruled for over a millennium by Iranian sovereigns, it remained predominantly Semitic speaking (with an important Greek speaking population) and it is unlikely that it ever had a considerable population of Iranian descent.

Almost all material of religious significance from key Parthian sites, such as Palmyra, Ashur, Hatra and Dura Europos, is Graeco-Semitic.[20] It is instructive that, among the hundreds of divine names mentioned in inscriptions, Iranian deities are almost totally absent. Even at Hatra, which was under Parthian rule for most of its history (unlike Palmyra and Dura Europos), all recorded divinities are of Semitic origin.[21]

Another region located beyond the initial limits of the Iranian world, but with exceptionally strong historical and cultural ties to Iran, is the Southern Caucasus (the modern republics of Armenia, Georgia and Azerbaijan). Probably during the sixth century BCE, the South Caucasus was incorporated into the Achaemenian Empire, and Armenia, Iberia (K'art'li) and Colchis were subjected to profound and long-term Iranian influence in material culture, architecture and religion.[22] It is not entirely clear, from either the Armenian or the Iranian sources, whether or not Armenia was considered part of *Ērānšahr*.[23] However, it is beyond doubt that culturally it was much more Iranian than any other land inhabited by non-Iranians and that it occupied a place of special importance for the Parthian and the Sasanian kings.[24]

2. *Historical Overview*

The chronological boundaries of this study are determined by the accepted periodization of the history of ancient Iran—from the appearance of the Iranian tribes on the historical scene until the Arab

20 The religion of Palmyra and Hatra was described in a recent study as "preponderantly Semitic, with notable Babylonian and Arab influences"; see Dirven 2011: 164. One exception is the title of the god Nergal and the dogs that accompany him in Parthian Hatra, that possibly show the influence of Iranian religious beliefs. See Dirven 2009. There is also limited evidence for the presence of Parthian language and culture at Dura Europos: Millar 1998.

21 Dirven 2011: 169.

22 On the Caucasus in the Achaemenian period, see Knauss 2005; Knauss 2006. Regarding Iranian elements in Georgian material culture, see Tsetskhladze 2001; Lordkipanidze 2001; Kipiani 2004.

23 See the discussion in Garsoïan 1985: X, 6–7, n. 17; XI, 29–35; Thomson 2004: 376. On the concept of *Ērānšahr* and its significance, see Gnoli 1989b.

24 See Garsoïan 1985: X who provides a *prolegomenon* to the study of Iranian elements in Armenian culture with an exhaustive bibliography. For a recent survey of the contribution of Armenian sources to the political history of the Sasanian Empire, see also Greenwood 2008.

conquest of almost the entire Iranian world.[25] The Iranians split from the semi-nomadic Indo-Iranian people (usually associated with the archaeological "Andronovo culture" located in the southern Ural region) at an uncertain date, perhaps early in the second millennium BCE. After that, speakers of Iranian languages migrated and dispersed over vast regions of the Eurasian steppes and Central Asia, entering the Iranian plateau (it is not yet definitely established whether they came via Central Asia or the Caucasus) and reaching the Zagros mountains in the west.

By 835 BCE, when Iranians were mentioned for the first time in Assyrian annals, Iranian principalities and chiefdoms were already firmly established in Western Iran, and the Medes, Persians and other Iranian ethnic groups were being formed from acculturation with autochthonous Hurrian, Elamite and other local populations of the Zagros region. Gradually growing in power and attaining a greater level of sophistication in their administration, organization and state institutions under the influence of Mesopotamian civilization and its Imperial cultures, they were able to defeat and ultimately replace the Assyrians and Babylonians as the hegemons of the Ancient Near East towards the middle of the first millennium BCE. The existence of a "Median Empire" has been questioned over the last few decades, with the suggestion that the Medes were, in fact, no more than a loose confederation of tribes. Be that as it may, it is the Persian Empire, ruled by two consecutive dynasties, the Teispid and the Achaemenian, that can be considered the first Iranian Empire.

In the sixth century BCE the Persians united almost all of the sedentary Iranian people and, for the first time, incorporated both Western and Eastern parts of the Iranian world into one political entity. The Achaemenian Empire remains to this day the largest Iranian Empire ever, and was a source of inspiration for many future Persian rulers. Faced with the unprecedented might of the Achaemenians, only the diverse Scythian tribes in the Eurasian steppes, of all the Iranians, were able to resist Persian expansionism and retain their independence.

The Macedonian conqueror, Alexander the Great, was the last king to rule the united Empire, and his death in Babylon in 323 BCE was followed by its rapid disintegration. In the middle of the third century BCE, Parthiena and Bactria broke from the Seleucid kingdom and attained *de facto* independence, once again politically separating the Eastern Iranian lands from the West. Parthiena was soon conquered by the nomadic Parni Scythian tribes, who assimilated into the local population and established the Parthian Empire in the second century BCE by crushing the Seleucids and capturing Mesopotamia.

In Sogdiana and Bactria, the Graeco-Bactrian kingdom was overrun by successive waves of Saka and Yuezhi nomads who, starting from the middle of the second century BCE, established on its ruins principalities ruled by rival clans. In the first century CE, the leader of the clan of the Kushans, Kujula Kadphises, subdued the other chiefdoms and laid the foundation for the Kushan Empire that ruled Bactria and parts of modern Pakistan and India until the third century CE. At the height of its power, the Kushan Empire formed the central link in the "Silk Road", mediating between China and the Parthian and Roman Empires. The Parthian and the Kushan periods are sometimes described as the "Iranian Renaissance", the period when Iranians again took power after the foreign, Hellenic "interlude". The Parthians and the Kushans were indeed Iranians, but not Persians. It was in Pars, the heartland of the Achaemenians that preserved many traits of Persian culture during the Hellenistic and Parthian periods, that the new Persian dynasty of the Sasanians was to arise.

It is likely that its founder, Ardašīr I, succeeded in uniting Mesopotamia, Western Iran and parts of Eastern Iran under Persian rule for the first time since the Achaemenians. It is in the Sasanian era

---

25 For a general introduction to the history of the ancient Iranian world, see the relevant entries in the *EIr* and Frye 1984, which, although dated, remains the only study that fully treats both Western and Eastern Iran in a balanced manner. For more recent useful surveys of the major periods of Iranian history and valuable case studies, see also two new *Oxford Handbooks* edited by Daryaee 2012 and Potts 2013.

that the Avesta was edited, written down and canonized.[26] In this period Zoroastrianism acquired its familiar and distinctive form, with the core Middle Persian Zoroastrian literature being composed and state-clergy relations being transformed.

In the East, starting from the third century CE, nomadic confederations of uncertain origin and mixed ethnic composition, known as Chionites, Kidarites and Hephtalites, established successive states bordering the Sasanian Empire, triggering complex and intense cultural exchange, trade and frequent warfare with the Sasanians. In the fourth century CE, a unique Sogdian civilization began to evolve in the valleys of the Zeravshan and the Kashka-darya rivers, beyond the northern borders of the Sasanian controlled area. In contrast to the superseding Imperial entities of Western Iran, Sogdian culture was created by independent or semi-independent city-states ruled by local lords. The urban population and merchants enjoyed a degree of political power unparalleled anywhere else in Iranian history.

In the seventh and eighth centuries the Sasanian Empire and the Sogdian principalities fell to the armies of the Muslim Arabs. The Islamic conquest and subsequent conversion of almost all Iranians to Islam (the Caucasian Ossetians are the only Iranians who are predominantly Christian), and their incorporation into the Caliphate, inaugurated a new era in the history of the Iranian world.

2. *Zoroastrian Texts and Iranian Iconography*

Like the study of Iranian religions in general, research into Iranian religious iconography has also been almost completely bound to the Avesta and Middle Persian Zoroastrian literature. Deities, images, animals and symbols have all been interpreted based on the descriptions found in these texts. However, the very relevance to all Iranians of the Avesta, Zoroastrian practices and other materials preserved in the Pahlavi texts is by no means self-evident.

This has not escaped the attention of those who have studied Iranian religious pictorial expressions. In 1972 Jacques Duchesne-Guillemin observed that "une sorte d'hiatus" exists between Iranian sacred texts and Iranian religious iconography.[27] It is instructive that, despite the fact that the Avesta is a "Sasanian book",[28] even for Sasanian culture, the evidence of the usage of the Avesta as a source of visual imagery is insignificant at best. Gherardo Gnoli observed that "the study of Sassanian iconography for interpretations designed to explain everything—or practically everything—in terms of the canons of the Zoroastrian religious tradition" is "an exaggerated and restrictive tendency".[29] Prudence O. Harper further stressed that "in Sasanian material culture the Zoroastrian presence is ambiguous, hard to define and difficult to recognize …",[30] and Albert De Jong has recently remarked regarding the Avesta that it:

> was not considered a source of narrative traditions or imagery. Its practical use in many areas of Sasanian culture, such as politics, propaganda, and belles lettres, would have been rather limited. The best way of seeing these texts is to see them as a collection of ritual texts in the heads of priests.[31]

Elsewhere, De Jong further observed that:

> The idea that the Avesta would be in any sense comparable to the Bible in Hellenistic Judaism or in Christianity, that is, a source of inspiration and stories for everyone to exploit, as a sacred book, is surely misleading.[32]

---

26 For the most recent discussion, see Panaino 2012: 79–84.
27 Duchesne-Guillemin 1972: 265.
28 Kellens 1998: 525.
29 Gnoli 1993/1994: 81.
30 Harper 2006: x.
31 De Jong 2009: 38.
32 De Jong 2005: 90.

This should not surprise us, since the extant Avestan texts were used only for rituals and educational purposes.[33] Unfortunately, such voices remain a minority. The "exaggerated and restrictive tendency" to read every Iranian image in terms of Zoroastrian literature is still being applied, not only to the subject matter of Sasanian art, but also to pre-Islamic pictorial expressions in general. In this study I have deliberately chosen to refrain from applying the term "Zoroastrian" to anything other than the variant of the Iranian religion associated with the Sasanian Empire and Middle Persian literature. There are several interconnected reasons for this stance. Despite tireless scholarly efforts, the main questions concerning the pre-Sasanian history of the Zoroastrian faith are still very inadequately answered.[34] The difficulties begin with the almost impenetrable mist over the personality of the Prophet Zoroaster himself, the nature of his teachings and alleged reforms and the place of his doctrine in the broader context of other Iranian cults. It would be pointless to review here the exhaustive, repetitive and inconclusive debates over the question of "Zoroaster's Time and Homeland", since this was recently accomplished in a masterly way by Shaul Shaked.[35] His arguments for the tentative dating of Zoroaster to the ninth or eighth centuries BCE appear convincing and do not contradict any of the very few established facts.[36] As for the prophet's homeland, we are on safer ground in placing him in Eastern Iran, perhaps even more specifically in the region of the Pamir Mountains.[37]

We know close to nothing of the early history, significance and transmission of the corpus of religious texts that would become the Avesta—the sacred canon of the Zoroastrian religion—before it was put into writing in the late Sasanian period, besides the fact that it was transmitted orally for a long period of time.[38] We are in near complete ignorance regarding the development and transformation of Zoroastrianism into the dominant religion in the Sasanian Empire and the extent to which the religious practices and beliefs of the Sasanian period reflect those of earlier periods.[39]

One of the few firmly established facts is the use of the calendar corresponding to the Avestan in the Aramaic documents from fourth century BCE Achaemenian Bactria.[40] This calendar was probably established by the Achaemenian kings within a century of their conquest of Egypt and it was directly modeled on the Egyptian calendar.[41] However, we have only indirect evidence for the Avesta in the Sasanian period. It is mentioned as a "book" only in the Islamic period and Sasanian royal inscriptions do not contain a single quotation from or clear reference to the Avesta.[42] One of the main difficulties is the absence of a clear set of criteria for what Zoroastrianism *is* that could then be applied to ancient Iranian religious sources.[43] For example, if we accept the view that "Zoroastrianism is the only religion

---

33 Skjærvø 2012: 5.

34 This is reflected also in "the absence of a generally recognized and accepted reliable history and description of early Zoroastrianism. Most twentieth-century descriptions of Zoroastrianism disagree on important points of chronology, location, and doctrine"; Skjærvø 2011b: 76–77. For an excellent survey of the history of Zoroastrianism, see Stausberg 2002–2004.

35 Shaked 2005.

36 Shaked 2005: 189.

37 Grenet 2005.

38 For an introduction to Avestan literature and its problems, see Kellens 1998; Shaked 2007; Hintze 2009.

39 In De Jong's words: "what we do not know is *what* the Avesta was in Western Iran in any period before the (late) Sasanian Empire"; De Jong 2005: 89.

40 Naveh and Shaked 2012: C3:2 and perhaps also C3:18.

41 For a recent discussion with references to previous literature, see Stern 2012: 174–191.

42 De Jong 2009: 32–33, 36. De Jong later wrote, "although there are numerous possible allusions to 'Avestan' ideas and expressions, there is not a single actual quotation from any Avestan text either in Old Persian or in Middle Persian inscriptions"; see De Jong 2010a: 538.

43 Skjærvø, in a recent contribution, defines Zoroastrianism as "the religion expressed in the (entire) *Avesta*" and goes on to argue that "the similarities between Achaemenid religion and Zoroastrianism are so numerous and fundamental that one must conclude that the Achaemenid kings, at least from Darius onward, were Zoroastrian"; see Skjærvø 2013b: 563. This line of argument, however, is not without its problems. The similarities between the Avesta and the Achaemenian inscriptions could be satisfactorily explained by their shared Iranian linguistic, cultural and religious background, in the same way that Judaism,

to recognize Ahura Mazdā as the supreme god",[44] the inevitable conclusion would be that only the Achaemenians and Sasanians were definitely Zoroastrians, while the people of Eastern Iran like the Bactrians and Sogdians were clearly not. Unless we have a coherent and commonly accepted definition of what is required in order to be considered a Zoroastrian, such attempts would serve no purpose. It seems best, therefore, to refrain from using the term "Zoroastrian" altogether prior to the Sasanian period.[45]

As noted by David Bivar, because Zoroastrianism is the best-known Iranian faith, it is natural to identify all forms of Iranian religions with its norms.[46] However, it is impossible to deny that not all Iranian religious expression accords with the Zoroastrian tradition. For instance, some aspects of the religious behavior of the three western Iranian dynasties, such as marrying foreign women, burying and caring for their diseased, directly contradict what is found in Middle Persian Zoroastrian literature.[47] Iranian religious life in antiquity undoubtedly encompassed many more activities and beliefs than those that have come down to us as part of the Zoroastrian canon. What is usually called "Zoroastrianism", in the pre-Islamic period, was "a fairly large range of cult and worship, which is hardly capable of systematic treatment".[48] Furthermore, the formation of the Zoroastrian "creed" and the definition of orthodoxy, as the agreed-upon norms and religious conventions and what is excluded from it, probably occurred only in the Islamic period.[49]

The Kushan, Sogdian and other Iranian religious traditions are certainly related to the religious worldview expressed in the Avesta, but these relations are best described not as "paternal", but as "fraternal", as variations within the broad pan-Iranian religious tradition. Even in Western Iran, the pre-Sasanian forms of Iranian religious teachings and cults were very diverse, and the initial writing down of Zoroastrian literature is probably responsible for the loss of the significant part of these teachings. Therefore, it would be more useful and, indeed, more correct to call them by the general and neutral terms "Iranian cults" and "Iranian religions" whose exact nature often eludes us, but of which Zoroastrianism, as it is known from the Sasanian period onward, was obviously a part.[50]

By now, it should no longer appear paradoxical that the Avesta and the later Zoroastrian writings are very inappropriate sources for the interpretation of pre-Islamic Iranian iconography. The Avestan texts, as preserved by modern Zoroastrianism, are undoubtedly only a small portion of the enormous corpus of pre-Islamic Iranian religious, cultic and mythological traditions (most of which were transmitted orally and were probably never written down). Therefore, even in the very few cases of correspondence between an artistic image and a literary description, one cannot necessarily presuppose a direct knowledge of the Sasanian Avestan texts underlying the creation of the image. It could instead reflect a common mythological background, only a specific variant of which was preserved in the Avesta.

The Sogdian version of the *Ašəm vohū* prayer, one of the four main prayers of Zoroastrianism, provides an excellent illustration. It is around three hundred years older than the oldest surviving manuscript of the Avesta. However, the Sogdian *Ašəm vohū* derives from some unknown source independent of the Sasanian Avesta.[51] This unequivocally indicates that other ancient Iranian sources with parallels in

---

Christianity and Islam appear much more fundamentally and substantially alike while they are undoubtedly different religions. See also the recent article by Kellens, who rightly emphasizes that "aucun document achéménide *connu* ne fait la citation *directe* d' un texte avestique *connu*"; Kellens 2013: 551.

44 Shaked 2005: 194.

45 See also the important discussion in Kellens 2013, esp. 552–553.

46 Bivar 1998: 5.

47 See the discussion and examples in De Jong 2010a: 533–536.

48 Shaked 1994a: 97.

49 Shaked 1994a: 98.

50 For a similar approach, see Tremblay 2006.

51 Sims-Williams suggests that it was preserved in Old Iranian from Achaemenian times. See Sims-Williams 2000: 9.

Avestan literature do not necessarily originate in a knowledge of the Avestan text as codified by the Sasanian and the Pahlavi Zoroastrian tradition.

Nevertheless, there is no alternative within the Iranian written tradition, so one is obliged to use the Zoroastrian canon because it provides the only written attestations of a genuine Iranian religious system recorded by the Iranian tradition itself. Without the accompanying text, the iconography usually remains silent and most attempts to identify Iranian gods are inevitably based on written sources. To understand the "secondary or conventional subject matter" and "intrinsic meaning" of the pictorial expressions, we have to combine them with themes and concepts transmitted through literary and oral sources.[52] However, while using the Avestan and Middle Persian texts to illuminate archaeological finds and visual imagery, one must always keep in mind their enormous chronological and contextual problems. In every case, it is necessary to substantiate their relevance to a particular culture and period. We should be careful when comparing images from different Iranian cultures belonging to different periods, and even more so when using textual evidence to interpret images where there is no definitely established geographical and chronological association between them.

In light of the above, one can appreciate why the situation in the study of the religions of pre-Islamic Iran and Central Asia differs considerably from many other civilizations of the ancient Near East and Classical Antiquity. Unlike Mesopotamian, Egyptian and Greek religions, for which there is an abundance of primary literary sources at our disposal, the importance of iconography for the study of the religions of the pre-Islamic Iranian world appears to be comparatively much more significant. This state of affairs with the Iranian written sources offers an unusual opportunity for the student of iconography, by turning the latter into a source of prime importance for Iranian religions.

52 Panofsky 1962: 6.

CHAPTER 2

WRITTEN SOURCES

1. *Inscriptions*

The earliest Iranian written sources at our disposal are the Old Persian Achaemenian royal inscriptions, which mention Ahura Mazdā, Mithra and Anāhitā.[1] However, these inscriptions give us no information regarding the appearance of the deities.

One of the most significant inscriptions, both for our present purpose and also for the study of Graeco-Iranian syncretism, is the bilingual Parthian-Greek inscription engraved on the bronze statue of Heracles. Discovered in 1984 at Seleucia on the Tigris, and dated to 151 CE (fig. 1),[2] the Greek inscription informs us that the image of Heracles has been brought from Mesene and placed in the temple of Apollo. Its importance, however, lies in the fact that, in the Parthian version of the text, Heracles is called *Warhagn* (Vərəθraγna) and Apollo—*Tīr*. This statue thus constitutes a rare case—one can be certain that the image, a pure Greek Heracles from an iconographic point of view, was identified with Vərəθraγna.

The Sasanian royal inscriptions provide little information regarding the appearance of gods.[3] Very much like their Achaemenian predecessors, the Sasanian kings proclaimed their devotion to Ahura Mazdā, with "Anāhitā the Lady" (*anahīd ī bānūg*) being mentioned once in the Paikuli inscription of king Narseh:

> *ud amā kū ān frawardag wēnom ud pad ohrmazd ud wispān yazdān ud anahīd ī bānūg nām az armen ō ērānšahr rōn wahēzom.*
>
> And then I saw that letter, in the name of Ohrmazd and all the gods and Anāhīd the Lady, we moved from Armenia toward Ērānšahr.[4]

The four inscriptions of the eminent Zoroastrian priest Kartīr, who played a major role in the religious and political administration of the Sasanian Empire in the second half of the third century CE, provide more valuable data.[5] In the longer inscriptions, where his *cursus honorum* is given, Kartīr proclaims that through his actions:

> *uzdēs gugānīh ud gilistag ī dēwān wišōbīh ud yazdān gāh ud nišēm āgīriy.*
>
> idols were destroyed and the dwellings of the demons demolished and the places (thrones) and the seats of the gods were established (§ 11).[6]

Of particular significance for our study is the account of Kartīr's visionary journey to Paradise, which is found in two of his inscriptions—Sar-e Mašhad and Naqš-e Rostam.[7] In this vision, Kartīr's *hangirb*[8] encounters six divine characters, which all appear to have definite anthropomorphic shape. Five of them

---

1 For a recent translation of the Old Persian inscriptions, see Lecoq 1997. See also the introduction in Huyse 2009: 73–84.
2 Bernard 1990b.
3 For a useful recent survey of the Sasanian inscriptions, see Huyse 2009: 90–102.
4 Paikuli 9.19, ed. and tr. by Humbach and Skjærvø 1983: 3.1., 35.
5 On Kartīr and his career, see Skjærvø 2011a; for a French edition of the inscriptions, see Gignoux 1991.
6 Following the arrangement given in Skjærvø 2011a.
7 On Kartīr's vision, in addition to Gignoux 1991, see also Skjærvø 1983; Grenet 2003c and Schwartz 2007.
8 Literally: "having the same body/form". This word should probably be understood here as Kartīr's *mēnōg* form.

are called "princes" (*šahriyār*) and carry the title "the color of dawn" (*spēdagān*).[9] The first prince, is mounted on a superb horse and holds a banner (*drafš*) (§ 25). The second sits on a golden throne and has scales (*tarāzūg*) in front of him (§ 27). The third also sits on a golden throne, but he is more superb than the first two. He holds a certain object, called **čayēn/čiyēn*,[10] that turns out to be a bottomless well (*čāh*) full of evil creatures (*xrafstar*) (§ 28). The fourth does not possess any specific attribute, but is described as the most superb of them all. He takes the hand of Kartīr's *hangirb* and leads him over the Činwad bridge (§ 28). Finally, the last prince points a finger at Kartīr's *hangirb* and smiles (§ 34). The other character that features prominently in Kartīr's vision, and who accompanies him on his journey to the hereafter, is a superb woman, coming from the East on a road that is luminous (*zan-ēw paydāg az xwarāsān ōrōn āyēd ... ud ān rāh kū rōšn*). She and Kartīr's *hangirb* take each other's hand (*awēšān āgenēn harw-dōnān dast*) (§ 26).

Moving to Eastern Iran, the first inscription that is relevant to our enquiry is the longest of those uncovered at the Kushan sanctuary at Surkh-Kotal (SK 4).[11] In this inscription, which commemorates the renovation of the temple during the reign of Kanishka, it is recorded that, when the temple ran out of water, "the gods withdrew themselves from their seat" (§ 3) and were "transported to the fortress of Lraf" (§ 4). The departure of the gods obviously refers to the temporary removal of the temple's cultic statues,[12] indicating that the Surkh-Kotal temple and probably also other Kushan temples were actual "houses of gods" in the sense that is known from the ancient Near East and especially from Mesopotamia.

In the first sentence of this inscription, the sanctuary is identified as κανηþκο οανινδο βαγολαγγο, which could mean "Kanishka's temple of (the goddess) Oanindo", although it could equally be translated as "the temple of Kanishka's victory" or as "the temple of victorious Kanishka".[13] Since the epithet "victorious" is also given to Kanishka in the Rabatak inscription, the latter reading seems preferable. It also seems unlikely that a major sanctuary like Surkh-Kotal was the temple of the goddess Oanindo, since she does not appear in the Rabatak list (see below) and therefore could hardly have been considered a goddess of great importance. It should be noted that the Rabatak temple was not named after a deity, not even after the great goddess Nana, but was rather called βαγεαβο "Bage-ab" ("God's Water"; line 8).[14] Furthermore, it is explicitly stated in the SK 4 that "the gods" had withdrawn from the temple. No special mention is made of Oanindo or, in fact, of any specific deity and nothing suggests that any one of these "gods" was more "elevated" than others.

This contrasts with the Rabatak inscription, which, undoubtedly, is the most important Iranian inscription recently discovered. Found in 1993 at the site of Rabatak, in the Baghlan province of modern Afghanistan,[15] it commemorates the construction of the still unexcavated sanctuary called βαγεαβο "Bage-ab" ("God's Water"), which was probably located at the same site. The Kushan king Kanishka, who is addressed in the inscription as "the righteous, the just, the autocrat, the god worthy of worship" (lines 1–2), claims that he "has obtained kingship from Nana and from all the gods" (line 2). The sanctuary itself was made for the "glorious Umma (ομμο)", "... the above-mentioned Nana (νανα) and the above-mentioned Umma, Aurmuzd (αορομοζδο), Muzhduwan (μοζδοοανο), Sroshard (σροþαρδο),

---

[9] Grenet 2003c: 10, translates *spēdagān* as "éclatant"; Skjærvø 2011d: no. 85, has "resplendent".

[10] Grenet 2003c: 11, translates it as "un mur de pierre sèches"; Skjærvø 2011d: no. 85, has "laddle".

[11] For the text with a French translation, see Lazard, Grenet and De Lamberterie 1984.

[12] Sims-Williams and Cribb 1996: 109.

[13] See the discussions in Lazard, Grenet and De Lamberterie 1984: 199–201 and Grenet forthcoming a, who favours the first option.

[14] Sims-Williams 2004/2008: 63.

[15] For the *editio princeps*, see Sims-Williams and Cribb 1996. For revised and updated editions, see Sims-Williams 1998 and especially Sims-Williams 2004/2008. See also Fussman 1998, Göbl 1999, Carter 2006 and Gnoli 2009. For a general survey of Bactrian inscriptions, see Huyse 2009: 105–112.

Narasa (ναρασαο) (and) Mihir (μιιρο)" (lines 9–10). Kanishka also "gave orders to make images (πιδγιρβο) of the same, (namely) of these gods who are inscribed hereupon, and he gave orders to make (images of) these kings ..." (lines 10–12). Between lines 9 and 10 there are traces of an additional interlinear inscription in smaller letters "... who in Indian is called Maaseno (Skr. Mahāsena) and he is called Bizago (Skr. Viśākha)". Mahāsena and Viśākha are generally considered to be manifestations of the Indian god of war and sacred wisdom also known under the names of Skanda, Kumāra and Kārrtikeya.[16] Joe Cribb commented in the *editio princeps* that it is not clear to which Iranian god the names Maaseno and Bizago were meant to relate.[17] Most scholars, however, believe that they refer to Sroshard.[18]

2. *The Avesta*

The Avesta and the Rig Veda, composed in closely related archaic Indian and Iranian languages, are our principal sources for Indo-Iranian religion.[19] Ever since they were translated into European languages, there has been an intensive and still very much inconclusive scholarly debate regarding the context that is reflected in these hymnic collections.[20]

The Avesta is a heterogeneous corpus of texts, compiled and edited by various authors during different periods and written in related eastern Iranian languages.[21] The oldest part of the Avestan corpus, the *Gāthās*, are composed in Old Avestan. They are usually attributed to the prophet Zoroaster himself and regarded as reflecting his teachings.[22] According to the now prevailing view, the Avestan texts were composed in Eastern Iran between the second half of the second millennium BCE and the Achaemenian period.[23] The Avesta was transmitted orally for many generations before being committed to writing during the late Sasanian period.[24] The Avestan texts that we possess now are in fact, liturgical, ritual texts independent from the Sasanian "Great Avesta" whose contents are described in the *Dēnkard*. They were set down as an instruction manual for the priests when the oral tradition was in decline.[25]

It is usually claimed that the cult of the Indo-Iranians was aniconic since the Avesta and the Rig Veda make no mention of either idols or cultic statues; furthermore, they provide no detailed anthropomorphic descriptions of the deities of the Indo-Iranian pantheon. The Iranian goddess Anāhitā, whose appearance is described in the Avesta in vivid anthropomorphic terms, is usually cited as the sole exception that proves the rule.[26] A careful reading of the Avesta and the Rig Veda, however, provides clear indications that other deities were also conceived anthropomorphically. One of the three principal deities in the Rig Veda, Agni, and some secondary deities possess certain anthropomorphic features such as hair, teeth, eyes etc.[27] Similarly, in the Avesta, a deity is usually described through one or two typical traits, *pars pro toto*, while its general appearance remains obscure.

16 Carter 2006: 354.
17 Sims-Williams and Cribb 1996: 85.
18 Carter 2006: 354; Gnoli 2009: 151; Grenet 2006/2010: 88.
19 On Indo-Iranian religion, see Gnoli 2006 with further references.
20 On the Avesta and related problems, see p. 6. On the relationship between Avestan and Vedic literature, see Shaked 2005; Shaked 2007.
21 For a recent introduction to the Avestan corpus, see Hintze 2009.
22 Hintze 2009: 20–25.
23 Cantera 2012: VII.
24 On the transmission of the Avesta, see also Kellens 1998.
25 Cantera 2012: XI–XII.
26 For instance, Grenet 2006/2010: 87.
27 Elizarenkova 1999: 498, 501.

The Avestan hymn dedicated to the *yazata* Tištrya has numerous epithets that relate to his visual appearance: "white", "shining" (which he shares with Māh and Ātar), "luminous" (shared with Aši), "beaming from afar with shining immaculate rays",[28] "visible from afar",[29] "sound-eyed",[30] and "radiant" (like Apąm Napāt, Aši, Anāhitā, Vərəθraγna and Yima).[31]

Sometimes the context clearly indicates that a deity was conceived anthropomorphically, although no explicit allusion to its visual appearance is provided. Thus *Vidēvdāt* describes Vohu Manah as enthroned on a golden throne when a soul of the righteous crosses the Činwad bridge.[32] The souls of the righteous are guided over the Činwad bridge by "that beautiful one, strong, fair of form, accompanied by two dogs at her sides".[33] This beautiful woman is certainly the Daēnā. In a Young Avestan text, *Haδōxt nask*, we find a more vivid and detailed description of the Daēnā, which appears to a righteous man on the third night after his death:

> His own *daēnā* appears in the form of a maiden, beautiful, queenly, white-armed ... as beautiful as the most beautiful of creatures ... (proclaiming) ... 'Youth of good thought, good words, good deeds, good inner self (*daēnā*) I am your very own inner self'.[34]

Many Avestan deities have anthropomorphic or zoomorphic incarnations. Tištrya has three visual manifestations. He is said to assume the shapes of "a radiant, shiny-eyed man of fifteen, tall, overpowering, powerful, of heroic talent",[35] "a bull with golden hooves",[36] and of "a beautiful white horse with golden ears and golden bridle".[37]

Vərəθraγna has ten incarnations: one abstract, a wind; seven zoomorphic—a bull, a stallion, a camel, a boar, a bird-of-prey (*vārayna*), a wild ram, and a wild goat; and two anthropomorphic—a fifteen-year-old youth and a man.[38] It is possible that the wild boar was considered his most important incarnation, since, in the *Mihr Yašt*, Vərəθraγna is described as a wild, sharp-tusked boar, flying before Mithra.[39] Also Aŋra Mainyu assumes the form of a horse on which Taxma Urupi travels around the world for thirty years.[40]

Mithra is described as having a thousand ears and ten thousand eyes.[41] In another place it is said that he has the sun instead of eyes.[42] Ahura Mazdā also has the sun instead of eyes[43] and possesses a unique epithet—*hukərəptəma*, "of fairest form".[44]

Mithra is also a charioteer and appears as:

> ... the skilful warrior who has white horses and pointed spears with long shafts, who shoots afar with swift arrows; ...[45]

---

28 Y. 8.2. ed. and tr. by Panaino 1995: 149–151.
29 Y. 8.4.
30 Y. 8.12.
31 Y. 8.13.
32 *Vd.* 19.27–32.
33 *Vd.* 19.30. tr. by Boyce 1984: 80.
34 *HN* 2.11. tr by Shaki 1996.
35 Y. 8.13, ed. and tr. by Skjærvø 2011d: 56; he shares this form with Vərəθraγna.
36 Y. 8.16. ed. and tr. by Skjærvø 2011d: 56.
37 Y. 8.18. ed. and tr. by Skjærvø 2011d: 56.
38 Abaev 1984.
39 Yt. 10.70.
40 Yt. 15.12, 19.29.
41 Yt. 10.7.82.
42 Y. 3.13; Yt. 7.12.
43 Y. 3.13; Yt. 7.12.
44 Y. 1.1; 26.2. See Boyce 1975a: 198.
45 Yt. 10. 102. ed. and tr. by Gershevitsch 1959: 122–123.

He is armed with spears and hatches,[46] but his favorite weapon is a mace.[47] It is noteworthy that the Indian Mitra is almost entirely deprived of warlike qualities, which are fulfilled by Indra, although in some cases Mitra does use a snare and arrows.[48] The chariot of the Avestan Mithra is accompanied by Rašnu on the right, and by the goddess Čisti who is "white herself, she wears white garments".[49] In addition to Mithra, some other Avestan deities also ride their own chariots. For instance, Vayu rides a golden chariot with golden wheels. He also has golden weapons and wears a helmet, crown, necklace, garments, girdle and shoes all made of gold.[50] The goddess Aši also drives a chariot. Her anthropomorphic appearance in the *Ard Yašt* is confirmed by the passage where she touches Zoroaster with both hands.[51] She is described as beautiful, tall, and strong.[52] In the *Hōm Yašt* the *yazata* Haoma appears before Zoroaster in the form of the "most handsome man in the whole material world".[53] His common epithets in the Avesta are "the golden-green one" and "golden-green-eyed".[54]

However, the most detailed and outstanding anthropomorphic description of any deity in the Avesta is that of the goddess Anāhitā in the *Ābān Yašt*:

> Displayed in the shape of a beautiful young woman, Ardwī Sūrā Anāhitā stands most powerful and high-born, well-shaped and girded high, upright and splendid in her brilliance, wearing a coat with long sleeves, with rich designs, embroidered with gold. Ever and again, carrying barsom in her hands, wearing square earrings, high and noble born Ardwī Sūrā Anāhitā would wear a golden brooch upon her beautiful neck and tighten her waistband to enhance her breasts. On her head she bound a golden crown with a hundred stars, eight crenellations, and rings like wheels and with inimitable, beautiful, well-made droplets. Garments of beaver fur she wore from three hundred beavers.[55]

3. *Greek and Latin Sources*

Due to the lack of Iranian sources, especially concerning cultic iconography, we must turn to their historic adversaries, the Greeks and Romans, who provide the majority of the available written evidence and often the only text with which we can supplement the material data.[56]

Herodotus, the earliest to report on Persian religious practices and beliefs in the Achaemenian period, famously stated that:

> I know that the Persians have these customs: it is not their custom to erect statues, temples and altars, but they even make fun of those who do, because—as it seems to me—they have not considered the gods to be of human form, as do the Greeks.[57]

Both parts of this statement, frequently repeated by other classical authors,[58] are problematic. The "father of history" was certainly wrong concerning the Persian conception of the divine, which was anthropomorphic.[59]

---

46 Yt. 10. 129–130
47 Yt. 10. 96.132.
48 Schmidt 2006.
49 Yt. 10.126, ed. and tr. by Skjærvø 2011d: 54.
50 Yt. 15.57.
51 Yt. 17.22.
52 Skjærvø 1987.
53 Y 9.1–2.
54 Boyce 2003.
55 Yt. 5.30.126–129, ed. and tr. by Skjærvø 2011d: 62–63.
56 The classical sources regarding Iranian religions have been assembled and analyzed by De Jong 1997, which is now the standard reference work (replacing Benveniste 1929).
57 Hdt. 1.131. For a commentary on this passage, see De Jong 1997: 92–96.
58 Diog. Laert. 1.6–8; Cic. *Rep.* 3.9.14; Clem. Al. *Protr.* 5.65.1; Epiph. *Adv. haeres.* 13.
59 Boyce 1982: 179; De Jong 1997: 95; Jacobs 2001: 90. For a detailed discussion of Iranian anthropomorphism, see Chapter 5.

He further continues and describes the Persian sacrificial rites thus:

> But it is their custom to go up to the highest summits of the mountains and sacrifice to Zeus, calling the entire vault of heaven Zeus. And they sacrifice to the sun and the moon and the earth and fire and water and the winds. Only to these, now, they have sacrificed from the beginning, but they have learnt, from the Assyrians and the Arabians, to sacrifice also to Ouraniē; the Assyrians call Aphrodite Mylitta, the Arabians Alilat and the Persians Mitra.[60]

Herodotus was also the first to shed light on the religion of the Scythians, stating that the Scythian pantheon consisted of:

> Hestia in particular, and secondly Zeus and Earth, whom they believe to be the wife of Zeus; after these, Apollo, and the Heavenly Aphrodite, and Heracles, and Ares. All the Scythians worship these as gods; the Scythians called Royal sacrifice to Poseidon also.[61]

In addition to their *interpretatio graeca*, Herodotus also gave the Scythian divine names:

> In the Scythian tongue, Hestia is called Tabiti; Zeus (in my judgment most correctly so called) Papaeus; Earth is Apia; Apollo Goetosyrus; the Heavenly Aphrodite Argimpasa; Poseidon Thagimasadas.[62]

Their etymologies, however, pose numerous problems and it has proved problematic to correlate them with the deities known from the Indo-Iranian and Zoroastrian traditions.[63]

Herodotus also provides us with particularly valuable information about Scythian rituals and the image of the Scythian god whom he calls Ares, but, unfortunately, he does not give his original Scythian name:

> … their sacrifices to Ares are of this sort. Every district in each of the governments has a structure sacred to Ares; namely, a pile of bundles of sticks … On this sacred pile an ancient akinakes (short sword) of iron is set for each people: their image of Ares. They bring yearly sacrifice of sheep and goats and horses to this akinakes, offering to these symbols even more than they do to the other gods.[64]

Other classical authors also mention the Scythian adoration of a sword.[65] Writing about the Alans, who succeeded the Scythians and Sarmatians in the Pontic steppes, the Roman historian Ammianus Marcellinus noted that:

> Among them no temple nor sanctuary is to be seen, not even a straw-roofed hut is visible anywhere; but according to a Barbarian custom, a naked sword is fixed in the ground and they respectfully worship it as god of war and protector of the regions through which they travel.[66]

A similar motif is attested in the epos of the Caucasian Ossetians, the descendants of the Alans.[67]

In the Hellenistic period, the Babylonian priest Berossus, writing in Greek, recorded that Artaxerxes II introduced the cult statues of the goddess Anāhitā to the temples of some major cities throughout the Achaemenian Empire, i.e. Babylon, Susa, Ekbatana, Persepolis, Bactra, Damascus and Sardis.[68] While this cannot be proved,[69] it finds some indirect support in Artaxerxes's royal inscriptions, where the goddess Anāhitā is mentioned for the first time.[70] Statues of Persian gods are mentioned twice in the

60 Hdt. 1.131. See De Jong 1997: 107–110.
61 Hdt. 4.51.1.
62 Hdt. 4.51.2.
63 See, for example, the discussions in Abaev 1962 and Bessonova 1983.
64 Hdt. 4.62.
65 See the references in Maenchen-Helfen 1973: 279 and Bessonova 1983: 46.
66 Amm. Marc. 31.2.23, ed. and tr. by Alemany 2000: 36–37.
67 Bessonova 1983: 46; Bessonova 1984: 5.
68 Clem. Al. *Protr.* 5.65.3. Images of gods among the Persians according to Herodotus and Berossus are discussed in Jacobs 2001.
69 Jacobs 2001: 90.
70 A^2Ha, A^2Sa, A^2Sd. Lecoq 1997: 269–275.

Historiae Alexandri Magni of the Roman historian Quintus Curtius Rufus. First, describing the royal chariot in the cavalcade of the Achaemenian army, Curtius notes that it was decorated with golden statues of Nin and Bel.[71] Second, he reports that, following the capture of Persepolis by the Macedonian army, Alexander permitted the images of the gods that were standing in the Achaemenian capital to be smashed.[72] These statements are questionable as sculpture rarely existed in Achaemenian art,[73] and, even if Curtius' description of the chariot is trustworthy, Nin and Bel are Babylonian divine names rather than Iranian.

Flavius Josephus, the Jewish historian of the first century CE, tells the story of two Jewish brothers, Anilaeus and Asinaeus, who became semi-independent local rulers in Parthian Babylonia.[74] This narrative contains numerous Iranian epic motifs and was probably composed by a Parthianised Babylonian Jew.[75] In this story, Anilaeus marries a gentile woman, the wife of a "certain Parthian". Entering his house, the woman:

> concealed the images of those gods which were their country gods, common to her husband and herself: now it is the custom of that country for all to have the idols they worship in their own houses, and to carry them along with them when they go into a foreign land; agreeable to which custom of theirs she carried her idols with her.[76]

This story follows the famous Biblical *topos* of gentile idol-worshipping spouse, who eventually brings downfall upon her Jewish husband.[77] Although her first husband is called a "Parthian", there is no means of knowing whether she was of Iranian or Semitic descent.

Strabo, also writing in the Roman period, repeats Herodotus' statements that Persians do not erect statues and altars, that they worship heaven as Zeus and the sun as Mithra and records their veneration of natural elements.[78] However, Strabo goes on to tell us that in Cappadocia there are numerous sanctuaries of Persian gods, including Anāhitā and Ōmanos, and that Magi in that land used to carry an image of the god Ōmanos in a procession.[79] Ōmanos is most probably the Greek rendering of the Old Persian form **Va(h)u-manah-*, Vohu Manah, the "Good Thought", one of the Aməša Spənta, "Life-giving/Bounteous Immortals", the beneficent divinities of Zoroastrianism. The same god is also mentioned by Strabo in another passage where he describes the temple of "Anaïtis and the gods who share her altar—Ōmanos and Anadatus, Persian gods" in the Pontic city of Zela.[80] The existence of a cultic statue of Vohu Manah is all the more significant, as it indicates that, in addition to gods that were easily identifiable with other Near Eastern and Greek deities, a typically Iranian abstract personification could also be represented anthropomorphically.

Clement of Alexandria quotes the account of Dino that the Persians and the Medes consider fire and water to be the only statues of the gods.[81]

The *topos* of Persian aniconism is found also in the *Lives and Opinions of Eminent Philosophers* of Diogenes Laertius, who informs us that the Magi:

> condemn the use of images, and especially the error of attributing to the divinities difference of sex.[82]

---

71 Curt. 3.3.11.
72 Curt. 5.6.5.
73 See p. 181.
74 Joseph *AJ*. 18.314–370.
75 Herman 2006.
76 Joseph *AJ*. 18.344. ed. and tr. by Whiston 1974.
77 See Herman 2006: 247, n. 5 and 6.
78 Str. 15.3.13.
79 Str. 15.3.15. De Jong 1997: 150–156.
80 Str. 11.8.4. For a discussion of this passage, see De Jong 1997: 150–156.
81 Clem. Al. *Protr*. 5.65.1. De Jong 1997: 305.
82 Diog. Laert. 1.6.

The second part of this statement is incompatible with the evidence of the Iranian written sources and iconography, where the majority of Iranian gods always appear as male or female.

A curious piece of information concerning the visual appearance of Iranian deities is found in the enigmatic passage of Philo of Byblos (c. 64–141 CE), where he cites "Zoroaster the Magus" who "literally says in the Sacred Collection of the Persians: 'God has the head of a hawk'".[83] This passage is more reminiscent of an Egyptian rather than an Iranian deity—such images are never found in Iranian iconography. Porphyry of Tyre (234–c. 305 CE), a compatriot of Philo, wrote that the famous Greek philosopher Pythagoras learned from the Persian magi that:

> … the god himself, whom they call Oromazes, resembles light with regard to his body and truth with regard to his soul.[84]

The connection between light and the body of Ahura Mazdā is in full accordance with Iranian written sources.

In the biography of Aurelian included in the *Historia Augusta*—a Latin collection of biographies of Roman Emperors of uncertain date and unknown authorship—the following curious story is preserved:

> Furthermore, when he [Aurelian] had gone as envoy to the Persians, he was presented with a sacrificial saucer, of the kind that the king of the Persians is wont to present to the emperor, on which was engraved the Sun-god in the same attire in which he was worshipped in the very temple where the mother of Aurelian had been a priestess.[85]

The reference here is undoubtedly to Mithra, who was indeed at the time depicted like the Roman Sol and, therefore, familiar to the future Roman Emperor.

An additional Latin source is the historian Ammianus Marcellinus whose work contains numerous important data regarding Sasanian society and customs. From Ammianus we learn that, in 164 CE, the soldiers of Lucius Verus captured the statue of Comaean Apollo from the Parthian capital of Seleucia on the Tigris—Ctesiphon.[86] It is interesting that the bilingual inscription on the bronze statue of Heracles/Vərəθraγna from Seleucia, dated to 151–150 BCE, mentions the temple of Apollo/Tīr in Seleucia on the Tigris.[87]

4. *Christian Sources in Armenian, Georgian, Syriac and Greek*

Christian sources written in Armenian, Georgian, Syriac and Greek contain many allusions to Iranian cults and deities. Armenia and Georgia are the only two Caucasian nations possessing their own distinctive written tradition and their hagiographical and historical writing should not be neglected. Approached critically, they reveal significant Iranian material that is not found elsewhere. In fact, the works of Armenian historians are the closest thing to genuine Iranian historical sources that we have.

Most deities of the Armenian and Georgian pre-Christian pantheons have Iranian names and, although there was probably local Caucasian influence, their Iranian component remained significant. Of particular importance for our purposes are the numerous references to cultic statues found in these texts.

---

83 Quoted in Euseb. *Praep. evang.* 1.10.52. See: De Jong 1997: 301, n. 193.
84 Porph. *Pyth.* 41. De Jong 1997: 255–256.
85 *Hist. Aug. Aur.* 5.5.
86 Amm. Marc. 23.6.
87 See p. 11.

1. *Armenian*

The Armenian sources are openly hostile towards the Sasanians and Zoroastrianism, even more so than their Greek and Syriac coreligionists.[88] Of the eight deities from the pagan Armenian pantheon that appear in these sources, six carry distinctively Iranian names, one is Semitic and one is presumably local Armenian/Caucasian.

The earliest source regarding Armenian pre-Christian religion is *The History of the Armenians* attributed to a certain Agat'angełos. His work, whose leitmotif is the conversion of Armenia to Christianity by St Gregory the Illuminator, was probably composed in the second half of the fifth century CE.[89] Although Agat'angełos dedicates considerable space to refutating idolatry, he provides little concrete information about the cults of pre-Christian Armenia, the visual appearance of their gods, or their forms of worship.[90] Agat'angełos' discussion of idolatry, and much of the detail concerning pre-Christian Armenian cults and idols, should be approached with caution on account of its use of Biblical images and motifs.[91] According to him there were ten sanctuaries in Armenia located in seven cities: three temples of the goddess Anahit, at Artashat, Erēz and Ashtishat; one of the god Tir near Artashat; one of Aramazd at Ani; one of Vahagn at Ashtishat; one of Mihr at Bagayaṙich; one of Nanē at T'il; one of Astḷik at Ashtishat; and one of Barshamin at T'ordan.[92] It is worth mentioning that one of the Armenian terms for temple, *mehean*, derives from the name of the god Mihr (Mithra).[93]

Armenian idols were made of a variety of materials. According to Agat'angełos', the statues set by king Trdat: "are of wood and some of stone, some are of bronze, and some of silver, and some of gold".[94] Little detail can be derived about the appearance and cult of these idols. The sole exception is the statue of Anahit in her famous temple in the village of Erēz (modern Erzinjan) where:

> … the king ordered Gregory to present to the altar of Anahit's statue offerings of crowns and thick branches of trees. But he did not agree to serve the worship of the gods.[95]

This statue was made of gold[96] and Agat'angełos ascribes to the goddess Anahit colorful epithets like "the Golden-mother" and "the Golden-born goddess".[97] Anahit has a very dominant presence throughout the whole work. Her usual epithet is "the lady" (*tikin*),[98] a title analogous to that used for the goddess in Sasanian Iran.[99] Anahit probably occupied an especially important position in the Armenian pantheon, possibly eclipsing even Aramazd himself, since she is at times named before him:

> … the great Anahit, who gives life and fertility to our land Armenia, and with her the great and noble Aramazd.[100]

She is distinguished among other gods:

> … unless you agree to offer worship to the gods, and especially to this great lady Anahit.[101]

---

88 Nina Garsoïan defines the attitude of the Armenian authors as "deep anti-Iranism": Garsoïan 1989: 51. See also Thomson 2004.
89 Thomson 1976: xvi.
90 Thomson 1976: xl–xli.
91 Thomson 1976: xl–xli.
92 Thomson 1976: 440.
93 Russell 1987: 264–265; Garsoïan 1989: 546. On the cult of Mithra in Armenia, see Russell 1987: 261–289.
94 Ag. 71.
95 Ag. 48.
96 Ag. 786.
97 Ag. 809.
98 Ag. 53, 59, 127.
99 On the cult of Anahit in Armenia, see also Russell 1987: 243–253.
100 Ag. 68.
101 Ag. 53.

She is also the only deity in the Armenian sources to have three temples, while all others, including Aramazd, had only one temple each.

Tir, another god whose epithets are reported by Agat'angełos, also had a temple in Armenia in the vicinity of Artashat. Tir is called "the interpreter of dreams", "the scribe of pagan learning" and "the secretary of Ormizd".[102]

In contrast to the later historian Movsēs Xorenac'i,[103] Agat'angełos did not identify any of the Armenian gods with Greek deities. In the Greek version of his *History*, however, the goddesses Nanē and Astłik are equated with Athena and Aphrodite respectively.[104] It is also noteworthy that, in the Armenian version, Nanē is called "the daughter of Aramazd".[105]

The next source to be considered is *The History of Armenia* attributed to P'awstos Buzand, which was probably composed in the latter part of the fifth century CE.[106] P'awstos confirms the information of Agat'angełos as to the existence of the temple dedicated to Vahagn-Vərəθraγna at Ashtishat, and identifies him with the Greek Heracles:

> … the shrines of the temple of Heraclēs, that is to say of Vahagn, at the place called Ašrišat …[107]

P'awstos obviously regarded the pre-Christian religion of Armenia as the "worship of demons" (*diwapaštut'iwn*) and linked with idol-worship:

> And after his [St. Nersēs] departure from this world, many districts of Armenia, and many people turned back to the ancient worship-of-demons, and they erected idols in many places in Armenia with the permission of King Pap … and so they erected many images and prostrated themselves before them.[108]

However, it is Movsēs Xorenac'i, commonly celebrated as the Armenian "father of history", who is our principal source of knowledge about the culture and religion of pre-Christian Armenia. Although most of his information regarding pagan Armenian religion is borrowed from Agat'angełos, Movsēs Xorenac'i furnishes it with his own valuable interpretation.[109] His work probably dates to the eighth century CE.[110]

The most important contribution of Xorenac'i to the study of the Armenian pantheon is his identifications of Armenian gods with Greek ones. Movsēs equates Anahit (Anāhitā) with Artemis, Vahagn with Heracles, Tir with Apollo, Aramazd with Zeus, Nanē with Athena, Mihr with Hephaestus and Astłik with Aphrodite.[111] In the *History* of Xorenac'i we find echoes of the tradition that idols were introduced to Armenia from the Graeco-Roman world by king Artashēs in the first half of the second century BCE:

> Finding in Asia images of Artemis, Heracles, and Apollo that were cast in bronze and gilded, he [Artashēs] had them brought to our country to be set up in Armavir. The chief priests, who were of the Vahuni family, took those of Apollo and Artemis and set them up in Armavir; but the statue of Heracles, which had been made by Scyllas and Dipenes of Crete, they supposed to be Vahagn their ancestor and so set it up in Tarawn in their own village of Ashtishat after the death of Artashēs.[112]
>
> He [Artashēs] also took from Hellas images of Zeus, Artemis, Athena, Hephaistos, and Aphrodite, and had them brought to Armenia.[113]

---

102 Ag. 778. On the Armenian Tir, see Russell 1987: 289–323.
103 See below.
104 Thomson 1976: lxiii.
105 Ag. 786.
106 Garsoïan 1989: 11.
107 PB 3.14.
108 PB 5.31.
109 Thomson 1980: 29.
110 Thomson 1980: 58–61.
111 Thomson 1980: 149, n. 7.
112 MX 2.12.
113 MX 2.12.

Xorenac'i's chronology seems defective, since he attributes the building of the temple in Armavir to Vaḷarshak (first century CE) who then erected "statues of the sun and moon and of his own ancestors".[114] However, it follows from his narrative that the idols, which were first housed in Armavir, were later transferred to Bagaran and finally installed by Artashēs in his new capital Artashat:

> He [Artashēs] erected in it [Artashat] a temple and transferred to it from Bagaran the statue of Artemis and all the ancestral idols. But the statue of Apollo he put up outside the city near the road.[115]

Additional statues were set up by king Tigran II (95–55 BCE):

> Tigran consented and raised the statue of Zeus Olympus in the fortress of Ani, that of Athena in T'il, the second statue of Artemis in Erēz, and that of Hephaistos in Bagayaṙich. But the statue of Aphrodite, as the beloved of Heracles, he ordered to be set up beside the statue of the same Heracles in Ashtishat.[116]

In front of the temples, Tigran set up altars[117] according to the Greek fashion. We may draw interesting parallels with the Oxus Temple at Takht-i Sangin where similar Greek altars were installed in front of the entrance.[118]

An additional reference to temples with statues of "Ormizd who is Aramazd" and Anahit is found in a seventh-century CE Armenian polemical text against iconoclasm.[119]

According to Xorenac'i, all these idols were destroyed by the Sasanian king Ardašīr I, after his victory over the Arsacid dynasty:

> He [Ardašīr] increased the cults of the temples and ordered the fire of Ormizd, which was on the altar at Bagavan, to be kept perpetually burning. But the statues that Vaḷarshak had set up as the images of his ancestors with those of the sun and the moon at Armavir, and which had been transferred from Armavir to Bagaran and then brought to Artashat, these Artashir broke up.[120]

We learn from this passage that the fire-cult and cultic statues were present in Armenian temples, which seem very similar to the temples of Hellenistic Bactria like Takht-i Sangin and Ai Khanum. It is not inconceivable that Parthian temples also followed similar patterns. Besides the already mentioned *mehean*, two additional terms, *atrušan* and *bagin*, are employed by Armenian authors for pre-Christian cultic places. These are usually interpreted as referring to "fire-temple" and "idol-temple", although the context does not always allow for such a differentiation, especially for the *bagin*.

Movsēs Xorenac'i also provides two interesting comments about the visual appearance of two Armenian gods. Regarding Aramazd, he reports that:

> There is no Aramazd safe among those wishing to hear that Aramazd exists; among the four or more called Aramazd is a certain bald Aramazd.[121]

The word "bald" (*kund*) has also been interpreted as "strongest", which perhaps makes more sense in this context.[122] Some medieval Armenian sources mention the "four-faced image" of Aramazd.[123] James Russell thinks that this description relates to the four days of the Zoroastrian month that are called after Aramazd,[124] but it is equally possible that these "faces" had a concrete rather than allegorical meaning, perhaps indicating that Aramazd in Armenia was believed to possess a number of incarnations.

---

114 MX 2.8.
115 MX 2.49.
116 MX, 2.14.
117 MX, 2.14.
118 Litvinskiy and Pichikyan 2000: 169–175.
119 Der Nersessian 1944/1945: 63–64.
120 MX 2.77, ed. and tr. by Thomson 1980: 225.
121 MX 1.31, ed. and tr. by Thomson 1980: 122.
122 Thomson 1980: 122, n. 1.
123 Russell 1987: 162.
124 Russell 1987: 162.

The second sentence is a unique fragment of a pre-Christian Armenian hymn in which the god Vahagn is described in the following manner:

> From the flame a red-headed young boy ran out. He had fire for hair, and had flame for beard, and his eyes were suns.[125]

This is the most detailed description of the visual appearance of an Armenian deity found in the written sources. It is intriguing and, from the perspective of the Iranian tradition, somewhat unexpected that this hymn attributes to Vahagn-Heracles a fiery, flaming appearance.

An additional Armenian source is Eznik Koghbac'i, dated to the fifth century CE, who provides valuable information on Zoroastrianism in his book *Refutation of the Sects*. In his account of the birth of the twins Ohrmazd and Ahriman, Eznik describes the first as radiant and fragrant and the other as dark and fetid.[126]

2. *Georgian*

Two collections of medieval Georgian texts, *The Conversion of K'art'li* (*Mok'c'evay k'art'lisay*) and *The Life of K'art'li* (*K'art'lis C'xovreba*), contain much material concerning the pre-Christian past, indicating that the religion of the ancient inhabitants of K'art'li, like that of their Armenian neighbors, was profoundly influenced by Iranian religious tradition. The texts that form *The Conversion of K'art'li* were probably written down between the seventh and the tenth centuries CE, while the *The Life of K'art'li* dates from around 800 to the fourteenth century CE.[127]

The Life of K'art'li lists six "idols", named Armaz, Zaden, Gac'i, Ga/Gaim, Ainina and Danina, which were introduced to Georgia by different kings who bear Iranian names.[128] *The Life of K'art'li* attributes the erection of Gac'i and Ga/Gaim to the first mythical ruler of K'art'li, Azon, who, according to the text, was appointed by Alexander the Great:

> Now Azon abandoned the religion given by Alexander, and he began to worship idols. He made two idols of silver, Gac'i and Gaim.[129]
>
> After this Azon forgot the faith given by Alexander, and made two silver idols, Gac'im and Gayim by name, which he worshipped.[130]
>
> And after him P'arnavaz became [king]. He erected a great idol on the ledge of a mountain and he gave it his [own] name Armazi. And he raised a wall from the bank of the [? Mtkuari] river, and he called [this fortress] Armazi.
>
> And after him Saurmag became king. He erected the idol Aynina along a/the road. And he began to build up Armazi.
>
> And after him Mirvan reigned. And he erected the idol Danina along a/the road, in front [? of Aynina], and finished building Armazi.
>
> And P'arnajob reigned and erected the idol Zadeni on a mountain. And he built [the Zadeni fortress].[131]

The identification of the gods that appear in the Georgian texts has been long a subject of intense debate. Some scholars have proposed deriving Armazi and Zadeni from the pantheon of ancient

---

125 MX 1.31.
126 EK 2.1.
127 *The Conversion of K'art'li* and the *The Life of K'art'li* are very complex collections of texts. I am following the division and chronology proposed by Rapp 2003: 56–57.
128 P'arnavaz (299–234 BCE), Saurmag (234–159 BCE), Mirvan (159–109 BCE), and P'arnajob (109–90 BCE). All the dates are according to Rapp 2003: 485–487.
129 *KC LK* 21.
130 *KC LK* Armenian version 20.
131 Rapp 2003: 259.

Anatolia.[132] However, perhaps already from the Achaemenian period, K'art'li was wholly within the Iranian cultural sphere and Iranian influence on K'art'velian material culture is unparalleled in scope.[133] Especially noteworthy for its profound Iranian connections is the sacred complex of Dedoplis Mindori in Georgia (second-first centuries BCE).[134] Some elements of the architectural layout of Dedoplis Mindori correspond to the "Iranian type" of Iranian temples.[135]

The Georgian texts also draw a portrait of a society whose culture, royal ideology, social structure and political organization are deeply rooted in Iranian tradition,[136] which even influenced the Georgian language.[137] As has already been noted, most of the K'art'velian kings and nobles that are known to us have distinctly Iranian names.[138] The Georgian chronicles also preserve lucid references to Zoroastrian customs, such as *xvaētvadatha* (next-of-kin marriages), and to the exposure of corpses practiced by the pre-Christian population of K'art'li.[139] This strongly suggests that the Georgian gods also have Iranian interpretations, which are in fact, readily available for most of them and seem to be the most cogent.

The first two "idols", Armazi and Zadeni, are probably a corruption of a single deity—the Iranian Ahura Mazdā.[140] This is confirmed by the fact that these two deities are almost always named together, e.g. in *The Life of St Nino*:

> And they were sitting there and praising their accursed gods, Armazi and Zadeni, and promising them sacrifices upon their return.[141]

In the Georgian capital Armaz, St Nino witnesses the ritual procession in which the king and queen approach an idol of Armazi that was erected on the top of a hill. The idol is described in meticulous detail:

> Behold, there stood a man, made of copper, a golden coat of mail upon his body and a golden helmet, and his shoulder-pieces were of silver and beryl, and he held in his hand a sharpened sword, shining brightly and swinging in his hand, so that if one were to touch it, he would be doomed to death.[142]

Unfortunately, there is no means of knowing whether this vivid anthropomorphic description of the cultic statue of Armazi may be taken as reflecting the actual appearance of a real idol. If this was the case, we could suppose that Armazi was a warlike deity. Movsēs Xorenac'i calls the Georgian Aramazd, destroyed by St Nino, the "god of thunder",[143] indicating that he may indeed have possessed some traits of a warrior thunder god. It is interesting that, unlike in neighboring Armenia, Armazi seems to have led the Georgian pantheon, perhaps adopted as such in the Achaemenian period under the influence of the Persian cult.

Next to the statue of Armazi, there were two additional idols:

---

132 Van Esbroeck 1990: 2708, with references. Rapp also maintained that "the names of the idols have ancient Anatolian and Near Eastern roots"; see Rapp 2003: 273; 278. However, in the article published in 2009, he reconsidered his position and wrote that "Armazi was almost certainly connected to the Zoroastrian supreme god Ahura Mazdā" and probably represented "a localized version of the Zoroastrian Lord of Wisdom": Rapp 2009: 671, n. 68, 675–676.

133 For references, see n. 22.

134 Gagošidze 1992.

135 See Shenkar 2011.

136 Rapp 2003: 113–118; and especially Rapp 2009. See also Gvelesiani 2008.

137 Rapp 2009: 660–661.

138 See Rapp 2009: 660, who lists some of them and their Iranian etymology.

139 *KC LK* 16–17 (Armenian version 17).

140 Marr 1902: 7, maintains that Zadeni is derived from *yazdān*.

141 *MK LN* 2.2.B.

142 *MK LN* 3.3.

143 MX 2.86.

> At the right hand was another idol, of gold, and its name was Gac'i, and at its left hand was an idol of silver, and its name was Ga, and these were gods to your fathers in Arian-K'art'li.[144]

These idols are mentioned again as standing on the summit of the mountains together with Armazi and Zadeni:

> And in the land of K'art'li were two mountains and on them, the two idols, Armazi and Zadeni: they breathed the odour of thousands of souls of firstborn youth, for their parents considered it a pleasant sacrifice to Armazi and Zadeni, by which they would avoid death forever. And thus it was until now. And there were the other royal idols, Gac'i and Ga. And one of the king's household was sacrificed to them, burned with fire, and the idol's head was powdered with his ashes.[145]

In his seminal study, Nicholas Marr interpreted Gac'i and Ga/im as Semitic divine names that were adopted and transformed by the Christian historians.[146] However, as we have already seen with Armazi and Zadeni, it is possible that Gac'i and Ga/im also derive from one Iranian deity that has been corrupted beyond recognition. It is not inconceivable that this could be Vərəθraγna, who, together with Aramazd and Anahit, formed the principal triad of the pantheon in neighboring Armenia. Moreover, Movsēs Xorenac'i refers to the existence of a statue of Vahagn in Georgia that was honored with sacrifices.[147]

The Life of K'art'li and *The Conversion of K'art'li* mention two additional idols, Ainina and Danina, which may also represent an altered form of a single Iranian divine name—that of the goddess Anāhitā, although it is also possible that they conceal two distinct goddesses—Anāhitā and Nana.[148]

In *The Life of St Nino* we find an additional deity, *i'trudzhan* (Chelishi codex) or *itrushana* (Shatberdi codex), who is called the "god of the Chaldeans and the enemy of Armazi".[149] The various Mesopotamian and Syriac identifications proposed for this deity by Marr are hardly convincing.[150] The Shatberdi codex probably preserves the more original form since, in the *Martyrdom of St Shushanik* (the oldest extant piece of Georgian literature dated to the late fifth century CE), we find another variant of the same word, yet in a different context. The husband of Shushanik, Varsken, who had converted to the Persian religion during his stay at the Sasanian court, is accused of having "rejected the True God and worshipped *atrošan*".[151] We find exactly the same term in the Armenian sources where it refers to a fire-temple/altar. It is probably a loanword from Parthian **ātarōšan*, which presumably means "place of burning fire".[152] Thus, a certain Armenian noble who denounced Christianity and converted to Zoroastrianism swore before the Persian king that:

> I shall first build an atrušan in my hereditary domain, that is to say, a house for the worship of fire.[153]

Therefore, the *itrushana* mentioned in the *The Life of St Nino* is not a Chaldean god, but simply the sacred fire of the Zoroastrian religion.[154] Thus we can easily understand the apparently meaningless sentence in *The Life of St Nino*, which seeks to explain the rivalry between Itrushana and Aramazi, by the fact that the latter "turned the sea back on him [on Itrushana]",[155] or, in the Armenian version, "overcame the other [Itrushana] with water".[156] What can be more effective to fight fire than water? It is worth noting

---

144 *MK LN* 3.3.
145 *MK LN* 2.4.
146 Marr 1902: 18–23.
147 MX 1.31. This information could originate from the story about Heracles borrowed from Eusebius: Thomson 1980: 123, n. 6.
148 Already briefly discussed by Marr 1902: 9.
149 *MK LN* 2.5; *KC LN* 91, 106.
150 Marr 1902: 25–28.
151 *Mart.Susan.* 2.
152 Boyce 1975a: 98–99. See also the discussion in Russell 1987: 482–495.
153 PB 4.23.
154 This interpretation was already suggested by Kekelidze 1936. I owe this reference to Mariam Gvelesiani.
155 *KC LN* 91.
156 *KC LN* Armenian version 48.

that, in the Armenian version of *The Life of St Nino*, Itrushana is called "the god of the Persians".[157] It is possible that the Armenian translator used a different Georgian manuscript which has not survived but which contained the correct Iranian association of Itrushana.

The "rivalry" between the Georgian god, Armazi, and the Persian sacred fire, Itrushana, reflects a common tendency in the Georgian texts, which not only differentiate between the ancestral religion of the Georgians (associated with idols) and the Persian religion (characterized by the fire-worship), but often set them against each other:

> He [king P'arnajob] built the castle of Zaden; and he made an idol with the name of Zaden and set it up at Zaden. He also began the construction of the city of Nelkarisi, which is Nekrisi, in Kaxet'i. After this he adopted the religion of the Persians, fire-worship. He brought from Persia fire-worshippers and magi and installed them at Mc'xet'a, in the place which is now called Mogut'a. He began openly to blaspheme the idols. Therefore, the inhabitants of K'art'li hated him, because they had great faith in the idols.[158]
>
> He built the citadel of (Z)adēn, erected an image at (Z)adēn, and built in Kaxet'i the city Nekrēs. After this he honoured the magi of the Persian religion, built for them a site which is now called Mogt'a, and established a fire-temple. The Georgians were angered and requested Varbak, king of Armenia, to give them his own son as king. 'For our king, they said, has forgotten the faith of his maternal ancestors, and serves his paternal religion'.[159]

In another place, Mirvan, son of king P'arnajob, says to the Georgians:

> Although I have been raised among Persians, yet I abide by the religion of your fathers. I believe in the gods who protect K'art'li ...[160]

Later, when the Persian king appoints his son Mirvan to rule over Georgians, he also promises them that:

> My son will observe both religions, the fire-worship of our fathers and the worship of your idols.[161]

Yet the Persian religion is also associated with idols in the Georgian texts. In the narrative on the exploits of king P'arnajob, the idol Zaden, built by him, seems to be related to the religion of the Persians and to "fire-worship". In the *Life of St Nino* (*The Life of K'art'li* version), the first Georgian Christian king Mirvan orders his son:

> Where you find those abominations, the idols of fire(-worship), destroy them by fire and make those who hope in them drink the ashes.[162]

St Nino finds in the capital Mc'xet'a the "magism and error of those people who worshipped fire ...",[163] but the magi are described as the adversaries of the chief idol of the city, Armazi:

> If anyone approached, he resigned himself to death and said: 'Woe to me if I have neglected the majesty of the great god Armazi, or we have allowed ourselves to speak with the Hebrews or to heed the magi'.[164]
>
> They trembled and said: 'Woe unto us. If we have failed in sacrifice or have sinned by speaking with a Jew or with magi, we shall be put to death by Aramazd'.[165]

The picture that emerges from the Georgian sources, therefore, is ambiguous and confused. Rapp suggests that the religion of pre-Christian K'art'li was a local form of Zoroastrianism,[166] which was

157 *KC LN* Armenian version 56.
158 *KC LK* 29.
159 *KC LK* Armenian version 27.
160 *KC LK* 31.
161 *KC LK* 65.
162 *KC LN* 130.
163 *KC LN* 88.
164 *KC LN* 89.
165 *KC LN* Armenian version 47.
166 Rapp 2009: 673, n. 76.

replaced by king P'arnajob with the Iranian version practiced by the Sasanians.[167] To the Christian authors of these texts, the Georgian ancestral religion was not identical with the Persian one, at least not under the later Georgian kings. Despite being headed by gods with Iranian names, the "idol-worship" of K'art'li is clearly set apart from the "Persian religion of fire-worshippers", although the latter also appears to be associated with idols.[168]

It seems that the religion of K'art'li, just like its material culture, was greatly influenced by Iranian civilization in the Achaemenian period. It is in this context that the "Georgian ancestral pantheon" with an "Iranian substratum" was formed out of a mixture of Iranian and local elements. It seems that the Georgians represented the Iranian gods, which were introduced to K'art'li by the Iranians or an Iranized ruling elite, in human form and the veneration of their idols, made of precious metals, played a central part in the Georgian cult. The distinction and later tension between the "ancestral Georgian" and Persian Sasanian religions probably reflect the differences that developed in each, both of which had similar Achamenian foundations. It is possible that they also reflect an attempt by the Sasanians,[169] to enforce Zoroastrianism in K'art'li as they tried to do in Armenia.

However, the attitude of the Georgian sources towards Persian religion is not always negative. We find magi living in their own district, in the K'art'velian capital Armazi, and seemingly practicing their own cult in a manner very similar to the Jews and other religious groups. Idolatry seems to lie at the center of the Georgian cult. Out of seven idols venerated by the ancient Georgians, according to *The Life of K'art'li* and *The Conversion of K'art'li*, four relate to Iranian tradition and probably refer to two deities (Ahura Mazdā and Anāhitā, or Ahura Mazdā and Nana), two are of uncertain etymology and origin, and one is also probably Iranian. It is noteworthy that, in the earliest Georgian historical source—*The Conversion of K'art'li* (which forms the core of the collection of texts bearing the same name, probably composed in the seventh century CE)[170]—information regarding the pre-Christian gods and cults of K'art'li is almost completely absent. We only find a group of unnamed idols that were surrendered by Georgian nobles to be destroyed.[171]

3. *Syriac*

Although Syriac sources provide very little information that is relevant to our subject, one hagiographic collection, *The Acts of the Persian Martyrs*, does give some useful information.[172] The potential of this source for the study of Zoroastrianism has not yet been fully realised, since there is still no critical edition of many sections,[173] few of which have been translated into a modern language.[174] Furthermore, no one has yet assembled the Iranian religious material that is preserved in *The Acts of the Persian Martyrs*.[175]

---

167 Rapp 2009: 668, n. 61.

168 However, this most probably reflects the monotheistic anti-idolic discourse rather than actual worship of divine statues by the Sasanians. For the discussion of this discourse, see Chapter Five.

169 King P'arnajob is estimated to have ruled from 109 to 90 BCE, more than 300 years before the advent of the Sasanian dynasty. Therefore, the attribution of the "religious reform" to that king could be an anachronism. Alternatively, it is possible that the entire chronology of the early K'art'velian kings, much of which is conjecture, should be revised.

170 Rapp and Crego 2006: 185.

171 Rapp and Crego 2006: 193.

172 For a recent overview of Syriac sources on pre-Islamic Iran, see Gignoux 2009. Jullien 2008 and Brock 2009 provide further bibliographic information for *The Acts of the Persian Martyrs*. A number of fragments referring to Zoroastrianism were assembled by Bidez and Cumont 1938: 93–137. Some individual Syriac texts were also discussed by Benveniste 1932/1933 and de Menasce 1938.

173 The non-critical edition is Bedjan 1890/1897.

174 Hoffmann 1880.

175 With the exception of Gray 1913/1914, which, however, only discusses the Greek texts.

In Syriac literature, Persian religion is generally associated with the worship of luminaries, the Sun, the Moon and other natural elements.[176] Sometimes the names of the "Persian" gods are mentioned in their Semitic form. Thus, during the great persecutions of Christians under Šāpūr II, the king ordered one of his generals, a recent convert to Christianity, to worship the Sun, the Moon, Fire, Zeus, Bel, Nebo and Nanai, "the great goddess of the world".[177] However, references to statues of Iranian gods are very rarely encountered.

The eighth-century author Theodore bar Koni states that, in the days of king Pērōz:

> an edict was issued against idols and their priests, that the religion of the magi alone may continue.[178]

It is not entirely clear whether the decree was directed against adherents of pagan Mesopotamian cults, "idolatrous" Iranians or Christians, but there is evidence of Christians being persecuted during the reign of Pērōz.[179] The last part of the sentence suggests that an attempt was made to suppress all non-Zoroastrian religions and cults. Theodore bar Koni is more famous for his account of the birth of Ohrmazd and Ahriman, which closely corresponds to the similar story found in the writings of the Armenian historian Eznik Koghbac'i.[180] Bar Koni also describes the newborn Ahriman as "gloomy and hideous" and Ohrmazd as "odorous and brilliant".[181] His description of Zoroastrianism contains a curious passage in which he writes that: the Earth was an adolescent virgin betrothed to Parisag (Av. *Fraŋrasyan*, MP. *Frāsiyāg*; NP. *Afrāsīāb*); fire was given the ability to speak and walked with Gounrap (Av. *Kərəsāspa*, NP. *Garšāsp*); Parisag was once a fish, an ant or an old dog; Koum (Av. *Haoma*) was a dolphin and a cock that swallowed Parisag; and Kiku'uz (Av. *Kauui Usan*, NP. *Kay Kāvus*) was a mountain ram.[182] Although the Earth convincingly alludes to the goddess Spəntā Ārmaiti, and Koum was recognized as the god Haoma, the exact source of these motifs is not clear as they are not attested in the extant fragments of Iranian mythology.[183]

Another largely neglected Syriac hagiographical text, which was produced in Sasanian Northern Mesopotamia and contains some information about Iranian religion, is the *Life of Mar Yāreth the Alexandrian*. It tells of Mar Yāreth's encounter with the "idols" associated with the "Magi".[184] Mar Yāreth and his disciple arrive in the village of Ragūlū, which is in the province of Beth Arbaye in Northern Mesopotamia, and which is said "to be very strong in Magianism (*mgūšūtā*) and in the stinking doctrine of idols (*ptakrē*)". In this village there was "a great house of idols" (*bēt ptakrē ḥad rabā*) that was adorned with "thirty-two images/statues/idols" (*ṣalmīn*) and where many priests (*kūmrē*) served. When the saint entered the temple, he found a villager and asked him about the "images". The man answered, "they are gods (*'alāhē*), whom all the earthly kings worship (*sāgdīn*)". Upon hearing this, St Yāreth proclaimed, "God forbids that the believing (i.e. Christian) kings should worship idols/statues" (*l-glipē sāgdīn*). He then prayed in front of the statues, which fell down upon the priests and killed them. The statues were then broken into pieces. Then, according to the well-known hagiographical *topos*, St Yāreth resurrected the priests, and all the inhabitants of the village, characterized as "pagans" (*ḥanpē*) and "Magians" (*mgūšē*), converted to Christianity.

---

176 Shaked 1994a: 90.
177 Shaked 1994a: 91.
178 Gero 1981: 16.
179 Gero 1981: 17.
180 See p. 22.
181 BK 11.13.
182 BK 11.13.
183 See the discussion of this passage in Benveniste 1932/1933: 192–204.
184 The Syriac text (according to the manuscript British Museum Add. 12,174, fol. 253^{v}–259^{r}) and the English translation were courteously provided by Sergey Minov, who is preparing a critical edition of this text.

Contrary to Theodore bar Koni, who clearly distinguishes between "idols and their priests" and the magi, the author of this text uses the terms "magi" and "pagans" interchangeably and it is impossible to establish whether this temple and its idols had anything in common with Iranian religion. It is noteworthy that the priests in the temple are not called "magi" but *kūmrē*. The same word *k'urm* in Armenia was also used to designate a pre-Christian priest.[185] The story of Mar Yāreth could be taken as another expression of the syncretistic Irano-Semitic cults of Late Antique Babylonia, but it could reflect the polemical intention of the author to combine the local "pagan" religion with the religion of the Persian rulers.

In the Syriac version of *The Alexander Romance*, Alexander the Great is credited with founding a temple in Samarkand that was painted with gold, decorated with precious paintings and dedicated to "the goddess Rhea whom they call Nani".[186] This description corresponds to the interior of Sogdian temples, which were adorned with beautiful paintings.

The Syriac hagiographical texts allude to idols in temples, presumably in an Iranian context. The authenticity of these sources, however, is often questionable and it is impossible to ascertain whether these temples and idols are indeed related to the Iranian cult. Furthermore, one has to keep in mind that accusations of "idolatry" are typical of monotheistic discourse. Labeling someone as an "idol-worshipper" does not necessarily imply that they actually used idols or were even polytheistic.[187]

It is to be hoped that scholars of Syriac will assemble and study the Iranian material contained in these texts. This would undoubtedly contribute to our understanding of the Iranian cult and the general religious situation in the Sasanian Empire and Late Antique Babylonia.

4. *Greek*

In the Greek *Acts of the Persian Martyrs*, there is a curious piece in the *Passion of St Acindynus* (who was martyred during the persecutions of Šāpūr II). It contains the story of an "idol of Zeus" in the temple (ναός), which fell to the ground when the saint, led by the king, entered the sanctuary.[188] Although ναός is a general word for temple in Greek, the context of the narrative suggests that this might have been a fire-temple. Zeus is a well-attested *interpretatio graeca* of Ahura Mazdā, so it could be that this text is unique in mentioning an idol in a Sasanian fire-temple. However, the date and historical value of this text are uncertain, since St Acindynus and his companions are not known from any other source.[189]

There is an interesting account regarding St Eugene of Trapezus who, in the late third century, destroyed a statue of Mithra that was standing on the "Hill of Mithra" in the Pontic city of Trapezus.[190] Although Western Mithraic mysteries are attested at Trapezus in the Roman period, the "Hill of Mithra" appears more appropriate for the cult of an Iranian god than the Roman Mithraic cult, which was usually celebrated in caves and subterranean sanctuaries.[191]

In his account of Heraclius' campaign against the Sasanians, Cedrenus, based on the story of Theophanes, thus describes a painting that Heraclius encountered at the fire-temple Ta<u>k</u>t-e Solaymān (Ādur Gušnasp—one of the three principal sanctuaries of Late Sasanian Iran):

> And after the conquest of the town of Gaznaca, where the fire-temple, treasure of Craesus king of the Lydes, and the false veneration of charcoal were located, when he entered there, (Heraclius) found the abominable image of Cosroes, his figure in the domed chamber of the palace, as though he were enthroned in heaven

185 Russell 1987: 299; Garsoïan 1989: 539–540.
186 Grenet 1995/1996b: 215–216.
187 On the polemical use of "idolatry" in monotheistic discourse, see Hawting 1999: 67–88.
188 Gray 1913/1914: 46.
189 Delehaye 1907: 407.
190 Boyce and Grenet 1991: 302.
191 Boyce and Grenet 1991: 302–303.

> and around it the Sun, the Moon and the Stars, to which ones (the Persian king) was paying a superstitious fear as he were serving the gods, and placed round angels bearing scepters to him. He (i.e. Cosroes), fighting against God, had arranged a machine which, from that place let drops of rain fall and produced sounds like that of thunders.[192]

Nikephoros also reports on the same episode:

> In one of these (temples of fire) it was discovered that Xosroes, making himself into a god, had put up his own picture on the ceiling, as if he were seated in heaven, and had fabricated the stars, the sun and the moon, and angels standing round him, and a mechanism for producing thunder and rain whenever he so wished.[193]

From these descriptions it seems that the painting in question was probably situated in the palatial and not in the sacred part of the temple. Matthew Canepa has suggested that the Byzantines might have confused the image of Ahura Mazdā for the image of the king,[194] although it could also be Vohu Manah, who is described in Kartīr's vision and in the journey of Ardā Wīrāz as seated on a golden throne.[195] While there are numerous images of enthroned kings, no representation of an enthroned deity is known from Sasanian art. It is more likely, therefore, that Ta*k*t-e Solaymān was indeed decorated with a painting depicting the Sasanian king.

5. *The Babylonian Talmud*

The Babylonian Talmud (*Bavli*) was edited in Sasanian Babylonia.[196] Although it contains little information regarding the earlier periods of Iranian history,[197] and despite the Talmudic sages' preoccupation with matters Roman rather than Persian,[198] the *Bavli* can still provide some insights into Sasanian religion. There are some references to Iranian mythological motifs,[199] but there are no descriptions of, or explicit references to, Zoroastrian deities, except for the mention of Ahura Mazdā and the Evil Spirit (*Sanhedrin 39a*) and the possible identification of Ahura Mazdā with a demon.[200]

Richard Kalmin has assembled the passages from the *Bavli* that mention idols and idolatry.[201] In contrast to its preoccupation with cultic statues in Palestine, the *Bavli* contains only sporadic references to them in Babylonia.[202] It would seem that idols were not usually present in Babylonian public spaces, so the rabbis did not encounter them unless they themselves took the initiative and sought them out.[203]

We thus find the story of Rav Menasheh encountering an idol of *Markolis* (Mercury) in a place called Bei Torta:[204]

---

192 Panaino 2004: 563–564.
193 Panaino 2004: 564
194 Canepa 2009: 148–149.
195 See p. 11–12 and p. 32.
196 The final redaction of the *Bavli* is now thought to have occurred in the sixth-seventh centuries CE; see Kalmin 2008: 641, n. 44. For a useful survey, see also Kamlin 2006a. The last few years have seen a renaissance in the field of "Irano-Talmudica", with an increasing number of scholars contributing to our understanding of Iranian and Jewish traditions under the Sasanian Empire. For example, see Herman 2005; Elman 2007; Secunda 2009; and the collection of articles in Bakhos and Shayegan 2010.
197 Krauss 1940: 27.
198 Krauss 1940: 90, 97.
199 See Kiperwasser and Shapira 2008; Kiperwasser and Shapira 2012; Kiperwasser and Shapira forthcoming; Kiperwasser forthcoming.
200 Kiperwasser forthcoming.
201 Kalmin 2006b: 103–121; Kalmin 2008.
202 Kalmin 2008: 632.
203 Kalmin 2008: 630.
204 B. *Sanhedrin* 64a.

> Said Rava bar Rav Yizhak to Rav Yehudah, "Behold there is a temple of an idol in our locality. When the world needs rain, [the idol] appears to them in a dream and says to them, 'Slaughter for me a man and I will bring rain'. They slaughter for it a man and rain comes".[205]

Another important reference records the existence of a statue in a synagogue:

> Behold the synagogue of Shaf ve-Yatev in Nehardea in which they had set up a statue (*andarta*), and Abuha de-Shmuel and Levi entered it and prayed in it and they did not worry about suspicion.[206]

It appears that this story is referring to the statue of the king rather than the image of a deity.[207] The rabbis mentioned in this story were probably active in Babylonia before the rise of the Sasanians, during the Parthian period.[208] The identity of other idols mentioned in the *Bavli* is unknown. In fact, it seems that they are most likely to represent Pagan deities of Greek or ancient Mesopotamian origin, such as Zeus, Ares, Aphrodite, Tammūz, Bel, Nergal Nabu and others,[209] rather than Iranian deities, evidence for whose worship in Late Antique Babylonia is very meager.

It is impossible to establish either the size of the Iranian population or the number of Zoroastrians in Sasanian Babylonia.[210] Not all Iranians were Zoroastrian, as many were converts to Christianity.[211] It seems that Zoroastrians were mainly associated with the administration and the military, so their numbers were probably limited.[212] Moreover, Mesopotamian "Zoroastrianism" was probably quite different from that attested in Middle Persian literature, being significantly influenced by the local Semitic religions.[213] The Iranian population appears to have been concentrated mainly in the major cities such as Ctesiphon.[214] Some Iranians also held estates in Babylonia, while others served as garrisoned troops.[215] Christian sources attest to the popularity of the "Magian religion" in the area around Arbela in the middle of the eighth century CE.[216] The sources suggest that, besides Ctesiphon, the main concentration of the Zoroastrian population was in the northern regions of Babylonia.

Magi are frequently mentioned by various sources,[217] but there is only limited evidence for the existence of fire-temples in Babylonia.[218] The Arab historian al-Masʿūdī refers to a fire-temple in *Astīniyā*, near Baghdad, which was established by the Sasanian queen Bōrān, and also notes the existence of numerous fire-temples in Iraq.[219] There were also fire-temples in Ctesiphon, Irbil and Sawād (near Sūrā).[220] However, it seems that the majority of Babylonians in the Sasanian period were ethnically and culturally Semitic and spoke Aramaic.

The *Bavli* refers to the magi even less than it refers to idols, and usually only negatively.[221] Despite its paucity of references to idols in Babylonia, the *Bavli* contains extensive polemics against idolatry,[222] which, according to Richard Kalmin, was merely "in the minds of the rabbis".[223] While there is no

---

205 B. *Avodah Zarah* 55a.
206 B. *Avodah Zarah* 43b.
207 Kalmin 2008: 638, n. 31.
208 Kalmin 2006b: 108.
209 Hämeen-Anttila 2006: 46–52. Some of these are mentioned in the incantation bowls.
210 Morony 1976: 41. For the distribution of the Iranian population in Sasanian Mesopotamia, see Morony 2005: Chapter 5.
211 Morony 2005: 280.
212 Morony 2005: 280.
213 Shaked 1997: 114–115.
214 See Morony 2005: 280.
215 Morony 1976: 46.
216 Robinson 2004: 98–100.
217 See Morony 1976: 41; Morony 2005: Chapter 10.
218 Morony 1976: 44.
219 Masʿūdī, vol. 2, 1412.
220 See Morony 1976: 44; Morony 2005: 283.
221 Kalmin 2010: 92–93 and references given in n. 52. See also Secunda 2005/2009.
222 Kalmin 2008: 639.
223 Kalmin 2008: 642.

doubt that such polemics are part of a late antique discourse common to Christianity, Islam and Zoroastrianism,[224] the possibility remains that the pagans of late antique Babylonia continued the traditions of ancient Mesopotamia. The majority of the population of Babylonia in this period seems to have been pagan, and there is evidence that pagan temples and shrines, which undoubtedly contained idols, continued to exist in the Babylonian countryside even into the Islamic period.[225] Therefore, it is likely that the situation with idol-worship in Babylonia was different to the Roman Near East in that, in Babylonia, idols were removed from the public sphere and kept in the temples, in accordance with millennia old Mesopotamian practice. This, rather than a "Sasanian iconoclasm" as proposed by Kalmin,[226] could be the main reason underlying the paucity of evidence for encounters with cultic statues in the *Bavli*.

Unlike Palestinian rabbis, Babylonian rabbis simply did not have the opportunity to encounter idols in baths or market places. As Kalmin mentions in passing,[227] contrary to the Graeco-Roman tradition, where statues were abundant in the public environment, in Babylonia anthropomorphic images of gods were confined to the temples in line with the ancient Mesopotamian practice, and the common people were able to see them only on special occasions and festivals. When the Mesopotamian gods were displayed outside the temples during the year, they were usually represented by a non-anthropomorphic symbol.[228] This explains why the rabbis devoted considerable effort to the polemics against idols, but only rarely encountered the objects of their attacks themselves.

6. *Zoroastrian Middle Persian Literature*[229]

Zoroastrian Middle Persian (Pahlavi) literature is a corpus of mainly theological texts containing Zoroastrian religious ideas, commentary on the Avesta and various ritual prescriptions. This literature was composed, or at least assembled and edited, in the Islamic period (chiefly in the ninth-tenth centuries CE).[230] It is not always clear, therefore, whether certain material reflects a genuine Sasanian context or the later setting in which the diminishing Zoroastrian community were living under oppressive Muslim rule.[231]

Middle Persian literature contains numerous anthropomorphic allusions to Zoroastrian deities. In the *Dēnkard* (7.3), Zoroaster sees Vohu Manah (Wahman) in the shape of a man:

> *ka az ān ul raft zardušt, ā-š mard dīd ka raft az *rapiϑwin-tar nēmag. ān būd wahman, ud ān awe sahist wahman pēškarb, ku pad-tan-cašm-tar bawēd, ud pēš-nēk, ku pad harw ciš pēš būd, ān awe sahist wahman cand ān ī 3-mard-nēzag bālāy …*
>
> When Zoroaster went up from there, he saw a man who was going from the southern direction. That was Wahman. Wahman seemed to him as one who has the form in front, so that he might be more visible to bodily eye, and as one who has goodness in front, namely, he was to the fore in everything. Wahman seemed to him to have the height of three spears of a man …[232]

Zoroaster also encounters Vohu Manah in a vision in the *Wizīdagīhā ī Zādspram*:

---

224 See p. 183ff and Shenkar forthcoming a.
225 Hämeen-Anttila 2006: 197.
226 Kalmin 2006b: 103–104; Kalmin 2008: 630, 638. For a discussion of the unsubstantiated theory of "Sasanian iconoclasm", see p. 183ff and Shenkar forthcoming a.
227 Kalmin 2008: 655.
228 See detailed disscussion on p. 180.
229 Transcriptions and translations of Middle Persian texts have often been modified either by me or by the *Middle Persian Dictionary Project*.
230 For a general survey of Middle Persian literature, see Cereti 2001.
231 Shaked 1994a: *passim*; Shaked 2008: 105.
232 *Dk.*(*M*) 624.8–12; Shaked 1971: 62.

ka-š az āb abar āmad u-š jāmag pōšīd ēg-eš dīd wahman amahraspand pad mard ēwēnag ī hu-cihr ī rōšn ī brāzyāg kē-š wars wizīmag dāšt ceōn wizīmag nīšān ī dōīh paymōzan-ē abrēšom homānāg būd paymōxt dāšt ke-š ne būd ēc brīn ud darz pad-eš ce xwad rōšn u-š būd bālāy nō andčand zardušt.

When he [Zoroaster] came out of the water, and put on his clothes, he then saw Wahman Amahraspand in the human form, handsome, shining and radiant, who had his hair divided, like what is divided is a sign of duality; he was wearing a dress like silk, in which there was no cut or seam, like it was light itself and his height was nine (times) as much as (that) of Zardušt.[233]

In the same text, Daēnā manifests herself as a beautiful woman[234] and Spəntā Ārmaiti (Spandarmad) appears in the form of a young girl:

u-š paymōxt dāšt rōšnīg paymōzan kē be frōgīhist ō wispān kustagān hāsar-+ē drahnāy ī ast +frasang-ē homānāg u-š pad mayān bast dāšt zarrēn kustīg ī xwad būd …

[She] wore a shining robe which radiated in all directions, for the distance of one *hāsar*, that is one parasang. And she was girded with a golden girdle …[235]

In the *Dēnkard*, Zoroaster sees Spandarmad who is "good from the front, good from the back and good all-around, beautiful in every place" (*hu-ōrōn ud hu-parrōn ud hu-tarist ku hamāg gyāg nēk būd*).[236]

Another reference to Vohu Manah's visual appearance is found in *Ardā Wīrāz Nāmag*, which describes the journey of the righteous Wīrāz to heaven and hell and his interaction with some Zoroastrian deities. During his extra-corporeal journey, Wīrāz is accompanied by Sraoša (Srōš) and Ādur, who are described anthropomorphically:

pad ān ī fradom šab man ō padīrag be mad srōš-ahlaw ud ādur-yazad … ud pas pērōzgar srōš-ahlaw ud ādur-yazad ān ī man dast frāz grift.

On the first night the righteous Srōš and the god Ādur came to meet me … Then victorious Srōš, the righteous and the god Ādur took hold of my hand.[237]

Wīrāz encounters his Daēnā who appears as a beautiful girl:

u-š ān ī xwēš dēn ud ān ī xwēš kunišn padīrag āmad kanīg kirb ī nēk pad dīdan ī hu-rust ku pad frārōnīh rust ēstēd frāz-pestān ku-š pestān abāz-nišast ī dagrand angust ke-š kirb ēdōn rōšn ceōn dīd hu-dōšag-tar nigerišn abāyišnīg-tar.

Then his own *daēnā* and his own deeds [came towards him] in the form of a girl, fine in appearance, well grown that is, she was grown in virtue, with prominent breasts that is, her breasts were uplifted, whose fingers were long, whose body was so luminous that (her) appearance was most pleasing and contemplating (her) was most seemly.[238]

When Wīrāz crosses the Činwad bridge (assisted by Mihr, Rašn, the good Wāy, Wahrām, and Aštād) he sees the god Rašn:

u-m dīd man ardā wirāz rašn ī rāst ke tarāzūg ī zard ī zarrēn pad dast dāšt ud ahlawān ud druwandān handāzēd.

And I, Ardā Wirāz, saw the just Rašn, who held in his hand a yellow golden balance, weighing (the deeds of) the righteous and the sinners.[239]

233 *WZ* 21.4.
234 *WZ* 31.5.
235 *WZ* 4.5–6.
236 *Dk* 7.4.58.
237 *AWN* 4.1, 3. In 5.4 and 11.7 the gods again take the hand of Ardā Wīrāz.
238 *AWN* 4.9.
239 *AWN* 5.3.

Vohu Manah, who is also undoubtedly anthropomorphic, rises from the golden throne to meet him:

> *ud pas ul ēstād wahman amahraspand az gāh ī zarrēn-kard. u-š ān ī man dast frāz grift pad humat ud hūxt ud huwaršt.*
>
> And then Wahman Amahraspand rose up from the golden seat. He took hold of my hand with good thoughts, good speech and good deeds.[240]

Wīrāz claims that he also saw the Aməša Spənta and other gods, but unfortunately does not provide more details on his experience:

> *u-m dīd hēm amahraspandān. u-m dīd abārīg yazdān.*
>
> And I saw the Amahraspands. And I saw other gods.[241]

Wīrāz is even honored with an audience with Ahura Mazdā himself:

> *ce-m rōšnīh dīd u-m tan ne dīd u-m wāng ašnūd u-m dānist ku ēn ast ohrmazd.*
>
> For I saw a light but did not see a body, and I heard a voice and I understood that it was Ohrmazd.[242]

This important sentence confirms that all the other gods appeared before Wīrāz in human shape. Moreover, it is to be understood that Ahura Mazdā also has a body that can be seen. The "position" of Wīrāz was just not "elevated" enough to enable this.

The prophet Zoroaster was able to see Ahura Mazdā. In a passage from the Middle Persian *Šāyast nē Šāyast*, based on a lost Avestan text, Ahura Mazdā is described as having a complete anthropomorphic appearance:

> *az abistāg gyāg-ēw paydāg ku zardušt pēš ōhrmazd nišast u-š wāz hamē xwast u-š ō ohrmazd guft ku-m sar ud dast ud pāy ud wars ud rōy ud uzwān ī tō ēdōn pad cašm ceōn ān-ez ī xweš ud wistarag ān dārēh ī mardōmān dārēnd. u-m dast dah tā dast ī tō be gīrēm. ohrmazd guft ku man mēnōg ī a-griftār hēm dast ī man griftan ne tuwān. zardušt guft ku tō a-griftār ud wahman ud ardwahišt ud šahrewar ud spandarmad ud hordād ud amurdād a-griftār ud man ka az pēš ī tō be šawēm ud tō ud awēšān-ez nē wēnēm ce ān kas ī ka-š wēnēm u-š yazēm az-eš ciš ham tō ud ān haft amahraspand yašt bawēd ayāb nē. ohrmazd guft ku šnawē ō tō gōwēm spitamān zardušt ku amāh harw tan-ēw dāyag-ēw ī xwēš ō gētīg dād ēstēd ke rāy ān xwēš-kārīh ī pad mēnōg kunēd pad gētīg andar tan ī awe rawāg kunēd. gētīg ān ī man ke ohrmazd hēm mard ī ahlaw ud wahman gōspand ud ardwahišt ātaxš ud šahrewar ayōšust ud spandarmad zamīg ud nāirīg ī nēk ud hordād āb ud amurdād urwar.*
>
> It is revealed by a passage of the Avesta that Zardušt was seated before Ohrmazd and was learning his word by heart and he spoke to Ohrmazd, saying "Your head and hands and feet and hair and face and tongue (are) visible to me even as those of my own, and you have such clothes as men have. Give me (your) hand, so that I may take hold of your hand". Ohrmazd said "I am an intangible spirit; it is not possible to take hold of my hand". Zardušt said "You (are) intangible, and Wahman and Ardwahišt and Šahrewar and Spandarmad and Hordād and Amurdād (are) intangible; and when I depart from before you, and do not see you and them also when I see that person and worship him, there is something (perceptible) of him should you and those seven Amahraspands be worshipped likewise or not?" Ohrmazd said "Listen. I say to you, oh Spitama Zardušt! Each one of us has given to the material world (*gētīg*) a foster-mother of his own, where by the proper duty which he makes in the spiritual world (*mēnōg*) is made current in the material world. (In) that material world of Mine, I, who am Ohrmazd, (preside over) the just man, and Wahman over cattle, and Ardwahišt over fire, and Šahrewar over metals, and Spandarmad over earth and virtuous woman, and Hordād over waters, and Amurdād over plants".[243]

240 *AWN* 11.1–2.

241 *AWN* 11.9.

242 *AWN* 101.6.

243 *ŠnŠ* 15.1–5.

In another Middle Persian text, the *Dādestān ī dēnīg*, written in the ninth century CE by the Zoroastrian priest Manūščihr, it is claimed that it is possible to see Ahura Mazdā in *mēnōg* "through wisdom and the power of similitude":[244]

> *18-om pursišn ān pursīd ku ruwān ī ahlawān ud ruwān ī druwandān ka be ō mēnōgān šawēnd +ēg-šān ohrmazd ud ahreman be abāyēd dīd ayāb ne? passox ēd ku ahreman rāy guft ēstēd ku-š gētīg nēst. ohrmazd-ez andar mēnōgān mēnōg pad ān ī gētīgīg ud ān-ez ī mēnōgīg +šnāyišnīg. kirb wēnišnīg spurr nē be pad xrad ud zōr ī hangōšīdag wēnīhēd. ī ceōn guft be ō spitāmān zardušt ka-š +dast-dahišnīh zāyist u-š guft ku: dast ī +mard ī ašō gīr ce-m pad tō xwēš dēn hu-cašm gīrišnīh ī and ku gīrē wēnē ān ke az ān ī man xrad ud xwarrah mehmānīh wēš abar. ruwān ī ahlawān ud druwandān pad ān ī mēnōgīg sōhišn ān gāh wēnēnd ke ohrmazd dīd ud sahēnd. ēdōn-ez ān ī ahreman +ham-zamān pad ān ī xrad ī-š dādār abar burd bārīgīhā be šnāsānd tā ohrmazd ud ahreman.*
>
> The eighteenth question: when the soul of the righteous and that of the wicked go to the spiritual world, is it possible for them to see Ohrmazd and Ahriman or not? The reply is this: it has been said of Ahriman that he has no material existence. Ohrmazd is indeed a spirit among the spiritual beings and deserves propitiation in the material as well as in the spiritual world. His form is not completely visible, but he is seen through wisdom and the power of similitude. As he (i.e. Ohrmazd) told Spitama Zardušt, when he (i.e. Zardušt) asked (him) to give him a hand, and he said: 'Grasp the hand of the righteous man (i.e. guide him), for when you grasp my religion with a good eye (generously), you see as much as you grasp, that which has more of my wisdom and splendor dwelling in him. The souls of the righteous and the wicked see through a spiritual sense the place which was seen by Ohrmazd, and they like it (?). Likewise in the case of Ahriman, by the wisdom which the Creator provided to them, they will at once discern between Ohrmazd and Ahriman.[245]

The thirteenth question in the same text addresses the visibility of the gods in general and Ahura Mazdā in particular:

> *u-š wahman amahraspand ō ohrmazd ī dādār handēmānēnēd ud az ohrmazd framān gāh ud mizd paydāgēnēd ān ī ohrmazd ō handēmān gāh pad ān ī wēnēd dānēd ud ayābed šād bawēd. ohrmazd ī weh dahagān dādār andar-ez mēnōgān mēnōg u-š mēnōgān-ez wēnišn ōh dīd ī mēnōgān abar gētīgan paydāg. be ān ī ka pad wuzurg-andēšīh ī dādār mēnōgān gētīgīg-wēnišnīhā paymōzēnd ayāb ō gētīgān mēnōg sōhišnīg wēnišn abyōzēnd enyā axw pad gētīg sōhišn mēnōgān dīd pad ān hangōšīdag tuwān ceōn ka tanīhā wēnēnd ī ke-š ruwān andar ayāb ka ātaxš wēnēnd ke-š wahrām andar ayāb āb wēnēnd ke-š xwēš mēnōg andar ast.*
>
> And Wahman the Amahraspand introduces him into (the presence) of Ohrmazd the Creator and by order of Ohrmazd he makes manifest his place and reward, (namely) a place in the presence of Ohrmazd, (and) he becomes glad through what he sees, knows and gets. Ohrmazd, the Creator of the good creatures, is indeed a spirit of spirits (*mēnōgān mēnōg*), and the beings of his *mēnōg* vision is (like) that which is manifest to the *gētīg* beings through watching the *mēnōg* beings. Except when through the great consideration of the Creator, the *mēnōg* beings are clothed in *gētīg* visibility, or when the *mēnōg* vision is joined to the *gētīg* beings, the self being (of men) can see the spirits through a *gētīg* sense by that similitude in just such a way as when one sees bodies in which there the soul, or when one sees fire in which there is Wahrām, or when one sees water in which there is its own spirit.[246]

In the *Pahlavi Rivāyat Accompanying the Dādestān ī Dēnīg*, which is probably dated to the late ninth or early tenth century CE,[247] Ohrmazd and Spandarmad are described as an affectionate, embracing couple:

> *ka zardušt pēš ohrmazd nišast ud wahman ud ardwahišt ud +šahrewar ud hordād ud amurdād ud +spandarmad pērāmōn ī ohrmazd nišīnēnd +a-š +spandarmad pad kanār nišīnēd u-š dast pad grīw āwurd estād. zardušt +be ō ohrmazd pursīd kū ēd ke pad kanār ī tō nišīnēd u-š ēdōn dōst hē ud ān-iz ō tō ēdōn dōst hē ne tō kē ohrmazd hē +az awe cašm be wardē ud ne awe az tō be wardēd ne +tō ke ohrmazd hē awe az dast be hilē ud ne awe tō az dast be hilēd. ud ohrmazd guft ēn spandarmad ī man duxt u-m kadag-bānūg ī wahišt ud mād ī dāmān.*

244 On the notion of *mēnōg*, see p. 188.
245 *Dd* 18.1–5.
246 *Dd* 30.3–5.
247 Williams 1990: 8.

When Zoroaster sat before Ohrmazd, and Wahman and Ardwahišt and Šahrewar and Hordād and Amurdād and Spandarmad are sitting around Ohrmazd, Spandarmad sits at his side, and she brought her hand (to be placed) on (his) neck. Zoroaster asked Ohrmazd: Who (is) this who is sitting at your side to whom you are so friendly, and she is also friendly to you in such a manner? Neither do you, who are Ohrmazd, turn your eyes from her, nor does she turn (hers) from you; Neither do you, who are Ohrmazd, let her from (your) hand, nor does she let you from (her) hand. And Ohrmazd said: This (is) Spandarmad, who (is) my daughter and the lady in charge of my Paradise, and the mother of the creatures.[248]

The Account of the Creation of the World found in the chapter 46 of the same text describes how Ahura Mazdā created different natural phenomena and creatures out of his own body. He created sky from his head, earth from his feet, water from his tears, plants from his hair and oxen from his right hand.[249]

Another Pahlavi text, the *Bundahišn*, provides some glimpses of the appearances of Vayu and Aŋra Mainyu (Ahriman):

way ī weh jāmag ī zarrēn ud sēmēn ud gōhr pēsīd ud ālgōnagān ud was rang paymōxt, brahmag ī artēštārīh dāšt ce abar raftār az pas ī dušmenān pad petyārag zadan ud dām pānagīh kardan.

The good Way donned a garment of gold and of silver, adorned with gems, red and of many colors, the costume of warriorhood, since his own duty consists in pursuing the enemies to smite Evil and to protect the creatures.[250]

Ahriman is said to have a frog-like (*wazaγ-kirb*) body[251] and that of "the frog, the vicious crab".[252] He also can take the shape of a "fifteen year old youth".[253]

The *Bundahišn* also describes the goddess Druwāsp as holding a horse on her limb:

u-š a-margīh ēn kū tan ī pasēn pad āmadan ud šudan ī xwaršēd bawēd. u-š arwand-aspīh ēn kū-š asp ī nēk abar druwāsp handām, čē druwāsp handām bārag dārēd. u-š rāyōmandīh ēd kū-š abzār was.

And his immortality is this, that the Future body will occur thanks to the coming and going of Xwaršēd. And his being of fast horses is this, that his good horse is on a limb of Druwāsp, as a limb of Druwāsp holds (his) destrier. And his richness is this, that he has much power.[254]

Middle Persian texts also contain numerous references to "idols" and "idol-worship".[255] According to the *Dēnkard*, it was the mythical evil dragon Dahāk, portrayed as active in Babylon, who incited people to idolatry (*uzdēs-parastišnīh*).[256] The *Dēnkard* states that "Wahrām fire represents goodness" and is "the adversary of the idols" (*ātaxš ī warahrān wehīh ud uzdēs petyārag*).[257] In the *Dādestān ī Mēnōg ī Xrad*, idol-worship is called the "eighth-worst sin".[258] It also contains the following prohibition against idol-worship:

az uzdēs-paristišnīh ud dēw-ēzagīh dūr pahrēz, ce paydāg ku agar kay-husraw uzdēszār ī pad war ī čēčist ne kand hād, andar ēn sē-hazārag ī hušēdar ud hušēdarmāh ud sōšāns ke jud-jud pad harw hazārag sar az awēšān ēk āyēd ke harw kār ī gēhān abāz wirāyēd ud mihrōdrujān ud uzdēs-paristān ī andar kišwar be zanēd, ēg petyārag ēdōn stahmag-tar būd hād ku rist-āxēz ud tan ī pasēn kardan ne šāyist hād.

---

248 *PhlRDd* 8.2–5.

249 *PhlRDd* 46. A similar account of Creation, albeit with some differences, is found in a passage by al-Jayhānī quoted by al-Shahrastānī. See p. 43–44.

250 *GBd* 3.4.

251 *IBd* 3.9; *GBd* 4.7 (*ān ganāg mēnōy kirb ī dīdan dēs wazaγ*).

252 *GBd* 27.1.

253 *GBd* 4.7.

254 *GBd* 26.67–68. tr. and ed. by Raffaelli 2014: 211. He also comments on this passage that "this sentence seems to refer to an iconographic portrayal of Druwāsp, perhaps taking its inspiration from a myth unknown to us, according to which this divine entity took care of the horses of Xwaršēd"; see Raffaelli 2014: 211, n. 15.

255 Some of these references were collected by Jackson 1914.

256 *Dk* 7.4.72. ed. and tr. by Molé 1967: 56.

257 *Dk (M)* 551.13–15.

258 *DMX* 35.

> Abstain from idol-worship and demon-veneration, because it is obvious that if Kay Husraw has not destroyed the idol-temple on the Lake Čēčist, during these three millenniums of Ušēdar and Ušēdarmāh and Sōšāns (each of) whom comes separately at the end of each millennium to rearrange the affairs of the world and to smite oath-breakers and idol-worshippers of the land, the adversary would have become stronger, that resurrection and the final embodiment would not be possible.[259]

The same text gives a description of Daēnā coming to meet the souls of the righteous in the form of a beautiful maiden:

> *u-š ān ī xwēš nēk-kunišn pad kanīg kirb ō padīrag āyēd, ī az harw kanīg ī pad gēhān hu-čihrtar ud weh, ud ān ī ahlaw ruwān gōwēd ku tō ke hē ke-m hagriz kanīg ī az tō hu-čihrtar ud weh pad gētīg ne dīd. pad passox paywāzēd ān kanīg kirb ku: az ne kanīg be kunišn ī nēk ī tō ham juwān ī hu-menišn ī hu-gōwišn ī hu-kunišn ī hu-dēn.*
>
> And that is his own good deeds coming to meet him in the form of a maiden that is more beautiful and better than any maiden in the world. And the soul of the righteous says: Whom can you be, I never saw a maiden in this world more beautiful and better than you? In answer, the form of a maiden replies: I am not a maiden, but your good deeds.[260]

From the following passage of the apocalyptic text *Zand ī Wahman Yasn*, it is clear that the idol-temple (*uzdēszār*) was considered an abode of the Evil Spirit and his demons:

> *frāz rawēd pišōtan ī wištāspān pad ham-ayārīh ī ādur farrbay, ud ādur gušnasp, ud ādur ī burzēnmihr ō uzdēszār ī wuzurg, nišēmag ī druwand gannāg mēnōg. xēšm ī xurdruš, ud hamāg dēwān, ud druzān, ud wad-tōhmagān, ud jādūgān ō ān ī zofāytom dušox rasēnd. be kanēnd ān uzdēszār pad ham-kōxšišnīh ī pišōtan ī bāmīg.*
>
> Pišōtan son of Wištāsp will go forth, in cooperation with Ādur Farrbay and Ādur Gušnasp and Ādur Burzēnmihr, to the great idol-temple, abode of evil Gannāg Mēnōg. Xēšm with the bloody club, all the *dēws* and demons, those of evil stock and the sorcerers will reach the deepest hell. They will destroy that idol-temple struggling together with the glorious Pišōtan.[261]

In the *Zand ī Wahman Yasn*, the idol-temple appears to be an antithesis of the good religion:

> *ud wāng kunēd mihr ī frāx-gōyōd ō pišōtan ī bāmīg ku, be kan, be zan ān uzdēszār ī dēwān nišēmag. raw ō ēn ērān dehān ī man ohrmazd dād abāz wirāy gāh ī dēn ud xwadāyīh … ud abar rasēd pišōtan ī bāmīg ud ādur ī farrbay, ud ādur ī gušnasp, ud ādur ī burzēnmihr ī pērōzgar be zanēd ān druz ī was-ōz, be kanēd ān uzdēszār ku nišēmag ī dēwān.*
>
> And Mihr of the wide pastures will cry to the glorious Pišōtan, "Raze, smite that idol-temple, abode of the *dēws*. Go to these Ērānian lands which I, Ohrmazd, have created (and) restore the status (of) religion and sovereignty" … And the glorious Pišōtan, the victorious Ādur Farrbay, Ādur Gušnasp and Ādur Burzēnmihr will arrive and smite those powerful demons, they will raze that idol-temple which is the abode of the *dēws*.[262]

The *Bundahišn* and other Middle Persian texts also preserve a story that Kay Khosrow destroyed an "idol-temple" (*uzdēszār*) at Lake Čēčist and established a fire cult in its place.[263] Lake Čēčist is usually identified with Lake Urmia and the temple built by Kay Khosrow with Ādur Gušnasp.

In the *Mādayān ī Hāzar Dādestān* (*The Book of a Thousand Laws*) we find traces of a legal persecution against idol-temples:

> *ēk ān ī ham pusānveh guft ku 1000 ādurōk ī mard ka dādwar pad gyāk ku uzdēs-kadag būd uzdēs az-eš kand nišāst ka-š sardār xvēšāvand ī pad nāmčišt ne paydāg būd mard ī pad warahrānīh ō dādgāh nišāst pad sardār dāštan.*

---

259 *DMX* 2.93–95.
260 *DMX* 2.125–130.
261 *ZWY* 7.26.
262 *ZWY* 7.36–37.
263 *GBd* 18.12; *IBd* 17.7; *Dk* (*M*) 599.1–2; *DMX* 2.95; *PhlRDd* 48.42.

> The same Pusānveh has also said the following: if a man sets up 1000 altars in the (very) place where there was an idol shrine—the idols having been destroyed ("dug out") there by a judge—without appointing a particular person from among his agnates as the guardian over these altars, then the man who has set up a Warahrān Fire should be considered the guardian of these altars.[264]
>
> *ud ān ī guft ku abar awe bay husraw ī kawādān mard-ē dandān nām būd mard-ē ādurtōxm nām būd pad zamīg hāwand pad uzdēs-cār dāšt ceōn pad framān ud dastwarih ī mowbedān uzdēs az-eš kand (ud) ādur(r)ōg-ē pad-eš nišāst.*
>
> It is also said, (that) under (our) late sovereign Husraw son of Kawād, one man named Dandān and another named Ādurtōxm held equal (lots) of land under an idol-shrine, when the temple of the idols was dug up from the place ("from there") by the order and with the sanction of the mowbeds, and a Fire-altar was set up there instead.[265]

The short, curious text *Shā-Wahrām* expresses a messianic hope for the advent of a ruler, from the line of the Kavis, who would free Iran from the Arab yoke, restore the Zoroastrian religion and allow the Zoroastrians to wreak their vengeance upon the Muslims: "we shall let the mosques fall down, we shall establish fires, we shall raze the idol-temples" (*mazgitīhā frōd hilēm, be nišānēm ātaxšān, uzdēszārīhā bē kanēm*).[266]

The *Kār-nāmag ī Ardašīr ī Pābagān*, one of the few non-priestly Pahlavi compositions, contains an odd story of Ardašīr's battle against the monster "Worm" (*kirm*) and his followers led by Haftōbād—the "Protector of the Worm".[267] The story is set in southern Pars along the Persian Gulf. The name "Haftōbād" may possibly provide an insight into the context of this tale. Walter B. Henning proposed that Haftōbād derives from **haftaxwa-pāta*, "The Guardian of the Seventh (part)", a title that can be traced back to the Achaemenian period.[268] This story appears to be a variant of the well-known Indo-European initiation myth of the dragon-slaying hero. In addition to the name Haftōbād, however, it contains some other curious details that might hint at its historical context. For example, the Worm is called an "idol" (*uzdēs*)[269] and his servants are constantly addressed as "idol-worshippers" (*uzdēsparistagān*).[270] Furthermore, we are told that the Evil Spirit made the Worm so powerful that "many people of (these) lands turned away from the religion of Ohrmazd and Amahraspands" (*hamōyēn mardōm ī kustagīhā az dēn ī ohrmazd ud amahraspandān wiyābān kard ēstēnd*),[271] and become idol-worshippers. It is clear, therefore, that the idolatrous followers of the "idol" Worm were not gentiles, *anērān*, adherents of foreign religions, but Iranians who have "abandoned" Zoroastrianism. The Worm was seen as a symbolic allusion to non-Zoroastrian Iranian cults, and the story as an echo of the suppression of such cults by Ardašīr I.[272]

Grenet has proposed the interesting explanation that this story might reflect religious beliefs surrounding the silk worm in China and Khotan, which were possibly transferred to the region of the Persian Gulf along with the silk itself.[273] I would add another proposal as to the origin of this enigmatic story. It is set in or around Elymais, where the Elamite-speaking population survived into Islamic times. One of the most prominent features of Elamite religious iconography is the serpent, which frequently serves as an attribute and the throne of an Elamite god.[274] There is every reason to suppose that snakes

---

264 *MHD* 94.4.
265 *MHD*, A 37.1–5. See also Macuch 1981: 220–221.
266 *ŠW* 2.
267 *KAP* 10–13.
268 Henning 1968.
269 *KAP* 10.4, 12.7.
270 *KAP* 12.7, 13.5, 13.13.
271 *KAP* 12.7.
272 Chunakova 1987: 30. For previous interpretations of this story, see Chunakova 1987: 93.
273 Grenet 2003b: 34.
274 Serpent imagery was widespread in Elamite art; see Root 2002: 176–178. On the Elamite "god with a serpent", see Trokay 1991.

played an important role in Elamite cults, and it is not improbable that some remnants of these cults continued into the Parthian period, hence the survival of the archaic title **haftaxwa-pāta*. It is possible, therefore, that the story of Ardašīr's battle against the "Worm" reflects the suppression in Pars of some Elamite cults that were associated with a snake.

7. *Manichaean Texts in Sogdian and Middle Persian*

A fragmentary Manichaean Sogdian text mentions temples with copper idols. It is not clear, however, where these temples are located:

> … northwards … a great mountain … on the skirts of the mountain there is a … place of the gods (*βaγistān*). In the temple there are many gods who are endowed with speech, but they are rather difficult to serve … on the flanks (?) of the mountain, upwards, … there are another two temples, one of gold, the other of silver. What gods there are in both those temples, they are set with all kinds of jewels, but they do not talk with men. Whoever satisfies the brazen gods who are in the temples …[275]

This is not the only reference to idols in the surviving Manichaean literature. A fragmentary Sogdian text mentions an idol (*yzδ'ys*) that Zarēr, the brother of Zoroaster's patron, had "at the foot of a tree".[276]

There are also a number of fragments of polemical texts against idol-worship in Middle Persian:

M 219 V:

> Seize the path of the gods …, the head of (?) akk these which are painted here. This is a place of worship of idols (*uzdēsčār*) which they call the house of gods. And by the (mere) name 'house of gods' they are lost. They run in droves. When one asks 'Whereto?', they say: 'To the house of gods for worship and devotion and offerings before them'. And the masters of the temples (*bašnbedān*)[277] call out: 'Come to the house of the gods!' And inside the house of the gods there are no gods. And those that are deceived cannot explain, for they have been intoxicated by the winds.[278]

M 174 II:

> … deceiving … the great (nobles?) who worship and … no … other than the knowledge of the gods […], nor the idol worshippers who worship the images, the gods of 'Lyinghood' (*uzdēsparistān kē paristēnd ō pahikarān ō bay ī drōzanīh*), nor the deceived teachings.[279]
>
> The worlds are amazed
> at the deceived idols (*uzdēsan*),
> the images (*pahikarān*) over
> the walls: wooden and stony.[280]

M 28 I:

> In the end they will be brought to shame
> all those who worship
> the idols (*uzdēsan*), on that last
> day, and they will go to
> destruction.[281]

275 Henning 1945: 473–474.
276 Sundermann 1986: 469.
277 Skjærvø 1995/1997: 241 translates "idol temples".
278 Skjærvø 1995/1997: 241 with some changes.
279 Skjærvø 1995/1997: 242.
280 Skjærvø 1995/1997: 242.
281 M 28 I. Skjærvø 1995/1997: 247.

The last verse is of special interest since it concludes a polemical hymn directed against Jews, Marcionites and Zoroastrians ("who worship the burning fire"), all of whom are included in the category of "those who worship the idols" who will be annihilated on the Day of Judgment.

The Manichaean texts also contain allusions to the visual appearance of certain divine figures. A fragmentary Sogdian text describes the journey of the soul of the just to Paradise and its encounter with a beautiful virgin, a personification of its deeds, undoubtedly modeled on the Zoroastrian Daēnā:

> And his own deed, the wonderful divine king's daughter, the virgin, appears to him, the eternal fruit (?), a drink, a flower garland around the head ...[282]

A Manichaean Sogdian tale about Caesar and the thieves indicates that the Sogdians probably also imagined *x^varənah* in anthropomorphic form:

> When the lights and lamps had been lit in the tomb, one of those thieves placed the diadem of majesty on his head and put on royal garments. He approached the coffin where the Caesar was lying, and spoke thus to him: "Hey, hey, Caesar, awake, awake! Fear not, I am your Farn! Now, besides I am the guardian Farn for (?) many thieves and jugglers (?)."[283]

8. *The Chinese Sources*

Chinese-Iranian diplomatic contact was first established by the end of the second century BCE by the Chinese envoy to the Yuezhi, Chang Ch'ien (Zhang Qian).[284] From the Kushan period, the Chinese became politically and culturally involved in Central Asia. Some of the numerous emissaries, missionaries and Buddhist pilgrims visiting Eastern Iran in the first half of the first millennium CE recorded their journeys, including accounts of the exotic customs and beliefs of the remote "western regions". This information is often hard to use due to the Chinese transcriptions of Iranian names. However, these sources provide some information on the visual aspect of eastern Iranian and especially Sogdian religion.

The Chinese referred to the religions practiced in the "western regions" by the term *xian*, which seems to designate a variety of religious practices and cults of the Turko-Sogdian population.[285] The "Geography of Shazhou", written before 640 CE, mentions a temple dedicated to the deity *xian*. Located east of the city Dunhuang in the county of *li*, it was decorated with religious paintings and twenty niches relating to the monthly festivals in honor of the principal deities of the Sogdians.[286] The same source also tells us that the fire-temple of *xian* contained innumerable manuscripts painted on silk.[287] Another seventh century CE text mentioning the *xian* fire-temple reports that it contained "countless images both moulded and painted".[288] Regrettably, only one *xian* deity is named in the Chinese sources. The chronicle *Liangjing xinji*, composed by Wei Shu in 722 CE, mentions a temple of a "heavenly god" whose name in Buddhist texts is *Moxishouluo*.[289] *Moxishouluo* is the Chinese transcription of the Indian Maheśvara, one of the names of Śiva identified with the Sogdian Wešparkar.[290]

---

282 This fragment was published by Henning 1945: 476–477. It is reproduced here according to the new translation given in Azarpay 2011: 65.

283 Henning 1945: 478–479. Grenet suggested that this tale is a late Sogdian translation of an original Parthian text reflecting Manichaean contact with the Palmyran court: Grenet 2001/2002: 207–208.

284 See the survey of China's relations with the pre-Islamic Iranian world in Pulleyblank 1992.

285 See Riboud 2005.

286 Riboud 2005: 74.

287 Riboud 2005: 80.

288 de la Vaissière 2005: 129.

289 Riboud 2005: 74.

290 See p. 154.

The "Chronicle of Beishi", a sixth century CE *Pei shih* (*History of the Northern Dynasties*), tells about the cult of the deity *Dexi*,[291] who was worshipped in all the lands to the east of the "western sea". *Dexi* was depicted by a fifteen foot high golden idol to which cattle and sheep were offered.[292] Unfortunately, no description of the visual appearance of this idol is given.

9. *Medieval Sources in Arabic and Persian*

Numerous allusions to cultic statues are found in Muslim sources written in Arabic and Persian. Al-Mas'ūdī (896–956 CE) writes that the idols originally housed in the great fire-temple of Eṣṭaḵr were removed, and the building was turned into the fire-temple.[293] The Muslim historian visited the ruins of the sanctuary and found it surrounded by a large temenos wall. This wall was decorated with skillfully carved anthropomorphic reliefs, which were interpreted by the locals as "images of prophets".[294] The ruins he described, however, probably did not belong to a Sasanian fire-temple, but to the Achaemenian platform of Persepolis. This can be deduced from his descriptions of typical Persepolitan columns and the "anthropomorphic reliefs" that seem to depict the famous tributary processions of people from the *apadana*. We are also told that, when king Vištāsp embraced Zoroastrianism, he removed the idols from a temple located near Isfahan, on the top of Mount Mārbīn, and converted it into a fire-temple.[295] Furthermore, the famous Sasanian sanctuary of Ādur Gušnasp (Taḵt-e Solaymān) was also transformed into a fire-temple.[296]

Al-Shahrastānī (1086–1153 CE) writes of the enmity between "idol-worshippers" and "fire-worshippers", and also states that some "idol-temples" were transformed by the latter into fire-temples.[297]

According to al-Ṭabarī (838–923 CE), when the Muslims conquered Ctesiphon they captured a statue embellished with precious stones.[298] In the Great Hall of the Sasanian palace (Ṭāq-i Kisrā), the Arabs found statues of men and horses, which they did not destroy but left intact. When the Great Hall was later converted into a prayer hall, the statues were still there.[299] Other Sasanian equestrian statues, made of silver and gold and embellished with precious stones, were also captured by the Arabs.[300]

Al-Ṭabarī is also an important source regarding the Arab campaigns in Transoxania, during which they captured numerous idols that were venerated by the local Iranian population. In the city of Paykand, the Muslims captured "innumerable gold and silver vessels" as well as idols made of precious metals. These were melted down together and presented to Qutaybah b. Muslim, who was governor of Khurāsān between 704/5 and 714/5 CE.[301]

After Qutaybah seized a fortress of the king of Shūmān, he returned to Kish and Nasaf and went to Bukhara. On his way:

> He stopped at a village in which there were a fire temple and a house of gods; in [this village] there were peacocks, and they called it "the Dwelling Place of the Peacocks" (*manzil al-ṭawāwīs*).[302]

---

291 Identified with the Sogdian deity Taxsīč (*txs'yc*), who has been compared with Tammūz; see Grenet and Marshak 1998: 9–10.
292 Belenitskiy 1954: 61; Grenet and Marshak 1998: 10.
293 Mas'ūdī, vol. 2, 1403.
294 Mas'ūdī, vol. 2, 1403.
295 Mas'ūdī, vol. 2, 1373. The same story is also reported by Shahrastānī, vol. 2, 1224.
296 Mas'ūdī, vol. 2, 1400.
297 Shahrastānī, vol. 2, 1224.
298 Ṭabarī, vol. 13, 39–40.
299 Ṭabarī, vol. 13, 23.
300 Ṭabarī, vol. 13, 28. See also Shalem 1994: 78.
301 Ṭabarī, vol. 23, 137.
302 Ṭabarī, vol. 23, 177.

The ancient name of this place was *Arfūd*.[303] This passage is interesting because al-Ṭabarī distinguishes between a "fire-temple" and a "house of gods". This does not seem to be the case with his account of the conquest of Samarkand, the most important Sogdian city, where only fire-temples are mentioned and are unambiguously associated with idols:

> Qutaybah made peace with them [inhabitants of Samarkand] in return for one hundred thousand slaves, the fire temples, and the adornments of the idols. He took receipt of that on the basis of which he had made peace with them, and he was brought the idols, which were despoiled and then placed before him; gathered together, they were like an enormous edifice. He ordered that they be burned, and the non-Arabs said to him, "Among them are idols the burner of which will be destroyed". Qutaybah said, "I shall burn them with my [own] hand." Ghūrak came, knelt before him, and said, "Devotion to you is a duty incumbent upon me. Do not expose yourself to these idols". Qutaybah called for fire, took a brand in his hand, went out, proclaimed "God is great," and set fire to them; [others then also] set fire [to them], and they burned fiercely. In the remains of the gold and silver nails that had been in them, they found fifty thousand *mithqāls*.[304]

Sogdian idols, therefore, were made of wood, upon which richly decorated garments were nailed using nails made of precious metals. This accords with a wooden idol from the Surkh Mountains in Tajikistan, which was clothed in the same fashion.[305] Furthermore, according to the account of Ibn A'tham, Qutaybah demanded from the inhabitants of Samarkand that they surrender "the decorations of the idols that were in the fire-temples".[306]

The Arabs encountered the veneration of idols in all the regions of Sogdiana. This practice undoubtedly continued into the Islamic period. In a famous trial, Ḥaydar b. Kāvūs, the local prince (*afšīn*) of the Sogdian principality of Ustrushana, was accused of apostasy and sympathy toward the pre-Islamic Iranian faith. Ḥaydar b. Kāvūs punished two Muslim fanatics who attacked a "house of idols" in Ustrushana, removing the idols and turning the shrine into a mosque. Bejeweled idols and richly ornamented "heretical" books were found in his house near Samarrā, and were used as material evidence against him:[307]

> In his residence was found a tabernacle (*bayt*) containing an image of a man, carved out of wood and covered with many ornaments and jewels and having in its ears two white stones with intricate gold filigree work over them.

An additional idol was also found and:

> a book of the Magians called *Z.rāwah* and many other books pertaining to his faith by means of which he used to worship his lord.[308]

Ustrushana is again linked with idols in al-Ṭabarī's account of the brother of Ḥanash (al-Jaysh) b. al-Sabal, ruler of Khuttal, who fled from the Arabs to Ferghana, and was sent back to Ustrushana with many idols.[309]

In his Persian translation of al-Ṭabarī, Abū ʿAlī Amīrak Balʿamī (fl. second half of the tenth century CE) ascribes the introduction of idolatry to Yima.[310] Seduced by the Evil Spirit, Yima set up five statues of himself, made of gold, silver and precious stones, and demanded that he be venerated as a god. After his death, the people, now used to idolatry, continued to worship the statues under different names.

Al-Balādhurī (ninth century CE) reports that the terms of the surrender of Samarkand to the Arab leader Qutaybah b. Muslim included:

---

303 Barthold 1968: 98–99.
304 Ṭabarī, vol. 23, 194.
305 See p. 112 ff.
306 Grenet 1999/2000: 175.
307 Ṭabarī, vol. 33, 187.
308 Ṭabarī, vol. 33, 200.
309 Ṭabarī, vol. 26, 31.
310 Balʿamī 63–65.

> the houses of the idols and the fire temples. The idols were thrown out, plundered of their ornaments, and burned, although the Persians used to say that among them was one idol with which whoever trifled would perish. But when Ḳutaibah set fire to it with his own hand, many of them accepted Islam.[311]

Al-Balādhurī also writes that, when the Arabs conquered al-Buttam (the mountainous region in the upper reaches of Zeravshan), they seized money and "idols of gold".[312] In the province of Zamīndāvar in eastern Afghanistan, the Arabs encountered a thriving cult of an enigmatic deity called "Zūn". His shrine was erected on a high place, called the "hill of Zūn", which housed his idol that was made of gold and decorated with rubies. The Arab commander, ʿAbd-al-Raḥmān b. Samora, captured the temple, cut off a hand from the idol and removed the rubies, which were set in its eyes, in order to demonstrate to the local ruler that it was powerless.[313] Al-Bīrūnī also mentions that the idol was made of gold and had sapphires for eyes.[314]

The tenth century traveler and geographer Ibn Ḥauqal describes wooden figures of elephants, camels, bulls and other wild animals, displayed beside each other in a square in Samarkand.[315]

Narshakhī (c. 899–959), in his *History of Bukhara*, reports that the Arab conquerors found a silver idol weighing 4,000 dirhams in a local temple in Paykand.[316] He also tells us that the inhabitants of Bukhara, who were converted to Islam by Qutaybah, continued to worship idols secretly. Qutaybah did not give up, however, but eventually succeeded in imposing Islam on the population, building mosques and eradicating the "precepts of the fire-worshipers".[317] It appears that Narshakhī did not differentiate between the veneration of idols and fire-worship. The grand mosque of Bukhara, transformed by Qutaybah from a temple, had gates adorned with images of idols, which were captured by Muslim townsmen from the "infidel" local landlords. Narshakhī writes that on these gates each of these landlords "made the figure of his idol".[318]

Other fire-temples in Bukhara were also transformed into mosques. Narshakhī gives a valuable account of the bazaar adjacent to one such former fire-temple, where idols were still sold in the Islamic period:

> In Bukhara there was a bazaar called the bazaar of [the day of] Mākh. Twice a year for one day there was a fair, and every time there was this fair idols were sold in it. Every day more than 50,000 dirhams were exchanged (for the idols). Muḥammad ibn Jaʿfar has mentioned in his book that this fair existed in his time, and he was very astonished that it should be allowed. He asked the elders and shaikhs of Bukhara the reason for this. They said that the inhabitants of Bukhara in olden times had been idol-worshippers. They were permitted to have this fair, and from that time they have sold idols in it. It has remained thus till today. Abu'l-Ḥasan Nīshāpūrī in his book "The Treasury of the Sciences," says that in Bukhara in ancient times was a king who was called Mākh. He ordered this market to be built. He ordered carpenters and painters to prepare idols each year. On a certain day they appeared in the bazaar and sold the idols, and the people bought them. When their idol was lost, broken, or old, the people bought another when the day of the fair came. Then the old one was thrown away. That place, which today is the grand mosque of Mākh, was a grove on the river bank. There were many trees, and the fair was held in the shade of those trees. That king came to this fair and sat on a throne in the place which is today the mosque of Mākh to encourage the people to buy idols. Everyone bought an idol for himself and brought it home. Afterwards this place became a fire-temple. On the day of the fair, when the people had gathered, all went into the fire-temple and worshipped fire. The

311 Balādhurī 189.
312 Balādhurī 195.
313 Balādhurī 144. On Zūn, see Bosworth 2002 and Bosworth 2008: 105–108.
314 Bīrūnī 65.
315 Ibn Ḥauqal 492.
316 Narshakhī 19.
317 Narshakhī 20.
318 Narshakhī 21.

> fire-temple existed to the time of Islam when the Muslims seized power and built a mosque on that place. Today it is one of the esteemed mosques of Bukhara.[319]

Previous commentators on this passage have noted how it represents a unique written account of a domestic, private cult centered on idol worship, and of the important place that idols occupied in the religious life of pre-Islamic Bukhara. It is also noteworthy, however, that the idol-bazaar predated the fire-temple, and that the fire-temple was later built in the same location, incorporating the idols and their sale into the fire-cult.[320] This contrasts with the accounts of historians writing about Western Iran. For instance, according to al-Masʿūdī, "idol-temples" were also transformed into "fire-temples", but this procedure necessarily accompanied the destruction of the idols. Selling idols on fixed dates indicates that these idols were intended for a special event and were probably connected with the cult of a major Bukharian god. Since the fair was held twice a year, it could be that it was established to celebrate the death and resurrection of a Sogdian fertility god, perhaps Taxsīč-Tammūz or Siyāvush, whose cult in Bukhara is reported by Narshakhī.[321]

Al-Bīrūnī (973–1048 CE), a native of Chorasmia, is another important source regarding pre-Islamic Iranian cultic traditions. While discussing the feasts of the Persians, he mentions a bull that draws a chariot of the Moon and has golden horns and silver legs.[322] This description accords with existing Sasanian visual representations of the Moon-god Māh.[323]

According to the *Tārīkh-i Sīstān*,[324] the Sistanian Zoroastrians had a fire-temple and a temple of the sun (*khvarshīd*) in 670 CE.[325] The same source also recounts a fascinating story of the negotiations between a local ruler and the Arab general Rabīʿ ibn Ziyād who, intending to inspire terror in the Iranians, ordered a throne of human corpses. The Sistanian leader was so astonished by the sight of Rabīʿ ibn Ziyād that he told his companions: "It is said that Ahriman does not appear in daylight. Here he is! There could be no doubt about it!"[326] The *Tārīkh-i Sīstān* also notes that Yaqūb bin Laʿyth as-Saffār sent fifty silver and gold idols from Kabul to the Caliph al-Muttamid (ruled 870–892 CE) to be thrown in Mecca under the feet of the faithful Muslims.[327]

The *Kandia* (*al-Kand*), a thirteenth century source on the history of Samarkand, reports that there were many idol-temples in Samarkand before the Arab conquest.[328] The city also housed an idol, set on the tower, which was seen from afar and drew numerous pilgrims who came to Samarkand to pay homage to it.[329] Qutaybah destroyed them and distributed the idols, which were made of precious metals and stones, among his warriors.[330] However, this description could have been inspired by ninth or tenth century speculative literature regarding the religion of the Sabians of Harran rather than by living testimony about local traditions.[331]

Some Islamic sources also allude to the anthropomorphic nature of Zoroastrian gods. In a passage by al-Jayhānī quoted by al-Shahrastānī, Ohrmazd is said to have created the world in the following manner:

---

319 Narshakhī 6.
320 For a contrary view, see Belenitskiy 1954: 60.
321 Narshakhī 4, 8. On Taxsīč-Tammūz, see Grenet and Marshak 1998: 9–10.
322 Bīrūnī 239–240.
323 See p. 98ff.
324 See Smirnova 1974: 22.
325 *TS* 93.
326 *TS* 82.
327 *TS* 216.
328 *Kandia* 249–250.
329 *Kandia* 250.
330 *Kandia* 249.
331 See Grenet 1999/2000: 176–177.

> I created the whole of this world from myself. I created the souls of the righteous from the hair of my head; the sky from my brain; nails and arms (?) from my forehead; the sun from my eye; the moon from my nose; the stars from my tongue; Srōš and the rest of the angels from my ear; the earth from the tendon of my foot.[332]

A dichotomy emerges, therefore, from the sources that describe the religious situation in western and Eastern Iran on the eve of the Muslim conquest. The Arabs encountered numerous idols and idol-temples in Eastern Iran, while statues are almost exclusively limited to the secular sphere in Western Iran. When idols and idol-temples are mentioned in a western Iranian context, they are, in fact, a reminiscence of a past that no longer existed, having been replaced by the fire-cult prior to the arrival of Islam.

It is also significant that, in general, Muslim authors do not distinguish between fire-temples and idols when describing the campaigns in Eastern Iran. For them, or for their sources, the veneration of idols and the fire-cult did not represent separate, opposing cultic practices. In Western Iran, the situation was apparently different, since al-Shahrastānī clearly distinguishes between idol-temples and fire-temples and records a confrontation between the practitioners of both cults.

10. The *Shāh-nāma*

The *Shāh-nāma* (*The Book of Kings*), the great national epic of Iran composed by Abū'l-Qāsīm Firdausī around 1000 CE, is a rich source for pre-Islamic Iranian tradition.[333] Firdausī's masterpiece, in which historical narrative is interwoven with legend (this is true even for the third, "historical" part of the poem), to a large extent predetermines the way Iranians perceive their pre-Islamic past and exerts considerable influence on scholarship.[334]

Firdausī probably based his poem on the *Xwadāy-nāmag* (*The Book of Lords*), a late Sasanian compendium of mythical and historical traditions, which he consulted in its New Persian prose translation. *Shāh-nāma* contains descriptions of the visual appearance of two divine personages originating in pre-Islamic mythology. The first is Ahriman, or Iblīs, as used interchangeably by Firdausī.[335] Ahriman appears before Ḍaḥḥāk as a human in the "shape of a well-wisher" (سان یکی نیکخواه) and seduces him to sanction the murder of his father.[336] Later, Ṭahmūrāth mounts Ahriman as if he was a "swift-going stallion" (تیزرو بارگی) and uses him to make a journey around the world.[337] The second is Surūsh, who appears numerous times in the poem as the divine messenger.[338] He is described as very fine looking, with long musky hair, a face like that of a *houri* (حور)[339] and having two wings.[340] He is sent to warn Siyāmak "in the form of a *pari* wearing a leopard skin" (بسان پری پلنگینه پوش),[341] and comes to the rescue of Khusrau wearing green clothes and mounted on a white horse.[342]

The *Shāh-nāma* also includes several allusions to idols and idol-worship. Isfandīār, commissioned by his father Guštāsp to spread the Zoroastrian faith, managed to convince many people to burn their

332 Shaked 1994b: 67.
333 See the introduction to the latest prose translation of the *Shāh-nāma* into English by Davis 2006. The material relating to Zoroaster and Zoroastrianism has been collected by Ghazanfari 2011.
334 This influence was not always a positive one. An excellent example is the notion of *far*(*r*); see p. 131ff.
335 See Ghazanfari 2011: 92–97.
336 *Shāh-nāma*, vol. 1, 46, b. 88.
337 *Shāh-nāma*, vol. 1, 36, b. 26–28.
338 Ghazanfari 2011: 82–92.
339 *Shāh-nāma*, vol. 1, 72, 277.
340 *Shāh-nāma*, vol. 4, 246, 1190.
341 *Shāh-nāma*, vol. 1, 23, b. 26.
342 *Shāh-nāma*, vol. 8, 144, 1903.

idols and to kindle fire in their place (بتان از سر گاه میسوختند به جای بت آذر برافروختند).[343] It is interesting that the Turanians, the epic enemies of Iran in the *Shāh-nāma*, are not associated with idolatry. Instead, the palace of Mīhrāb, king of Kābūl and the father of Rūdāba, is described as "the house of idol-worship" (خانه ی بت پرستان),[344] and they are said to be of a "different faith and way" (نه هم دین و هم راه بود).[345] This possibly reflects the influential cults with rich anthropomorphic imagery, encountered by the Arabs in Afghanistan, which persisted well into the Islamic period.

343 *Shāh-nāma*, vol. 5, 154, b. 842.
344 *Shāh-nāma*, vol. 1, 85, b. 309.
345 *Shāh-nāma*, vol. 1, 185, b. 314.

CHAPTER 3

ICONOGRAPHIC PANTHEON

1. *Ahura Mazdā*

Ahura Mazdā ("Lord Wisdom/The Wise Lord", literally "the All-Knowing (ruling) Lord"[1]) was the god of the prophet Zoroaster and remains the principal deity worshipped in modern Zoroastrianism.[2] It is uncertain whether he was an Old Iranian deity who probably originated in the times of Indo-Iranian unity or was the original creation of Zoroaster.[3] Ahura Mazdā was venerated not only in Achaemenian and Sasanian Iran, but also in Kushan Bactria, among early medieval Sogdians and perhaps also by other Iranian peoples.[4]

1. *Western Iran*

The first image of Ahura Mazdā created by the Iranians is probably the Achaemenian "Figure in the Winged Ring", which is undoubtedly the most significant divine image to emerge from Achaemenian art and is one of its most well known and recognizable manifestations.[5] This figure is found in countless variations in almost every form of media, including rock-reliefs, seals, bullae and satrapal coinage. It makes its first—and most detailed and elaborate—appearance on the victory relief of Darius I carved at the rock of Behestūn (fig. 2).[6] The following description and discussion will therefore focus on the Behestūn Figure. The figure floats above the procession of defeated rebel-leaders and is shown in full profile looking left toward the king (fig. 3). The upper, anthropomorphic part of its body emerges from the winged ring, while the lower part is replaced by a bird's tail. It holds a ring in his left hand and raises its right hand with an open palm in a gesture of blessing. The figure is bearded and wears a Persian robe and a high tiara embellished with a star symbol enclosed in a circle.[7] The headdress was presumably also adorned with horns, today no longer visible. The image certainly portrays a transcendental being. In the

---

[1] Skjærvø 2011d: 13.

[2] On the name of Ahura Mazdā, see Boyce 1975b: 37–40 and Skjærvø 2002: 402–403.

[3] For the view that Ahura Mazdā is the creation of Zoroaster, see Gnoli 1980: 199–203 and recently Kreyenbroek 2008/2012: 48–50 with references. The structure of his name, typical for dual Zoroastrian abstractions, is a serious argument in favour of his Zoroastrian origin: Shaked 1987: 239. His name, written in Akkadian as ^{d}*Assara* ^{d}*Mazaš* is probably mentioned for the first time in Assyrian documents of the eighth-seventh century BCE (in the list of gods originating from the library of Assurbanipal III R pl. 66, Kol.9.Z.24), see Boyce 1982: 15; Boyce 1987; Dandamaev and Lukonin 2004: 321. Around the same period we find also theophoric names incorporating *mazda*: cited with references in Boyce 1982: 15; and possible evidence for worship of a deity named *bagmaštu(m)* or *bagmastu(m)* on the Armenian plateau—a region of intense Irano-Hurrito-Urartan contacts, which was interpreted as **Baga-Mazdā*: Grantovskiy 1998: 31–33; 345–349.

[4] It is possible that other deities formed with *mazdā-* existed among Scythians. Humbach and Faiss 2012: 6, have recently suggested that the component *masadas* in the name of the Scythian god Thagimasadas (associated by Herodotus with Poseidon) derives from *mazdā* and the name itself could mean "supervisor of the waves". Another Scythian personal name that probably contains the same component is Oktamasades, interpreted by the German scholars as the "supervisor of the well-cleared ways": Humbach and Faiss 2012: 7.

[5] On the "Figure in the Winged Ring", see Boyce 1982: 103–105; Root 1979: 169–178. For the most recent and detailed discussions, consult Merrillees 2005: 115–117 and especially Garrison 2011: 47–51; Garrison prepublication: 25–40.

[6] On the relief of Darius at Behestūn, see Luschey 1968 and Root 1979: 58–61.

[7] This is the only Achaemenian monument featuring this type of headdress. On all other representations, its headgear mirrors that of the king.

ancient Near East, a wing, attached to a human or beast served as a symbol of the divine or supernatural, and winged beings are widespread in Achaemenian art.[8]

Since the Achaemenian symbol is obviously based on the iconography of the Assyrian god in the winged ring, usually identified as Aššur,[9] and often appears above Achaemenian royal inscriptions that mention Ahura Mazdā, it has usually been thought to represent the highest god of the Achaemenian dynasty.[10] However, some scholars have preferred to identify this symbol as a *fravaši*—"the pre-existing soul",[11] of the king.[12] Others have interpreted the figure in the winged ring as *x*ᵛ*arənah*, the god-given glory, divine favor, and fortune guiding the ruling dynasty.[13]

Each theory has its own merits and weaknesses. The identification with a *fravaši* can be dismissed, since in Zoroastrian scriptures they are always referred to as being female.[14] Both the *fravaši* and the *x*ᵛ*arənah* hypotheses seem to have been at least partly influenced by the tendency in modern Zoroastrianism to consider Ahura Mazdā as an abstract transcendental Supreme Being, who has no anthropomorphic shape. This inclination is understandable, considering the centuries during which Zoroastrians existed as an oppressed minority under Muslim rule with its intolerance of anthropomorphic representations of the divine as well as the Christian Protestant influence of the nineteenth and twentieth centuries. However, it seems that in antiquity the situation was entirely different.[15] For instance, in the Sasanian period, Ahura Mazdā was depicted in anthropomorphic shape on the rock reliefs of the Persian kings.[16]

Perhaps the most active critic against the identification of the Achaemenian symbol as Ahura Mazdā has been Alireza Sh. Shahbazi, but his arguments are difficult to accept.[17] The fact that in later periods in Commagene, under the Kushans and the Sasanians, Ahura Mazdā was depicted in a fully anthropomorphic shape, significantly different from the half-human Achaemenian figure in the winged ring, is not a persuasive argument.[18] One should not expect a continuation of Achaemenian

---

8 Merrillees 2005: 114, Figs. 12b, 15–18.

9 Root 1979: 172; Lukonin 1987: 96; Panaino 2000: 39. According to some, the Assyrian symbol could also be a representation of Shamash: Green 1995: 1838; Collon 2001: 79–80; Ornan 2005b: 212–213; Ornan 2009: 101–102 and even that of the war-god Ninurta: Green 1995: 1838. Black and Green 1992: 38, reject the identification with Aššur and insist on Shamash. It might be useful here to bring Raede's conclusion that the Assyrian god in the winged disk "could then represent high godhead under various names—Shamash, Ashur, possibly Ninurta, Nabu or other gods, or even several at once.": Raede 1995: 232. For additional references to studies on the iconography of Aššur and the identification of the Assyrian symbol with Shamash, see Holloway 2002: 170, n. 298.

10 For example Ghirshman 1954: 160–161; Root 1979: 172; Lukonin 1977: 96; Lecoq 1984: 325; Vanden Berghe 1988: 1514; Dandamaev and Lukonin 1994: 342–343; Boardman 2000: 146; Jacobs 2001: 85; Briant 2002: 248 and many others.

11 Skjærvø 2011d: 18.

12 Unvala 1930. On *fravaši*, see for example Boyce 2002: 195–199. Calmeyer 1975 proposed that it could symbolize the δαίμων of the royal ancestor of the king. Undoubtedly, δαίμων would be the most appropriate and natural *interpretatio graeca* of *fravaši*.

13 See Shahbazi 1980: 199–147; Boyce 1982: 103–105; De Jong 1995: 906–907; Huff 2004: 601–602; Curtis 2008: 137 and also Jamzadeh 1982. On the *x*ᵛ*arənah* see p. 131. Recently, Mark Garrison has drawn attention to the Elamite concept of *kitin*, which essentially has a very similar meaning and significance in Elamite ideology as the *x*ᵛ*arənah* in Iranian ideology, but has an advantage of attestation in the Achaemenid period in which *x*ᵛ*arənah* is lacking: Garrison pre-publication: 36–37. Every deity was thought to possess his own *kitin*, which was also given a visual representation of an emblem, kept in a special room within the temple: Koch 1995: 1965. An additional interesting suggestion belongs to Bruno Jacobs, who reaches the conclusion that the winged figure in the ring represents both Ahura Mazdā and the Sun god who enjoyed a shared position of the highest deity in the Achaemenian cult: Jacobs 1991. The sun symbolism of the figure in the winged disk was also noted by Moorey 1979: 221 among others.

14 Shahbazi 1974: 137–138.

15 For the discussion of Iranian anthropomorphism see Chapter Five.

16 These observations were already made by Duchesne-Guillemin 1966: 91, n. 8.

17 Shahbazi 1974: 138–144. See also his recent emotional attempts to defend his theory: Shahbazi 2003/2004: 77–78.

18 Shahbazi 1974: 143–144.

artistic traditions and ideology in Commagene or in Kushan Bactria. The Sasanian Ahura Mazdā, as elaborated below, was probably at least partly inspired by the Achaemenian image. Moreover, contrary to what Shahbazi maintains,[19] in Iranian art Ahura Mazdā was never depicted as a Zoroastrian priest, but rather, in most cases, as a duplicate of the king. Shahbazi's observation that the identification of the Achaemenian figure in the winged ring is based on an unproven assumption that the Assyrian figure represents Aššur is, however, more difficult to dismiss. Certainly, this symbol is not labeled on the Assyrian reliefs. Nevertheless, it has been shown that several centuries before the Assyrians adopted this symbol, the winged ring was already employed to represent important deities in the Near East.[20] Because of great similarities and constant visual association between the Assyrian figure and the king, it is probable that the figure symbolized the highest god and not ordinary members of the pantheon. Aššur is therefore the most likely candidate for the Assyrian symbol.

The Achaemenian figure in the winged disk is carved on the Behestūn relief, on royal tombs of Naqš-e Rostam, and numerous times on the walls of Persepolis. Interestingly, the figure occurs only rarely in Persepolitan glyptics and appears mostly with two categories of scenes, labeled by Garrison as "devotional" and "heroic encounter", that both have ideological connotations.[21] It undoubtedly depicts a concept of great importance for the Achaemenians. However, *x^varənah* is not mentioned even once in the Old Persian inscriptions—their main protagonists are the king himself and his patron deity Ahura Mazdā. Furthermore, until the late Sasanian period there is no evidence that *x^varənah* was an important component of Iranian royal ideology and legitimate kingship.[22]

Jacob's comparison with the Sun god seems much more relevant, taking into account the evident solar symbolism of the figure in the winged ring. However, Old Persian inscriptions contradict the idea that Ahura Mazdā shared his position as the head of the Achaemenian pantheon with any other deity.[23] It has been suggested that the winged ring without the human figure, which also features frequently in Achaemenian glyptics, could be considered as a representation of the Sun god.[24] However, it appears that the winged ring should be regarded as an "aniconic version" of the figure in the winged disk.[25] That the two symbols are basically one and the same, is apparent in the cylinder seal from the famous Oxus treasure where the winged disk is shown twice in the same composition—combined with the human figure and separated from it (fig. 4). We must therefore conclude that there is insufficient reason to doubt that the figure in the winged ring represents Ahura Mazdā. This identification suggests itself and reflects the available iconographic and textual evidence in the best way possible.[26]

The winged ring with a human bust probably originated in Neo-Assyrian art in the first quarter of the ninth century BCE.[27] Later on, it appears both in monumental art, where it is found in six separate scenes on the reliefs in the throne room of the North Western palace at Nimrud and in small artifacts such as cylinder seals.[28] However, in all the Assyrian monumental representations, the figure in the winged ring

---

19 Shahbazi 1980: 119.

20 See Ornan 2005b.

21 Garrison 2011: 48–49.

22 See p. 131ff. The symbolic meaning of the figure in the winged ring as a divine source of legitimacy of Darius' rule is beyond doubt. It is explicitly stated in the inscription that Darius is the king by the grace of Ahura Mazdā and that Ahura Mazdā has granted him the kingdom (DB § 5). The bestowing of royal power by the deity upon a ruler is not found in the Avesta and is a characteristic trait of Mesopotamian kingship and ideology: Gnoli 1974: 163–164.

23 De Jong 1997: 306, n. 211.

24 Lukonin 1977: 97; thinks that it was probably taken to symbolize the "Sun-god Mithra".

25 On aniconism, see Chapter Four.

26 Lecoq 1984: 325. See also recent evaluation of all theories and discussion by Finn 2011: 225–227 who reaches similar conclusions.

27 Its first occurrence is probably on the glazed tile of king Tikulti-Ninnurta II (890–884 BCE): Ornan 2005b: 211, Fig. 2.

28 For an in-depth discussion of this symbol in first millennium BCE Assyrian art, see Ornan 2005b: 211–217.

always faces the same direction as the king. In contrast, on the Behestūn relief, Ahura Mazdā faces the king and is rendered on a much larger scale than any images of Aššur.[29]

In the ninth century BCE, the Assyrian figure of the deity in the winged ring begins to appear in the art of neighboring Urartu.[30] In some cases, the Urartan deity is shown in full anthropomorphic shape, holding a bow or a ring and standing on a bull.[31] Regretfully, there is no scholarly consensus over the identity of this Urartan god, who was often identified in the past as Haldi, the chief deity of the Urartan pantheon.[32] Ursula Seidl has demonstrated convincingly that the figure in the winged ring from Behestūn is closer in its details to the ninth century BCE Urartan examples than to the later Assyrian ones, and it is possible that the Achaemenians borrowed it via Urartan mediation.[33]

Many features of the Behestūn relief are remarkably similar to the Neo-Assyrian royal reliefs.[34] It has also been pointed out many times that the theme of royal victory combined with divine investiture that is carved on the rock of Behestūn derives from earlier predecessors, and most notably the relief of Anubanini, king of Lullubi (around 2017–1794 BCE).[35] The same theme would become the focal point of Sasanian monumental art almost 700 years after Darius. Interestingly, on all representations after Behestūn, the horns—the most characteristic and important Mesopotamian visual symbol of divinity—were abandoned for the image of Ahura Mazdā.

Ahura Mazdā was the patron god of the dynasty, at least starting with Darius I. This, however, does not necessarily imply that he was also the supreme Persian god. In fact, the data of the Persepolis tablets do not attest to his exclusivity or superiority and seem to suggest that he was not in fact the most important deity worshipped in the Persepolis area, being overshadowed by a god of Elamite origin, Humban.[36]

The Achaemenian Ahura Mazdā did not vanish after the conquest of most of the Iranian world by Alexander of Macedon. His image continued to be employed during the Hellenistic and the Parthian periods by the local Iranian dynasts of Pars, who enjoyed a certain degree of autonomy and minted their own silver coinage, bearing their title, *frataraka*, written in Aramaic script.[37] It is undoubtedly significant that no representations of Ahura Mazdā are found in official Parthian art. Originating, as they did, in the eastern Iranian nomadic milieu and carrying distinctive Iranian theophoric names,[38] the Arsacids did not create any visual images of indubitably Iranian divinities and were generally ignorant of Achaemenian art and culture. Thus, the iconographic repertoire of Parthian coinage and sculpture

---

29 Root 1979: 211–212. It is also noteworthy that while on the Behestūn relief the figure of Ahura Mazdā is different from that of Darius in several aspects, at Persepolis he is already depicted in exactly the same garments, headdress, and pose as the king: Lukonin 1977: 96.

30 Eichler 1984: Type 1.1. On the representations and symbols of Haldi, see now: Zimansky 2012.

31 See, for instance, Seidl 1980.

32 Eichler 1984: 72. However, see Calmeyer 1983: 183; who is skeptical about the existence of anthropomorphic representations of Haldi and proposes that he was often venerated without a cultic image. See also D'yakonov 1983.

33 Seidl 1994: 122–127.

34 Root 1979: 215. For a discussion of the Assyrian influence on the Achaemenian culture, administration and art, see Dandamaev 1997.

35 For example, see Calmeyer 1994: 137; Root 1995: 2621; although some graphical formulae and conceptions expressed at Behestūn can be traced as far back as the Old Akkadian period: Westenholz 2000: 122; Feldman 2007. For the relief of Anubanini, see Vanden Berghe 1984: no. 1. The prominent role that Mesopotamian heritage has played in the formation of Achaemenian royal art has been long acknowledged by scholars. See, for instance, Calmeyer 1994.

36 From some 250 texts recording cultic activities, only 10 texts record the supply of offerings for Ahura Mazdā, while 26 are concerned with offerings for Humban: Henkelman 2008: 216. Ahura Mazdā also occupies only the eighth place in the list of the cumulative value of the popular offerings in Persepolis tablets expressed in barley: Henkelman 2011: Tab. 1.

37 This title is usually translated as "rulers" or "governors". On *frataraka* and their coinage, see Frye 1984: 158–162; Boyce and Grenet 1991: 110–116; Wiesehöfer 1994: 101–136; Wiesehöfer 2001; Panaino 2002a; Wiesehöfer 2007; Potts 2007: 272; Callieri 2007: 115–146; Haerinck and Overlaet 2008; Curtis 2010; Wiesehöfer 2010a.

38 In fact, Ahura Mazdā is attested as a component in the personal names of the inhabitants of Old Nisa. See, for instance, Diakonoff and Livshits 2001: nos. 600:3; 306:3.

is wholly Graeco-Roman,[39] adopted from the sedentary Hellenistic population that they came to rule, disregarding the Western Iranian Achaemenian legacy, including the image of Ahura Mazdā as the figure in the winged ring.

The first fully anthropomorphic representation of Ahura Mazdā appears in Western Iran simultaneously with the rise of the Sasanian dynasty on three rock-reliefs attributed to the first Sasanian king, Ardašīr.[40] The relief at Fīrūzābād is probably one of the earliest (fig. 5).[41] Its composition is asymmetric; it shows Ardašīr, a page holding a fly-whisk, and three dignitaries depicted on the right side of the scene facing the sole figure of Ahura Mazdā standing in the left part of the relief. There is a strict hierarchy in the size of the individuals. The king and the god are the largest figures of equal dimensions, followed by three courtiers and the page who barely reaches the king's shoulder. Ahura Mazdā is portrayed here as a bearded man, wearing a high mural crown tied with a diadem, holding a rod in one hand and a diadem in another. The king reaches out for the diadem and makes a gesture of adoration towards the god. A noteworthy and unique detail of this relief is the fire-altar placed between the king and his heavenly patron.

The composition of the second relief, located at Naqš-e Rajab can be divided into four distinct pairs (fig. 6).[42] Two central figures of Ardašīr and Ahura Mazdā, two smaller figures standing behind the king that are usually identified as a page and the crown prince Šāpūr, two dwarfish personages between the *šāhān šāh* and the god, and a pair of female characters on the right edge of the relief. The latter clearly do not belong with the composition. Their backs are turned on Ahura Mazdā, and one of the women makes a gesture of homage toward someone left out of the relief. In addition, the two female figures are separated by a pole or half-frame from the main scene. They were probably carved later than the main relief, as was also the case with the portrait and the inscription of the high priest Kartīr adjacent to the relief from the left.[43] For an unknown reason this scene was never finished and it is possibly the latest of Ardašīr's reliefs, the carving of which was interrupted by his death. The internal chronology of the rock-reliefs of the first Sasanian monarch is still controversial as they are characterized by a variety of stylistic features with no clear and undisputable typology or development.[44]

Ahura Mazdā is represented in royal garb, wearing a crenellated crown and a diadem, holding a rod and extending a beribboned ring to the king. Ardašīr, in his distinctive *korymbos* crown, raises his left hand, gesturing with bended forefinger, while his right hand grasps a diadem together with the god, as distinct from his other reliefs where King of Kings is shown only reaching for it. This may reflect Ardašīr's confidence in his achievements and divine patronage and can perhaps be considered as an additional argument for this relief being made at the end of the king's rule.[45]

---

[39] Curtis 2007 has argued recently (and a similar view was also expressed by Cribb 2007: 362), that it conceals Iranian divinities and conceptions. However, this assumption goes far beyond the available evidence and there is no sufficient iconographic or textual data to support the *interpretatio Iranica* of pure Greek and Roman motifs on these coins. We know for certain that in the Parthian Empire Iranian gods could indeed be equated with their Greek counterparts, but so far the bronze statue of Heracles-Vərəθraγna from Mesene remains the only unquestionable testimony to this phenomenon. See p. 11. Invernizzi 2005: 76 has also argued that the statues from Nisa, whose iconography is Greek, "are intended to represent Iranian gods in Greek guise". Also notable is the proposal of Fabrizio Sinisi to interpret one variant of Tyche found on Parthian coins as the image of Nana. For the discussion, see p. 118.

[40] On the Sasanian investiture, see also studies by Göbl 1960 and Ghirshman 1975.

[41] Hinz 1969: 119–123, Taf. 56; Schmidt 1970: 125; Vanden Berghe 1984 no. 51; Luschey 1987: 377; Vanden Berghe 1988: 1521. The reliefs of Ardašīr I are discussed in detail in Hinz 1969: 115–145. For a more recent overview, see also Luschey 1987.

[42] Hinz 1969: 123–126, Taf. 57–59; Schmidt 1970: 123–125, Pl. 96; Vanden Berghe 1984: no. 52; Luschey 1987: 377–378; Vanden Berghe 1988: 1522–1523.

[43] Schmidt 1970: 131, Pl. 98.

[44] Luschey 1987: 377.

[45] Thus, Schmidt 1970: 125, basing on stylistic features, thinks that this relief is later than the others attributed to the first Sasanian king.

Two diminutive individuals, placed between the king and his god, and standing less than half of their size, are the most enigmatic characters of the relief. A small figure of similar size is also found on the relief of Narseh at Naqš-e Rostam. The left character at Naqš-e Rağab wears a *kulāf* tied with a royal diadem and raises his right hand with a pointed forefinger in the same gesture as the "crown-prince Šāpūr" standing behind the king, but unlike "Šāpūr" the left hand of the small figure is not hidden in the long sleeve of his garment, but is freely suspended along the body. Unfortunately, the second figure is badly effaced and the details of his appearance are barely visible. He seems to possess a short, accurately cut beard. He is probably naked and his head is uncovered—a most unexpected feature for an Iranian noble, let alone king or deity. In one hand he holds an unidentified battered object and in another—a staff. It may be that the carving of this rod was not completed, and it is thought to represent not a *barsom*, but a club.

The third relief of Ardašīr I, carved under the Achaemenian tombs at Naqš-e Rostam, is remarkable for its exceptional technical quality and the relief is of paramount significance for the study of Iranian religious iconography (pl. 2).[46] This equestrian investiture is executed in a very high relief, superseding in this aspect all other known Sasanian examples. Two imposing equestrian figures identified by the trilingual inscription[47] as Ardašīr (on the left), and Ahura Mazdā (on the right), dominate the composition. They are disproportionally large comparing to the realistic, but undersized mounts. The king and his god wear long garments falling dawn in pleats and a cloak, fastened on the chest. The shape of their beards and headdresses is, however, different. Ardašīr has a short, accurately cut beard and wears a scull-cap crowned with a *korymbos* and tied with a diadem with long, flying ends. The beard of the highest Zoroastrian god has a square form, reminiscent of Achaemenian prototypes and he wears a mural crown and a diadem. In his left hand Ahura Mazdā holds a rod and with his right hand offers a diadem to the king. Ardašīr reaches for the diadem, bending his left arm, with his hand clenched in a fist with a pointed forefinger. A page standing behind Ardašīr holds a fly-whisk over his head. The hooves of Ardašīr's horse trample a prostrate figure unanimously identified with the last Parthian king, Artabanus IV, while under the horse of Ahura Mazdā lies a bearded, bareheaded man with writhing snakes instead of hair and the pointed ears of an animal.

Although al-Ṭabarī records that Ardašīr's grandfather, Sāsān (and probably also his descendants), was a custodian of the temple of Anāhitā at Eṣṭaḵr,[48] it is significant that on all his reliefs Ardašīr chose Ahura Mazdā and not Anāhitā as the god bestowing royal authority upon him.

One of the two rock-reliefs probably carved by Šāpūr shortly after his accession to the throne located at Naqš-e Rağab (fig. 7) presents a scene of an equestrian investiture, doubtless modeled on the Naqš-e Rostam relief of his father.[49] However, it is different from the latter in several aspects; here Ahura Mazdā occupies the left side of the relief while the king is depicted on the right. The god also loses his rod and has only a diadem in his right hand, and no defeated enemies are shown under the hooves of the horses. The faces of the figures are badly damaged, but the crenellated crown of the god, lacking a royal *korymbos* but covering luxuriant curls of hair is nevertheless clearly visible.

The last of the Sasanian equestrian investiture reliefs carved by Wahrām I follows the pattern of the visual representations of investiture established by his grandfather Ardašīr at Naqš-e Rostam, which was slightly modified and "canonized" by Šāpūr I at Naqš-e Rağab (fig. 8).[50] Ahura Mazdā, on the left,

46 Hinz 1969: 126–135, Taf. 60–68; Schmidt 1970: 122–123, Pls. 80–81; Vanden Berghe 1984: no. 53. Luschey 1987: 379; Vanden Berghe 1988: 1523.

47 Schmidt 1970: 123, Pl. 82; Back 1978: 282. The inscription on the divine horse in Middle Persian, Parthian and Greek reads "this is the image of the god Ahura Mazdā (Greek version: Zeus)".

48 Al-Ṭabarī vol. 5, ed. and tr. by Bosworth 1999: 4. See also Chaumont 1958; Chaumont 1965: 171.

49 Schmidt 1970: 125–126, pl. 99; Vanden Berghe 1984: no. 56; Vanden Berghe 1988: 1524–1525.

50 Schmidt 1970: 128–129; Herrmann 1981: 11–20; Vanden Berghe 1984: no. 62. No convincing explanation for the discontin-

who wears an uncovered crenellated crown adorned with a diadem and offers a diadem, is minutely copied from the reliefs of Šāpūr. One interesting detail of the relief of Wahrām I is that the figure of the king is larger than the image of the god because of his tall *korymbos* (extending beyond the relief panel). This trait, observed here for first time in Sasanian, and perhaps even Iranian, art would be later fully developed at Ṭāq-i Bustān. Wahrām reaches for the ring with his right hand while his left hand rests confidently on the hilt of his long sword.

The figure of the defeated enemy under the horse of Ahura Mazdā is missing, as on the relief of Šāpūr I at Naqš-e Rajab. Wahrām's mount tramples the unidentified adversary, who was probably added later under Narseh after the main panel was completed.[51] The relief also carries an inscription but the image of Ahura Mazdā is not labeled as it is on the relief of Ardašīr at Naqš-e Rostam.

In sharp contrast to the partially anthropomorphic god of the Achaemenians and the *frataraka*, the Sasanian Ahura Mazdā has a fully human shape from the very beginning.[52] This indicates a departure from the earlier prototype, although the Sasanians were probably familiar with the Achaemenian image of Ahura Mazdā (represented on the coins of the *frataraka*).[53] The appearance of Achaemenian motifs in Sasanian art is not surprising, as Pars was unique in preserving elements of the Achaemenian heritage during the Hellenistic and the Parthian periods.[54] Thus, it seems that the image of the highest Zoroastrian god was recreated under the first Sasanian king, drawing inspiration, and employing artistic and stylistic motifs from the Achaemenian art preserved in their native Pars.[55]

However, there is more. The Iranian written sources provide clear and unambiguous evidence that Ahura Mazdā was perceived in anthropomorphic terms. Already in the Avesta and throughout Middle Persian literature, the highest Zoroastrian god was thought to possess a complete human form in *mēnōg*, which could be seen and perceived only by chosen individuals possessing extraordinary qualities.[56] The case of Wīrāz, who was honored with an audience by Ahura Mazdā, but was able to hear only his voice and see the light,[57] is exemplary. Zoroaster, for instance, saw Ahura Mazdā in a completely anthropomorphic form, identical in his physique and clothing to a human being.[58] The light that Wīrāz saw is often associated with the visual manifestation of Ahura Mazdā not only in Iranian, but also in foreign sources, for instance, Porphyry of Tyre.[59]

---

uance of the motif of the investiture under Wahrām II have been proposed, although Lukonin 1969: 112, attributes it to the religious and political activities and influence of Kartīr.

[51] For the identification of this figure, see Herrmann 1981: 19.

[52] The recent suggestion by Overlaet 2013 that the investing figure on the Naqš-e Rostam relief originally depicted a priest or a king-priest is impossible to accept for a number of reasons that cannot all be discussed here. It completely ignores the millennia-old tradition of rock-reliefs in Mesopotamia and Elam showing the divine investiture, to which the Sasanian reliefs undoubtedly belong. The *barsom* that Ahura Mazdā holds in his hand is not an exclusive instrument of priests as Overlaet maintains (p. 324), but it was certainly also used by laymen, kings and, most importantly, by gods in the Avestan texts.

[53] Contrary to what Lukonin 1977: 162, claims. The art and the ideology of the Sasanian state were formed in Pars. In a certain sense, the Sasanian kings were the descendants of the *frataraka* and drew heavily on their legacy. Gariboldi 2004: 41, for instance, stresses that on the coinage of the king of Pars we can find "the cultural, religious and artistic roots of all the characteristic motifs of the Sasanian coinage".

[54] Lukonin 1977: 139. Although it remains a debated issue, the Sasanians probably did not preserve their own genuine historical memory and knowledge (independent of the Graeco-Roman tradition) of the Achaemenian dynasty: Yarshater 1971. For a different opinion, see Shahbazi 2001, who advocates that the early Sasanians did possess some memories of the Achaemenians, and Daryaee 2006a, who largely accepts Shahbazi's considerations.

[55] See a recent article by Canepa 2010 surveying the elements of the Achaemenian legacy of Pars and its importance in the creation of Sasanian royal ideology and art.

[56] On the notions of *mēnōg* and *gētīg*, see p. 188.

[57] See p. 33.

[58] See p. 33.

[59] See p. 18.

Finally, the last "prince the color of dawn", described in Kartīr's vision as pointing a finger at the priest's *hangirb* and smiling, is most probably Ahura Mazdā himself.[60] This apparently provides us with both literary and iconographic evidence that in the third century in Sasanian Iran Ahura Mazdā was perceived as a fully anthropomorphic divinity. The iconographic data, and literary and epigraphic sources present a coherent picture of the appearence of Ahura Mazdā fully realized in human form from the dawn of the Sasanian era.

On all three reliefs of Ardašīr I, the highest Zoroastrian god is given two attributes, the rod and the beribboned ring. The rod that Ahura Mazdā holds in his left hand seems to be a *barsom* (Av. *barəsman*), a bundle of twigs used in the Zoroastrian liturgy. The beribboned ring in his other hand is most probably a diadem, like that worn by the king and by the god himself. Archaeologists and art historians have exhaustively discussed the symbolism and the significance of this second object. It is often claimed to represent a royal *x^varənah*,[61] which is unlikely, as no pre-Islamic Iranian text is known to make this association.[62] From the Hellenistic period, the diadem became a necessary element in the Western Iranian royal headdress and it seems that for the Iranian kings it held the same symbolism as it had for their Seleucid predecessors—the most important visual element of royal authority and a symbol of kingship.[63] Taken together, however, the *barsom* and the diadem represent a remarkable visual parallel to the "rod and ring" held by some gods in ancient Mesopotamia as a symbol of their divine power.[64] Whether the Mesopotamian rod and ring owe their origin to the measuring rod and line is not entirely clear, but they are never held by a mortal—only by a deity.[65] Although Ahura Mazdā keeps the *barsom* and the ring separate, while in Mesopotamia the rod and the ring were always held in the same hand, there can be little doubt that the same millennia-old Mesopotamian concept of delegating divine power and authority to the king is represented on the Sasanian reliefs.[66]

Such symbolism was probably inspired by Mesopotamian and Elamite visual representations, as well as the Behestūn relief, still visible in Sasanian times.[67] For instance, the seventeenth century BCE Elamite relief from Kurangun, in which the bearded god wearing a horned headdress presents to the male worshipper a rod and a ring[68] and the rock-relief of Anubanini, king of Lullubi, in which the goddess Ištar

---

60 See p. 11–12.

61 For example, see Shepherd 1983: 1081, 1087; Vanden Berghe 1988: 1514; Abka'i-Khavari 2000: 43; Azarpay 2000: 68; Rose 2005 and a bibliographical survey down to 1984 in Tanabe 1984: 29, n. 4. Shepherd 1972 argued that the ribbons of the Sasanian diadem derive from the Graeco-Roman world and have "sacred" meaning. Choksy distinguished between two types of ring/diadem and maintained that the beribboned diadem represents royal glory bestowed by the gods, Iranian *x^varənah*, and that the plain ring/diadem is the symbol of victory: Choksy 1989: 128–129. This interpretation is difficult to accept since the plain ring in the Mesopotamian and Achaemenian tradition, even when it appears in the triumph scenes (reliefs of Anubanini and Darius the Great at Behestūn), is inseparable from the bestowal of divine power and legitimacy by the deity upon the victorious monarch. It is also clear that beribboned and plain rings were used interchangeably by both deities and mortals and were in all probability considered variants of the similar object sharing the same meaning. Even on the coin of Wahrām II, studied by Choksy 1989: Pl. 10.1; the bust on the obverse holds a beribboned diadem while the figure on the reverse (both figures are identified by Choksy as Anāhitā) extends a plain ring. Therefore, it seems that the so-called "plain ring" is simply a reduced representation of the royal diadem.

62 Thus in Narseh's Paikuli inscription, the crowning of a king with a diadem is mentioned several times as symbolizing royal authority, but no connection with the *x^varənah* is drawn: Humbach and Skjærvø 1983 § 4, 6, 35, 51.

63 For instance, the Arsacid kings were at times portrayed on coins without their tiara, but never without a diadem: Olbrycht 1997: 53.

64 Van Buren 1949: 449; Root 1979: 173. See especially the recent study by Slanski 2007.

65 Van Buren 1949: 434, 449. Slanski 2007, suggests that the rod and ring are surveying tools for laying straight lines that symbolize righteous, god-given kingship.

66 For a recent survey of scholarly discussion of the Sasanian investiture, see Kaim 2009: 404. The profound influence of the Mesopotamian civilization on Achaemenian and Iranian ideology, kingship and religion is discussed in Gnoli 1974; Gnoli 1988; Panaino 2000.

67 However, see Kuhrt 2010: 92, who writes that the ring that Ahura Mazdā holds at Behestūn "seems peculiar to the Iranian sphere" and is unrelated to the Mesopotamian royal symbols.

68 For the latest discussion of this relief, see Potts 2004.

bestows royalty and power upon him symbolized by a ring.[69] It appears that the original Mesopotamian plain ring gradually became associated during the Hellenistic period with a royal diadem.

Aside from the relief of Darius the Great at Behestūn, scenes of investiture never feature in Achaemenian art, but compositions in which rulers are granted a diadem or wreath appear in Western Iran in the Parthian period.[70] In the Pahlavi texts, a monarch awards nobles with the *kulāf ud kamar* (a high cap and a belt).[71] According to Kartīr's inscriptions, he was invested with *kulāf ud kamar* by the king.[72] In the Cologne Mani Codex, Šāpūr I was crowned by the "great (royal) diadem" (διάδημα μέγιστον)[73] and a diadem is also mentioned several times by Narseh in his Paikuli inscription.[74] The portraits of Sasanian seals suggest that Persian nobles and functionaries of high rank also wore a diadem;[75] and Armenian kings were crowned with a "diadem" (*patiw*) which was also an attribute and indicator of the rank of nobility in Armenian society.[76] Iconographic motifs frequently have multiple meanings rather than single, exclusive ones. Without a doubt, in both Parthian and Sasanian art (especially on seals and on silver vessels) not all scenes depict the investiture of a mortal by the deity. It is possible that by the Parthian era, the diadem—merged with a Greek wreath—had come to symbolize the granting of authority and power in general, perhaps a covenant between the king and his vassal or a husband and his wife.[77]

It is noteworthy that in Mesopotamia and in Achaemenian Iran equestrian figures are never found involved in this act. In the Avesta as well, Ahura Mazdā never appears as a horseman.[78] The reliefs from Commagene are also situated entirely within the "Mesopotamian" tradition of foot investiture.[79] The equestrian investiture seems to have been introduced in the Parthian period,[80] although it is possible that it already had prototypes in Scythian art.[81] Parthian coins depict both enthroned and mounted

---

69 Vanden Berghe 1984: no. 1; Vanden Berghe 1988: 1512–1513.

70 Examples of the handing over of a ring in Parthian and Sasanian art are listed in von Gall 1990: 102–106. See also pre-Sasanian graffiti from Persepolis: Callieri 2003. Most of the themes current in the Sasanian reliefs are already present in the Parthian reliefs, see Vanden Berghe 1987: 248–252. Notable examples in monumental art are the stele of Artabanus IV and Kwasak from Susa: Kawami 1987: 48–51, no. 5; two reliefs at Sar-e Pol-e Zohab in Khuzestan where investiture is probably depicted: Kawami 1987: no. 4; and especially the relief from Hung-e Yar Alivand, also in Khuzestan: Vanden Berghe and Schippmann 1985: 39–42, Fig. 2; Kawami 1987: no. 51. On the latter, two horsemen are shown facing each other and one probably holds a ring.

71 Von Gall 1990: 107. The exilarch, the leader of Babylonian Jewry, received a special belt called a *qamar* from the Sasanian king as a sign of his authority and high rank. See Herman 2012: 76–81.

72 Gignoux 1991: 68.

73 Sundermann 1990: 295. See also the discussion in Chaumont 1979.

74 Sundermann 1990: 297.

75 See also Procop. *Pers.* 1.17.26–30 who records an episode in which a defeated Sasanian general was punished by the king in the manner that: "… he took away from him a decoration which he was accustomed to bind upon the hair of his head, and an ornament wrought of gold and pearls. Now this is a great dignity among Persians, second only to the kingly honor". On the symbols of honor bestowed by the Sasanian monarchs on their subjects, see also Rose 2001: 46–47.

76 PB 3.11, 4.2, 5.37.

77 Ghirshman 1970: 179, thought that it represented a "present for a marriage", offered on the occasion of the festival. Its relation to the Avestan concept of "contract", personified by the god Mithra, was also proposed. See Kaim 2009.

78 De Jong 2006: 238.

79 On the cults of Commagene and their connections with Iranian religions, see Duchesne-Guillemin 1978; Boyce and Grenet 1991: 314–353; Waldmann 1991; Jacobs 2000.

80 Kawami 1987: 147.

81 The so-called "investiture scene" on a Scythian rhyton from Karagodeuakhsh kurgan is frequently quoted in the discussions of the origin of images of investiture in Iranian art: Rostovtzeff 1922: 104; Artamonov 1961: 73–76; Ghirshman 1964: 359, Fig. 465; Bessonova 1983: 115–116. Two horsemen in Scythian attire are shown facing each other, their horses trampling beheaded enemies. One holds a rhyton and a scepter/spear while the other raises his right hand in a gesture of greeting, blessing or adoration. His left hand is not preserved and it is impossible to establish what he originally held in it. This scene has been interpreted as a divine investiture with the deity being identified as Ahura Mazdā based on the Sasanian reliefs: Ghirshman 1964: 359, Fig. 465, and Mithra (Scythian Goetosyrus): Bessonova 1983: 116. However, there is no certainty that the Karagodeuakhsh rhyton indeed represents divine investiture; and of course, any identifications with Ahura Mazdā should be *a fortiori* dismissed.

figures of the king receiving a diadem from Tyche or Nike,[82] emphasizing the complex nature of the Arsacid dynasty that successfully combined their nomadic heritage with the administrative structure created by their predecessors and the sedentary traditions of the populations that they came to rule.[83] In all probability, the equestrian investiture reflects the culture of nomadic, horse-breeding Scythians and Parthians, in contrast to the foot investiture of sedentary Mesopotamians and Achaemenians. In the Sasanian era, both the "Western-foot" and the "Eastern-equestrian" investiture, the legacy of Mesopotamians and Parthians respectively, were fused together within one artistic and ideological tradition.

However, in sharp contrast with their Parthian predecessors, the Sasanian kings receive the diadem from the hands of Ahura Mazdā, and not Tyche or Nike. If Ahura Mazdā was ever venerated by the Parthians, he was certainly not the supreme source of royal legitimation as he had been for the Persian dynasties—the Achaemenians and the Sasanians.

Some elements of the image of Ahura Mazdā as produced under the first Sasanians, such as a crenellated tiara, the shape of the beard and the treatment of other facial features may go back to Achaemenian art,[84] ultimately deriving from Mesopotamia. A crown with crenellations is worn by royal figures on the Assyrian reliefs.[85] Darius, Xerxes and Artaxerxes II are depicted on their tomb reliefs wearing crenellated crowns[86] and in a slightly different form, closer to the Sasanian types, it appears also on coins of certain *frataraka* rulers of Pars during the Hellenistic period.[87] In the Parthian period, Tyche on the reverse of the coins wears a classic *corona muralis*.[88] A crown with stepped crenellations, a continuation of the Achaemenian type, is worn by the marble female head, probably a portrayal of Tyche or a Parthian queen, found at Susa and dated to the late first century BCE.[89] On one of his coin types, Ardašīr I himself wears a mural crown.[90] It is on this portrait of the king that the representation of Ahura Mazdā on Sasanian reliefs is probably based.[91] Among several types of crowns worn by Ardašīr, the crenellated crown was perhaps chosen because of its archaic, Achaemenian associations.[92]

In a legend on his coinage, Ardašīr I is addressed as *mazdēsn bay ardašīr šāhān šāh ērān kē čihr az yazdān*.[93] The exact translation of this title and its implications have been discussed at length by philologists and historians alike.[94] Grammatically *bay* can be understood here as "Lord",[95] but also as

---

[82] Calmeyer 1979: Fig. 2.7, 2.9 (enthroned) and Fig. 2.10 and 2.11 (mounted). The earliest evidence comes from the coins of Pacorus I (ca. 39 BCE.): Curtis 2004. There can be little doubt, however, that the concept of Tyche offering a diadem to a king, was adopted from the depictions of Greek and Roman Nike crowning kings, deities and heroes with a wreath, probably already in the Hellenistic period. Nike crowning a ruler with a wreath appears on a coin of *frataraka* Vādfradād: Lukonin 1977: 114–115; Boyce and Grenet 1991: 115.

[83] Olbrycht 1998: 76. Another element of Arsacid culture linked to their nomadic heritage is the introduction of a trouser-suit as royal attire. This outfit, associated with Iranian nomads, signifies a sharp departure from the royal garb of sedentary Near Eastern people, including the Achaemenians: Curtis 1998: 67.

[84] See recently Canepa 2010: 577–578.

[85] Azarpay 1972: 109.

[86] Calmeyer 1993: Fig. 13. For a study of the crenellated crown in Iran, citing many examples, see Vanden Berghe 1978: 137–143. It was possibly perceived as a dynastic crown of the Achaemenians and crenellations were probably regarded as a symbol of protective and sacred power: Henkelman 1995/1996.

[87] Peck 1993: 410, Fig. 18.

[88] See references in Vanden Berghe 1978: 140, n. 34.

[89] Peck 1993: 412, Pl. XVII.

[90] Alram and Gyselen 2003: Type V.

[91] Lukonin 1969: 48.

[92] Gyselen 2010a: 73 associates the mural crown with a concept of divine protection, embodied by Tyche.

[93] This legend appears on the coinage of all Sasanian kings until Ardašīr II.

[94] Sundermann 1988; Panaino 2004: 560; Alram and Gyselen 2003: 186–190; Alram, Blet-Lemarquand and Skjærvø 2007: 30–37; Daryaee 2008: 66; and especially the recent in-depth lengthy article by Panaino 2009a. See also a discussion of the titulature of the Sasanian kings in Huyse 2006.

[95] See Sims-Williams 1989; Panaino 2009b: 339–340.

"divine" as this word also means "god/divinity";[96] and *čihr* was variously translated as "image/seed/origin/essence/aspect/nature".[97] Therefore, the whole title can be translated "the divine Mazda-worshipping Ardašīr/Mazda-worshipping Lord Ardašīr, king of kings of the Iranians, whose image/seed/origin is from the gods". If *čihr* here is to be understood as "image/form/visible appearance",[98] referring to the physical appearance of the king given the shape of the gods, than the whole title could be read "formed in the image of the gods/a visible manifestation (deriving) from the gods".[99] This provides yet more support for the idea that the king was considered a representation of Ahura Mazdā in *gētīg*.[100]

According to the Zoroastrian scriptures, every divinity has its *gētīg* manifestation—or even a number of them. Divinities were always believed to possess a human form in *mēnōg*, but were not always represented in this way in *gētīg*.[101] Thus, the Aməša Spənta ("life-giving/bounteous immortals") are represented by various natural elements and Ahura Mazdā by humankind.[102] It would therefore be natural to conceive and visually present Ahura Mazdā as a mirror image of the Sasanian king—the best and most perfect human being, possessing superior physical and moral qualities.[103] The Achaemenian kings were probably also considered to be an "image" of Ahura Mazdā[104] although they never call themselves *baga* ("god")[105] and they were never perceived as a living gods, only as mortal delegates of the divine on earth.[106] The designation of the Iranian king as a "god" (θεός) first appears during the reign of

---

96 In the Greek version of the trilingual inscription at Naqš-e Rostam both king and Ahura Mazdā are called θεός: Back 1978: 281–282; see also Alram, Blet-Lemarquand and Skjærvø 2007: 33–34.

97 See Panaino 2009a.

98 This interpretation is preferred, for instance by Alram, Blet-Lemarquand and Skjærvø 2007: 37. However, see Shaked 2008: 115 n. 3; who remarks that "the use of the preposition *az* 'from' practically excludes any translation except 'origin'". This is also confirmed by the parallel Greek text that has γένος ("lineage, stock, kin, family") for *čihr*. Also Huyse prefers to translate *čihr* as "Abstammung": Huyse 2006.

99 Panaino 2009a: 232–233.

100 Panaino 2009a: 238.

101 On aniconism in Iranian religions, see Chapter Four.

102 Shaked 1971: 81–82.

103 Because of his possession of a material, corporeal form, the Sasanian king could only be considered a mortal man, not one of the *yazdān*. He was only god's earthly representative in *gētīg* and because of this he possessed the attributes of divine power and divine rights to the throne, but was not considered a living god and worshipped as such himself. However, it should be emphasised that the king was the most exalted among all mortals and the line separating him from the divine appears to be very thin. We know that the Magi who guarded the tomb of Cyrus received sheep, wheat, wine and horses to sacrifice for the dead king (Arrian (6.29.7)) and Theopompus reports that during the banquets, a special table was set in honor of the δαίμων of the living Achaemenian king (Athenaeus (6.60)). Four documents from the *Persepolis Fortification Archive* make mention of allocation of provisions to the "servants" attending the tombs (*šumar*) of the members of the royal dynasty: Henkelman 2003. It is plausible that certain cultic activities were also involved, and probably points to the veneration of the deceased ancestors: Rollinger 2014: 193–194. According to Ammianus Marcellinus, Arsaces was deified after his death and placed among the stars. Therefore, he and his successors were called "brothers of the Sun and Moon" Ammianus Marcellinus (23.6.5). This information is regarded by some scholars as unreliable and related to the Sasanians rather than to the Arsacids: Drijvers 1999: 198. However, it is interesting to note in this connection, the depiction of the multi-rayed star (sun?) and a crescent moon symbolically placed on either sides of the portrait of the king on the coin of Orodes II: Koshelenko and Gaibov 2010a: 192, Fig. 4a–b. A figure worshipping before the star and the moon is shown on coins of one of the *frataraka* rulers: Gariboldi 2004: 42, Fig. 11. It therefore seems likely that kingship in Western Iran already had some connections with astral symbolism before the Sasanian period and the information provided by Marcellinus could indeed be considered trustworthy. Šāpūr I ordered an animal sacrifice "for the soul" (*pad ruwān*) as well as for the souls of his relatives and even of other nobles: ŠKZ 33–34. See Panaino 2009a; who underlines the parallels between and the common nature of these Achaemenian and Sasanian rituals. It is also well known that Sasanian kings established royal fires through which the king could be venerated.

104 Plut. *Vit. Them.* 27.3.

105 Panaino 2004. It should also be noted that in neither the Achaemenian royal inscriptions nor in Zoroastrian literature, is Ahura Mazdā called a "king", but only a "lord/sovereign"; OP. *xšaϑriya* and Av. *xvatāi*: Hultgård 1993: 7, n. 17. This further emphasizes the distinction between the king and the god that probably existed in Western Iran.

106 Kellens 2002: 448.

the Arsacid dynasty, undoubtedly inherited from the Seleucid titulature.[107] Unfortunately, most Parthian kings issued coins with Greek legends, and therefore their Iranian titular terminology remains largely unknown to us.

The concept of *kē čihr az yazdān* is most strikingly represented on early Sasanian reliefs. By placing the king on the same footing as the god it is symbolically demonstrated that he is the earthly, *gētīg* delegate of Ahura Mazdā, but he is not identical with him. Thus, they are depicted as being the same size and wearing similar garments, but with different crowns in order to break what would otherwise be a perfect likeness. Such "egalitarian" relations between the king and the deity are not found in earlier Western Iranian art. On later Achaemenian monuments, the god mirrors the image of the king. However, the Achaemenian kings never depicted themselves on the same level as Ahura Mazdā,[108] and the same holds true also for their *frataraka* successors in Pars.

The creation of the first fully anthropomorphic image of Ahura Mazdā in the Sasanian period was not accidental but connected to the glorification of the institute of kingship and the persona of the Sasanian monarch. Tallay Ornan, who analyzed the unexpected appearance of the anthropomorphic gods on the rock reliefs of the Assyrian king Sennacherib, which is exceptional for the Assyrian monumental art of the period, argued that "the adoption of the anthropomorphic rendering of deities was to bring together divine and royal images in order to increase the status of the king by demonstrating his physical proximity to the gods and, more importantly, his likeness to the divine".[109] This is undoubtedly also correct in the case of Ardašīr. The invention of the human-shaped Ahura Mazdā by the first Sasanian monarch was to serve the purpose of elevating the king to a semi-divine status and to liken him to the god.

In Eastern Iran the institute of kingship and royal ideology developed in a remarkably different way. The Kushan kings, in addition to *βαγο*, were also called "worthy of divine worship" (βαγ[η]-ζνογο)[110] and their statues were installed in the temples as evidenced from Surkh-Kotal and Rabatak inscriptions.[111] This seemingly confirms that unlike in Western Iran, the Kushan kings were subject to full divinization.[112] While we do not possess similar evidence for Western Iran,[113] in Armenia, we have indications that royal statues were erected in temples and stood among the idols of gods.[114] This important issue should be elaborated at length elsewhere, but for the purposes of this study we may conclude that while in Western Iran (basing on Achaemenian and Sasanian evidence), the king was considered the "living images of the gods"[115] among the Kushans he was fully divinized. Despite this disparity, in both parts of the Iranian world the figure of the king was considered a visual manifestation of the god.

Another important characteristic of the Sasanian image of Ahura Mazdā is that in most cases he is shown alone, without the retinue that accompanies the king on some reliefs. On two late Sasanian reliefs at Ṭāq-i Bustān, Mithra and Anāhitā are depicted as his companions[116]—the same divinities invoked in the Achaemenian royal inscriptions centuries earlier, but it is important to note that they are placed behind the king, forming *his* retenue. It is undoubtedly significant that the Aməša Spənta, which are of

---

107 Koshelenko and Gaibov 2010a.
108 Huff 2008: 39.
109 Ornan 2007: 165.
110 See discussion of this title in Panaino 2009b.
111 See p. 12.
112 Panaino 2009a: 214. See also Mukherjee 1988: 313–322, who argues that the Kushan kings were deified, and worshipped in temples by means of their cultic statues during their lifetime and after death. For a different view, see Verardi 1983: 280, who argues against the deification of Kushan rulers.
113 However, we now have evidence from a tablet dated to the first year of Xerxes that offerings were made in Babylonian temples to the statue of Darius. See Rollinger 2014: 194.
114 See p. 19.
115 Panaino 2009a: 234.
116 See p. 70 and p. 104.

paramount importance in the Zoroastrian tradition as the assistants and the helpers of Ahura Mazdā, are completely absent from Sasanian art and are never invoked in Sasanian royal inscriptions. Perhaps the abstract personifications of the Aməša Spənta were less popular with the laity and the secular elite, who found it easier to devote themselves to the more "concrete" and more comprehensible Anāhitā and Mithra.

Sasanian Ahura Mazdā possibly appears not only on rock-reliefs, but also on coins. The second Sasanian king, Šāpūr I introduced a new type of reverse on his coins—two personages flanking the fire-altar (fig. 9).[117] They are dressed in royal attire and hold a staff or a spear in the right hand,[118] while the left hand rests on the hilt of a sword. On the majority of issues of Šāpūr I these individuals wear a simple, uncovered mural crown, while on some coins the crown is supplemented with a royal *korymbos* (globe of circles covered with fabric).[119] On two types of Ōhrmazd's I coins the figures are portrayed facing the altar for the first time.[120] However, in those cases the scene is different, probably representing an investiture of the king by male and female deities—Mithra and Anāhitā. Under Wahrām I, the figures once again face away from the altar (fig. 10). However, unlike the "attendants" on the coins of Šāpūr I they usually wear different crowns, only few types being identical.[121] From the reign of Narseh, the figures always face the altar. In some cases, these "attendants" are indistinguishable, in others they may differ by the type of their crowns and the length of the staves they carry. Starting from Xusrō I, the figures are always depicted frontally, leaning on their swords.

The identification of these "attendants" presents a serious challenge. The coins of the *frataraka* showing a worshipper in a gesture of adoration before an enigmatic structure[122] are usually considered in this connection as a possible source of inspiration. However, a composition that includes two figures placed on both sides of a structure is already found in the Achaemenian period.[123] Since these Sasanian "attendants" are dressed in royal garments, they cannot be priests,[124] but might rather represent an image of a king or/and a deity.[125] The possibility that they symbolize a "dual image of the king in the role of the guardian of the sacred fire"[126] cannot be ruled out with certainty, but such duality is not characteristic of Sasanian art and these "attendants" often wear different crowns.[127] Their position, with their backs turned to the fire-altar, could be taken to express the idea of protection, the safeguarding of the sacred fire,[128] but these observations do not bring us any closer to discovering the identity of these figures, since potentially, king, deities and priests could all be represented in this role.

---

117 Göbl 1971: 18–19; Alram and Gyselen 2003: 191–193; Gyselen 2010a: Fig. 4; Schindel 2013: 835.

118 Some scholars identify it as a scepter: Alram and Gyselen 2003: 191, n. 39.

119 Alram and Gyselen 2003: 193, Fig. 2b; Gyselen 2010a: Fig. 6. This exclusive detail of the royal headdress was interpreted as having a religious significance and connected to the *x^{v}arənah*: Azarpay 1972: 114; Canepa 2009: 193; reflecting the heavenly claims of the Sasanian kings: Von Gall 1984: 188; or as a symbol of the "glory and power of Persian kingship": Peck 1993: 414. See also Herzfeld 1939: 104–107. There is, however, not a single text explaining the symbolism of this important royal element and therefore its significance and meaning remains obscure.

120 Gyselen 2010a: Figs. 16, 17. According to the proposal by Gyselen 2010a: 78, this change in design was inspired by Roman coins.

121 See Gyselen 2010a: 78–79; Gyselen 2010b: 193–195.

122 For a recent evaluation of various interpretations proposed for this structure, see Potts 2007.

123 For instance, a seal from Persepolis (PFS 11*): Garrison 2000: 141, Fig. 18. This scene is strikingly similar to the reverse design of Sasanian coins and provides yet another example of the continually growing corpus of evidence for the remarkable continuity of Achaemenian artistic tradition in the Sasanian period.

124 As proposed by Göbl 1971: 18.

125 See recently Soudavar 2009: 419–420, who argues that the left figure is the image of a king and the right is that of a deity.

126 Alram 2008: 21. See also Alram and Gyselen 2003: 192 and n. 49 for references to other studies sharing this opinion.

127 Excluding, perhaps, a curious symmetrical representation at Ṭāq-i Bustān of Šāpūr III standing next to his father Šāpūr II: Schmidt 1970: 137–138; Fukai and Horiuchi 1972 Pl. LXVI–LXXIII; Vanden Berghe 1984: no. 80.

128 Alram and Gyselen 2003: 191.

The reverse of coins of Wahrām I, where the figure to the left of the altar is always wearing a royal radiate *korymbus* crown specific to this king,[129] suggests that the left "attendant" is most probably the image of the king himself. The right "attendant" on the coins of Wahrām I in most cases has an uncovered mural crown,[130] although on a certain type the crenellations are stretched so that they resemble spikes similar to those forming the radial crown of the king.[131] Two gold coins from the mint of Merv, which were struck with the same reverse die, provide conclusive evidence that the figure of the left "attendant" is indeed that of a king. The same die was used twice, first to strike the reverse of the coin of the Kushano-Sasanian king Ōhrmazd II and then for the coin of Šāpūr II.[132] For the second coin, the die was reworked to make the figure of the left "attendant" wear a crown of Šāpūr II instead of that of Ōhrmazd II.[133]

The identity of the righthand figure is far more difficult to establish.[134] It is tempting to regard the twin figures on the reverse of the Sasanian coins as images of a king and his *mēnōg* prototype, Ahura Mazdā.[135] The types where the "attendants" have different crowns seem to reinforce this assumption, while those where they are shown with exactly the same crown weaken it.[136] On all Sasanian reliefs—the only media where we find unquestionable visual representations of Ahura Mazdā—the god wears an uncovered crenellated crown. However, both "attendants" occasionally have crowns topped with a royal *korymbos*, which is usually worn by the king.[137] Given the inadequate state of our knowledge of Sasanian iconography due to the paucity of relevant textual evidence, we cannot rule out the possibility that Ahura Mazdā could also have been depicted with the royal *korymbos* crown in the later period.[138]

Perhaps this is the case with the small bust on the obverse of the coins of Jāmāsp facing the king (fig. 11). It is bearded, wears a mural crown topped with a *korymbos* and extends a diadem.[139] Since the bust clearly invests the king with a diadem, it is most probably an image of a deity. The beard and the crenellated crown, characteristic of images of Ahura Mazdā on Sasanian reliefs, support the suggestion that this particular bust depicts the chief Zoroastrian god,[140] despite the addition of the exclusively royal *korymbos* to his crown. Therefore, we may suggest that contrary to his canonized representation in monumental art, Ahura Mazdā could occasionally be depicted on coins wearing a crenellated crown topped with the *korymbos*.

---

129 Gyselen 2010a: Figs. 18, 19.

130 Gyselen 2010a: Fig. 18.

131 Gyselen 2010a: Fig. 19.

132 Cribb 1990: 166; coins no. 62 and no. 63.

133 Cribb 1990: 166.

134 Thus, after evaluating various possibilities, Gyselen cautiously concludes that no single interpretation is available for the right "attendant" who could have had multiple meanings and might have represented various individuals under different circumstances: Gyselen 1990: 254; Gyselen 2010a: 79.

135 Lukonin 1969: 68; Trever and Lukonin 1987, *passim*. Schindel 2004: 29, considers the left figure to represent the king and the right to be the image of Ahura Mazdā. However, in his recent review of Sasanian coinage he seems to favor the possibility that both figures represent the king. See Schindel 2013: 835.

136 Some types of Šāpūr I, where both figures have similar uncovered crenellated crowns could perhaps be explained as reflecting the ambition of Šāpūr I to make his image identical to that of the god. He was one of the most powerful and significant Sasanian monarchs and achieved the impressive military triumphs over the Romans. See Alram, Blet-Lemarquand and Skjærvø 2007. It is possibly not accidental that he chose a crenellated crown as his primary type, since it was worn by Ahura Mazdā on the investiture reliefs of his father and was probably closely associated with the supreme Zoroastrian god. Another speculative possibility is that the right "attendant" represent Šāpūr's father Ardašīr I, who also had this type of crown. For the types of Šāpūr's I crowns, see Alram and Gyselen 2003: 190, Fig. 1b.

137 For example on one type of Wahrām I: Gyselen 2010a: Fig. 20.

138 Especially from the fifth century CE, when the royal crowns become stereotyped and lose their individuality.

139 Schindel 2008: Pl. I; Fig. 1.I.

140 Göbl 1971: 51; Göbl 1983: 328; Tanabe 1993: 68; Göbl 1999: 159; Schindel 2008. Alternatively, Curtis 2008: 142 proposes to identify it as the personification of the royal *x*ᵛ*arənah*. However, this suggestion is not supported by any textual or iconographic evidence.

The cult of Ahura Mazdā spread beyond the initial borders of the Iranian world to Commagene, Armenia and K'art'li (Eastern Georgia). In Commagene we find his depiction as Zeus (fig. 12). In Armenia, there was a temple of Aramazd in Ani where his idol stood.[141] This idol was probably not unlike the Greek statues of Zeus from Asia Minor. The idol of the K'art'velian Armazi, who was the principal deity of pre-Christian K'art'li according to the sources, is described in meticulous anthropomorphic detail as an armored warrior made of copper and adorned with precious stones.[142]

2. *Eastern Iran*

In Eastern Iran it is possible to identify just one unquestionable representation of Ahura Mazdā—in the royal art of the Kushan kings—and two others: the Graeco-Bactrian statue from Ai Khanum and one of the deities in the art of the Sogdian city-states, whose identification is uncertain.

The fragments of an acrolithic statue from Ai Khanum belong to one of the few monumental cultic statues known from the Iranian world. They were uncovered by the *Délégation Archéologique Française en Afghanistan* (*DAFA*) in the principal temple of the Graeco-Bactrian city of Ai Khanum in Bactria (fig. 13).[143] The temple itself, known in scholarly literature as the "Temple with Indented Niches" was erected on a three-stepped podium within a wide *temenos* on the main street of the city, close to the palace and belonged to the "Mesopotamian type" of Iranian temples.[144] All that was preserved of an enormous acrolithic statue, which once stood in the cultic niche in the back wall of the central hall, are marble fragments of a male foot and a hand.[145] The length of the front part of the beautifully modeled foot is 27 cm, indicating that the statue was probably three times the size of a man. The fingers are sculpted in a "pure Greek" naturalistic style and a winged thunderbolt decorates the sandal. The left hand of the statue, as evidenced from the only preserved fragment, grasped an object, perhaps a scepter.

Although the style of the surviving fragments, and especially the thunderbolt decorating the sandal, suggest that they belonged to a statue of Zeus,[146] the fact that the statue was housed in a temple of the "Mesopotamian type"[147] has led scholars to propose a syncretism between the Greek and Oriental deities.[148] Different candidates for the deity venerated in the form of the Ai Khanum monumental statue have been put forward. However, new textual evidence, which has recently become available, suggests a return to the original identification with Zeus-Ahura Mazdā, as originally proposed by Paul Bernard.[149] This evidence comes from the fourth century BCE Aramaic documents found in Bactria, which have been translated and edited by Shaul Shaked and Joseph Naveh. One of these documents, which mentions a "libation for the temple, to Bel",[150] ambiguously indicates that the cult of the Mesopotamian Bel

141 See p. 19.

142 See p. 23.

143 For the most recent summary of the excavations of Ai Khanum carried out by *DAFA* and their results, see Bernard 2009. For a useful popular survey, see also Bernard 2008.

144 Also known as *temple à redans* and *temple à niches indentées*. The final publication exists only for the small finds from the temple: Francfort 1984. For preliminary reports, discussion and evaluation of its architecture and finds, see Bernard 1970: 321–348; Bernard 1971: 414–432; Bernard 1989; Bernard 1990a: 51–53; Downey 1988: 65–73; Hannestad and Potts 1990: 93–95; Pichikyan 1991: 239–243; Boyce and Grenet 1991: 165–171; Litvinskiy and Pichikyan 2000: 283–289; Bernard 2008: 92–93; Shenkar 2011; and especially the recent important article by Martinez-Sève 2010; who is currently preparing the final report on 'The Temple with Indented Niches', to be published in the *MDAFA*.

145 First publication: Bernard 1969: 338–341; See also Pichikyan 1991: 245–246.

146 Bernard 1990a: 53. However, see Francfort 2012: 122–123, who argues that the statue did not necessarily represent Zeus and was possibly even female.

147 On the Iranian temples of the Mesopotamian type, see Shenkar 2011: 126–133.

148 Downey 1988: 73.

149 Bernard 1974: 298. In his later publications, Bernard adopted the identification with Mithra proposed by Grenet. See, for example, Bernard 2008: 93.

150 *zwtr' 'l bgn' lbyl* (זותרא על בגנא לביל): Naveh and Shaked 2012: C1:37.

existed in Bactria as early as the Achaemenian period. The identification of the Greek Zeus with the Semitic Bel and the Iranian Ahura Mazdā is a well-known phenomenon also attested in the western regions of the Achaemenian Empire.[151]

Because of the inscription, the identification of the deity labeled Ōoromozdo (ΩΟΡΟΜΟΖΔΟ) portrayed on the four rare coins of the Kushan king Huvishka with Ahura Mazdā is certain.[152] On two of them, the name of the deity is given in full and on other two, it is abbreviated as Ōrom (ΩΡΟΜ).[153] On the type with the full legend, the god is facing left, draped in Greek style clothes—a tunic, and a cloak (fig. 14). In his left hand, he holds a spear or a staff and offers a diadem with his right hand. Ōoromozdo is bearded and has a nimbus surrounding his head. It is impossible to determine whether he has a headdress as it was left off the field. The style of the figure on the type with a short legend appears less "Greek" in terms of its garment and proportions, and the god does not hold a diadem in his right hand (fig. 15).[154] Since the figure on this type is preserved in full length, one can clearly see the *polos* that the deity wears on his head. His iconography is remarkably distinct from both the Achaemenian figure in the winged disk and the image created under the Sasanians. Like most Kushan deities, the figure of Ōoromozdo was probably inspired by Hellenistic and Roman iconography, although he does not appear on the first Greek issue of Kanishka. If he had done, he would be probably have been called "Zeus". The distinctive *polos* the deity is wearing indeed hints that his image may be modeled on Zeus[155] or on Kushan Sarapis, although this cannot be demonstrated with certainty.

Ahura Mazdā also appears in the Bactrian Rabatak dedicatory inscription, where he is mentioned third in the list, in the slightly different form αορομοζδο.[156] It is clear from the inscription (line 12) that his statue (as well as those of the other gods) stood in the still unexcavated sanctuary located at the site of Rabatak in Bactria; and it is clear now that statues of various Kushan deities were also placed in the other Kushan temple of Surkh-Kotal.[157]

As far as the iconography is concerned, many deities on Kushan coins are indisputably gods of investiture, bestowing royal authority by means of a beribboned diadem.[158] However, a complex question arises as to the extent to which the deities portrayed on coins reflect the "royal pantheon" of the Kushans and the general religious situation in the Kushan Empire. We can be confident that the frequency of occurrence of a certain deity on coins does not reflect his or her position in the Kushan pantheon, as it generally does not agree with the hierarchy of the Rabatak list of gods.[159]

The first triad of gods according to lines 9–10 of the Rabatak inscription consists of Nana, Umma, and Ahura Mazdā. The third place occupied by Ahura Mazdā in the Rabatak inscription does not accord with his extremely rare appearance on Kushan coins, and it is noteworthy that on the coins of Kanishka he does not appear at all. It cannot be said with certainty whether the hierarchy of deities of the Rabatak list imitate most venerated deities in the Empire, a pantheon of the ruling dynasty, or perhaps, personal preferences of Kanishka and Huvishka.[160] It is also probable that deities mentioned in the Rabatak inscription reflect those that were locally popular in Bactria, rather than in the whole Kushan empire.[161]

151 See Shenkar 2011: 129.

152 Rosenfield 1967: 83–84, Fig. 9; Göbl 1984: Ōoromozdo I.

153 However, see Bracey 2012: 200–201, who suggests that the deity labeled ΩΡΟΜ could be an image of Sarapis with an erroneous legend.

154 Göbl 1984: Ōoromozdo II.

155 Especially Zeus-Bēlos on the coins of Seleucia on the Tigris, see Grenet 1991: 148, Pl. LIX Figs. 3–4

156 See p. 12–13.

157 Sims-Williams and Cribb 1996: 109. On the temple of Surkh-Kotal, see Fussman 1983.

158 Cribb 1990: 174; Göbl 1999: 159.

159 For instance, one of the most popular deities on coins, Oešo, is not mentioned at all in the Rabatak inscription.

160 This last possibility is favored by Grenet forthcoming a. Gnoli 2009: 142, considers them to be the "protective divinities of Kaniška and of the Royal Household".

161 Carter 2006: 355.

Another possible representation of Ahura Mazdā in Kushan Bactria is a painted terracotta panel, showing a worshipper in the presence of a Zeus-like deity. This panel is part of the group, assumed to have been found in Afghanistan, that is currently kept in the Metropolitan Museum of Art in New York and in various private collections.[162] On stylistic grounds, their provenance can be placed in the region of Balkh and Dilberjin in Bactria.[163] Martha L. Carter dates these panels to the middle of the second to the middle of the fourth century CE and suggests that they originally decorated inner walls of a Kushan sanctuary.[164] The panel in question depicts on the left a worshipper in Kushan dress with his hands clasped in a gesture of adoration (pl. 3). He is facing a deity of the same size, who wears a red tunic and a white mantle. The god is bearded and has long, curling hair. In his right hand, he holds a partly preserved unidentified object (a *vajra*?). He is nimbate and wears a diadem and what seems to be a short *kalathos*. If his headdress is indeed a *kalathos*, than the god depicted on this panel could be either Ōoromozdo or Sarapis, both of whom are depicted with this headdress on Kushan coins.[165]

Despite the existence of representations of Ahura Mazdā both in Sasanian Iran and in Kushan Bactria, it is interesting to note that Ahura Mazdā does not appear on Kushano-Sasanian coins and no relevant legend is attested with his name. Therefore, it is impossible to state definitely whether he was included in their pantheon.[166]

It is appealing to connect the Bel from the Aramaic documents of the Achaemenian period, the "Zeus" from Ai Khanum, and the Kushan Ōoromozdo to a continuous, uninterrupted tradition of worship of Ahura Mazdā, who was merged with Bel and later Zeus in Bactria, spanning the Achaemenian and Kushan periods. However, the only definite image of Ahura Mazdā in Eastern Iran is the Kushan Ōoromozdo.

Despite the wealth of Sogdian religious iconography, it is extremely difficult to recognize visual representations of Ahura Mazdā.[167] Boris Marshak identified the Sogdian Ahura Mazdā as the elephant-rider from the paintings of the "Red Hall" at Varakhsha,[168] on the series of terracottas depicting the beardless male figure holding a cithara and on the mural from the northern wall of the northern shrine of Temple II at Panjikent.[169] This identification is apparently based on the following suggestions and assumptions. Since some Uigur Buddhist texts employ the name *Xurmuzda* for Śakra/Indra, and Sogdian Buddhist texts call the god Indra "Āδβāγ" (*"δδβγ*, *"δβγ*, or *'δδβγ*), meaning "The Great God", Helmut Humbach postulated in an influential article that in the Sogdian language, "Āδβāγ" was used instead of "Ahura Mazdā", whose name was taboo.[170] Based on this, Marshak identified the Sogdian personage riding the elephant, which is the *vāhana*— the vehicle of Indra, or enthroned on the elephant-throne, as Indra-Āδβāγ-Ahura Mazdā.

162 Carter 1997. For a discussion of the other panels, see p. 136 and p. 155–156.

163 Carter 1997: 582–583.

164 Carter 1997: 583, 585. Tigran Mkrtchev, who is preparing a detailed study of the panels, suggests that they be dated to the first quarter of the third century CE (personal communication). It is tempting to speculate that they might originate from the recently pillaged site of the Kushan temple at Rabatak.

165 Mention should also be made of two busts of deities wearing *kalathoi* from Gandhāra, kept in a private collection, and a necklace worn by a statue of Bodhisattva which shows a bust of a bearded god wearing a *kalathos*: Carter 1999/2000. Likewise in these cases, it is impossible to establish whether they depict Ōoromozdo or Sarapis.

166 Tanabe 1991/1992: 60.

167 Although his name is attested in Sogdian onomastics. See Livshits 2010: 242.

168 Belenitskii and Marshak 1981: 31–34; Marshak 1999: 181; Maršak 2000: 159; Marshak 2009: 38. For publication of the paintings, see Shishkin 1963: 152–158 (description); 204–205 (discussion) Tab. VI–X.

169 Marshak and Raspopova 1994/1996: 195–198. One of the terracottas from Panjikent (Fig. 16) depicts this deity seated on a throne supported by elephant protomes. This identification is accepted by Grenet 2006/2010: 92 and by Mode 1991/1992; who thinks that another image of "Āδβāγ-Ahura Mazdā" decorated one of the altars depicted on the mural in room III/6 at Panjikent: Mode 1991/1992: 183, Fig. 3. It is also embraced by other scholars, for instance Carter 2002: 272.

170 Humbach 1975a: 400–401.

There are several difficulties with these arguments. Sims-Williams has pointed out that Āδβāγ is an epithet not exclusive to Indra; it has also been applied to the Manichaean "Father of Greatness".[171] Most recently, Antje Wendtland has discussed in detail the Sogdian Buddhist, Manichaean and other texts mentioning Xurmuzda and Āδβāγ.[172] She noted that in Sogdian texts these names are attested only as the designation of the Manichaean "Primal Man", and stressed that the identification of Āδβāγ with Indra in Buddhist texts does not necessarily prove that these deities are identical.[173] However, two Sogdian documents describing Zoroaster's ascension to Heaven and his dialogue with Āδβāγ, which echo Zoroastrian Middle Persian literature, leave no doubt that in this case Āδβāγ replaces Ahura Mazdā.[174] The same tendency of replacing the name of a deity with his title is also attested in the case of Mithra, who is never referred to in Sogdian onomastics by his name but always as "Baga" ("the God").[175] Therefore, we may assume that some Sogdians called Ahura Mazdā by the name "Āδβāγ" and sometimes associated him with the Indian Indra, as they did for other Sogdian deities.[176]

Returning to Sogdian iconography, except for the elephant, neither the rider from the "Red Hall" nor the cithara players on the terracottas demonstrate any attributes of Indra, or Ahura Mazdā as he is known from Sasanian and Kushan iconography.[177] One should also note the absence of the third eye, mentioned as the characteristic trait of Āδβāγ in the Buddhist text *Vessantara Jātaka* 913–921.[178] This trait, however, would only have significance in the Buddhist context. In order to explain the discrepancy between the image of the cithara player and the expected appearance of Ahura Mazdā, a complex explanation was proposed—perhaps too complex to sound convincing: the crown is the expression of royalty, the sword, of might, and the cithara is taken from the Christian image of King David.[179]

The only possible image of Indra-Āδβāγ-Ahura Mazdā seems to be the left figure on panel D. X. 3. uncovered by Aurel Stein in the Buddhist shrine (D. X.) at Dandan Uiliq at Khotan (fig. 16).[180] The deity in question has a third eye on his forehead and holds a *vajra*, a distinctive attribute of Indra. His depiction together with two other unmistakably Sogdian divinities, Nana and Wešparkar, provides us with the necessary context to identify him as Indra-Āδβāγ-Ahura Mazdā exactly as attested by the above-mentioned literary evidence. His appearance (the third eye, the absence of an elephant-throne) and attributes (the *vajra* and not the cithara) clearly indicate that the Sogdian Ahura Mazdā has nothing in common with the figure from the "Red Hall" of Varakhsha or the cithara-player of the Sogdian terracottas.

Therefore, we must conclude that at present only one single image of Ahura Mazdā is known from the rich Sogdian religious iconography, and it comes from Khotan, not from the Sogdian heartland. We

171 Sims-Williams 1983: 138.

172 Wendtland 2009.

173 Wendtland 2009: 123–124.

174 See Grenet and Azarnouche 2007/2012: Appendix 1.

175 Sims-Williams 1991. The original meaning of the word *baga* is "distributor, dispenser", from the root *bag* "to distribute, allot". The meaning "god" is a later development securely attested for the first time in Achaemenian royal inscriptions, see Sims-Williams 1989.

176 In this context it is also worth mentioning the copper coin of the Indo-Greek king Eucratides I with a legend "the city god of Kapiśa" which shows an enthroned Zeus with an elephant protome: Mac Dowall 2007: Fig. 9.37. If the elephant here is to be taken as an allusion to Indra, this coin could be an indication of an early assimilation of Zeus with Indra. We have already discussed the evidence for possible identification of Zeus with Ahura Mazdā on the Ai Khanum material; and it is not impossible that the Sogdian Ahura Mazdā-Āδβāγ was identified with Indra via the mediation of Indo-Greek Zeus.

177 Marshak himself admits that the face of a beardless god with a cithara on the terracotta from Panjikent is too young for Ahura Mazdā and "would better suit Mithra or Tir, who were linked with Apollo": Marshak and Raspopova 1994: n. 36.

178 Wendtland 2009: 120. Although Belenitskii and Marshak 1981: 33, wish to see the third eye on the preserved part of the forehead of the elephant-rider from the "Red Hall", this must remain hypothetical.

179 Grenet 2006/2010: 92.

180 Stein 1907: 259–261.

can only speculate as to whether this reflects the fact that Ahura Mazdā did not occupy a prominent place in the Sogdian pantheon headed by the goddess Nana.

3. *Conclusions*

In summary, we can state that four iconographical traditions of visual anthropomorphic representation of Ahura Mazdā existed in the Iranian world. The earliest was developed under the Achaemenians in Western Iran and followed the Mesopotamian and Urartan prototypes. This tradition was not completely abandoned after the death of Darius III, as it frequently appears on the *frataraka* coinage and probably contributed to the recreation of an image of the god in the Sasanian period.

The second representation of Ahura Mazdā was created independently in the East by the Kushan kings. It was based on Graeco-Roman models, perhaps the images and cultic statues of Zeus (-Belos?), who may have been associated with Ahura Mazdā in Hellenistic Bactria. This Kushan Zeus-type Ahura-Mazdā probably did not survive the Kushan Empire itself, and it did not exert any visible influence on contemporary or future neighboring cultures.

In Sasanian dynastic monumental art, eight images of the highest Zoroastrian god are known from the royal rock-reliefs. Ahura Mazdā obviously had a special significance as a deity of imperial investiture and as the source of imperial legitimacy in Sasanian Iran. Out of nine rock-reliefs showing investiture, only Narseh at Naqš-e Rostam is granted divine royal power by the goddess Anāhitā. An additional image of Ahura Mazdā possibly appears as an investing deity on the coins of king Jāmāsp, and it is likely that he was also occasionally represented as the right-hand "attendant" on the reverse of Sasanian and Kushano-Sasanian coins from the reign of Šāpūr I until the downfall of the Sasanians in the seventh century CE. The distinctive feature of the Sasanian Ahura Mazdā is that he always appears bearded and wears a crenellated crown. On the rock-reliefs the crown is always uncovered, while on coins the royal *korymbos* crown was probably also used. The fourth image of Ahura Mazdā, shaped under the influence of the iconography of Indian Indra, is recognizable on the unique Sogdian plaque from Khotan.

If the frequency of the appearance of Ahura Mazdā in visual art is to be taken as an indirect indicator of the popularity of this deity, the inescapable conclusion is a clear predominance in the veneration of Ahura Mazdā among the people of Western, as opposed to Eastern, Iran. This probably reflects the fact that in Western Iran, at least from the Achaemenian period onward, Ahura Mazdā was the principal deity and the patron of the ruling dynasty (with the possible exception of the Arsacids), while in Eastern Iran he was possibly only an ordinary member of the pantheon of Bactrians, Sogdians and other Eastern Iranian peoples. The Parthian "gap" in the imagery of Ahura Mazdā should probably be viewed in this light.

It is noteworthy that even in Western Iran Ahura Mazdā, unlike Mithra or Māh, does not seem to appear in unofficial art forms, such as seals or silverware. Several possible interpretations can be proposed for this phenomenon. It is reasonable to assume that Ahura Mazdā was closely associated with the institution of kingship, and his *mēnōg* representative—the king—was naturally interested in the creation of images that would emphasize his divine legitimacy. We can further speculate that as the highest god (a position he occupied in Western Iran), Ahura Mazdā was possibly considered to be "remote" and unattainable by the common people, who would instead have directed their prayers and affection to less "elevated" deities, such as Mithra, who served the concrete functions of providing light, fertility and wealth.

2. *Airyaman*

The Avestan deity Airyaman (MP. Ērmān), whose very name means "friend, companion", was the personification of friendship already in the Indo-Iranian pantheon and continued to play this role in the Zoroastrian tradition.[181] In the latter, Airyaman also becomes a *yazata* of healing and is entrusted with an important eschatological task in the *frašegird*—the final renovation of the world. Airyaman is also known in Manichaeism.

1. *Western Iran*

A deity associated with healing is usually one of the most venerated divinities in any polytheistic pantheon. However, there are no indications that Airyaman was ever visually represented in Western Iran.

2. *Eastern Iran*

Airyaman is also unattested in the Kushan pantheon and there is no evidence that he was known in Bactria. His only image in Eastern Iran, and in fact, in the entire Iranian world, was identified in a fragmentary wall painting from Panjikent labeled by the inscription naming the god. The fragments of this painting were discovered in the northern wall of Temple's II portico (X/13).[182] It depicts a deity facing left, dressed in a polychrome pants, broad tiger skin cloak and leaning on a bow. Unfortunately, only his legs were preserved with a one-word Sogdian inscription identifying the character as "Aryaman". Next to it is another fragmentary inscription containing the word *δaxme* "grave". In front of the god, a large golden shield is painted decorated with a figure of a dancer.

Aryaman is one of only two deities in Sogdian art to be labeled by the accompanying inscription, indicating that this practice existed in Sogdiana. A bow is an unexpected attribute to be associated with the god of healing. However, the Sogdian Airyaman could also have possessed additional characteristics and personalities that are unknown to us, different from the Avestan god. Furthermore, even the Avestan gods not directly associated with warfare usually carry weapons as a symbol and sign of their prowess and status.

3. *Conclusions*

To date, only one unique image of Airyaman has been identified in Iranian iconography—in the painting from Panjikent where the god is depicted with a bow. Unfortunately, the poor preservation of the painting prevents us from learning more about the visual appearance of Sogdian Airyaman.

3. *Anāhitā*

One of the central female deities in the Zoroastrian tradition, Anāhitā (MP. Anāhīd), has its origins in the Avestan pantheon where she is called *arəduuī sūra anāhitā*—a tripartite epithet usually translated as "moist, mighty, undefiled".[183] In the Avesta Anāhitā is essentially a water goddess.[184] Warfare and erotic love are never associated with Anāhitā in the Avesta, where only her healing function is attested.[185] Of all the Avestan gods, her anthropomorphic description in Yt. 5 is the most detailed and expressive.[186]

---

[181] Boyce 1985b.

[182] Marshak 1995/1996: 306; Shkoda 2009: 77–78.

[183] Boyce 1975b: 71. Skjærvø translates "the lofty, life-giving, unattached/unblemished (heavenly water)"/unattached. See Skjærvø 2002: 400 and Skjærvø 2013a. Kellens 2002/2003: 321–323 proposes "competent/straight, strong, unattached". See also a recent article by William Malandra who suggests that "originally the name meant "Unboundedness," i.e., "Innocence, Guiltlessness," but once it had become hyper-corrected in Old Persian and Avestan to Anāhitā it was understood to mean "Faultless."": Malandra 2013: 108.

[184] Boyce 1975b: 73.

[185] Yt. 5.15.1; Kellens 2002/2003: 319.

[186] See p. 15.

Before discussing the iconography of Anāhitā, it is important to address the widespread trend in scholarly literature to identify (often without any discussion) every divine feminine image coming from the Iranian world with Anāhitā. Needless to say, in most cases such identifications are unsubstantiated and there is no corroboration for this in the available sources.[187] Another tendency, also frequently encountered, is the automatic identification of Anāhitā with another great goddess of the Iranian world, Nana.[188] This issue is far more complex than it is usually acknowledged. In fact, no compelling material (iconographic or epigraphic) evidence exists for the identification of Anāhitā with Nana.[189] It is widely known that in ancient polytheistic religions, deities sharing similar natures, functions and attributes were not always assimilated or merged, but often coexisted side by side without absorbing one another.

1. *Western Iran*

Before making her first appearance in the inscriptions of Artaxerxes II,[190] the early history of Anāhitā is shrouded in the mists of time. Since she is the only female deity invoked in Achaemenian royal inscriptions, it is plausible to assume that she was also the most important goddess in the Achaemenian royal pantheon at least from the time of Artaxerxes II onwards. After the fall of the Achaemenians and until the rise of the Sasanians, we have no archaeological or epigraphic evidence for her worship in Iran, although there is no reason to suspect that it ever ceased.

Female images are never found in Achaemenian monumental art, but are occasionally depicted on gems and finger rings.[191] The most remarkable examples, which are sometimes considered to represent goddesses, originate from the famous "Oxus treasure" and depict female figures wearing crenellated crowns.[192] In addition, one golden plaque dated to the Achaemenian period from the Mir Zakah hoard found in Eastern Afghanistan in 1992 shows a regal female figure holding a bowl and wearing a crenellated crown.[193] Three further examples of high-ranking women, seated or standing and wearing a spiked crown are carved on three Graeco-Persian seals kept in the Peshawar Museum.[194] Although the divine nature of these regal women cannot decisively be ruled out, the iconography of these seals does not exhibit any specific divine attributes and could in fact portray Achaemenian queens or noble women.

It is possible that in the Achaemenian period, crenellated crowns were reserved not only for royalty, but were also extended to the nobility.[195] Moreover, on the Pazyryk carpet, not only noblewomen, but also the smaller-sized, and definitely subordinate figures of maidservants standing behind them carrying a towel, are depicted wearing crenellated crowns.[196] However, one enthroned lady on the large felt carpet from Pazyryk holding a branch and facing a rider who seems to pay her homage, might indeed be a goddess based on the Scythian parallels from southern Ukraine.[197]

Two well-known Achaemenian seals are usually chosen to illustrate visual images of the goddess Anāhitā.[198] The first is the seal originally from the De Clercq collection, which shows an enthroned

---

187 This is rightly criticized, for instance, by Shahbazi 1983: 261; Frye 1984: 231, n. 101; Pugachenkova 1987: 86; Kellens 2002/2003: 318.

188 For instance, Tanabe 1993: 84–85, along with many others.

189 See p. 116–117.

190 A^2Ha, A^2Sa, A^2Sd.: Lecoq 1997: 269–275.

191 See Lerner 2010: 153 who lists the available examples and also Brosius 2010a: 141, n. 3.

192 Dalton 1964: nos. 38, 104, 103. For instance, Kuz'mina 2002: 220–235, identifies them as the images of Anāhitā.

193 Grenet 2010: Pl. 8.

194 Callieri 1997: nos. 4.1–3.

195 Goldman 1991/1992: 100, n. 32.

196 Rudenko 1970: Fig. 139; Barkova 2009: Figs. 3–7. Although it is also probable that this nuance reflects a misunderstanding of Achaemenian iconographic principles by provincial artisans, see Lerner 2010: 160.

197 See p. 86 ff.

198 For instance, Briant 2002: 253–254, Fig. 37.

woman receiving an offering of a dove. The woman is shown in a royal dress, holding a flower in her hand and wearing an unusually complex headdress, which consists of a "ribbed", perhaps feathered, tiara and a long veil drawn over it which falls down her back (fig. 17).[199] Facing her, there is a smaller figure of an attendant offering a dove. Behind him or her, a typical Achaemenian incense burner is placed, and further to the right a standing female figure in a crenellated crown is depicted. She is also veiled and shown holding an unidentified object in her hand. Two important features single this seal out among other representations of high-ranking Achaemenian women: the dove and her unusual "ribbed" tiara covered with a veil. The dove is traditionally connected with various Near Eastern goddesses[200] and this unique headdress is sometimes also understood as an indication of her divine nature.[201] If we accept the interpretation of the scene on this seal as a presentation of an offering to a goddess, which is by no means certain,[202] Anāhitā would naturally be the leading candidate for the identification of the enthroned goddess given the apparent Iranian context of this seal.[203] However, other goddesses coming from Iranian and even non-Iranian backgrounds cannot be ruled out *a priori*.

The second cylinder seal was found in 1882 at the site of ancient Gorgippia (modern Anapa) on the Northern shore of the Black Sea (fig. 18). The often reproduced seal, attributed to the group of "Graeco-Persian" gems produced in Anatolia in the fourth century BCE, depicts two individuals.[204] On the left side, a man wearing a Persian robe and a crenellated crown raises his hands in adoration towards a divine female figure before him. The goddess is standing on a lion—an attribute that makes her divine identity unquestionable. She is fully draped and surrounded by rays projecting out of her body as spikes. Like the male character, she also wears a crenellated crown. In her left hand the goddess holds a scepter while her right hand is raised in a gesture of blessing. The divine character of the female figure is beyond doubt. Her portrayal is remarkably close to the distinctive iconography of the Mesopotamian Ištar, as she is known from ninth-eighth centuries BCE Urartan and Assyrian art.[205] However, the goddess on the Gorgippia seal differs from the Urartan and Assyrian examples in one aspect—the Achaemenian crenellated crown she wears. The crown and the worshipper standing before her in Persian royal insignia, tempt one to find an *interpretatio iranica* for the goddess. Indeed, she is most often cited as the Achaemenian image of Anāhitā.[206]

It is an oft-repeated convention that Achaemenian Anāhitā was influenced by the cult and the visual representation of the great Mesopotamian goddess Ištar.[207] However, the evidence for such influence is not compelling and for the most part, late and indirect.[208] While the existence of such influence cannot be ruled out—and is moreover even probable given the enormous popularity of Ištar in the ancient

---

199 Lerner 2010: 159, calls it a "fluted tiara" and emphasizes that this headdress is "unique among female depictions of the period".

200 Moorey 1979: 224. A women engraved on one ring from the Oxus Treasure has a dove perched on her hand, see Dalton 1964: Pl. XVI 104.

201 Lerner 2010: 159.

202 See Brosius 2010a: 143–148, who interprets the iconography of this seal as an audience of the high-ranking woman.

203 Lerner 2010: 159. Curiously, Judith Lerner did not rule out the possibility that the goddess on the Gorgippia seal also represents Anāhitā, although she has a "regular" crenellated crown and not the unique headdress of the woman from De Clercq seal, see Lerner 2010: n. 18.

204 Boardman 1970: no. 878; Boardman 2000: 165, Fig. 5.19.

205 The closest parallels are the depictions of Ištar on a silver medallion from Zinjirli, see Möbius 1967: Fig. 1; Ornan 2001: Fig. 9.14; and on Neo-Assyrian seal of Nabu-uṣalla, see Ornan 2001: Fig. 9.16. On the iconography of Ištar, see Seidl 1976/1980; Cornelius 1989: 59–61. For a general discussion of goddesses standing on lions in ancient Near Eastern art, see also Strawn 2005: 194–199 with references.

206 Most recently Compareti 2007: 209–210; Grenet 2006/2010: 87, Fig. 1.

207 For instance, see Panaino 2000: 37–38.

208 It is interesting to note that the seal from Gorgippia is always invoked in these discussions to illustrate the evident impact of the iconography of Ištar on the Iranian goddess, as if the identity of the female deity depicted on this seal as Anāhitā is firmly established.

Near East—we do not possess any firm confirmation that Anāhitā was assimilated with Ištar already in the Achaemenian period, and furthermore it is unlikely that she would acquire her iconography in its entirety. It is interesting to note that in Roman Anatolia (the region from which this seal originates) the goddess Anaitis was identified with Artemis and her visual representations were based on portrayals of Anatolian Artemis.

The goddess on the Gorgippia seal also has little in common with the Avestan description of Anāhitā,[209] who was never specifically associated with a lion (a standard mount and attribute of the goddess Nana).[210] Therefore, in the Iranian milieu, Nana would be the most plausible and natural candidate for a goddess standing on a lion. Although it must be noted that in all known images of Nana with a lion (which are late and originate from Eastern Iran), the goddess is always depicted seated on the beast, never standing on it. Nonetheless, we must not exclude the possibility that this is Ištar herself, shown venerated by the figure in Persian royal dress on this seal. Moreover, this interpretation seems preferable. There is nothing unusual or surprising in Iranians worshipping foreign deities and we should not presuppose that every such case necessarily requires an *interpretatio iranica*.

No images of Anāhitā are known from the Iranian world in the Hellenistic and Parthian periods. This is in sharp contrast with the abundant evidence from Asia Minor where the worship of Anaitis existed in a form of a "quasi-independent cult".[211] In Asia Minor, Anaitis commonly assumes the iconography of Artemis of Ephesus, and there were cultic statues of her installed in temples and depicted on coins.[212] However, it is not clear what Anaitis shared with the cult of the Persian Anāhitā besides her name. The name of Anāhitā is attested on two tesserae from Palmyra[213] where she is also invoked in the dedicatory inscription on a column drum dated to the 18 CE.[214] In Armenia, Anāhitā was also identified with Artemis and we have many allusions to her statues made of precious metals that stood in Armenian temples.[215] Unfortunately, no description of these statues has survived, but Movsēs Xorenac'i writes that they were brought to Armenia from Asia Minor.[216] Therefore, we can assume that these statues resembled the iconography of Anaitis from Asia Minor. Her worship in the Caucasus probably extended further north to the realm of K'art'li.

The earliest representation of Anāhitā in Western Iran dates only from the Sasanian era. One of the two reverse types on the coins issued under the Sasanian king Ōhrmazd I[217] depicts two figures turned toward the fire-altar placed between them (fig. 19).[218] The left character wears royal regalia and a crown similar to that of the king. On the right side of the altar, there is a female figure in a long folding dress wearing an uncovered mural crown. Both characters hold a long rod in their hands, which could be either a sword, or more probably, a *barsom*. In a recent article, Rika Gyselen has suggested that the appearance of Anāhitā is linked to the images of Tyche on contemporary Roman coins.[219] The connection with Tyche strengthens the impression that the female on the coins of Ōhrmazd I is likely to be a goddess, and not a queen. This conjecture is also supported by the fact that on other types of coins of Ōhrmazd

---

209 See p. 15. The only element indicating the possible influence of Mesopotamian iconography is her crown, incorporating "seven towers/palaces" (*ašta.kaošda*) in Yt. 5.128: Panaino 2000: 38, n. 16. Turreted crowns were generally worn by queens in first millennium BCE Assyrian and Elamite art, see Álvarez-Mon 2010: 58–61, Pl. 23, 24b.

210 Ael. *NA*. 12.23 mentions tame lions that were kept in a "shrine of Anaïtis" in Elymais. However, it seems that in fact he refers to the goddess Nana, rather than Anāhitā, see Boyce and Grenet 1991: 47–48; De Jong 1997: 274, n. 94.

211 Boyce and Grenet 1991: 66.

212 On the cult and imagery of Anāhitā in Asia Minor, see Reding-Hourcade 1983; Boyce and Grenet 1991: 211–235.

213 Ingholt, Seyrig and Caquot 1955: nos. 166, 167. On n. 166, the bust of the goddess is also depicted.

214 Kaizer 2002: 159.

215 See p. 19.

216 See p. 20.

217 On Ōhrmazd I and his reign, see Weber 2007.

218 Lukonin 1969: 170; Göbl 1971: II, 2; Gyselen 2010a: 78, Fig. 17.

219 Gyselen 2010a: 78.

I, Mithra in his distinctive radiate crown offers a diadem to the king.[220] Contrary to Mithra, the goddess is shown here not with a diadem of investiture, but holding a rod, which is probably a *barsom*. This object is an attribute of Ahura Mazdā and Mithra on Sasanian rock-reliefs, and therefore it is not wholly surprising to also find it in the possession of Anāhitā. Moreover, in the *Ābān Yasht*, Anāhitā is described as holding a *barsom*.[221] This could be one of the rare cases in Sasanian art where the image of the divinity appears to have something in common with his/her Avestan description.

Another female figure often understood as Anāhitā is found on the coins of Wahrām II.[222] The design of this type of reverse of Wahrām's II coins is copied from that of Ōhrmazd's I, with one main modification—the replacement of the male figure in radiant crown with a female figure (fig. 20). She wears a long dress, and a bonnet ending with the head of an animal or bird (eagle and beaver according to Choksy;[223] eagle or falcon according to Gyselen).[224] Following the model set by Ōhrmazd I, the female extends a diadem to the king who is separated from her by a fire-altar and receives the diadem with a hand raised in adoration. The full analogy with Mithra on the coins of Ōhrmazd I confirms the divine nature of the woman. Although she is not wearing a crenellated crown, the female on Wahrām's II coins should most probably also be identified as Anāhitā, the only goddess from the rich Zoroastrian pantheon involved in the other investiture scenes in Sasanian art and mentioned in Sasanian royal inscriptions.

Anāhitā also features in Sasanian monumental art, where two or possibly three examples of her sculptured representation were identified.[225] She is shown offering a diadem of investiture to a king on two Sasanian reliefs, Narseh's at Naqš-e Rostam and that of Xusrō II at Ṭāq-i Bustān. The relief of the Sasanian king Narseh carved at Naqš-e Rostam is the only relief of this king and it also marks a return to the investiture on foot (fig. 21), which had not appeared on Sasanian rock reliefs since Ardašīr I.[226] The composition is asymmetrical and consists of five figures. In the right part of the relief, the king receives a diadem from a female figure wearing an uncovered mural crown. With his left hand, Narseh grasps the hilt of a sword and the left hand of a woman is concealed in a long sleeve of her dress. Between them stands a small figure, similar to those portrayed on the relief of Ardašīr I at Naqš-e Rağab. His head is highly abraded, but the flying ribbons of the diadem indicate that he is probably a member of the royal family.[227] Two courtiers raising their right hands in gestures of adoration are carved behind the king (the figure of one of them was left unfinished).

The investiture relief in the upper panel of the large grotto at Ṭāq-i Bustān exhibits the last investiture scene found in Sasanian monumental art (fig. 22).[228] It follows a similar composition scheme to that first encountered on the relief of Šāpūr II/Ardašīr II located at the same site. The king in full royal insignia is portrayed in the center, flanked by two figures usually identified as Ahura Mazdā and Anāhitā. The king is generally thought to be Xusrō II, the last great Sasanian ruler. Theoretically, he could be anyone from Pērōz (under whom this type of elaborate winged crown first appears), until the last Sasanian king.[229]

220 See p. 102–103.
221 See p. 15.
222 For the most recent and detailed discussion with references, see Gyselen 2010b: 207–209.
223 Choksy 1989: Pl. 10.1,5,7 and Pl. 10.6.
224 Gyselen 2010b: 207.
225 Bier 1983, argued that the sculptured building block found at the site of Eṣṭaḵr could also represent Anāhitā, but from the preserved fragments depicting left buttocks, a hand and a thigh, it is impossible to say anything more definite other than that it belonged to a female figure.
226 Herrmann 1977: 9–11, Fig. 2, Pl. 8–14a; Vanden Berghe 1984: no. 75. According to the suggestion by Weber, the relief was probably carved after 298 CE. See Weber 2010.
227 He is identified as a "prince" by Herrmann 1977: 11.
228 Schmidt 1970: 138–139; Fukai and Horiuchi 1972: III–XXXIII; Vanden Berghe 1984: no. 81. The most detailed description of this monument is found in Movassat 2005.
229 For instance, see von Gall 1990: 100, who favors Pērōz, and Tanabe 1984: 40; Tanabe 2003, who prefers Ardaxšīr III. For an additional survey of the various opinions, see Movassat 2005: 9–19.

Nevertheless, the candidature of Xusrō II seems most appropriate, taking into account his military achievements and the fact that the hairstyle of the king resembles that on the coins of Xusrō II.[230] All the figures are shown *en face* and placed on bases resembling the pedestals of statues. The figure of the king visibly towers above the smaller figures of the deities, and the sophisticated crown of the *šāhān šāh* overshadows the uncovered mural crown of Ahura Mazdā, although they both wear similar garments.[231] The god, depicted to the right, holds a diadem outstretched toward the king in his right hand. In his other hand there is a perforation probably intended for an object which is now missing—perhaps a *barsom* made of metal.[232] An unusual feature of his visual appearance is his pointed beard, more reminiscent of portraits of Syrian Christian saints than of images of Ahura Mazdā on earlier Sasanian reliefs.[233]

A female figure to the left of the king wears an uncovered crown consisting of a wide hoop decorated with a stylized tree motif.[234] Beneath the crown she has a royal diadem with a double row of pearls. With her right hand she extends a diadem toward the king and in her left hand she holds an ewer from which she pours a stream of water. Just below the investiture scene, a large figure of an equestrian warrior turned to the right, whose entire body is covered by armor, is carved in high relief.[235] The rider is nimbate and in addition to the helmet, he wears a badly damaged headdress that was probably originally a crenellated crown. He carries a long lance and a small round shield.

Although the female figure is identified by an inscription in neither of the two reliefs, her appearance in royal attire with an uncovered crown and the obvious parallels with other reliefs of Sasanian investiture performed by Ahura Mazdā leave no reasonable doubt that this is the depiction of Anāhitā, the favorite patron-goddess of the Sasanian dynasty.

An additional portrayal of Anāhitā in Sasanian monumental art could be a separate panel with a female bust wearing an uncovered crenellated crown carved at Dārābgird in Pars. A small panel (0.5 m.) depicting a female bust was discovered at this site in 1975 by Vanden Berghe.[236] It was carved 1.03 m. below the left corner of the well-known Sasanian relief from the same site, which illustrates the triumph of a Sasanian king over Roman emperors (fig. 23).[237] This small panel is obviously unrelated to the main triumphal relief[238] and its precise dating and purpose is therefore unclear.[239] Stylistically, it could be said to belong to early Sasanian art and was probably carved as a part of an uncompleted relief in the late third century CE. The bust is shown in frontal view, but the head is turned to the left in full profile (fig. 24). The woman wears a large crown composed of three crenellations and her hair is divided into three parts. Her crenellated crown is plain, not topped by a globe of hair, or covered by fabric. Such unusual crowns are never encountered on Sasanian reliefs in particular and in monumental art in general and are found only on coins. Therefore, it is possible that the carving of the crown was not completed.

The traditional interpretation of these Sasanian female images as Anāhitā was contested by Alireza Shapour Shahbazi, who argued that the woman on Narseh's relief at Naqš-e Rostam was not a goddess,

---

230 Herrmann and Curtis 2002.

231 See the detailed descriptions of the figures of the king and Ahura Mazdā in Movassat 2005: 21–24, 43–44.

232 Overlaet 2013: 317, Pl. 14.

233 Harper 1999: 317.

234 Movassat 2005: 46–48.

235 Movassat 2005: 62–64.

236 Vanden Berghe 1978.

237 Vanden Berghe 1984: n. 58. There is no consensus over the identity of the Sasanian king, who is identified either as Ardašīr I or Šāpūr I. See Levit-Tawil 1992 and Herrmann 1996, with references to scholars arguing for both possibilities.

238 There are no parallels for such isolated small reliefs outside the larger ones among Sasanian rock-reliefs, therefore the speculations by Levit-Tawil 1992: 197–199, are hardly convincing.

239 Vanden Berghe 1978: 146, suggests that it could have been executed under Ardašīr I, Narseh, Ōhrmazd II or Šāpūr II. Levit-Tawil 1992: 201–202 concludes that it is contemporary with the main relief.

but his wife, Šāpūrduxtak.[240] To support his proposal he put forward three arguments: 1) since the woman on Narseh's relief conceals her hand in the sleeve of her dress, which Shahbazi interprets as a gesture of subordination, she could not be a goddess, but only a mortal woman; 2) she wears the same mural crown with three crenellations as the woman on the Dārābgird relief, which Shahbazi also identifies as Šāpūrduxtak; 3) a female figure depicted on the reverse of the coins of Wahrām II offering a diadem to the king is also a queen (another Šāpūrduxtak, spouse of Wahrām II) since she has a sleeve covering her hand and is specifically named in a legend on one coin type.

It should be noted immediately that on some issues of Wahrām II belonging to this type it can be clearly seen that the hand of the female figure offering a diadem to the king is not hidden in a sleeve, and even her fingers are clearly visible.[241] Doubts as to whether the act of covering one's hand with a sleeve necessarily represents humility have been raised by Arcangela Santoro. She considers the fragments from Xenophon describing this custom at the Achaemenian court (on which much of Shahbazi's argument is based) to be a late interpolation and also shows that there is no reliable iconographic data to support the idea that Achaemenian ceremonial required one to hide one's hands in sleeves in the presence of the king.[242] In sources from the Sasanian period, and in the Middle Persian literature, this pose is not mentioned. The only Sasanian pose of subordination documented both in texts[243] and in art[244] is crossed arms clasped to one's chest. Moreover, on the reliquary of Kanishka, the Kushan king is shown wearing a long *kaftan* with a long sleeve covering his left hand.[245] Abolala Soudavar also noted that a Kushan king, Vima Kadphises, hides his left hand in a sleeve on his coins.[246] At least in the Kushan mileau, any notions that this pose might have portrayed humility and subordination are quite clearly refuted. Furthermore, the longsleeved *kaftans* worn by Central Asian people until the modern period indicate that hiding one's hand in a sleeve is not a sign of subordination, but rather an element of dress originating in Central Asia as a means of protection in the cold climate and presumably no special meaning was assigned to it.

A female figure on the coins of Wahrām II is in all probability Anāhitā, and not his queen, since she is clearly shown bestowing sovereignty upon the king by offering him a diadem. A depiction of radiant Mithra performing exactly the same act of investiture on the other type of Wahrām's II reverse, puts her divine nature beyond reasonable doubt. Moreover, it has now been demonstrated, contrary to what Shahbazi maintained after being misled by Vladimir Lukonin,[247] that the name of Šāpūrduxtak does not appear on any of Wahrām's II coins.[248]

Shahbazi's interpretation has gained support among some scholars,[249] and was recently embraced by Weber, who further argued that the relief represents not the investiture of Narseh, but the symbolic ceremony of return of his *x^{v}arənah* celebrated within his family circle.[250] Her additional iconographic arguments against identification of the female figure with Anāhitā also deserve to be addressed and can be summarized as follows: 1) the passing of the ring of investiture is not in the center of the composition; 2) the figure of the king is the largest and dominates the scene; 3) Narseh hands over the ring to her and not the reverse.

240 Shahbazi 1983.
241 Curtis 2008: 140–141, Fig. 6; Gyselen 2010b: 208.
242 Santoro 2005: 290–291.
243 Literally "hands in armpits" (*dast ēr-kaš*). *Xusraw ī Kawādān ud rēdag-ē* 1, ed. and tr. by Azarnouche 2013. See also Herman forthcoming who cites Talmudic and Syriac evidence for this gesture.
244 Trever and Lukonin 1987: no. 9.
245 See p. 99.
246 Soudavar 2012: 8–9.
247 Lukonin 1969: 107, 177.
248 Weber 2009: 583–584, with references.
249 For instance, see Brosius 2010b.
250 Weber 2010.

The investiture scenes on the Sasanian reliefs are not necessarily situated in the center of the composition. Thus, the relief of Ardašīr I at Fīrūzābād is asymmetric and is shifted even more to the margin than Narseh's. The figure of Narseh appears larger only because of the high *korymbos* and we can see here the beginning of the tendency in Sasanian rock reliefs to augment the figure of the king, making him larger than even the gods. This trend culminates in the relief of Xusrō II at Ṭāq-i Bustān, where the king clearly overrides Ahura Mazdā and Anāhitā. I also fail to see that the female figure is holding the ring in any special manner. It seems that the grasp of her hand corresponds exactly to the manner in which Ahura Mazdā holds the ring on other Sasanian reliefs. It is also significant and certainly not accidental that the small figure placed between the king and the female figure, making a gesture of adoration towards the latter, unequivocally identifies her as the most elevated and high-ranking character in the composition.

Weber goes on to produce a rather odd argument that since Narseh laid claim to the investiture relief of his brother Wahrām I he already possessed one investiture relief and did not need another. In answer, one should only recall that Šāpūr I left two investiture reliefs and Ardašīr I, three.

The attribution of this relief to the second phase of the reign of Narseh also does not necessiatate a new interpretation, as Weber insists, since investiture reliefs were carved at various stages of a king's rule and not only on his enthronment, e.g. the reliefs of Ardašīr I. It is hardly a coincidence that the only king to mention Anāhitā in his inscription is Narseh in Paikuli.[251] He is also the only Sasanian king depicted receiving the diadem of divine kingship not from Ahura Mazdā, but from the queenly woman. Before seizing the Sasanian throne in a successful *coup d'état*, Narseh was the King of Armenia. It is tempting to suggest that during his stay in Armenia, where Anāhitā probably enjoyed extraordinary popularity,[252] Narseh became personally devoted to the cult of the goddess, which is reflected both in his relief and in the Paikuli inscription.

Unfortunately, unlike Ahura Mazdā, Anāhitā is never labeled in Sasanian art and does not have any distinctive attribute exclusive to her, such as the radiate crown of Mithra. It appears that the principal obstacle lying behind this debate is the claim that in the absence of an inscription, it is impossible to distinguish between Anāhitā and a Sasanian queen, one possible reason being that the representation of Anāhitā was presumably based on that of a queen, in the same manner as the visual image of Ahura Mazdā reproduced the image of a king. However, Ahura Mazdā by no means mirrors the king; the most significant iconographic distinction is his uncovered crenellated crown, as distinct from the royal crown covered by a *korymbos*. It is instructive that the female personage on the reliefs of Narseh, Dārābgird and on the coins of Ōhrmazd I is wearing an uncovered crown and therefore should be most probably identified as a divinity. Moreover, there is no certainty that Sasanian queens ever wore a crenellated crown, uncovered or topped by a *korymbos*. On two seals, which constitute the only cases where the queenly identity of the depicted women is verified by inscription, the queens have other types of headdresses.[253]

One possible example of a Sasanian queen wearing a crenellated crown is found on a seal formerly in the M. Foroughi collection.[254] The seal depicts a female bust facing to the right. Her torso is turned in a three-quarter view and the head is shown in full profile. She wears an unusual combination of a *kulāf* with earflaps and a crown with three large crenellations.[255] Aside the fact that such busts in

---

251 See p. 11.
252 See p. 19–20.
253 On the headdresses of Sasanian royal women, see Peck 1993.
254 Ghirshman 1962: Fig. 294b.
255 A similar headdress is also found on another seal (Gignoux and Gyselen 1982: 20.55, and with the queen on the coin of Wahram II (without crenellation)). See Gyselen 2004: no. 158. Ardašīr I wears a lavishly decorated *kulāf* of the same type on some of his early issues: see Alram and Gyselen 2003: Type II.

the Sasanian sigillography always portray individuals, this seal probably depicts a Sasanian queen. It should be emphasised that the woman on this seal wears a covered crenellated crown, unlike the female personages on the Sasanian reliefs and on a coin of Ōhrmazd I who has an uncovered mural crown, which was perhaps reserved for Anāhitā. Whether or not the crenellated crown was indeed exclusive to Anāhitā, it seems that the goddess had other types of crowns as well. At Ṭāq-i Bustān she wears a crown without crenellations, but decorated with floral motifs. On the coins of Wahrām II she has a bonnet ending with an animal head. Of course, since these goddesses are not labeled, their identification as Anāhitā is not indisputable—they could also represent other female divinities from the rich Zoroastrian Sasanian pantheon. However, given the prominent place occupied by Anāhitā in the Zoroastrian pantheon, her role as a patron of the Sasanian dynasty and the fact that she is the only goddess mentioned in Sasanian royal inscriptions, it is reasonable to assume that it was she who was chosen to be depicted in the most representative media of royal Sasanian propaganda: monumental rock-reliefs and coins.

These representations are not only found on coins and monumental reliefs; almost all media of Sasanian art are abundant with depictions of female figures. The tendency to relate them automatically to Anāhitā has attracted much criticism in the past, and is now largely abandoned by the specialists. Such feminine personages can be divided into three categories:

(1) Young women holding a flower are a popular iconographic theme on Sasanian seals.[256] It has been suggested that they depict Daēnā,[257] or are related to marriage.[258]
(2) Female figures that frequently appear on Sasanian silverware, especially on vases and ewers, are also often associated with the goddess Anāhitā.[259] These women are depicted in free postures, moving, or perhaps even dancing. As a rule, they are nude or draped in transparent dress and given various attributes; fruits, beribboned rings, musical instruments, animals, children, caskets, scarves, flowers, and birds being the most frequent.[260] They are never crowned, but some have a nimbus surrounding their heads.[261] The absence of crowns and royal garments renders their interpretation as Anāhitā improbable[262] and their interpretation as "priestesses"[263] can also be confidently rejected, as in the Iranian world, priesthood was generally reserved for men.[264] However, their adornment with a nimbus evidently indicates that they depict not merely "dancers" or "musicians",[265] but probably individuals of some cultic significance.[266] The most cogent interpretation (although by no means conclusive) is that they derive from Graeco-Roman Dionysiac maenad-like figures[267] that

---

256 For instance, see Gignoux and Gyselen 1987: AMO 10.1–10.6; IBT 10.1, 10.2; MCB 10.2.

257 Azarpay 1976a; Tanabe 1984: 45; Gnoli 1993/1994. This interpretation is considered possible by Gyselen who likewise rejects the idea that these female figures are related to Anāhitā or her cult, see Gyselen 1995a: 140, n. 141.

258 Brunner 1979: 49.

259 Shepherd 1980; Chaumont 1985.

260 See the catalogue of these figures and their attributes compiled by Shepherd 1980: 63.

261 For instance, Trever and Lukonin 1987: no. 18–20.

262 Even the female figure on the so-called "Stroganoff ewer" (Smirnov 1909: no. 79) despite being fully draped could not represent Anāhitā, as postulated by Ringbom 1957: 15; Trever and Lukonin 1987: 99–100; Marshak 1998: 86; Marshak 2002a: 142; Malek 2002: 30, n. 19, since she has no crown.

263 Orbeli and Trever 1935: xx; Pugachenkova 1952: 56; Ettinghausen 1972: 6.

264 Although the Avesta and Middle Persian Zoroastrian texts hint that women could participate and perform certain rituals. See De Jong 2003b; Hintze 2012: 53–54.

265 As interpreted, for instance, by Pugachenkova 1987: 86–87, who nevertheless does not deny the possibility of their association with some ritual activity connected with the feast.

266 Marshak 2002a: 142.

267 Although Duchesne-Guillemin 1974: 151–153, probably goes too far with the suggestion that they are nymphs, part of the escort of Artemis who was, in his opinion, subject to syncretism with Anāhitā. See also Abdullaev 2005: 237–238, Figs. 29–33, who interprets them as maenads and female figures symbolizing fertility.

were probably connected to festivals and personifications of months and seasons.[268] It is possible, however, that no special "Iranian" meanings were assigned to these female "dancers" who visually conveyed the concepts of feasting, fertility and wealth; and that their representation on prestigious silver vessels was mostly decorative.

(3) A scene with a naked woman carried by a giant bird and feeding it with a bunch of grapes is depicted on a silver plate from the Hermitage Museum[269] and is also found on the Sasanian seals.[270] Despite being interpreted by Lukonin as an illustration of the Avestan myth of Anāhitā coming to rescue the boatman Pāurva,[271] it has been convincingly shown to originate from a Buddhist story of the abduction of a married woman by a Bodhisattva in the form of a Garuda bird.[272] The Sasanian version of this myth was probably different since in the Buddhist version the woman resists her abduction, but in Sasanian iconography she is shown feeding the bird. Be that as it may, the woman in this scene does not portray Anāhitā.

Outside the official, royal art, a unique rendering of Anāhitā may be found in a female figure flanked by fishes on a stone receptacle uncovered in 1941 in the environs of Bīšāpūr (fig. 25).[273] The excavator, Roman Ghirshman, who dated it to the end of the fourth or beginning of the fifth century CE, interpreted the receptacle as an ossuary, but this seems unlikely. All sides of the receptacle are decorated with reliefs, which are unfortunately only partially preserved. They depict: 1) two winged horses facing in opposite directions; 2) a character seated frontally on a broad *takht*, wearing a *kaftan* and a crescent-shaped pendant. His left hand grasps the handle of an object, which is not preserved; 3) the lower part of a standing character wearing a long garment; 4) a woman figure, rendered *en face* and holding a circular object in her right hand.[274] Two fishes are carved to her left and right. Since one side of the receptacle carries the image of the chariot of Mithra, this female is also most likely a divinity. The fishes unequivocally allude to her association with water, and, therefore, Anāhitā appears the most suitable candidate. Unfortunately, it is impossible to identify the two remaining characters on this curious object.

2. *Eastern Iran*

Berossus in a famous passage lists Balkh among the cities where Artaxerxes II installed the statues of goddess Anāhitā.[275] However, the earliest evidence that has survived of her worship in Eastern Iran is found only several centuries later on the coins of Kushano-Sasanian kings Ardašīr I, Ardašīr II(?) and Ōhrmazd II. These coins are of unique importance, since this is the only example, except for the coinage of Asia Minor, where we find the visual representation of Anāhitā labeled by an inscription.

This "Kushano-Sasanian Anāhitā" falls into two completely distinct and unrelated iconographic types. The reverse of a coin of Kushano-Sasanian king Ardašīr I shows a female figure seated frontally under an arch. In her right hand she holds a ring and in her left hand, a spear (fig. 26).[276] The loose ends of her girdle are suspended, terminating with balls. She is nimbate and wears a composite crenellated crown, which seems to consist of three large projections. The legend to the right of the female figure is very fragmentary and difficult to read even on the best-preserved specimens. The tentative reading

268 Harper 1971; Harper 1983: 1120, n. 2; Marshak 1998: 86; Marshak 2002a: 141; Harper 2006: 127.
269 Trever and Lukonin 1987: no. 22.
270 Gignoux and Gyselen 1987: KP 20g.
271 Trever and Lukonin 1987: 89–90; Loukonine and Ivanov 2003: 90.
272 Azarpay 1995.
273 Ghirshman 1948.
274 Ghirshman 1948: 293.
275 See p. 16.
276 Göbl 1984: no. 1028; Cribb 1990: no. 16.

is *a*[*n*](*x*)[*y*]*t ZY* [*M*](*RWTA*) "Anāhitā the Lady". The Bactrian engraver who worked on this coin was probably unfamiliar with the Middle Persian script and/or copied the legend from a very bad prototype.

On the coins of his successor Ardašīr II, the king is shown in a pose of adoration before a figure of a female deity to his right, which perhaps depicts a cultic statue (fig. 27).[277] Her body is shown *en face*, and her head is turned towards the king. She holds a scepter topped by a globe in her left hand and with the other hand she presents the king with a tall crown decorated with ribbons. This crown resembles those of the Kushan kings Kanishka and Huvishka. The headgear of the goddess herself closely matches that of the female figure on the coin of Ardašīr I and although they have different dress and attributes, there can be no doubt that the same divinity is depicted on both coins, reflecting perhaps two different cultic statues which existed in Kushanshahr. Unfortunately, the Middle Persian inscription, which would confirm the identification of the goddess, is illegible. Here the goddess has the same attributes, but instead of the diadem, she offers a tall beribboned crown of the Kushan kings. It is interesting to note that in Sasanian art the deities are never shown presenting the entire crown, but only a diadem. It seems that for the Sasanians the diadem was a sufficient symbol of delegated divine royal power.

The third type of Kushano-Sasanian Anāhitā is found on the scythate gold coin of king Ōhrmazd II minted in Balkh. It portrays a king facing a seated figure of the goddess to the right (pl. 4).[278] The king raises his right hand in a gesture of adoration, holding a spoon in his left hand with which he places an offering on the head of a bird set between the two. The depiction of the bird, which here replaces the fire-altar usually shown on other coins of Ōhrmazd is unique. The smoke rising from the bird's head perhaps indicates that this is a depiction of a real altar worked in the form of a bird. The goddess sits on a stool, and offers the king a diadem with her right hand. In her left hand she holds a bow. She wears an unusual trapezoid headdress, widening at the top (a degenerate *kalathos*?) with a veil or a chin strap attached to it and a diadem whose ribbons are shown flying behind her back. There is a Middle Persian inscription identifying the king as Ōhrmazd and the goddess as *an'xyt ZY MROTA*, "Anāhitā the Lady".

This composition of a king worshipping before a goddess has a possible Kushan prototype. On one rare type of copper coins depicting Nana, there is a figure kneeling before her.[279] The fact that these coins have Middle Persian and not Bactrian inscriptions betrays direct Sasanian influence. Moreover, the same formula "Anāhitā the Lady" is also employed in Narseh's Paikuli inscription. Anāhitā does not feature in the Kushan pantheon and is not attested as a theophoric compound in Bactrian personal names. Therefore, it seems that her worship was imported to Bactria from Sasanian Iran after it came under the domination of the Western Iranian kings.

The coins of Kushanshah Ardašīr I appear to be roughly contemporary with the first probable image of Anāhitā in the West, on the coin of Ōhrmazd I,[280] although they are remarkably distinct and it is unclear whether there is a Sasanian influence/inspiration behind the creation of the Kushano-Sasanian Anāhitā or whether it was a parallel development. Be that as it may, in the subsequent decades of the third century CE, the development of the iconography of Anāhitā diverged in the East and West. In the Sasanian Empire, Anāhitā was always represented investing the king and had three variants of her crown and three attributes: a *barsom*, a diadem, and a ewer. The Kushano-Sasanian Anāhita had two types of crown and a spear, a diadem and a bow as her attributes. If the goddess in the Northern chapel of Temple II at Panjikent also represents Anāhitā, to her attributes in Eastern Iran we may also add a banner and a sistrum.[281]

---

277 Göbl 1984: no. 1029.4; Cribb 1990: no. 17.
278 Cribb 1990: no. 5.
279 Rosenfield 1967: 85; See p. 120.
280 The absolute chronology of the Kushano-Sasanian rulers is debated. See Cribb 1990; Grenet, Lee, Martinez and Ory 2007: n. 17.
281 See below.

The images chosen by the Kushano-Sasanians to depict the great Western Iranian goddess are quite different from her representation on Sasanian reliefs. Only Anāhitā as depicted on the coins of the two Ardašīrs shares features with the Sasanian goddess. The crown and the diadem link her with Anāhitā on the relief of Narseh. However, the spear, a clear warlike attribute, is unknown in Western Iran despite allusions in literary sources to Anāhitā as a warlike goddess. Anāhitā on the coin of Kushano-Sasanian Ōhrmazd II is completely different from the Sasanian imagery. The bow may also indicate her bellicose aspect or may possibly be an allusion to the adoption of some traits from Artemis. It is also possible that the bow is present here as the most important symbol of rulership and power that it was among Iranian nomads. Contrary to Anāhitā's image on the Sasanian reliefs and coins where she is always shown performing the act of symbolic investiture, on the coin of Ōhrmazd II a real cultic scene is probably represented depicting a king performing a sacrifice before the statue goddess. It is conceivable that these Kushano-Sasanian coins were based on depictions of the real cultic statues of Anāhitā, which were erected in her temples, following the Kushan traditions.

A possible explanation for the unusual iconography of Anāhitā on the coin of Kushano-Sasanian Ōhrmazd II was put forward by Grenet and Marshak, who proposed that here she assumed the appearance of one type of Kushan Nana who is depicted holding a bow.[282] However, all other elements in the figure of Anāhitā on the coin of Ōhrmazd II are completely different, especially the headdress, which finds no immediate parallels. Another curious feature of the scene on the coin of Ōhrmazd II is an altar in the form of a bird. It is perhaps noteworthy that on one image of Sogdian Nana from Ustrushana she is depicted holding a staff ending with a golden figure of a bird.[283] This may serve as an additional argument in favor of Grenet's and Marshak's proposal, bringing closer together this image of Anāhitā with Nana. However, this evidence is still not conclusive.

We have already seen that in Roman Asia Minor and in Armenia, Anāhitā was associated with Artemis.[284] This therefore can be taken as an additional indication that this image originates in the West rather than being a Bactrian creation.

Both images of Kushano-Sasanian Anāhitā have little in common with the Avestan description of the goddess,[285] whose very relevance beyond the circle of the Sasanian-Zoroastrian clergy is questionable. Neither spear nor bow—her attributes on these coins—are mentioned in the Avestan hymn dedicated to the goddess. The artisan who created these images and the ruler who ordered and approved it, were certainly relying on other sources and conceptions, perhaps also incorporating different elements from various local goddesses.

It is difficult to explain why there are two images of Anāhitā in the same cultural *mileux* and probably produced within a relatively short period of time of some sixty-one years, that are so distinct from one another. Any proposed explanation would necessarily be speculative, but perhaps some of the reasons could involve the existence of two distinct statues of the goddess and the difference between the types of coinage. While the copper coins of two Ardašīrs were in wide circulation, the gold coin of Ōhrmazd II had rather prestigious significance and their issue was obviously limited.

It is likely that the worship of Anāhitā had already spread from Bactria to Sogdiana in the early Kushano-Sasanian period, since we have an attestation of the personal name Nāhītāk at the Topraq-Qal'a documents in the neighboring Chorasmia dated to the third century CE.[286] However, contrary to the situation in Bactria, among the Sogdians we do find names with the theophoric component

282 Grenet and Marshak 1998: 8.
283 See below.
284 See p. 69 and p. 20.
285 See p. 15.
286 Livshits 2004: 191.

"Anāhitā".[287] Although, as in the case with Ahura Mazdā, there is no definite representation of the goddess in Sogdian art, the best candidate for the Sogdian representation of Anāhitā is the goddess depicted on the wall painting from the northern chapel of the Temple II (I. 5/6) in Panjikent (fig. 28).[288] It portrays an enthroned goddess in three-quarters view to the left. She has a double nimbus and wears an elaborate crown of three projections topped with small spheres. Additional floral and spherical elements are integrated into the crown. The goddess is dressed in splendid garments, adorned with jewelry, and ribbons of the diadem are shown flying behind her back. She is seated on the zoomorphic throne supported by two winged hybrid creatures resembling dogs or dragons. In her raised hands, she holds a sistrum and a banner. A smaller figure of a donor with a portable altar is depicted to her left and a female figure carrying a necklace is painted on the right side of the seated goddess. This painting is characterized by the presence of Hellenistic elements and techniques, which disappear in later Sogdian art as well as some Sasanian influences; for instance, a typical Sasanian pose. This combination of Hellenistic and Sasanian elements probably betrays the influence of the Kushano-Sasanian tradition of Bactria and, according to Marshak, is based on Kushano-Sasanian prototypes of the fourth century CE.[289]

A careful study of the mural has revealed that the original intention of the artisan was to depict the goddess holding a sword, which was later replaced with other attributes. Another possibility is that this painting was originally intended to depict a different goddess with different attributes.[290] The figure of the goddess under the arch, her pose, garments, and crown are remarkably similar to those of Anāhitā on the coin of the Kushano-Sasnaian king Ardašīr I. Her attributes, however, are different. Instead of a diadem and a spear, the Panjikent goddess holds a banner and a sistrum. Another significant detail of her image is the zoomorphic throne. It is noteworthy that in the Avesta Anāhitā's mantle is made of beaver's (Av. *baβra*) fur. In the Middle Persian texts this animal is called a "water dog" (MP. *sag ī ābīg*). Therefore, Grenet has proposed that these winged dogs represent the notion of the "water dog".[291] It is, however, more probable that this composite creature depicts one of the flying fantastic monsters that in Sogdian art conveyed a notion of *farn*.[292] It is curious that the painter originally intended to depict the goddess holding a sword. Could this be an echo of the spear held by Anāhitā on the coin of Ardašīr I?

Based on the striking similarity between the goddess from Temple II in Panjikent and Anāhitā on the coin of Ardašīr I, Grenet suggested that this wall painting from Panjikent portrayed the Iranian goddess.[293] Marshak, who was the first to draw attention to the resemblance between the two goddesses, subsequently also cautiously raised the possibility of this being an image of Anāhitā.[294]

As far as the artistic and the epigraphic material is concerned, there is no evidence for the worship of Anāhitā in Eastern Iran before the Sasanian conquest of the Kushanshahr. Even in the later epoch, when the worship of Anāhitā was brought to Bactria by the Sasanians and subsequently adopted by the Sogdians, she was unable to rise above the status of secondary female divinity whose functions are completely unknown to us and was certainly in the shadow of the great goddess of Eastern Iran—Nana. It appears that the inability of Anāhitā to hold ground in Central Asia can be explained by her failure to compete with the extremely dominant cult of the local water divinity, Oxus, whose veneration is attested

---

287 Lurje 2010: nos. 94, 95. It is noteworthy that these inscriptions date from the fourth-sixth century CE and in the later period Anāhitā is not attested in Sogdian texts or personal names.

288 Belenitskii and Marshak 1981: Fig. 34; Shkoda 2009: 72, Fig. 112.

289 Marshak 2009: 13.

290 Marshak 1999: 177.

291 Grenet 2002a: 208.

292 See p. 139.

293 Grenet 1996: 388; Grenet 2001/2002: 210; Grenet 2002a: 208.

294 Marshak 1999: 183. But see the recent article by Azarpay who suggests that this is the earliest image of the Sogdian *daēnā* in Azarpay 2011: 58, 75.

almost uninterruptedly from the Achaemenian period until the Muslim conquest. There was probably no room and no need for another, foreign divinity, patron of waters.

3. *Conclusions*

Three distinct iconographic types of pictorial anthropomorphic representation of Anāhitā have been identified in the Iranian world: two Kushano-Sasanian types, one of which possibly had continuation in the Sogdian art, and Sasanian queenly Anāhitā depicted as the goddess on investiture in rock-relief and on coins.

No image of Anāhitā seems to exist in Achaemenian, Hellenistic or Parthian art in Iran. All candidates for the representation of a goddess, such as the queenly woman figure from the De Clercq seal, are speculative and should be regarded as such. Despite her huge popularity in Western Iran and on the western periphery of the Iranian world (Asia Minor and Caucasus), very few images of Anāhitā are known from Western Iran and all of them date from the Sasanian era. It is reasonable to assume that her representations would have existed in the Parthian, and perhaps also in the early Sasanian period, but we do not possess any examples. Only after the worship of Anāhitā was introduced by the Sasanians to Bactria, do we find the first certain images of the goddess depicted on Kushano-Sasanian coins. If the reading of the inscription is correct, the earliest representation of Anāhitā appears already under the kings Ardašīr I and Ardašīr II.

Kushano-Sasanian Anāhitā seemingly possesses a warlike aspect not found in Sasanian iconography. The Sasanian governors of Kushanshahr created two types of anthropomorphic images of the great Western Iranian goddess and it is likely that these images reproduce cultic statues, which were placed in Bactrian temples according to the tradition inherited from the Kushans. It is plausible that they were partly inspired by western conceptions in which Anāhitā was equated with Artemis and by the statues of local, Bactrian divinities. It remains enigmatic why these conceptions did not influence the iconography of Anāhitā in Western Iran itself.

The first Sasanian image of Anāhitā appears on a coin of Ōhrmazd I where the goddess is depicted wearing a crenellated crown and holding a *barsom*. Wahrām II placed the image of the goddess on the reverse of his coins, depicting her holding a diadem, like on the coin of Kushanshah Ōhrmazd II, but wearing a different type of headdress—a bonnet. Narseh introduced the image of Anāhitā to the monumental rock-reliefs, replacing Ahura Mazdā as the bestower of kingship, which probably reflects his personal devotion to the goddess. Another image of Anāhitā in the Sasanian rock-reliefs, which was unfortunately left unfinished, could be a female bust wearing an uncovered crenellated crown at Dārābgird. Typologically it belongs to the same type as the Anāhitā on the relief of Narseh at Naqš-e Rostam. The third Sasanian type of Anāhitā, again assuming the role of a secondary deity, appeared toward the end of the Sasanian dynasty at Ṭāq-i Bustān.[295] If the female figure on the casket from Bīšāpūr indeed portrays Anāhitā, it would constitute the only image of the goddess from non-official art. The presence of the fishes—her special attribute—is unique to this image and is not found on her other representations both on the Sasanian reliefs and in Eastern Iran.

We may conclude that the Avestan description of Anāhitā, despite its outstanding anthropomorphism and expressiveness, had no (or at best, very little) impact on even the creation of the Sasanian image of the goddess. Only her crenellated crown and the *barsom* can be linked with the "seven towers/palaces crown" from the Avestan hymn.[296] It is, however, much more probable that the crenel-

295 Note the suggestion of Callieri who observed that almost all Sasanian reliefs were carved near water and proposed that while Anāhitā was depicted in human shape only three times, "she is actually always present-represented by the aquatic element according to the old traditions", see Callieri 2006: 344.

296 See p. 15.

lated crown of Anāhitā was adopted from Ahura Mazdā. Unlike Ahura Mazdā, an uncovered crenellated crown is not the only headdress of Anāhitā. On the coins of Wahrām II she wears a bonnet ending with an animal head, on the Kushano-Sasanian coin of Ōhrmazd II she has a *kalathos*-type hat, and Anāhitā on the Ṭāq-i Bustān relief wears a calotte decorated with leafs. This indicates that, unlike Ahura Mazdā, no canonical crown was created for the goddess.

4. *Aŋra Mainyu*

Aŋra Mainyu (MP. *Ahriman*), "the Destructive Spirit", is the chief adversary and antithesis of Ahura Mazdā and the embodiment of evil forces of darkness in the Zoroastrian tradition.[297] He is the head of the *daēvas* and his dwelling is in the north. It is interesting to note that according to the Zoroastrian scriptures, unlike Ahura Mazdā, Aŋra Mainyu does not have a *gētīg* existence.[298]

1. *Western Iran*

Aŋra Mainyu does not appear in Achaemenian inscriptions, but references to him "must have existed" in the lost works of Aristotle and his followers.[299] In the later period, Aŋra Mainyu is mentioned in the important testimony of Plutarch.[300] Only in the Sasanian era do we find both explicit references to Aŋra Mainyu (e.g. in Kartīr's inscriptions) and his visual representations. It is undoubtedly significant that Sasanian Ahriman was depicted on the rock-reliefs in a complete anthropomorphic shape, the only tribute to his wicked, corrupted nature being his snake-headed hair and animal ears.

The Armenian historian Eznik Koghbac'i and the Syriac author Theodore bar Koni describe Ahriman as being dark and fetid in contrast with the radiant and fragrant Ahura Mazdā, but this seems to be the only difference in their appearance.[301] The story preserved in the *Tārīkh-i Sīstān* seems to confirm that Aŋra Mainyu was conceived by the Iranians in human form.[302] Firdausī too did not hesitate to portray his Ahriman/Iblīs as a human being seducing Ḍaḥḥāk. This anthropomorphism of the Evil Spirit is rather surprising. Given the fact that Ahura Mazdā manifests himself in *gētīg* as mankind, one would expect his antithesis to be imagined in completely inhuman, monstrous shape. We must remember, however, that both of these sources date from the Islamic period.

One of the visual manifestations that Aŋra Mainyu assumes in Pahlavi literature is that of a fifteen year old youth, but the Evil Spirit on the relief of Ardašīr I at Naqš-e Rostam is a bearded man, hardly inspired by Zoroastrian texts and notions. Moreover, in *Bundahišn*, the form of Ahriman is not associated with a snake, but is rather said to be frog-like.[303] In fact, the image of the Sasanian Ahriman is reminiscent of the images of demons in Sogdian art. It can be surmised that the decision to portray Ahriman in anthropomorphic form for the first time at Naqš-e Rostam stemmed from the symbolical symmetry of the relief itself. The anthropomorphic figure of Ahura Mazdā, which mirrored the king, "required" the figure of the fallen adversary that would emulate the defeated Parthian king. It is interesting to note that out of the eight Sasanian rock-reliefs showing investiture by Ahura Mazdā, only at the Naqš-e Rostam relief of Ardašīr I and probably on the Bīšāpūr relief of his son, Šāpūr I, is Aŋra Mainyu represented as a visual illustration of the final triumph of Ahura Mazdā.

297 Gray 1929: 176–180; Duchesne-Guillemin 1985.
298 Shaked 1967.
299 De Jong 1997: 313.
300 Plut. *De Is. et Os.* 46–47. See De Jong 1997: 157–205.
301 See p. 22 and p. 27.
302 See p. 43.
303 See p. 35.

The equestrian relief of Šāpūr I at Bīšāpūr (fig. 29)[304] is even more badly abraded than Šāpūr's relief at Naqš-e Rajab, but it is also definitely based on the Naqš-e Rostam relief of Ardašīr I and is even closer to the prototype. The horses, depicted here more proportionally, trample the defeated foes. The mount of the King of Kings (to the right) stands over the body of the Roman Emperor Gordian III and it is to be assumed that under the hooves of Ahura Mazdā's horse lies the same figure with snake-headed hair, which was depicted under the god's horse at Naqš-e Rostam. With his right hand, Ahura Mazdā offers Šāpūr a diadem while his left hand is empty. The face of the god is badly disfigured. A new feature in this relief, which does not appear in the other investiture reliefs, is a figure of a kneeling individual, probably Philip the Arab, placed between the king and the god.

2. *Eastern Iran*

Numerous demonic representations have survived in Sogdian art, and portrayals of the demon-king Ḍaḥḥāk with snakes rising from his shoulders were discovered at Panjikent and at Bunjikat palace, at Ustrushana.[305] However, to date, no representations of the Bactrian or Sogdian Evil Spirit have come to light.

3. *Conclusion*

Aŋra Mainyu is the only deity from the entire pre-Islamic Iranian iconography whose image is found only in Western Iran. His portrayal was created by the Sasanian artisans for a specific purpose, to form the symmetrical imperial message conveyed by Ardašīr's Naqš-e Rostam relief. Since no comparable monuments of imperial propaganda which place the king on the same footing as a god, existed in Eastern Iran, there was apparently no need to depict the Evil Spirit. The fact that Ahura Mazdā was not the highest god in Eastern Iran and the paucity of visual representations of the principal Zoroastrian deity with whom Aŋra Mainyu is inseparably coupled, probably also contributed to his absence.

5. *Apąm Napāt*

Apąm Napāt ("Son of Waters") was probably an important Indo-Iranian divinity, but his position in the Avestan pantheon is not entirely clear.[306] Although no hymn in the Avesta is dedicated to him, from the fragmentary invocations in the Yašts and from allusions in Middle Persian literature, it can be deduced that he was probably one of the principal Iranian gods whose importance faded due to certain historical developments. Boyce has suggested that Apąm Napāt was in fact the title of a great Indo-Iranian divinity, Varuṇa, whose complete absence from the Iranian religious tradition was always difficult to explain.[307] Apąm Napāt, as his name implies, was obviously connected with water, and he is said to watch over the *x*ᵛ*arənah*, which was perhaps originally his distinctive attribute.[308] He also possesses a curious title, *bərəzant* MP. *Borz/Borǰ*, ("The High One").[309] It is also possible that in some Iranian cults, Apąm Napāt was venerated as a creator-god.[310]

304 Herrmann 1983: 7–11, Fig. 1, Pl. 1–8d; Vanden Berghe 1984: no. 59; Vanden Berghe 1984: 1525–1526.
305 Belenitskii and Marshak 1981: 67–68, Fig. 33. Marshak and Negmatov 1996: Fig. 40.
306 See Boyce 1987a; Boyce 2001: 250–255.
307 Boyce 1981; Boyce 1993/1994: 37; Boyce 2001. His additional epithet according to Boyce was *baga*.
308 Oettinger 2009.
309 Boyce 1987a.
310 Boyce 1987a.

1. *Western Iran*

There is no image of Apąm Napāt from the iconography of Western Iran and no potential representation of the god has been identified.

2. *Eastern Iran*

The only image that might possibly represent Apąm Napāt is that of a seated adolescent god on a wall painting discovered in a private house XXII, room 1 in Panjikent. It depicts a seated deity facing a three-headed standing god on a blue background (fig. 30).[311] The latter also has three pairs of hands and wears an ornamented breastplate and shoulder straps in the form of a wild beast with a wide-open mouth (fig. 31). Among his attributes, only a trident, a blowing horn, and a sword are clearly distinguishable. The central head of the figure has a moustache, the left one is juvenile/feminine, and the right head has distorted, animal-like, demonic features. The central and the left heads wear elaborate Indian-style headdresses. All three heads have a third eye and a flaming nimbus. The foot of the god has a Sogdian inscription *wšpr*(*kr*).

The three-headed god faces another character, seated with his legs crossed. Although the face of this figure is damaged, he too has an adolescent appearance since he has a disproportionally large head and his haircut is characterized by long locks, which in Panjikent art are reserved only for women and children.[312] His entire figure is surrounded by flames in which fish and tritons are visible. The young god wears a typical Sogdian garment, but has no weapons or any specific attributes. His right hand is placed on his waist and the left hand is extended toward the three-headed god with an open palm. Above his head are fragments of a flying creature, perhaps a giant bird, deduced by Grenet to represent the mythical bird Chamruš, associated with Apąm Napāt in *Bundahišn*.[313] This wall painting is dated to the first half of the eighth century CE.

Because of the Avestan connections with water and fire, the seated adolescent god was proposed to represent the Sogdian Apąm Napāt. The fact that the god is depicted seated before the standing Wēšparkar may indicate his more elevated status in relation to the latter. We may even speculate about his important place in Sogdian religion where he perhaps retained some of his "original" functions of a creator-god. It is also very interesting to note that on Kushano-Sasanian coins, Oešo (who is known as Wēšparkar in Sogdian) is called βορζοανδο ιαζαδο/βαγο βορζανδο in Bactrian and *Burzāwand yazad* in Middle Persian, which derives from the same root as *bərəzant*, an epithet of Apąm Napāt. It is even more intriguing that both these deities are painted together here, providing material for speculations about a close association between these two divinities.

3. *Conclusions*

The origins, history and place of Apąm Napāt in the Iranian cults are obscure. Unfortunately, iconography appears to be of little help. The only probable representation of Apąm Napāt in Iranian art appears to be a seated god from Panjikent. If this is indeed the unique image of Apąm Napāt, it seems to correspond to the Avestan description of the god as a fire burning within the water and could be one of the few cases of correspondence between the Avestan text and the visual image. The link between Oešo, Wēšparkar and Apąm Napāt is promising and deserves to be fully investigated elsewhere based on the literary evidence as well.

311 Marshak 1990: 307–308; Grenet 2006/2010: 92.
312 Marshak 1990: 308.
313 Boyce 2001: 254.

6. *Aši*

Aši (MP. *Ard, Ahrišwang*), whose name is derived from an Avestan noun meaning "thing attained, reward, share, portion, recompense", was probably an Old Iranian goddess, a personification of fortune and recompense.[314] Aši is the daughter of Ahura Mazdā and Spəntā Ārmaiti and the sister of the Aməša Spənta. In the Avesta she is described as beautiful, tall, and strong, and has epithets such as "luminous" and "radiant".[315] In one passage, she is said to touch Zoroaster with her hands.[316] One of her common epithets is *vaŋ^{v}hī* "good". She is also often associated with Mithra and drives his chariot.[317]

1. *Western Iran*

There are no visual representations of Aši from the Iranian plateau, although she is attested in one personal name from the Achaemenian period.[318]

2. *Eastern Iran*

The only anthropomorphic image that most probably depicts Aši is the Kushan goddess called "Ardoxšo" ("The Good Aši"), (ΑΡΔΟΧϷΟ) who appears for the first time on the coins of Kanishka I.[319] She is the most popular deity found on the reverses of the later Kushan kings, sometimes to the exclusion of all other gods. Robert Göbl divides the representations of Ardoxšo into nine iconographic types.[320] Although Ardoxšo, like other Kushan gods, had no predecessor on the first "Greek" issue of Kanishka I, she is undoubtedly modeled on Tyche-Fortuna as she is portrayed on Hellenistic and Eastern Roman coins. Her essential attribute is a cornucopia, which is present on all types. Other attributes include a tree branch, a diadem and a tall Kushan royal crown. On some issues, Ardoxšo is standing in profile (pl. 5), while on the most common types she is depicted frontally seated on a throne (fig. 32).

The image of Ardoxšo is the most common reverse design on the coins of the Kushan Empire. However, it is very difficult to derive any conclusions as to her position in the hierarchy of the Kushan pantheon, since she is absent from the Rabatak divine list.[321] Gerard Fussman has suggested that Umma, who leads the Rabatak gods together with Nana, may be an epithet of Ardoxšo.[322] If the French scholar is right, this would place Ardoxšo, together with Nana, as one of the prominent divinities of the Kushan pantheon. This forms a striking contrast to the Zoroastrian tradition in which Aši is a minor divinity, emphasising once again the breach between the religion reflected in the Zoroastrian scriptures and the pantheon of the Kushans. It is noteworthy that together with Pharro, Ardoxšo is the only divinity to be frequently depicted in freestanding Gandhāran sculpture.[323] This couple, symbolising fecundity and prosperity, was probably one of the most important elements of Kushan imperial ideology and propaganda. This fact underlines yet again the significance and the popularity of Ardoxšo in the religious life of the Kushan Empire. Possible additional evidence for the importance and functions of the goddess

314 Boyce 1976b: 65–66; Schlerath and Skjærvø 1987.
315 See p. 14.
316 See p. 15.
317 Yt. 10.68.
318 Tavernier 2007: 539.
319 For a discussion of the proposal of Francfort, who seeks to identify Ardoxšo with Oxus and supports different etymology of her name, see p. 129. On Ardoxšo, see also Callieri 2002.
320 Göbl 1984 Ardoxšo 1–9.
321 See p. 12–13.
322 Fussman 1998: 587. Grenet 2012b: 18, translates Umma as Iranian "highest/supreme" and identifies her with Scythian Tabiti whose attributes, according to the French scholar, are a mirror and drinking horn. However, the Scythian goddess with these attributes is probably not Tabiti, but Aphrodite-Argimpasa.
323 Quagliotti 2003.

is supplied by a Manichaean Middle Persian text where she is referred to as *bg'rdwxš* (the goddess Ardwakhsh) and is called the "guardian of the border".[324]

It is not clear whether Ardoxšo was worshipped in Sogdiana and represented in Sogdian art. It is reasonable to assume that the immensely popular image of Kushan Ardoxšo did not vanish into oblivion without leaving any trace and would have exerted some influence on the neighboring Sogdian pantheon, perhaps becoming a member of it. Furthermore, Ardoxšo was probably also known in Chorasmia as it appears from the name of a village *Ardaxūš-mēϑan*.[325]

According to Marshak, the iconography of the alabaster statue of a seated woman found at Panjikent is very close to representations of the Kushan Ardoxšo as she is portrayed on the coins of Kanihska III.[326] This statue of a seated female was discovered in room 11, situated in the northwestern corner of the courtyard of the Temple II (fig. 33).[327] The statue is 31.4 cm high, made of alabaster and her garments are painted in blue, green, and red. She was found in the stratum dated to the beginning of the eighth century CE, but this statue obviously belongs to an earlier period since her iconography derives from Hellenistic tradition and there are no visible Sasanian and Indian influences.[328] Therefore, this sculpture should probably be dated to the earliest period of Temple II existence, the fifth century CE.[329] As proposed by Valentin Shkoda, the statue was portable.[330]

Grenet also interpreted as Aši a goddess mounted on a ram, who is frequently paired in Sogdian art with a god seated on the throne supported by camel protomes (whom Grenet identifies as Vərəθraγna).[331] His main argument is based on a passage from the Avesta where the ram is described as a protector of the goddess Aši.[332]

It has also been suggested that a deity seated on a throne supported by rams on two groups of Sogdian ossuaries from the Kashka-darya region represent Aši. The first group consists of two Sogdian ossuaries, dated to the sixth-seventh century CE, with identical decoration, which were discovered in 1976 near the village of Sivaz in the Kitab district of modern Uzbekistan.[333] The scenes on the ossuaries are quite complex and consist of several anthropomorphic and animal figures divided in two registers (fig. 34). The left part of the upper register is dominated by a beardless character, flanked by two crouching figures playing on musical instruments. He wears a winged crown and holds a fire-altar in his left hand and a rod resembling a scepter. The figure sits on a carpet with his right leg tucked beneath him and two rams facing the opposite directions are depicted just below. Krasheninnikova's suggestion, that the rams form a zoomorphic throne,[334] is probably correct, and it is one of the characteristic features of the iconography of Sogdian deities. However, the god is depicted too high above the animals and there is no visual connection between them.[335] In the right corner, a larger figure is shown with both legs tucked beneath, raising the right hand in a gesture of blessing and holding a scepter (or perhaps a ladle for libations).[336] It is difficult to determine if this individual has a short beard.[337] A length of cloth stretches from his right arm and connects with the hand of a smaller kneeling figure to the left. Between them, a

324 Grenet forthcoming a.
325 Lurje 2004: 209–210.
326 Marshak 1999: 180.
327 Shkoda 2009: 71, with references to earlier publications.
328 Marshak 1999: 180.
329 Marshak 2009: 12, dates it "not later than the fith C. CE.".
330 Shkoda 2009: 98–99.
331 Grenet 1993: 157–159. For the description of these paintings, see p. 138–139.
332 Yt. 17.55–56.
333 Grenet et al. 1993: 52–55.
334 Grenet et al. 1993: 54.
335 Grenet et al. 1993: 62. Marshak 1999: 185, suggests that these are sacrificial animals.
336 As proposed by Grenet 2009: 108.
337 Grenet 2009: 108.

crouching naked figure in a bonnet is depicted. In the lower register, to the right of the rams, there are depictions of a priest wearing a *padām* performing a ritual, a fire-altar, and a saddled horse.

The second group is represented by the fragments of three stamped ossuaries bearing similar decorations which were found in 2012 at Yumalaktepa, five kilometers to the south-east of Shahr-i Sabz.[338] The composition is in fact a more "detailed" version of the scenes found on the Sivaz ossuary and is schematically divided into two registers, although it probably can be read continuously (pl. 6). It is also possible that it shows different scenes combined together by a common subject, like some murals from Panjikent. Overall, ten human figures are represented in this composition. In the upper right corner, a figure is shown seated cross-legged and flanked by two servants facing outside and holding a fly swatter. His right hand is raised in a gesture of blessing with one finger pointing upwards and the left hand suspended along the body. To the left of this group, a male figure is depicted holding scales in his left hand. In the left pan a small nude figure of a boy is shown "attached" in the unnatural diagonal position.

The left part of the upper register is occupied by a second group of one main figure and two attendants. The central character is sitting in the typical Sogdian pose with one leg tucked beneath on the zoomorphic throne formed by two rams and covered with a carpet. His left hand is raised in a similar gesture with a pointed finger and in his right hand he holds a cornucopia. The headdress is effaced, but it appears that he wears a crenellated crown. The attendants play a harp and a lute. Immediately below the figure with the scales, a priest is shown standing before a square object, wearing a *padām* and holding a *barsom*. A saddled horse is placed just behind him. In the center foreground, a female figure is shown kneeling facing left. Her left hand is hidden in the long sleeve of her coat and in her right hand she holds a round object.

The deity seated on the throne supported by rams on the Yumalaktepa ossuaries, holds a cornucopia, a distinctive attribute of the Kushan Ardoxšo and probably wears a crenellated crown. She might represent here the "good reward" granted to the deceased in Paradise.[339] In the Avesta, Aši is often associated with Sraoša and Vohu Manah, forming a sort of "triad".[340] We may speculate that in Sogdian religion this triad was rather Aši—Rašnu—Vohu Manah (if the identification of the latter is sound). The corresponding divinity on the Sivaz ossuary wears a winged crown and holds a fire-altar although he also mounts a throne supported by rams. An image of a goddess holding a cornucopia and perhaps belonging to the same type as Kushan Ardoxšo is also known from a Sogdian terracotta found at Zartepa.[341] In addition, the figure holding a cornucopia (no. 4) from Biyanajman and Miankal ossuaries may also depict the Sogdian Aši.[342]

3. *Conclusions*

Despite her description as an anthropomorphic goddess in the Avesta, it appears that there were no attempts in Western Iran to represent Aši. In Eastern Iran, she was probably a prominent member of the Kushan pantheon and her iconography was based on that of Tyche, reflecting the idea of abundance that she personified. Her later history is vague and insufficiently understood. Several divine images from Sogdian art discussed above could be representations of Sogdian Aši if we suppose that she also kept her Kushan attribute—the cornucopia—in Sogdian art. However, the evidence for that is not compelling.

338 Berdimuradov, Bogomolov, Daeppen and Khushvaktov: 2012.
339 "You appoint reward for deed and word: bad for the bad, good reward for the good": Y. 43.5.
340 Schlerath and Skjærvø 1987.
341 Abdullaev 2003: 26.
342 See p. 170 ff.

7. *Argimpasa*

The Scythian goddess Argimpasa (or Artimpasa) belongs to the third level of the hierarchy of the Scythian gods as described by Herodotus[343] and she is equated by him with Aphrodite Ourania.[344] The etymology of her name is not entirely clear, although it is most probably Iranian.[345]

1. *Western Iran*

No representation of Argimpasa has been uncovered on the Iranian plateau.

2. *Eastern Iran*

Argimpasa-Aphrodite is usually identified with the most popular divine character in Scythian art—an enthroned queenly woman depicted with a man facing her.[346] There are several variations of this composition on numerous Scythian objects. First to be considered is the golden diadem, found in the Sakhnovka kurgan in modern Ukraine that depicts ten individuals—nine male and one female—involved in various activities, such as playing musical instruments, pouring wine, and drinking (fig. 35).[347] Especially intriguing are the two figures on the far left. A bearded Scythian grasps a kneeling, half-naked man by his hair and prepares to stab him with a dagger. His "victim" appears to hold a ram's head in his hands. The central figure is that of an enthroned queenly woman wearing a tall headdress and a veil, which falls down her back. In her hands she holds a mirror and a vessel. Behind her stands a servant with a fly-whisk. A bearded male armed with a bow and holding a rhyton is kneeling before her. The diadem is probably dated between 350–300 BCE.

A series of small golden plaques found in many Scythian kurgas, such as Nosaki,[348] Chertomlyk and Oguz[349] also depict an enthroned female figure portrayed in full profile (fig. 36). These plaques were probably part of the headdress decoration.[350] The goddess wears a long garment and her head is covered with a veil. In her left hand she holds a mirror. Facing her is a figure of a young man drinking from a rhyton. This individual does not wear a belt and—unusually for representations of Scythian men—is unarmed. From the Merdzhany kurgan comes a golden fragment of a facing of a silver rhyton depicting a frontally enthroned queenly woman holding a small vessel in her right hand (fig. 37).[351] Her throne is placed between a tree and a horse's skull on a stick. Approaching her is an equestrian with a rhyton in his raised right hand.

Perhaps the most intriguing and complex scene is found on the gold plaque from Karagodeouashkh kurgan. It is divided into three registers and was originally part of the conical female headdress.[352] In the upper register, a standing female figure is depicted dressed in a chiton and a himation. Below her, there is a beardless, bareheaded frontal character riding a chariot. The lower register contains images of five figures, a woman flanked by two young men and two additional figures stand behind her (fig. 38). The central female character wears a tall conical headdress and grasps the upper part of a rhyton handed to

343 Raevskiy 1977: 121; Ustinova 1999: 68.
344 Hdt. 4.59. See Ustinova 1999: 75–87, with references to previous literature.
345 Humbach and Faiss 2012: 7–8, suggest that *Argim-pasa* is derived from OIr. *ṛgant-pāϑra-* "protection of the rushing (waves)". See also Ustinova 1999: 75–76, who cites several previous suggestions.
346 See the detailed discussion in Bessonova 1983: 98–155; Ustinova 1999: 113–122.
347 Reeder 2001: no. 40.
348 Reeder 2001: no. 41.
349 For the full list with references, see Reeder 2001: 148, n. 2.
350 Bessonova 1983: 98–99.
351 Artamonov 1961: 62; Bessonova 1983: 112.
352 Bessonova 1983: 107–111; Ustinova 1999: 123–127.

her by a man on her left. The second man holds a vessel. It is not entirely clear whether the standing figures are young males or females. All the figures are shown frontally, unlike the other scenes with the seated goddess, which are always rendered in profile.

The Scythian goddess usually wears a veil and her most common attributes are a mirror and a small vessel. Given the incredible popularity of this scene in Scythian art it would be natural to identify the goddess as Tabiti-Hestia, the head of the Scythian pantheon according to Herodotus. However, the seated goddess is clearly modeled on the iconographic type of a Greek Aphrodite.[353] Therefore, it appears that she is best understood as Argimpasa-Aphrodite. The individual facing her is always male, at times juvenile or bearded, unmounted or equestrian. His constant attribute, present in each case and characterizing this scene as essentially cultic, is a rhyton. The plaque from the Karagodeouashkh kurgan demonstrates an unusual variation of this composition with two male protagonists instead of one, and two additional characters of uncertain sex. Both the rhyton and the vessel are also present here, but are offered to the goddess by the men flanking her. The semantics of these scenes and the identity of the male figure(s) have been subject to much debate. The man has been interpreted as a king, hero or goddesses' paredrus and the whole composition has been explained as the adoration of the goddess, a divine investiture or a sacred marriage.[354] The definition of this scene as a veneration of Argimpasa-Aphrodite by a mortal seems preferable. The male characters lack any divine attributes and on the Sakhnovka diadem the Scythian kneeling before the goddess also does not have any attribute that would associate him with a deity and does not differ in any aspect from other figures, which are clearly mortals. If these scenes indeed depict the adoration of Argimpasa-Aphrodite, then the two figures on the back stage on the Karagodeouashkh plaque could perhaps be *enareis*, the effeminate, transvestite soothsayers of the Scythians, described by Herodotus.[355]

3. *Conclusions*

The seated goddess with a male adorant is undoubtedly the most popular divine image in the Scythian art. She should most probably be identified with Argimpasa-Aphrodite. This example clearly demonstrates that the divinity most frequently reproduced in art was not necessarily the head of the pantheon. All images of Argimpasa-Aphrodite, with all variations, render the same scene—the veneration of the seated goddess. Some of her most common representations are based on the Greek Aphrodite while the rest have different features. Unfortunately, besides the clue that is provided by her equation with the Greek goddess of love, nothing else can be said about her functions.

8. *Arštāt*

The goddess Arštāt (MP. *Aštād*, "Justice") is closely associated in the Avesta with Mithra and Rašnu and Yašt 18 is dedicated to her.[356] However, no description of the goddess is found in the Avesta and her epithets do not shed any light on her visual appearance.

1. *Western Iran*

There are no indications that Arštāt was represented in Western Iran in the Achaemenian, Hellenistic or Parthian periods. In the Sasanian era, there is solid evidence that she was imagined in human form,

353 Bessonova 1983: 99–100.
354 See the references in Ustinova 1999: 114–115.
355 Hdt. 1.105; 4.67.
356 Gray 1929: 136–137; Gnoli 1987.

since she is mentioned in the *Ardā Wīrāz Nāmag* among other deities helping Wīrāz cross the Činwad bridge.[357] However, even during Sasanian rule, there are no images that can be interpreted as that of Arštāt in Western Iran.

2. *Eastern Iran*

Pictorial representations of Arštāt are known only from Eastern Iran. The earliest is the Kushan Rišto (PIÞTO) created for the Kushan numismatic pantheon. Rišto is depicted on the gold coins of Huvishka assuming the iconography of Athena-Roma (fig. 39).[358] She wears a Greek helmet, heavy body armor and carries a spear and a large round shield. Although her image is clearly based on the iconography of Athena-Roma, Athena does not appear on the "Greek" issue of Kanishka, unlike some other Kushan gods, i.e. Helios/Miiro and Selene/Mao. Her absence from the Rabatak inscription makes it impossible to establish the place of Rišto in the Kushan divine hierarchy.

This tradition of visual representation of Arštāt continued in the Kushano-Sasanian period, in two fragments of wall paintings from Dilberjin located in northern Afghanistan, some forty km. from the city of Balkh. The first fragmentary painting (6.5 × 1.75 m) was discovered on the northern wall of room 12 of the complex adjacent to the northeastern section of the city-wall, close to the so-called "Dioscuri Temple".[359] A group of five characters of different sizes is pictured on a pink background (fig. 40). The central figure is larger than the rest and depicts a female seated frontally on the throne painted in yellow. She has a yellow nimbus surrounding her head and wears a blue cloak and a helmet of the same color depicted schematically, with two "tassels" on the end. Long curling hair is shown falling on her shoulders and ribbons fly behind her back. In her right hand the goddess holds an object, which is impossible to identify because the poor state of preservation. The excavator, Irina Kruglikova, notes that this object has a rounded or oval top and proposes that it could be a mirror.[360] Her left hand rests on a circular object which is most probably a shield decorated with a *gorgoneion*. The goddess on the painting is flanked by four figures of attendants, three of similar size, smaller than her and one dwarfish character, second from the right. Kruglikova dates the paintings to the Kushano-Sasanian period.[361]

The second wall painting depicting a female head wearing exactly the same helmet as the goddess in room 12 was found in the room 16 of the same complex at Dilberjin (fig. 41).[362] All walls of this room were decorated with murals and the excavators distinguished three stages of paintings. This fragment belongs to the central section of the northern wall. It shows two female heads, one in three-quarter view, and the second in profile. The latter is 30 cm. high, suggesting that the whole figure could be as high as 180 cm.[363] The female figure portrayed in profile wears a helmet of the Graeco-Bactrian type with two "tassels" on the ends and a large earring. A pinkish nimbus surrounds her head. In the eastern corner of the northern wall, another fragment depicting a procession of twelve male donors was uncovered.[364] The whole composition was therefore probably that of the cultic procession of adorants directed towards a deity or a group of deities portrayed in the center of the wall, only a small fragment of which—the head of a helmeted goddess—has survived. These paintings are dated by the excavators to the early Kushan period.[365]

---

357 See p. 32.
358 Göbl 1984, Rišto; Grenet 1984: 258–621
359 Kruglikova 1976: 96–100. On the "Dioscuri Temple", see Shenkar 2011: 124–126.
360 Kruglikova 1976: 97.
361 Kruglikova 1976: 88.
362 Kruglikova 1979.
363 Kruglikova 1979: 127.
364 Kruglikova 1979: 123–127.
365 Kruglikova 1979: 141–142.

The paintings showing the goddess wearing a degenerated Greek helmet and (in one case) holding a shield with a *gorgoneion* is clear evidence that Arštāt was venerated in Kushano-Sasanian Bactria and her iconography followed that of the Kushan Rišto.[366]

While Rišto from Kushan coins and from the Dilberjin murals appears as an independent divinity, Grenet identifies the female winged figure accompanying the chariot of the Bāmiān Mithra and carrying a shield with a *gorgoneion* as Arštāt. This painting, which once decorated the soffit of the niche of the Small Buddha at Bāmiān, before it was blown up by the Taliban in 2001, depicted a youthful god standing in a chariot drawn by four white horses (fig. 42).[367] The entire figure of the god, almost down to his knees, was encircled in a crenellated nimbus. Surrounding his head, there was an additional plain nimbus. Unfortunately, the upper part of the head was not preserved and it is unknown which headdress the god originally had. He was armed with a spear and a sword. On the both sides of the chariot, flanking the driver, two juvenile or feminine, nimbate winged figures were depicted. Both wore a helmet; the left figure had a shield decorated with what seems to be a *gorgoneion* and the right figure was armed with a bow and arrow. The position of the right hand of the first figure indicates that the original intention of the artisan was to depict an object in it, perhaps a spear, as Grenet has suggested,[368] which was not, however, painted. Directly above them, two half-human, half-bird figures with priestly attributes such as a *padām*, torch and a libation spoon attached to the belt were painted. In the upper corners of the painting, two wind-genies were shown, holding floating scarves over their heads. This painting was probably executed in the second half of the sixth century CE.[369]

Although not explicitly described in the Avesta as flying by Mithra's side, Arštāt is nevertheless his companion.[370] Grenet's suggestion therefore seems possible.[371] In a recent article, Grenet has also proposed that in this painting Arštāt represents the nocturnal light.[372] It is noteworthy that *ριϸτο* is probably also attested as a compound in a Bactrian name from the sixth century CE.[373]

Although no confirmed image of Arštāt is known from the Sogdian paintings, the goddess was probably also venerated in Sogdiana since her name is attested in the Sogdian onomasticon.[374] In the suburbs of Bukhara there was a village called **'st'βγn*, which Olga Smirnova has proposed to reconstruct as **'št'δβγn* "temple of A(r)shtad".[375] A possible Sogdian representation of Arštāt could be a fragmentary sixth century terracotta from Samarkand.[376] This identification is based on the preserved shield with the image of a *gorgoneion*.

3. *Conclusions*

There are solid indications that in the Sasanian period, Arštāt—like other deities—was imagined in Western Iran as an anthropomorphic being. This, however, was not expressed in the visual record. All her known representations were created in Eastern Iran. The earliest is the Kushan Rišto based on the iconography of Athena, who shared her main trait as the goddess of Justice. Unlike many Kushan gods, it appears that the image of Arštāt did not vanish from Bactrian art after the Sasanian conquest. Her representations at Dilberjin are recognizable thanks to her attributes, a Greek helmet and a shield with

366 She was first identified as Athena-Arštāt by Grenet 1987b.
367 Grenet 1993: 153–156; Grenet 1993/1994.
368 Grenet 1993/1994: 89.
369 Grenet 2006.
370 Yt. 10.100.
371 Grenet 1993/1994: 90–91.
372 Grenet 2003a: 39.
373 Sims-Williams 2010: n. 397.
374 Sims-Williams 1991: 177; Lurje 2010: no. 182.
375 Smirnova 1971: 98.
376 Grenet 1993/1994: 90.

a *gorgoneion*. It seems that from Bactria, her worship penetrated Sogdiana, where we find terracotta female figurines with attributes similar to those of Arštāt. It is plausible that they were the subject of a popular cult, but no pictorial representations of Arštāt are currently known from any other media of Sogdian art.

9. *Ātar*

Ātar (MP. *Ādur-Ātaš*) is a deity of fire, which also acts as his visual manifestation.[377] It is generally accepted that his cult stems from the veneration of the hearth fire among Indo-European people.[378] In the Avesta, Ātar is often addressed as "the son of Ahura Mazdā",[379] but no descriptions of his visual appearance are found or can be derived from his epithets.

1. *Western Iran*

The veneration of fire is one of the most celebrated and frequently remarked upon stereotypes of Iranian cults to be found in foreign written sources.[380] It is, however, unclear whether these references allude to the worship of Ahura Mazdā or of other gods by means of fire, or to the veneration of the god Ātar himself.

Ātar is attested in Iranian personal names in the Achaemenian period,[381] and from the Sasanian period, we have clear evidence that Ātar was perceived as an anthropomorphic divinity. This can be deduced from the *Ardā Wīrāz Nāmag* where Ādur accompanies Wīrāz on his journey and speaks to him[382] and from Theodore bar Koni, who mentions that fire possessed an ability to speak and was walking with the Avestan hero Kərəsāspa.[383] Unfortunately, these sources do not describe the visual appearance of the god, and there are no hints as to whether Ādur was in any way different from other gods encountered by Wīrāz. There are no references in the text to him possessing a flaming nimbus or flaming himself.

There are no indisputable visual representations of Ātar in Western Iran, although there are several divine images that may depict him. These include a flaming bust emerging from the fire-altar found on Sasanian and Kushano-Sasanian coins and seals. The bust on Sasanian coins appeared early in the fourth century CE on the reverse of the coins of Ōhrmazd II,[384] and continued to be reproduced until the reign of the king Balāš (fig. 43). The bust is shown both *en face* and in profile. It is bearded, has a typical Sasanian haircut, and does not wear a crown or a diadem. The flaming torso on the reverse of Kushano-Sasanian coins is attested for the first time on the coins of Ōhrmazd I and continues until the reign of Wahrām (fig. 44).[385] It shows a deity emerging from the fire-altar decorated with royal ribbons. The entire upper part of the body faces left. The god is bearded and flames come from his head and shoulders. In his left hand he holds a long spear and offers a diadem with his right. On one type of Ōhrmazd I, the god is labeled in MP. *Burzāwand yazad*.[386]

---

377 See Gray 1929: 66–70; Boyce 1989.
378 Boyce 1989: 1.
379 For references, see Gray 1929: 66.
380 For a review of the Greek and Latin sources, see De Jong 1997: 344–350.
381 Tavernier 2007: 539.
382 See p. 32.
383 See p. 27
384 Göbl 1971 V, 1,3; Gyselen 2000: Fig. 15.
385 Cribb 1990: nos. 24–27.
386 Cribb 1990: no. 24.

The bust in flames on the fire-altar is found on two Sasanian seals. The first seal depicts it in frontal view surmounted on a fire-altar (fig. 45).[387] It is beardless and has a juvenile appearance. Ribbons are depicted flying behind him and flames rise directly from his head. The altar is flanked by the symbols of a star and a moon crescent. The second seal kept in the *Bibliothèque nationale de France* generally shows a similar composition to that on the previous seal, but there are numerous nuances in iconography (fig. 46).[388] The fire-altar is of a different type, the haircut is short and the flames also rise from the shoulders rather than from the head alone. The ribbons of the diadem are also absent. The inscription on the seal is read by Shaked as "Mangarēn-Ādur, the man in charge of the Mithra-ritual (of) Shāpūr. Trustworthy".[389]

It is notworthy that on coins the bust is always bearded and at times wears a crown, while on seals it is beardless and bareheaded. In the late Sasanian period, a curious design of a bust surrounded by a nimbus of flames is portrayed on gold and silver issues of Xusrō II (fig. 47).[390] It is shown *en face* on both types, and has a feminine, youthful appearance, which makes its biological sex uncertain. It wears a diadem with two flying fillets depicted almost perpendicularly and two buckles of hair lie on the shoulders. On gold coins, the hair is tied in a bow. It should also be noted that the physiognomy is quite distinct on the two types of coins, although in all probability they represent the same individual.[391] Although on this occasion the bust is shown without an altar, it is possible that the coins were intended to depict the same divinity shown on seals.

Unfortunately we cannot be certain whether all these busts represent one god or a number of different deities. The Kushano-Sasanian coins, for instance, demonstrate that various gods were depicted emerging from the fire-altar. However, the association with a fire-altar and the fact that these deities are not rendered with a simple nimbus or tongues of flame rising from their shoulders, but rather with their entire head and shoulders aflame, suggests that at least some might indeed be representations of the fire-god Ātar.[392] There is additional evidence that appears to support this identification. Ātar is attested 159 times in Sasanian personal names, which makes him the most popular deity to appear in the Sasanian onomasticon, leaving behind Mithra with 120 occurrences, Māh with 93 and Ahura Mazdā with 53. Together, these four deities constitute more than 30% of Sasanian personal names.[393]

It is certainly not accidental that the same Mithra and Māh are the only gods to be definitely identified on Sasanian seals—the only medium of Sasanian art not subject to the control of the royal court and therefore reflecting the preferences of the people. If names can be taken as any indicator of the place of a god in popular religion, it seems plausible to suggest that the common devotion to Ātar must have been reflected also in unofficial art; on seals alongside the other popular gods, Mithra and Māh. Therefore, I am inclined to believe that the bust on the fire-altar on Sasanian seals indeed represents the fire-god Ātar.

The image of a naked, flaming youth, leaning on a pedestal on one Sasanian seal may also represent a unique, fully anthropomorphic variant of the same deity. The youth is standing in a free pose and is executed in a "hellenizing" style (fig. 48).[394] He is standing cross-legged, leaning with his left hand on a

387 Gignoux and Gyselen 1982: no. 20.79.

388 Gignoux 1978: no. 3.4; Gyselen 1993: no. 20.I.8.

389 Shaked 1995: 248.

390 These coins and the depiction of the bust in flames have been discussed numerous times. The most recent and detailed studies which should now be consulted are Gyselen 2000 and Mosig-Walburg 2009.

391 Interestingly, this bust was copied on early Muslim coins of Zāvulistān, see Gyselen 2010c: 237.

392 See the discussion on the identification of the bust in flames, with references to previous literature, in Gyselen 2000. An additional proposal is brought forward by Yamamoto 1981: 70, who suggested that the bust could represent a reigning king. Schindel 2004: 23, also believes that the bust in flames is the image of a king.

393 Gignoux 2005: 38.

394 Gyselen 1993: 10.B.16.

column-like pedestal and holds an unidentified object in his right hand. His beardless head is encircled in flames. The inscription reads *ardādar dibīr* "Ardādar the scribe". A very similar figure resting its left hand on a similar pedestal is also depicted on two Gandhāran seals.[395]

2. *Eastern Iran*

Ātar appears as a theophoric component in some Parthian names in the ostraca from Nisa,[396] but no Parthian pictorial representation of the fire god has yet been recognized. The Kushans created the only definite anthropomorphic image of Ātar in Iranian art—the god Athšo (ΑΘÞΟ) who replaces ΗΦΑΙϹΤΟϹ on the coins of Kanishka,[397] and continues to be represented under Huvishka.[398] On two main types Athšo is depicted facing left and holding tongs and a diadem (fig. 49) or facing right and holding tongs and a sledgehammer (pl. 7). On the first type, Athšo wears a diadem, has a long beard and tongues of fire rise from both of his shoulders. The most remarkable feature of the second type is that not only his head, but the entire upper part of his body, is encircled in flames. This is a feature unique only to Athšo among all the Kushan deities. His visual appearance and attributes are entirely borrowed from the Greek god Hephaestus.[399] On the first Greek issue of Kanishka, the god is called "Hephaistos", but renamed "Athšo" on subsequent Bactrian issues and in some cases the Bactrian legend was struck over the Greek one.[400] Similar to Pharro and Ardoxšo, whose images are found in the Buddhist art of Gandhāra, the iconography of Athšo also probably influenced that of Vishvakarman in Gandhāran art.[401]

A flaming bust on the fire-altar was most probably employed first by Ōhrmazd II for the reverses of his coins. It seems that in a very short period, it was adopted in Kushanshahr, starting with Ōhrmazd I. The Kushano-Sasanian god did not simply imitate the Sasanian handless prototype, but their coins show the entire upper part of the body emerging from the altar and holding a diadem and a spear, on one coin labeling the god as *Burzāwand yazad*.[402] He is therefore a continuation of the deity Oešo/Vayu and unrelated to Athšo.

The existence of the anthropomorphic image of Ātar in Sogdian iconography is doubtful. Kazim Abdullaev has proposed to interpret a god on a terracotta plaque found at the site of Chilek, 30 km to the north of Samarkand, as a Sogdian Ātar assimilated with Šahrewar.[403] This plaque depicts a beardless seated male deity in a characteristic Sogdian pose with one leg tucked beneath (fig. 50). He is wearing a winged crown surmounted by a moon crescent. One hand is placed on the hilt of the sword and another holds pincers. Tongues of fire are shown above the left shoulder. Under his right arm there is an oval object resembling a shield or a mask. The plaque is dated to the sixth century CE.[404] The tongs indeed bring him together with Kushan Athšo, the only god who has pincers as his main attribute. However, all other attributes of the god from the Chilek plaque are entirely different and some of them he shares not only with Kushan Šaoreoro, but also with other deities from the Sogdian and Kushan pantheons. Nevertheless, the tongs are unique to Kushan Athšo and clearly indicate a connection with fire. Marshak has suggested that this could be an image of the personified Ādur

395 Ur Rahman and Falk 2011: nos. 06.04.01, 06.04.02.
396 For example, Diakonoff and Livshits 2001: no. 721:5.
397 Rosenfield 1967: 77, no. 91.
398 Rosenfield 1967: 76; Göbl 1984: Atšo 1–3.
399 See Tanabe 1995/1996: 186.
400 Tanabe 1995/1996: Fig. 14b.
401 Tanabe 1995/1996: 185.
402 Cribb 1990: no. 24.
403 Grenet et al. 1993: 49–53.
404 Grenet et al. 1993: 52.

Gušnasp.[405] It seems more plausible, however, that the Chilek god is in fact the image of a Sogdian god of fire, who preserved the tongs as a main attribute from Athšo (originally deriving from Greek Hephaistos).

The attributes of character no. 3 from Biyanajman and Miankal—a fire-altar and a shovel—are fully fitting for Ātar.[406] The third, fiery god from a fragment of an incense burner from Jartepa II, could also be a Sogdian Ātar.[407]

3. *Conclusions*

It is clear from the literary sources that in Sasanian Iran Ātar was considered to possess a human shape in *mēnōg*. In *gētīg* his obvious visual manifestation was fire itself. It seems that the bust in flames placed on the fire-altar on some Sasanian coins and seals was an attempt to represent an anthropomorphic image of the god, as he in fact existed in *mēnōg*.

In Eastern Iran, Ātar (Athšo) was an important member of the Kushan numismatic pantheon and his iconography followed that of Greek Hephaistos. The bust on the altar on Kushano-Sasanian seals, where it is labeled, does not represent Athšo, but other divinities. In Sogdian art two possible representations of Ātar have been identified, but unfortunately neither is certain.

10. *Daēnā*

The meaning of the term *daēnā* (MP. *dēn*) can be interpreted as "the sum of man's spiritual attributes and individuality, vision, inner self, conscience, religion",[408] and most commonly reflects the notions of "one's religion".[409] Skjærvø, however, has proposed that the Avestan *daēnā* should rather be understood as "a mental faculty that 'sees' in the other world" and the Middle Persian *dēn* as "the totality of the (oral) tradition".[410] In a recent study, Alberto Cantera translates *daēnā* as "vision" and also argues that the Middle Persian *dēn* can often keep this meaning.[411] In the Avesta, Daēnā is referred to as the daughter of Ahura Mazdā and Ārmaiti,[412] while in the Aramaic inscription from Arebsun (Cappadocia) she is addressed as "the sister and the wife of Bel".[413] Bel here most probably represents the Aramaic translation of Ahura Mazdā.

Daēnā is the representation of one's actions in this world. She is the divine being whose anthropomorphic descriptions are the most common in Iranian literature. Moreover, the descriptions of her visual appearance are very similar and consistent both in the Avesta and in various Middle Persian texts.[414] Daēnā comes to meet the soul of the deceased at the Činwad bridge and, depending on his righteousness or wickedness, she manifests herself either as a beautiful maiden, or as an old, ugly woman. This idea and imagery was apparently so influential that it had an impact on Manichaean and even on Muslim thought.[415]

---

405 Marshak 1995/1996: 304.
406 See p. 170 ff.
407 See p. 101.
408 Shaki 1996.
409 For a recent survey of the concept of *daēnā* in Zoroastrianism with a comprehensive list of references to previous studies, see Azarpay 2011: 54–56.
410 Skjærvø 2011c: 334–335.
411 Cantera 2013: 129–131.
412 Y. 17.16.
413 Lemaire 2003: 146–152.
414 See p. 14 and p. 36.
415 Sundermann 2008: 160–162; Shaked 1990: 28–29.

1. *Western Iran*

Daēnā's flamboyant anthropomorphic descriptions in Zoroastrian literature and especially her appearance in Kartīr's inscription,[416] unambiguously indicate that Daēnā was imagined anthropomorphically in Western Iran at least from the third century CE and suggest that she was also often thus represented. However, no confirmed image of Daēnā has been identified from Western Iran. One reason appears to be a complete absence of eschatological scenes, especially crossing the Činwad bridge, in Western Iranian art,[417] where Daēnā would have been represented. Gnoli has identified the image of a young woman holding a flower, common on Sasanian seals, as that of Daēnā.[418] His suggestion is supported by the inscription appearing on one of these seals: *kunišn ī frāzrōn weh* ("the action that comes forward is good"). Here, the action can refer to Daēnā. Moreover, the flower in her hand may be an allusion to the sweet-scented plants that Daēnā walks among in *Ardā Wīrāz Nāmag*.[419] Such female images are very similar to the Achaemenian era representations found on seals manufactured in the so-called "Graeco-Persian" style.[420] Most recently, Grenet, accepting Gnoli's identification, has further proposed to recognize the image of Daēnā on three additional Sasanian seals. Two of the seals show male and female busts facing each other, and the third depicts a standing woman feeding a rooster.[421]

Another Sasanian image that has been proposed to portray Daēnā is found on the rock-relief at Tang-i Qandil.[422] This unusual relief, thought to represent a rare example of Sasanian unofficial art, depicts a woman dressed in a garment with long folds covering her feet and with a topknot on her head. She offers a flower to a princely figure followed by a dignitary holding a ring. The arguments that these female figures holding a flower, as well as their Achaemenian "predecessors", represent any divinity, let alone Daēnā in particular, are not sufficiently convincing. Furthermore, none of the figures are crowned—an important characteristic of Iranian divinities—and no images come from a funerary context, where one would most naturally expect to find the representation of Daēnā.

An additional possible image of Sasanian Daēnā is found on a seal in the British Museum, which depicts a scene of a banquet featuring a reclining male figure and a female standing before him.[423] If Gyselen's interpretation of this scene as a funerary feast is sound, the female figure could be Daēnā.[424]

2. *Eastern Iran*

Identifying the image of Daēnā in Eastern Iran is an even more complicated task. There are many candidates but no certain representations. Daēnā is absent from the Kushan pantheon, our "anchor" of Eastern Iranian religious iconography, but her possible image is found on a seal said to come from Gandhāra, which in fact could be of an Eastern Sasanian, perhaps more specifically Kushano-Sasanian, manufacture (fig. 51).[425] The seal depicts a tall, noble female figure accompanied by two dogs. She offers a jar to a male character of the same size who approaches her leading another, smaller figure into her presence.

---

416 See p. 11–12.
417 In fact, the only representation of the Činwad bridge in Iranian art is found on the Sino-Sogdian stone sarcophagus of Wirkak, influenced by Manichaean concepts and ideas. See p. 95.
418 Gnoli 1993/1994: 82.
419 *AWN* 4.15.
420 See also Azarpay 2011: 56–57, for a recent discussion of the possible representations of the Sasanian Daēnā.
421 Grenet 2013: 202–204. His interpretation is based on the inscriptions that appear on the two seals and contain the word *ruwān*: *Farr-Ohrmazd ī huxēm ruwān wēn-man* "Farr-Ohrmazd of a good-natured soul, see me!", *Bōxt-ruwān Wahrām humihr* "Wahrām, (be) blessed, faithful".
422 Grenet and Zhang Guangda 1996: 184, n. 10.
423 Gyselen 1995b.
424 Gyselen 1995b: 254.
425 Ur Rahman and Falk 2011: no. 05.01.11. For detailed treatment and argumentation, see Shenkar forthcoming b.

These two characters wear unusually short pants and a transparent long dress, which are probably attempts to represent underwear. From depictions on Sogdian ossuaries, which are mass-produced objects, we know that the soul of the deceased was shown naked. The depiction of the two characters on the seal in underwear probably means that they are actually in the *mēnōg* state—dead or on their extra-corporeal journey—but at the same time the scene conforms to the minimal standards of modesty.

One of Daēnā's distinctive attributes in the Avesta is the two dogs that accompany her. In the *Vīdēvdāt* 19.30 and in its Middle Persian translation, she is described as "having two dogs".[426] The jar which the lady holds and offers to the two approaching characters is not attested for Daēnā in Zoroastrian sources. However, a fragment of a Manichaean Sogdian text does mention a vessel with a drink as one of her attributes.[427]

There is much more room for speculation when one comes to Sogdian art. The concept of *dēn* is possibly attested in Sogdian personal names[428] and it is logical to assume that her image would be found among the wealth of Sogdian divine representations. Azarpay has recently argued that the enthroned goddess from the northern chapel in the Temple II in Panjikent may represent Sogdian Daēnā.[429] However, it is more likely that this goddess is the unique Sogdian rendering of Anāhitā.[430]

As already noted above, one would expect to find representations of Daēnā first of all in funerary contexts. The Sogdian ossuaries carrying figural decorations should therefore prove the most rewarding objects for the study. Grenet has already proposed to recognize Daēnā in the frontal female figure depicted on the ossuary from Changi, near Tashkent (fig. 52)[431] and as a kneeling figure in the upper register of the ossuary from Sivaz.[432] It seems that additional female figures that appear on Sogdian ossuaries may also allude to Sogdian Daēnā. On some Sogdian ossuaries, like that from the Krasnorechensk necropolis[433] or that from Sarytepe, formerly kept in the Samarkand museum (fig. 53),[434] a group of feminine "guardian" figures appears frontally with their hands crossed on their chests.[435] However, this pose in Sasanian art usually characterizes subordinate figures and appears inappropriate for a deity. It is also noteworthy that the figures on the Samarkand ossuary wear typical Sasanian garments and have Sasanian headdresses of round buckles lying on their shoulders.

The unique depiction of the crossing of the Činwad bridge is found on the eastern side of the Sino-Sogdian sarcophagus of Wirkak (579 CE).[436] Based on the account of the journey of the soul after death as recorded in the Zoroastrian scriptures, it is to be expected that Daēnā, who comes to meet the soul at the bridge, would feature prominently as one of the main protagonists in this composition. Indeed, she has been recognized in the winged, crowned female depicted in the center of the right panel, just below the god Wēšparkar.[437] However, it has been convincingly argued that this figure probably depicts not a Zoroastrian Daēnā, but a Manichaean Virgin of Light.[438]

---

426 Miguel-Angel Andrés Toledo has recently challenged the fact that the dogs are actually mentioned in this passage. According to him, the Av. *spānauuaiti* "having two dogs", could be a corruption in the transmission of Av. **spānahŋuuaiti* "endowed with sanctity". See Andrés Toledo 2013: 14–15. However, even if this suggestion is correct, another passage from the *Vīdēvdāt* (13.9) certainly attest to the belief in the two dogs guarding the Bridge where Daēnā is supposed to meet the souls.

427 See p. 39.

428 Lurje 2010: nos. 141, 813, 1285, 1411.

429 Azarpay 2011: 58–60.

430 See p. 78.

431 Grenet and Zhang Guangda 1996: Fig. 3.

432 Grenet 2009: 107. For the description of the ossuary, see p. 84–85.

433 Pugachenkova 1994: Fig. 3.

434 Pavchinskaya and Rostovzev 1988.

435 Grenet 1996: 386, suggest that they could be images of "prayers" or of *fravaši*.

436 Grenet, Riboud and Yang Junkai 2004: 276–278.

437 Grenet, Riboud and Yang Junkai 2004: 282–283.

438 Azarpay 2011: 63–66.

A drawing on paper from Dunhuang kept in the *Bibliothèque nationale de France* dated to the ninth-tenth centuries CE and showing a pair of seated goddesses was interpreted as the images of the "good Dēn" and of the Sogdian goddess Nana as the personification of the "bad Dēn" (fig. 54).[439] The goddess on the right side is four-armed, holding solar and lunar disks and her attributes are a wolf, a snake and a scorpion. The left goddess holds a miniature figure of a dog on a plate and a flower. Based on these attributes, the left goddess could indeed be Dēn. The right goddess is closer to Nana as she is shown in Sogdian art, while her identification as the "bad Dēn" is interesting but not confirmed.[440]

3. *Conclusions*

Daēnā presents one of the most interesting and challenging cases for students of Iranian iconography. On the one hand, there is a rare abundance of written sources describing her physical appearance and at the same time, there are also many possible and even probable candidates, but on the other hand, none of them is certain. We are unable to definitively identify any image of Daēnā in Western Iran although the women holding flowers on Sasanian seals are probably the strongest candidates.

In the East, we do find the appropriate context for the representation of Daēnā—on Sogdian ossuaries—but the evidence is still inconclusive. Perhaps the most interesting case is that of the seal showing a lady with two dogs. If the proposed interpretation of the scene on this seal is accepted, its subject and even some minor details appear remarkably consistent with the beliefs expressed in Zoroastrian texts, which is a noticeable rarity for ancient Iranian iconography. It would also mean that the notion of the *daēnā* as the personification of good deeds accompanied by two dogs and her anthropomorphic representation was known in the eastern Sasanian domains.

11. *Drvāspā*

The goddess Drvāspā (Av. Druuāspā, "possessing solid horses") is the Avestan patron of horses.[441] In the Avesta she is a divinity of minor importance and Yašt 9, dedicated to her, largely reproduces the hymn to the goddess Aši. This fact led Boyce to suggest that Drvāspā was originally an epithet of Aši, which only later developed into an independent deity.[442]

1. *Western Iran*

There is no evidence that Drvāspā was visually represented in Western Iran during any period.

2. *Eastern Iran*

Like the majority of known representations of Iranian gods, Drvāspā appears for the first time on Kushan coins as Lrooaspo (ΛΡΟΟΑCΡΟ). Lrooaspo is depicted on the gold coins of Kanishka and Huvishka (fig. 55).[443] The god stands in profile alongside a horse facing right. On one type he is shown with a nimbus surrounding his head and devoid of any other attributes. On the second, he does not have a nimbus, but wears a diadem with flying ribbons and extends another diadem with his hand. Unlike some deities of the Kushan numismatic pantheon, Lrooaspo was not known under a Greek name on the first minting of Kanishka. However, the most striking feature of Lrooaspo is that he is male, while the Avestan Drvāspā

439 Grenet and Zhang Guangda 1996.
440 See the in-depth discussion by Azarpay 2011: 66–75.
441 See Kellens 1996.
442 Boyce 1975b: 82.
443 Rosenfield 1967: 78–79; Göbl 1984: Arooaspo 1.

is female. This disparity in sex can possibly be explained by differences between Kushan religious notions and Avestan tradition rather than be due to a simple confusion. It is easy to envisage the same divinities being perceived not only as having different functions, but also being of different sex. Despite the change of sex, Lrooaspo clearly retains his role as a patron of horses, since he is depicted standing with a horse.

No other certain visual depiction of Drvāspā has come down to us from the pre-Islamic Iranian world. In Sogdiana Drvāspā is attested in personal names[444] and it has been proposed that a goddess holding a figure of a horse from the wall painting at Temple I, Panjikent constitutes a Sogdian image of the patroness of horses.[445] This figure was reconstructed from the fragments of murals discovered in the fill in the southwestern corner of the temenos wall of Temple I (fig. 56).[446] These paintings originally depicted a group of divinities and several much smaller figures of mortals. The goddess holding a small figure of a horse was part of the composition, consisting of at least six deities and attendants that unfortunately did not survive. Only parts of her upper body and head surrounded by a large ornamented nimbus are preserved. The figure of the horse is indeed an appropriate attribute for Drvāspā. However, given the almost complete absence of Sogdian religious texts, animals often depicted with various Sogdian divinities can rarely serve as a firm and reliable tool for their identification.[447] But in this case, the passage from *Bundahišn* describing Drvāspā holding a horse on her open palm, provides a remarkable parallel to this image and therefore both the Pahlavi text and the Sogdian image might indeed have a common Iranian myth about Drvāspā behind them.[448]

Another possible representation of Drvāspā is a male figure who was also reassembled from numerous fragments of murals uncovered in the fill in the same corner of the temenos wall of Temple I.[449] The best preserved fragment depicts a figure with an elaborately decorated horse (fig. 57). He has a moustache, a nimbus and a flaming halo, which probably surrounded his entire figure and tongues of fire rise from his left shoulder. The man has a sword attached to his belt and holds a lasso (?). On the left hand, there are traces of a poorly preserved Sogdian inscription *y'z(t?) ... 'spy(?)*, which can be translated as "a god with a horse" (?).[450] The original reconstruction of the excavators, Marshak and Raspopova, shows a male character standing before the horse that corresponds exactly to the pose of the Kushan Lrooaspo.[451] However, in the excavations report from season 2002 they claim that their first impression was erroneous and that he is actually mounted on the horse.[452] Nevertheless, if the suggested reading of the inscription on his left hand as "a god with a horse" is correct, this epithet is virtually identical with the name of Drvāspā and therefore the identification of this god with Sogdian Drvāspā is also possible.

3. *Conclusion*

Drvāspā was seemingly not depicted in Western Iran. Her only certain image is that of the male god Lrooaspo portrayed on Kushan coins. Despite the change of sex, Lrooaspo is undoubtedly the "patron of horses" as is the Avestan Drvāspā. It seems that the goddess holding a horse from Panjikent is also to be identified with Drvāspā.

---

444 Lurje 2010: nos. 438, 439.
445 Shkoda 2009: 76; Grenet and Azarnouche 2007/2012: 164.
446 Shkoda 2009: 76.
447 Grenet et al 1993: 65.
448 See p. 35 and n. 254.
449 Shkoda 2009: 76.
450 Shkoda 2009: 76.
451 Grenet notes that the position of this god in front of the horse "is reminiscent of Druwasp (LROOASPO) on Kushan coins". However, since he identifies the goddess with a figure of a horse from Temple I as Drvāspā, he prefers to see the god before the horse as "Wahrām or Tištrya": Grenet and Azarnouche 2007/2012: n. 25.
452 Marshak and Raspopova 2003: 45.

12. *Māh*

The moon god Māh ("moon") is never described as having a human shape in the Avesta or in Middle Persian literature.[453] Even his epithets do not contain any anthropomorphic allusions. Despite this fact, Māh is probably one of the most popular and often depicted divinities in Iranian art.

1. *Western Iran*

The veneration of the moon among Persians is noted already by Herodotus,[454] and the name of the Moon god appears as a compound in some six Old Persian proper names,[455] and in Parthian names from Old Nisa.[456] However, the first and the only image of Māh known from Western Iran is the Sasanian seal from the *Staatliche Münzsammlung* in Munich, which shows a symbolic representation of the moon god (Māh) riding a chariot drawn by two bulls (fig. 58).[457] The frontal bust of the god has a typical Sasanian haircut, beard, and garments decorated with stars. The crescent moon rises like horns behind his head. The chariot is represented by two wheels and the whole composition is surrounded by vine scrolls and stars. The iconography of this seal is very similar to another Sasanian seal formerly in Berlin that depicts a chariot of Mithra and on the seal formerly in the collection of Mohsen Foroughi that shows a male figure riding a chariot drawn by two fantastic birds.[458]

In the Avesta and Middle Persian literature, Māh is never described as a charioteer. The motif of the bull chariot was borrowed from the Graeco-Roman iconography of the moon-goddess Selene.[459] It is noteworthy that as late as the tenth century CE, al-Bīrūnī mentions a Moon chariot harnessed to a fabulous bull while discussing the feasts of the Persians.[460]

Unlike his astral companion Mithra, Māh never appears in Sasanian monumental art. On seals his image also seems to be less popular than that of the sun god and is attested only once.[461] However, he is one of only three or perhaps four deities depicted in Sasanian unofficial art (seals). It is certainly not accidental that Māh also features prominently in Sasanian personal names with ninety-three occurrences, making him the third most popular god in the Sasanian onomasticon.[462] As with Ātar and Mithra, both iconographic data and the evidence of personal names confirm the special place and popularity these three deities enjoyed in the "popular pantheon".

The cult of Māh is not directly attested on the periphery of Western Iran, at least not under his own name. However, Men, a moon god from Asia Minor who was also depicted with a crescent behind his shoulders just like Māh, is portrayed in this manner on coins from Roman Lydia and Pisidia and on other monuments from the Roman period.[463] It is possible that both the name and certain elements in the cult of Men are of Iranian origin and that he was introduced by Iranian settlers to Asia Minor and assimilated into the Phrygian cult.[464]

---

453 For references to Māh in the Avestan and Pahlavi texts, see Gray 1929: 87–89.
454 Hdt. 1.131.
455 Tavernier 2007: 541.
456 For instance, Diakonoff and Livshits 2001: nos. 207:5; 444:6, 537:7.
457 Harper 1978: no. 74.
458 See p. 103 and p. 145.
459 For a discussion of the frontal chariot motif, see p. 103.
460 See p. 43.
461 See below.
462 Gignoux 2005: 38.
463 Van Haeperen-Pourbaix 1983: Figs. 1–4.
464 Van Haeperen-Pourbaix 1983.

2. *Eastern Iran*

In Eastern Iran, the image of the Moon god appears for the first time on the coins of Kanishka. Mao (MAO) is the third most popular deity on the coins of that king and on those of Huvishka (fig. 59; pl. 8).[465] He replaced Selene (CAΛHNH) following the "reform of Kanishka", when the Greek names of the gods on the first issue of Kanishka were changed to their Bactrian names.[466] Göbl divides the images of Mao into ten types.[467] The essential attribute of Mao, found in all types, is a moon crescent behind his shoulders. Other attributes include a staff, a sword, and a diadem. All these attributes (except for the moon crescent, which is also attested with Manaobago) are among the most commonly used by all deities in the Kushan numismatic pantheon. He wears a diadem and a standard Kushan princely outfit. It is worth noting that Mao is never depicted with a nimbus.

Despite his popularity on coins, Mao is absent from the Rabatak inscription. His image, like those of many other Kushan deities is directly inspired by the Graeco-Roman prototypes. The crescent behind his back is also found on Graeco-Roman images of Selene, and in Palmyra, the local Moon god, Aglibol, is rendered with a radiate halo and a moon crescent just behind his head or on top of it. At least on one relief Aglibol is also shown wearing armor.[468] This relief, dated to the first century CE, and similar objects depicting Aglibol, could also have contributed to the formation of the Kushan Mao travelling east all as far as Bactria.

Images of Mao in Kushan Bactria were not limited to coinage alone. His representation is also found on the so-called "Kanishka reliquary", a gilded bronze Buddhist reliquary excavated in 1908 in the Buddhist stupa at Shāh-jī-kī-Dherī, Peshawar.[469] It probably dates to the second half of the second century CE.[470] One of the sides of the casket shows Kanishka between the Moon god (to the left) and the Sun god (to the right) (fig. 60). Mao is depicted with his characteristic crescent moon behind the back, holding a torque or a plain ring in his right hand and placing his left hand on the pommel of a sword. The image of Mao here corresponds almost exactly to his iconography on Kushan coins.

The tradition of representation of the moon god was probably continued after the Sasanian conquest as demonstrated by the silver plate with the moon chariot from the Hermitage. It was part of a hoard containing several items of Sasanian and Byzantine silverware found in 1907 near a village of Klimova, in Russia's Perm district.[471] It is therefore frequently referred to as the "Klimova plate" (pl. 9).[472] It depicts a chariot composed of two parts with two riders drawn by four bulls. The first anthropomorphic figure is shown standing frontally in the lower part of the chariot under an arch and holding a bow and arrow. He is beardless and wears a *kaftan* and a *kulāf*. The second figure sits on a broad, flat throne placed inside a huge crescent that forms the upper part of the chariot. He is seated cross-legged, leaning on a long sword. His dress, hairstyle, and *kulāf* are similar to those of the first individual, but he has a crescent behind his back. To his left, an axe on a long shaft is depicted. Two cupids fly above the bulls, holding the bridles and the whip. The plate is dated by Kamilla Trever and Vladimir Lukonin to the seventh century CE. According to Harper, it exhibits "essential differences from standard Sasanian imagery and the style is unparalleled on Sasanian works of art" and was made "somewhere east of Iran".[473] It was probably created in Sasanian-ruled Bactria and shows extensive Sasanian influence, since depictions

465 Rosenfield 1967: 80–81.
466 Rosenfield 1967: 98.
467 Göbl 1984: Mao 1–10.
468 Colledge 1986: Pl. XXIVb.
469 See Errington 2002.
470 Errington 2002: 106.
471 Trever and Lukonin 1987: no. 15.
472 E.g. Harper 1979: 61.
473 Harper 1979: 61.

of Māh riding a chariot (as well as Mithra and perhaps other deities) appear on Sasanian seals. On this plate, there is, however, an additional interesting attribute—an axe on a long shaft—which is not found together with the Moon god in other examples. This attribute, as well as the cushions, is probably connected to royal symbolism. A similar depiction of a king, seated cross-legged between cushions and holding an axe, was found in Panjikent (50/XXIII, eastern wall).[474] This fact strengthens the connection of the plate with the Eastern Iranian world and suggests that Māh is represented here as the cosmic ruler.

The image of Māh is found in Bactria again only in the seventh century Buddhist monastery at Fondukistan seventeen kilometers northeast of Kabul.[475] The monastery was traditionally dated to the seventh century CE, but is now believed to have been built around 700 CE or in the early eighth century CE.[476] In niche K a fragment of a wall painting was uncovered by the French archaeologists, depicting two standing figures (fig. 61).[477] The left figure is shown standing frontally with a head slightly bowed to the left and legs crossed. He has a long sword and a small round shield attached to his left hand. The character wears a *kaftan* and a crown consisting of three crescents and has large, oval earrings. He is nimbate and has a crescent moon behind his back. The second figure is also painted *en face*, but his head is turned to the right. He has a moustache and a red nimbus. Unlike the figure on the left, he is heavily protected in a scale armor shirt. He carries a long sword attached to his belt, but in another hand he holds an object resembling a mace. Although too considerable an amount of time has lapsed to suppose direct continuation, the similarity with the Kushan Mao and especially with Palmyran Aglibol, is remarkable. Like the latter, the god from Fondukistan is also rendered in full anthropomorphic shape and is armed with a sword. Māh is yet another example of an Iranian deity appropriated by local Buddhist art, like Mithra from Bāmiān.[478]

It was, however, the third type of Māh which would go on to became a popular representation of the god in Sogdiana, where several personal names containing the theonym *māh* are also attested.[479] Judging by the personal name *Māhak* from the Topraq-Qal'a documents, the Moon god was also worshipped in Chorasmia.[480] However, no representations of Māh are currently known from this region. In the rich iconography of the Sogdian city-states Māh was reduced to the symbolic representation of a human head mounted on a crescent moon and locked within a sphere, which is usually held by the goddess Nana together with the sun disk. Such images are known from Panjikent and Ustrushana. The sex of these personifications is not readily distinguishable. In some cases, like that of a painting from Panjikent dated to the first half of the eighth century CE, the Moon divinity appears to be female. It is shown as a bust in three-quarter view facing left and mounted on a crescent moon (pl. 10). It has a headdress resembling a turban and two long plaits.[481] The context of this image is not clear, but according to Marshak it was placed among similar depictions of other celestial bodies that probably had a magical meaning. Pavel Lurje has suggested that this goddess be identified as the deity *xšwm* known to us from Sogdian and Bactrian names.[482] According to Sims-Williams, the name of this divinity derives from "growing moon".[483]

474 Marshak 2002b: Fig. 65.

475 Hackin 1959: 49–59; Litvinskiĭ 2001b, thought that the architectural features of the stupa and the style of decoration suggested an even earlier date and D'yakonov 1954: 149, linked the iconography and style of the Fondukistan paintings to the murals of Panjikent.

476 Novotny 2007: 32.

477 Hackin 1959: 57–58.

478 See p. 89. On Iranian motifs in Buddhist art, see also Scott 1990.

479 Lurje 2010: 639–650.

480 Livshits 2004: 191.

481 Marshak 2009: 7.

482 In a paper presented at the conference "Pre-Islamic Past of Middle Asia and Eastern Iran", which took place at the Hermitage Museum, Saint Petersburg, 23.10.2013–26.10.2013. For the names, see Lurje 2010: nos. 212, 1356; Sims-Williams 2010: no. 558.

483 Sims-Williams 2010: no. 558.

Another Sogdian representation of Māh, which possibly owes something to the distant Kushan Mao and may be iconographically close to the Moon god from Fondukistan, is the god in the second medallion from a bronze plaque in a form of a crescent found at the Sogdian fortress of Jartepa II, located between Samarkand and Panjikent. This plaque is dated to the end of the seventh or the beginning of the eighth century CE.[484] It probably once decorated the lower part of an incense burner and depicts four medallions containing busts (figs. 62–63). The first bust from the left is a beardless feminine figure wearing a high crown and holding a plant in her bended right hand.[485] A triangular object rising from her shoulder possibly represents a tongue of fire (although in the third medallion, the flames are rendered differently). The excavators believe that she originally wore a mural crown,[486] but the upper part of the head is badly damaged and it is impossible to be certain. The character in the next medallion is beardless and has a headdress which widens towards the top. He is characterized by a large crescent moon attached to his back.[487] The third medallion contains the image of a juvenile figure who holds a fire-altar in his right hand. Tongues of fire rise from his left shoulder.[488] The last bust has no attributes, but has a long beard and a crown with astral symbols and a nimbus of dots.[489]

Like the Kushan Mao, the god in the second medallion has a crescent attached to his back, but also wears a high crown—a headdress otherwise attested only on the Fondukistan painting. It is noteworthy, however, that while the Kushan Mao is never shown nimbate or with tongues of fire, in Panjikent the personification of the moon always has these two attributes.

3. *Conclusions*

To summarize, three distinct iconographic types of the moon god can be identified. In Western Iran the only image of Māh rendered as a bearded charioteer appears on the Sasanian seal from the *Staatliche Münzsammlung* in Munich. The composition's conceptual origin is probably to be sought in Graeco-Roman art, but all the iconographic elements and its style are Sasanian. The Kushano-Sasanian Māh from the Klimova plate is a continuation of the Sasanian moon-charioteer transmitted to Bactria, but here he is depicted beardless, possibly reflecting an Eastern Iranian tradition in which the moon god never had a beard. However, the earliest image of the Iranian Moon god is the Kushan Mao whose echoes are probably to be found in Fondukistan and influenced the subsequent development of the third, Sogdian type.

The most characteristic attribute of Māh, which facilitates his identification, is a large crescent moon, usually attached to his back. It is to be noted, however, that the crescent behind the back is not an exclusive attribute of Māh, but is also found in Manaobago and even on one Bactrian image of Nana. In the Kushano-Sasanian and later Bactrian representations, Māh possibly also had a warlike aspect. This can be deduced from the axe that is associated with Māh on the Klimova plate, and, even more so, from the god's appearance at Fondukistan where he is shown as an armored warrior. The headdresses of Māh are also worthy of mention. He wears a variety of headdresses and does not possess any single, distinctive crown like his astral colleague Mithra. The Sasanian charioteer is bareheaded, the Kushan Mao has only a diadem, the enthroned Māh from the Klimova plate wears a *kulāf* and the Sogdian moon god from Jartepa II has a high, elaborate crown.

All images of the moon god, except for that on the Sasanian seal, are beardless indicating that in the East Māh was probably perceived as a young, juvenile god. In Sogdian art, when the Moon deity is

484 Abdullaev and Berdimuradov 1991: 64.
485 Abdullaev and Berdimuradov 1991: 65–66.
486 Abdullaev and Berdimuradov 1991: 71.
487 Abdullaev and Berdimuradov 1991: 66–67.
488 Abdullaev and Berdimuradov 1991: 67–68.
489 Abdullaev and Berdimuradov 1991: 68–69.

paired with Mithra, he is most probably Māh. However, when depicted as female the suggestion by Lurje to identify her as *xšwm* appears quite convincing.

13. *Mithra*

Mithra (MP. *Mihr*) was undoubtedly one of the most important Indo-Iranian and Iranian deities. His name derives from the noun *mitrá* "contract" with the meaning "covenant, agreement, treaty, alliance, promise" and it is generally agreed that the original function of Mithra was the personification of the notion of "contract".[490]

In the Avesta, Mithra does not yet appear in his more familiar role as the Sun or the Sun god, a position occupied by another deity—Xwaršēd—although he is closely associated with it. The endowment of Mithra with the solar functions is in fact a later development, which can perhaps be placed in the Achaemenian period.[491] However, the earliest certain identification of Mithra with the Sun appears in Strabo.[492]

1. *Western Iran*

David Bivar has developed the theory that "Mithraism" was a state religion of the Median kingdom and has associated a great deal of Iranian imagery with Mithra and "Mithraic religion".[493] His theory, however, has not gained acceptance. Despite the fact that Mithra is a popular compound in Achaemenian personal names and is mentioned by Artaxerxes II in his royal inscriptions, no indisputable visual representations of the god exist from the Achaemenian period. However, several candidates for his portrayal have been proposed, and it may therefore be useful to mention at least one of them here—the radiate Apollo on the coins of the Lycian dynast Mithrapata (c. 385 BCE) who was interpreted as Mithra because of the name of the ruler, which contains the god's name.[494]

No image of Mithra is attested in Iran in the Parthian period. This corresponds to the general picture of the almost complete absence of depictions of Iranian deities in Arsacid Iran. It is noteworthy that numerous images of the (Semitic) Sun god are known from Parthian Mesopotamia, notably from cities like Palmyra and Hatra. A radiate divinity was also popular in Elymais and appears on the coins of Susa. Unfortunately, the sex of the deity is unclear and hence he or she is usually identified as Nana, based on the historical sources that attest to the popularity of Nana in Susa.[495] However, on the rock-relief at Tang-i Sarvak II (NE side) dated to the second century CE[496] (fig. 64), the seated deity with a radiating crown appears to have a moustache and could therefore be Mithra, or perhaps a Semitic Sun god popular in neighboring Mesopotamia. A radiate bust also features on the reverse of the coins of the king of Pars, Manučihr I (first half of the second century CE).[497] A similar rayed nimbus is a distinctive attribute of Mithra in later Iranian art. However, no coins of other *frataraka* seem to depict deities and therefore the identification of the figure on the coins of Manučihr I as Mithra must remain conjecture.

The first definite portrayal of Mithra in Western Iran dates from the Sasanian period—a male figure wearing a rayed crown on the reverse of the coins of Ōhrmazd I. As on the first reverse type of this king,

---

490 Schmidt 2006.
491 De Jong 1997: 286.
492 De Jong 1997: 128–129.
493 Most fully described in Bivar 1998.
494 Shahbazi 1985: 504–505.
495 See the discussion on p. 117.
496 Kawami 1987: 89.
497 http://www.parthia.com/pdc_peus386_4.htm

which shows a female figure, the figures of the "attendants" are also placed on the both sides of the altar facing it (fig. 65).[498] The left character again has all the insignia of the king of kings, but instead of holding a rod, he raises his right hand in a gesture of adoration. On the other side of the altar, a male figure wearing a rayed crown is extending a diadem. His other hand rests on the pommel of the sword.[499] Mithra is shown here offering a diadem to the king standing in a pose of adoration on the other side of the fire-altar. This design is evidently borrowed from contemporary Roman coins minted in Samosata that depict Sol.[500]

Mithra is the most popular deity to appear on Sasanian seals. There are four images of the god, two of them depicting a symbolic representation of Mithra riding his solar chariot. According to Bernard Goldman this motif, which shows a frontal chariot of the Sun god with the wheels splayed out in side view in opposite directions, seems to have originated in a Western Asian environment not long before the beginning of the present era. It had become popular in Roman art by the third century CE, spread into Europe, and was then brought back into the Sasanian Empire.[501] Goldman concludes that the Sasanians probably adopted this motif from the Eastern Roman provinces.[502] One seal formerly kept in the *Kaiser Friedrich Museum* in Berlin, but now lost, depicts a frontal bust of a beardless god riding a chariot schematically represented by two wheels and drawn by two winged horses (fig. 66).[503] The god wears a diadem, but no ribbons are shown and he is enclosed in a radiate nimbus. A seal from the *Cabinet des Médailles* in Paris shows a frontal bust of the god (fig. 67). He has no beard or headdress, two globes of hair fall on his shoulders, and a rayed halo surrounds his head.[504] The seal has an inscription identifying the image as *mtry yzdty* "the god Mithra". This is the only known case in Western Iran where the image of this god is identified by an inscription. It is also notorious for the fact that unlike most other representations of the god, here Mithra does not have a round nimbus, but rays of light project directly from his head. The god's headdress is the same as that worn by the god on the Ṭāq-i Bustān relief. The third seal shows the upper part of a body of a figure emerging from a four-wheeled cart decorated with a lion's head (fig. 68).[505] It is beardless and wears a diadem whose ends are shown flying behind the shoulders. The head of the god is surrounded by a rayed nimbus. In one hand he holds a spear and in the other hand an object which is difficult to identify, but by analogy with other examples, it is likely that he grasps the hilt of a sword.

Unlike reliefs and coins, designs on seals were not subject to administrative control and were not an instrument of royal propaganda. Rather, this unofficial medium reflects the preferences of the individual owners of these seals. Therefore, Mithra probably enjoyed a wide popularity with functionaries, nobles and priests, perhaps even being the most popular deity in Sasanian society. The popularity of Mithra among the population of the Sasanian Iran is also supported, albeit indirectly, by the fact that names with the theonym *mihr* are the second most common among personal names with 120 occurrences (after Ātar with 159 occurances).[506] Literary sources also appear to confirm these observations. In Middle Persian literature Mihr is an important eschatological figure and a judge, frequently referred to as the head of a triad of deities consisting of himself, the goddess Anāhīd and Ohrmazd,[507] and it appears

498 Lukonin 1969: 170; Göbl 1971: II, 1; Gyselen 2010a: 78, Fig. 16.
499 Gyselen 2010a: 78, has proposed that his appearance as well as that of the female figure on the first type is linked to the images of Sol and Tyche from contemporary Roman coins.
500 Gyselen 2010a: Figs. 13, 14.
501 Goldman 1988: 88.
502 Goldman 1988: 94.
503 Ghirshman 1962: 243.
504 Gignoux 1978: 62, no. 1972.1317.45, pl. XXII, 6.84; Gyselen 1993 20.G.4.
505 Gignoux and Gyselen 1982: 10.9.
506 Gignoux 2005: 38.
507 Shaked 1994a: 93.

that he was a prominent god in the Western regions of the Sasanian Empire.[508] However, in apparent distinction from his place in popular worship, Mithra was never in a position to challenge the primary place of Ahura Mazdā in royal Sasanian ideology and art. If the story recorded in *Historia Augusta* can be trusted,[509] the images of Mithra decorated not only seals, but also Sasanian silver plates. The existence of such plates is certainly probable given the fact that the Kushano-Sasanian Klimova (?) plate depicts a chariot of Māh.

Another possible image of the chariot of Mithra in Western Iran adorns the stone casket from Bīšāpūr.[510] One of the narrow sides of this object shows a partially preserved representation of two winged, raised horses, which were probably a symbolic rendering of the chariot of Mithra, as it is depicted on seals.

The image of radiate Mithra at Ṭāq-i Bustān is the only image of the god on monumental rock-reliefs (fig. 69). This remarkable relief represents the investiture on foot, which saw a revival in Sasanian monumental art under Narseh.[511] However, the composition of this relief is original and departs from the first "foot investiture" scenes of Ardašīr I at Fīrūzābād and Naqš-e Rağab. In terms of style it is noteworthy that the figures are represented not in full profile, as before, but in three-quarter profile. In addition, as far as the iconography is concerned, there are several important innovations. The king is portrayed in the center, reaching for the diadem offered to him by Ahura Mazdā, who stands to the right in royal attire with his usual crenellated uncovered crown. Both the king and the god stand on the body of a defeated enemy, who is probably to be identified with the Roman emperor Julian the Apostate.[512] Behind the king, on a giant lotus flower, stands Mithra wearing a rayed crown and holding a *barsom* in his both hands. The relief at Ṭāq-i Bustān is, in fact, the first occasion in which a second deity, in addition to Ahura Mazdā, appears in the investiture scene on the rock-reliefs of the Sasanian kings. (Although Mithra here is not an investing deity himself, but merely "assists" Ahura Mazdā.) It is not clear why the Sasanian sovereign depicted at Ṭāq-i Bustān (be it Šāpūr II or Ardašīr II) did not "confine himself" to Ahura Mazdā, but added an additional divinity—Mithra. The lotus flower on which Mithra is standing was used as a symbol by the Kushano-Sasanian dynasty[513] and this perhaps points to Eastern connections or sources of inspiration. An interesting idea was expressed by Dominique Hollard, who supports the identification of a defeated enemy under the feet of Ahura Mazdā at Ṭāq-i Bustān and the Sasanian king as the Roman emperor Julian the Apostate. He suggests that Mithra was depicted here because Julian relied on the protection of Sol-Mithra in his campaign against Persia.[514] At Ṭāq-i Bustān, Mithra has a beard, while on the Sasanian seals the god is always depicted beardless. An additional detail is a *barsom*—an attribute unattested with any other image of Mithra in the Iranian world. On other Sasanian reliefs, a *barsom* is commonly held by Ahura Mazdā, and perhaps it had special significance in the context of symbolizing the divine investiture.

---

508 Shaked 1994a: 92.

509 See p. 18.

510 See p. 75.

511 The identity of the king depicted on this relief is subject to scholarly debate. Some have opted for Šāpūr II: Lukonin 1969: n. 22, 146–150; Vanden Berghe 1984: no. 79; Vanden Berghe 1984: 1529; while others prefer Ardašīr II: Schmidt 1970: 137; Ghirshman 1975: 125; Shahbazi 1987; Harper 1999: 315; Herrmann and Curtis 2002; Fukai and Horiuchi 1972 Pl. LXXIV–XCII; Rose 2005; Canepa 2009: 108–111 and 287–288: n. 64, 65; or Ardašīr III: Tanabe 1984: 40. All sides have put forward various stylistic and historical arguments but it seems that if the defeated foe is indeed Julian the Apostate, then the Sasanian king must be Šāpūr II. According to Calmeyer 1977: 187–188 and Shahbazi 1987, this relief depicts an investiture of Ardašīr II by his brother Šāpūr II, but this interpretation seems highly improbable, since on all other Sasanian royal rock-reliefs the king is invested by a deity; and only on the Salmās relief of Ardašīr I do he and his son probably invest local rulers who are clearly shown as inferior to the Sasanians. See Vanden Berghe 1984: no. 54.

512 See Hollard 2010: 156–157.

513 Grenet 2003a: 36.

514 Hollard 2010.

It is possible that the winged horses—a common motif on Sasanian seals—could also be an aniconic representation of Mithra and reproduce an aniconic version of the chariot, where the bust of the god and the wheels are altogether omitted.[515] One seal with protomes of two winged horses carries the inscription *dād-burz-mihr aspbed ī pahlaw panēh ō burzēn-mihr* "Dād-burz-mihr, a Parthian aspbed, protection in (the Fire) Burzēn-mihr", apparently adding weight to this suggestion,[516] although it should be noted that on this seal the horses are facing each other as opposed to their positions in representations of the solar chariot.

Although Mithra was undoubtedly worshipped in Armenia, the existence of his idols is not explicitly recorded by in Armenian sources. However, one of the Armenian terms for sanctuary—*mehean*—derives from the name of this god and we may safely conclude that statues of Mithra existed in these temples. It is noteworthy that Movsēs Xorenac'i identifies Armenian Mihr not with Helios or Apollo, but with Hephaestus.[517] This may signify that Armenian Mihr had a profoundly manifested fiery aspect, but was not directly associated with the Sun.[518] It is therefore not clear whether the statue of the sun erected by king Vaḷarshak at Armavir was, in fact, an idol of Mihr.[519] The Georgian sources do not refer to Mithra and therefore the existence of his cult in K'art'li cannot be confirmed.

2. *Eastern Iran*

As in Western Iran, the beginnings of the pictorial representation of Mithra in the Eastern Iranian world have been sought in the Achaemenian period. To cite just one example, it was proposed that the statuette of a nude youth wearing a tiara from the Oxus Treasure is the image of Bactrian Mithra dated to the Late Achaemenian period.[520] This suggestion is based primarily on the shape of the tiara, which is similar to that of Mithra from Commagene (fig. 70).

Herodotus and Strabo record that the Scythian Massagetae worshipped the sun as their only god.[521] Unfortunately, there is no means of knowing whether the "sun" here refers to Mithra, or possibly to some other deity derived, for instance, from the Iranian Xwaršēd. Be that as it may, there is no certain representation of Mithra from Scythian or Saka art, although depictions of the solar chariot of "Mithra-Helios" have been recognized on objects from Bosporus. The golden plaque from Gorgippia dated to the end of the first century BCE or the beginning of the first century CE, shows a Sun god wearing a rayed crown, riding a quadriga, and holding a whip in his right hand.[522] The chariot is rendered symbolically by two wheels; the sign of a crescent and a six-pointed star are depicted above the god's head. A silver detail of a horse harness from the Fedulovo hoard (which was probably manufactured in Bosporus) portrays a frontal bust of the Sun god in a radiate crown, riding in a chariot represented by two opposing protomes of horses (fig. 71).[523] These objects are usually connected by scholars with the Aspurgiani tribes of presumably Sarmatian, Iranian descent.[524] Therefore, they have been interpreted as visual representations of Mithra-Helios.[525] However, the place that Mithra possibly occupied in the Scythian and Bosporan pantheons is anything but clear and the interpretation of the solar rider as Mithra is conjectural. The god from the Fedulovo hoard is remarkably similar to Sasanian images

515 There are numerous examples. See for instance Gyselen 1993 40.1–40.18.
516 Gyselen 2003 Pl. 4d.
517 See p. 20.
518 On Armenian Mihr, see Russell 1987: 261–289.
519 See p. 21.
520 Carter 2005.
521 Hdt. 1.216; Strab. 9.513. On the horse in Scythian art and religion, see Kuz'mina 2002: 46–74.
522 Saprykin 1983: Fig. 1.
523 Saprykin 1983: Fig. 3.
524 Saprykin 1983: 70.
525 Saprykin 1983.

of the chariot of Mithra and especially to the seal that was formerly kept in the *Kaiser Friedrich Museum* in Berlin and to the bulla from Ak-Depe uncovered by Soviet archaeologists in 1963–1978 at the site of Ak-Depe (Southern Turkmenistan). Among fragments of over one hundred bullae there were seven imprints of a seal depicting a bust in a chariot drawn by horses (fig. 72).[526] The bust is shown frontally with his rayed crown around his head and locks of hair falling to his shoulders. The chariot is symbolically rendered by two rampant horses flanking the god and by two connected wheels below it. On one sealing it is possible to read the inscription [...] (*s*)*p dpywr W mgwy p'tyn,* "(... as)p, scribe and mage, (son of) Frayen". We may therefore assume that this seal was in the possession of a mage. Based on the stratigraphy, the sealings have been dated to the late sixth or the first half of the seventh century CE.[527]

Mithra is the most popular theophoric component in personal names from Old Nisa, far superseding all others. However, no Parthian image of the god is known. It is often thought that the earliest evidence for the influence of Iranian Mithra on the iconography of Greek deities is the rayed nimbus around the head of Heracles on the coins of the Graeco-Bactrian king Demetrius II.[528] Later, a radiate halo appears as an attribute of a Zeus-like figure on the coins of king Heliocles I (ca. 145–130 BCE) (fig. 73). Under the kings Amyntas and Hermaeus (ca. 95–70 BCE), he acquires a tiara. The tiara and nimbus were understood as an allusion to Mithra and taken as evidence that in Eastern Iran, Zeus was identified with the Iranian solar god.[529] A more likely candidate for the "Graeco-Bactrian Mithra" is Helios riding a quadriga on the coins of Plato (145–140 BCE) (fig. 74). The Iranians would have obviously "read" this image as Mithra, but there is no evidence that it was perceived by the Greek overlords as anyone other than Helios. It also should be noted that the first certain images of Iranian Mithra postdate these coins by some three hundred years, being themselves modeled on Graeco-Roman images of Sol-Helios and perhaps also on the representations of Mesopotamian and Syrian solar deities, such as Palmyran Malakbel.

The first image of Mithra in Eastern Iran is also commonly associated with the nameless Kushan king who minted coins bearing only his title "Soter Megas" ("The Great Savior").[530] The obverse of the coins of this ruler shows a diademed and nimbate bust facing right and holding an arrow (fig. 75). It is beardless and has a Greek appearance. Specialists have yet to reach a consensus whether Soter Megas was a son and successor of Kujula Kadphises (Vima Takto) or a military leader, perhaps of Greek origin,[531] who usurped the throne and held it for some fifteen years (c. 92/97–110 CE), but failed to establish a dynasty.[532] Besides his name, the coins of Soter Megas also pose additional problems. Although the iconography of the bust on the obverse indeed seems to be that of the solar Apollo on the coins of Hellenistic kings and on those of their nomadic successors, the obverse was usually reserved for the ruler's portrait, while the reverse typically depicted an image of a deity.[533] This holds true for all coins of the Graeco-Bactrian rulers (with the exception of the aforementioned coin of Hermaeus), for the issues of the Kushan kings and in fact, for most Iranian coins in general.[534] If Soter Megas was indeed a Greek, he may have depicted himself as Apollo with a rayed royal diadem, in similar fashion to Alexander portrayed as Heracles. Even if this bust represents Apollo, there is no certainty that he was understood as Mithra, although this would obviously be a natural interpretation for Apollo in the Iranian cultural sphere. One should also note the close similarity between this image of Apollo and the rayed bust on the coin of Manučihr I, king of Pars.

---

526 Gubaev 1971; Lukonin 1971; Gubaev, Loginov and Nikitin 1996, Sealing 1.3.
527 Gubaev, Loginov and Nikitin 1996: 55. Earlier Lukonin 1971: 51, proposed to date the bullae to the fifth-seventh c. CE.
528 E.g. Staviskiy 1977: 157.
529 Grenet 1991; Boyce and Grenet 1991: 162–165.
530 E.g. MacDowall 1975: 146–147; Grenet 2006.
531 Bopearachchi 2008: 45.
532 See the discussion in Bopearachchi 2008: 44–45 and Bopearachchi 2012: 128–133.
533 Mac Dowall 2007: 233.
534 Errington and Cribb 1992: 48–49.

The first unquestionable portrayal of Mithra in Eastern Iran and indeed in the entire Iranian world is the Kushan Miiro (MIIPO) who replaced HΛIOC on the coins of Kanishka as the second most popular reverse design, and also continued to be used on the issues of his successor Huvishka (figs. 76–79; pl. 11).[535] Miiro is one of the most popular gods to appear on Kushan coins and he concludes the Rabatak god list.[536] His statue was kept in the sanctuary at Rabatak and probably in other Bactrian Kushan temples as well. Göbl has divided all representations of Miiro into eleven types, with the last type being that of the Kushano-Sasanian king Ardašīr I. Like most other deities of the Kushan numismatic pantheon, Miiro is shown standing in full profile, facing right or left. Most of his attributes are common to the other gods depicted on Kushan coins: a spear, a sword with a pommel shaped in the form of a bird's head, and a diadem. On three types,[537] Miiro makes a gesture of blessing/benefaction, which he shares with another astral deity—Mao. An unusual and unique attribute shared by Miiro and his astral companion Mao is the torque that he holds on type 3. Miiro wears a diadem like many other Kushan deities, but has a distinctive rayed nimbus, emphasizing his solar character. It is, however, interesting to note that on one type (no. 7) Miiro has only a plain nimbus.

David Mac Dowall has argued that Miiro "ultimately stems from Zeus-Helios of the barbarous Heliocles type coins, the radiate solar Zeus of Hermaeus' issues, and the radiate bust found on coinage of the nameless Soter Megas".[538] However, there is no reason to distinguish the image of the Kushan Miiro from representations of other gods in the Kushan numismatic pantheon. Most of them were undoubtedly created at the same time (during the reigns of Kanishka and Huvishka), as a single group, mostly following Roman prototypes. In this respect Miiro is no different from other Kushan deities. All of his attributes, with the exception of the unusual torque in place of the expected diadem and radiate halo, are common to other gods and goddesses. There appear to be no grounds for deriving Miiro from the images on the coins of Heliocles, Hermaeus and Soter Megas, whom he does not even resemble.

An unusual image of Miiro is found on the "Kanishka reliquary",[539] where he flanks the Kushan king together with the Moon god Māh. Miiro extends a diadem to Kanishka, and appears to be wearing a headdress resembling a Phrygian cap—an element not found on his coin portraits where he is depicted wearing only a diadem. It is noteworthy that the only other occasion on which Iranian Mithra is depicted with such headdress is found on the other end of the Iranian world, in the kingdom of Commagene on the upper Euphrates. Here, Mithra, identified with no less than three Greek gods—Helios, Apollo and Hermes—shakes hands with the local king Antiochus I (62–37 BCE).

Fortunately, the Kushan tradition of labeling deities on the reverses of their coins was not abandoned after the Sasanian conquest of Bactria. Two coins of the Kushano-Sasanian king Ardašīr I minted in Balkh depict the enthroned Mithra offering a diadem and grasping a sword. The god is shown in three-quarter view facing right (pl. 12).[540] He extends a diadem with his right hand and his left hand grasps the hilt of a long sword placed between his knees. The Bactrian legend reads BAΓO MIYPO, "The god Mithra". The god sits on a throne with a high back. He is bearded, wears a diadem with ribbons falling down his back and his head is surrounded by a rayed nimbus. His dress, pose, and in particular his hairstyle, are typically Sasanian. A diadem and sword are also the typical attributes of the god on the Kushan coins. However, the Kushano-Sasanian portrayal of Mithra is utterly different and reveals direct Sasanian influence, especially in the rendering of the dress and the hairstyle. The composition

535 Rosenfield 1967: 81–82; Göbl 1984: Miiro. See also Mac Dowall 1975: 148–149.
536 See p. 12–13.
537 Göbl 1984: Miiro 1, 2, 8.
538 Mac Dowall 1975: 142.
539 See p. 99.
540 Cribb 1990: nos. 14, 15.

of enthroned deity is also never found in Sasanian art and apparently reflects a local, Bactrian tradition. One may speculate that this composition reproduces real statues of Mithra that stood in Bactrian temples. A further image of Mithra from Kushanshahr is the "Sasanian" Mithra on the coin of Kushano-Sasanian king Ōhrmazd I, minted in Merv, and copied from the coins of the Sasanian king Ōhrmazd I (pl. 13).

A Sasanian seal manufactured in one of the Sasanian-dominated regions of Eastern Iran and now kept in the British Museum shows the god rising from a mountain, which has been convincingly interpreted as an allusion to Mount Harā, from which Mithra, according to the Avestan passage, "surveys the whole material world".[541] The god is shown as a frontal bust on top of a mountain, represented by a pyramid of round rocks. He is beardless and does not wear a crown, only a diadem indicated by the flying ribbons. The god turns his head three-quarters towards a worshipper standing frontally and stretching his hands in a gesture of adoration before the deity. The god holds a short spear in one hand and is entirely encircled in a nimbus with projecting, spiked rays. His other hand probably rests on the hilt of a sword, as Grenet has suggested.[542] The headdress or hairstyle of the worshipper involves two thin ribbons or pigtails. At waist level, two thin ribbons with forked ends appear on either side. The seal may be dated to the late fourth or fifth century CE.

Although an association with the Avestan myth of Mithra appears plausible, the iconographic convention employed here by the Sasanian artisan in fact corresponds to depictions of the Mesopotamian Sun-god Shamash, who is sometimes shown emerging from a mountain.[543] The stance, the attributes, and the floating ribbons of the god on this seal are also similar to the Sasanian seal of Mithra in a four-wheeled cart. Therefore, this type of Mithra, later elaborated at Bāmiān, was probably imported from Western Iran. It is also possible that the worshipper depicted on the British Museum seal standing before Mithra is a priest, since his headdress is similar to one of the types attested among mages on Sasanian seals[544] and the double ropes that are depicted on both sides of his body probably represent the sacred girdle, *kustig*.

Like other Iranian deities included in the Kushan pantheon, such as Mao, the image of Mithra is also found in a Buddhist context in Bactria, on a wall-painting from Fondukistan. Here, Mithra has a moustache and a red nimbus, but most noteworthy is his appearance as a fully armored warrior-god, holding a sword and probably a mace, which is his favored weapon in the Avesta. Another representation of Mithra connected with Buddhist remains is the painting from Bāmiān. This painting, described as "the daily epiphany of Mithra as described in the *Mihr Yašt*", is the most elaborate version of the solar chariot of Mithra found in Iranian art, and is an extended version of the scene shown on the British Museum seal.[545] While it is clear that the figure of the god on both monuments is based on the same—probably Sasanian—prototype, the compositions and the meaning they were intended to convey are essentially different. The Bāmiān painting depicts a well-known (albeit the most detailed) composition of Mithra riding his solar chariot, whereas the British Museum seal shows the god rising from Mount Harā. Nevertheless, and rarely for ancient Iranian art, both compositions seem to agree with the Avestan passages.

A remarkably similar chariot of Mithra accompanied by two characters is depicted on a seal said to be found in Gandhāra (fig. 80).[546] The seal carries a Kharoṣṭhī inscription *arjuṇasa* "Of Arjuna". The pose and the attributes of the god—and the attributes of the two other charioteers—are almost identical to

541 Yt. 10. 51; Callieri 1990: 84; Grenet 2003a: 37–38.
542 Grenet 1993/1994: 87.
543 Callieri 1990: 84; Ornan 2005a: 39.
544 Gyselen 1990: Fig. 2.D.
545 Grenet 2006.
546 Ur Rahman and Falk 2011: no. 06.08.02. For a detailed discussion, see Shenkar forthcoming b.

those in Bāmiān. The most significant difference is that on the seal the head and shoulders of Mithra are surrounded by a plain nimbus, whereas on all other representations of the god in Iranian art he is always shown with a radiating nimbus—his distinctive attribute.[547] This variation, however, could be explained by the unsophisticated and schematic execution of the seal, and perhaps also by the fact that it was manufactured in the Indian cultural sphere. Additional evidence for the identification of the god on the seal with Mithra is provided by the inscription. Apart from the famous archer hero of the *Mahābhārata*, Arjuna was also the name of one of the Pārata kings who ruled over the area centered in the town of Lorarai in northwestern Pakistani Balochistan between c. 125–300 CE, according to the chronology proposed by Pankaj Tandon.[548] However, at certain periods their rule extended to southern Arachosia with Kandahar serving as their capital.[549] Of the fifteen personal names of rulers attested on the coins of Pāradān, thirteen are Iranian.[550] Six have the theophoric component *mira* (mithra) in their names, which seems to suggest the close association of the royal dynasty with the cult of Mithra. It is possible that this seal was actually owned by an individual devoted to Mithra who lived during under the later Pāratarājas or even after the disintegration of their rule in the fourth century.

The unique painting of Doḵtar-e Nōšervān discovered in 1924 in one of the niches of the rock-cut complex in the Ḵolm valley of northern Afghanistan, which probably dates from the beginning of the eighth century CE, has also been argued to represent Mithra.[551] It is badly damaged, but an image of an enthroned deity seated under an arcade can be traced in the center of the painting (fig. 81). The god, who is depicted frontally, wears unusual heeled shoes and has a long sword placed between his legs.[552] The throne is supported by two protomes of an ungulate animal, possibly a horse or a ram. The deity has an elaborate composite crown consisting of a frontal lion's head with large, curved horns, placed between a pair of wings. This hybrid headdress has parallels on Sasanian seals.[553] The head of the god is encircled in a tripartite nimbus from which the figures of animals emerge—four from each side. On the right side, there is an elephant, probably a goose,[554] a lion, and a bull, and on the left side, a ram and an ibex. The pose and sword of the deity correspond to Sasanian and Sogdian examples, while the zoomorphic halo, which is unattested in Iran, is reminiscent of that of Viṣṇu on some Indian monuments.[555] This god is probably the only one preserved from a much larger composition of several divine figures placed under arches that is well known from Sogdian ossuaries,[556] and it is therefore possible that he was not the most important deity depicted in this shrine.

The association of the Doḵtar-e Nōšervān god with Mithra is based on the presumed identification of the Sogdian god who sits on a throne supported by the foreparts of two horses as Mithra.[557] However, roughly contemporary images of Mithra from Fondukistan located not far from Doḵtar-e Nōšervān, and a slightly earlier painting from Bāmiān, are completely different. It is well known from Arab sources[558]

---

547 The only other exception is one type of Miiro on Kushan coins. See p. 107.

548 Tandon 2012: 34.

549 Tandon 2012: 43.

550 Tandon 2012, p. 27.

551 See Mode 1992; Klimburg-Salter 1993; Grenet 1995; Mode 1996; Compareti 2008: 137, n. 21 with references to previous studies.

552 The only parallel to heeled shoes that I am aware of is found on the standing figure on the Elymaean relief at Hung-i Kamālvand. See Vanden Berghe and Schippmann 1985: 43–46.

553 Grenet 1995: 116–117.

554 The interpretation of Grenet 1995: 110. Klimburg-Salter prefers a horse.

555 Loth 2003: 56–57, fig. 38. Grenet 1995, interprets the animals as astral and zodiac symbols. See also Grenet and Pinault 1997: 1052–1053.

556 For instance, the ossuaries from Biyanajman and Miankal.

557 Grenet 1995: 108. The French scholar has recently changed his opinion in favor of identification with Zūn. For the discussion, see below.

558 See p. 42.

and Bactrian documents from the kingdom of Rōb, that a deity called Zūn was the most important god in this region in Late Antiquity. It is therefore also possible that it is Zūn who is depicted at Doḵtar-e Nōšervān.[559]

In Sogdian onomastics Mithra was not usually referred to name, but was simply known as "Baga" ("the God").[560] However, it is interesting to note that Mithra is attested under his own name in the Chorasmian documents from Topraq-Qalʿa and Koi-Krylgan-kala.[561] Only two definite images of Mithra belonging to two different types are known from Sogdian art. The first is a sealing (no. 338) that was part of a unique assemblage of 411 bullae uncovered from the ruins of the Sogdian citadel of Kafir-Kala, some 11.7 km. from Samarkand.[562] The bullae are most probably dated to the early eighth century CE.[563] The sealing depicts a standing deity facing right with the body in three-quarter view and the head in profile (fig. 82).[564] His head is encircled in a rayed nimbus. The god offers a diadem to a male worshipper standing before him that carries a spear. The god on the Kafir-Kala sealing is very similar to the Miiro on Kushan coins.[565] In fact, the similarity is so striking that from a purely iconographic point of view one would place them in the same period and cultural milieu. However, their archaeological contexts are separated by half a millennium and they were found in neighboring, but nevertheless different, geographical areas. Be that as it may, there can be little doubt that Mithra from Kafir-Kala is a direct descendant of the Kushan Miiro. Furthermore, it is quite possible that this sealing was actually made by a Kushan-period seal, which was still in use in the Sogdian era.[566]

The second example is the representation on a fragment of a wooden frieze (2 m. long, 0.6 m. high) from Panjikent VII/11 decorated with carvings of two figures beneath arches (fig. 83).[567] Under the first arch from the right, there is a depiction of an enthroned figure. The state of its preservation is poor and only the zoomorphic throne composed of two gryphons can be seen clearly. The second arch contains a schematic representation of a charioteer. This individual is shown frontally with his head rendered in three-quarter view and turned to the left. He wears what appears to be a crenellated crown. His left leg is tucked beneath and with his left hand he holds a bridle. It is not clear what he originally had in his raised right hand, but it was perhaps a whip. The chariot is symbolically represented by two rampant horses and two wheels depicted below them. At first glance the image on the Panjikent frieze appears to follow a Sasanian type of symbolic representation in which Mithra rides his solar chariot (as in the image on the bullae from Ak-Depe). However, there are significant differences which point to a specifically Sogdian adaptation of the image. The wheels symbolizing the chariot are not depicted between the horses and the bust of the god as on Sasanian seals and at Bāmiān, but are placed below and to the side of the horses. The figure of the god also departs from the Sasanian examples. Mithra is shown here in a typically Sogdian posture with one leg tucked beneath, which is borrowed from Indian art, and it is noteworthy that the bridle that he holds with his left hand and a crenellated crown on the god's head are unattested on other images of the solar god. Another distinctive feature of this wooden relief is the depiction of horses without wings, unlike that found in Sasanian art. This detail is important for the identification

---

559 Grenet 2006. See p. 130 for further discussion of the Doḵtar-e Nōšervān painting and the proposed identification between Zūn and Oxus.

560 Sims-Williams 1991. The original meaning of the word *baga* is "distributor, dispenser", from the root *bag* "to distribute, allot". The meaning "god" is a later development securely attested for the first time in Achaemenian royal inscriptions. See Sims-Williams 1989.

561 Livshits 2004: 191.

562 Cazzoli and Cereti 2005.

563 Cazzoli and Cereti 2005: 137.

564 Cazzoli and Cereti 2005: 153–154.

565 Especially Göbl 1984 Miiro 7.

566 However, see also Compareti 2013: 136–137, who believes that this seal is a Sasanian import.

567 Belenitskiy 1973: 35.

of the Sogdian god on a throne supported by the foreparts of horses whose representations are known from Panjikent and Ustrushana.

The god on the horse throne from Panjikent is depicted on a painting excavated in 1972 on a sidewall in one of the private houses.[568] He is depicted seated cross-legged on a large throne supported by two horses (fig. 84). A long sword is placed on his knees. Only the lower part of his body is preserved and other details are lost. The huge deity from Ustrushana is painted in the center of the western wall of the "Small Hall", in front of the entrance, seated on a zoomorphic throne (fig. 85).[569] He is depicted *en face* in a slightly relaxed pose, leaning on his right elbow. The god wears jewelry and richly embellished garments. Especially noteworthy is an image of a winged horse that decorates one cuff of his dress. In his right hand he holds a scepter or a similar object and his left hand is placed on the hilt of a sword shaped in the form of a dragon's head. A short dagger attached to his belt has a hilt in the form of a griffon's head. The upper part of the painting is badly effaced and a fragment of a pointed beard is all that survives from the god's face and head. His throne is supported by two protomes of horses.

Both these deities are usually identified by specialists as Mithra.[570] Unfortunately, on all images of the Sogdian god only one of his attributes—a sword—can be easily recognized. The second object that he holds in his right hand is not preserved on the painting from Panjikent, but on the huge figure of the god from the western wall of the "Small Hall" at Ustrushana, it seems to be a kind of scepter. Below, I suggest that this god might in fact be Oxus.[571]

In the surviving fragments of the paintings from the "Small Hall" at Bunjikat, Ustrushana, the kingly figure in the chariot drawn by winged horses is found no less than five times on the northern, southern, and eastern walls. The two best-preserved images are on the northern and eastern wall. This male figure on the northern wall is depicted in the middle of the second register seated cross-legged in a chariot drawn by winged horses (fig. 86).[572] The chariot carries a tent-like rectangular construction with a triangular roof topped by a crescent combined with another element resembling a quadrifoliate flower. Exactly the same combination of symbols are also found atop a winged crown worn by the character. He has a short, accurately cut beard, a thin linear hint of a moustache, and wears a yellow-golden *kaftan*. In his right hand, the charioteer holds an object resembling a mace, or perhaps a short scepter. His left hand is not preserved. A dagger and sword are attached to his belt. A second well-preserved image of the same individual is painted on the eastern wall leading a group of heavily armed equestrians, facing the goddess Nana in the left corner of the lower register (fig. 87).[573] The chariot is drawn by winged horses and its decorations and the facial features of the rider are identical to those on the northern wall (fig. 88). There are, however, several significant differences. Here, the character is kneeling instead of sitting cross-legged; the crown is replaced by a helmet, although still surmounted by a crescent and "quadrifoliate flower"; he wears complex armor, is armed with a sword and a dagger and holds a long spear in his hand (Sokolovskiy proposes that this could be a trident instead);[574] And his right open palm is turned towards Nana in a gesture of greeting or adoration.

The excavators interpreted this character as the divine warrior-king.[575] He is undoubtedly the main protagonist of this cycle of paintings, and seems to lead the gods in their struggle against demons.

---

568 Belenitskii and Marshak 1981: 70.
569 Sokolovskiy 2009: 32–34.
570 Grenet 1993/1994: 87; Marshak 1999: 183; Grenet 2006. The identification by Negmatov 1984: 150–151 of him as the deified king, the ancestor of the ruling dynasty, was convincingly refuted by Shkoda 1980: 60–63; Shkoda 2009: 82–83.
571 See p. 130.
572 Sokolovkiy 2009: 42–43.
573 Sokolovkiy 2009: 46–47.
574 Sokolovkiy 2009: 47.
575 Negmatov 1984: 153; Skolovskiy 2009: 46.

This fact alone is sufficient to also identify him with the huge god on the horse throne depicted in the center of the western wall in the "Small Hall". It is also noteworthy that a scene from the same cycle, featuring a hero in a chariot and the goddess Nana engaged in a fight against demons, is apparently also found in Panjikent III/6. These paintings probably reproduce a Sogdian myth, which was well known to contemporaries, but unfortunately remains a complete mystery to us. On the two best-preserved examples the Ustrushana heroic charioteer does not have a nimbus—a common iconographic attribute of the divine in Sogdian art. However, it is important to note that the other unquestionably divine figures that feature in the decoration of the "Small Hall", Nana and Wešparkar, also do not have a nimbus. In addition, a nimbus surrounding the head of the huge god on the western wall of the "Small Hall" is in fact a hypothetical reconstruction and is not grounded in remaining fragments of the painting itself. These observations seem to put the divine nature of the figure in the chariot with the winged horses beyond reasonable doubt.

Discussion of possible Sogdian representations of Mithra would not be complete without mentioning the unique wooden statue found in 1979 by three schoolchildren in a cave in the Surkh Mountains near the villages of Zeravshan and Sarvoda in modern Tajikistan (fig. 89).[576] The statue is made of birch wood and is one m. high. It depicts a naked male figure with carefully modeled mustache and genitals (fig. 90). Although found naked, the holes and the remains of nails indicate that it was originally draped and had shoes, one of which was discovered in the same cave. The right hand of the male figure originally grasped an object, perhaps a scepter, part of which, topped with three figures of goats, was found together with the statue.[577] Additional items including nine mirrors, chainmail armor, remains of the scabbard of a sword, a dagger and a brass plaque in the form of a crescent moon combined with a sun that was originally attached to his headdress, were also discovered hidden in the cave during further investigations by the archaeologists. They were undoubtedly part of the same hoard and some of the items belonged to the original attire of the statue, which was probably adorned with elaborate garments, dressed in chainmail and armed with a sword and dagger. Because of the brass plaque with the combined crescent moon and sun disk image originally attached to his headdress, it has been proposed that this statue depicted Mithra.[578] However, this symbol is a common feature on the crowns of various Sogdian divinities and is not specific to Mithra.

Curious evidence for a possible statue of Mithra in Eastern Iran is found in the works of Varāhamihira, an Indian astronomer active in the early sixth century CE, who tells us of the "Maga", priests of the solar cult who were brought to India by a local king to serve in his newly built temple to a sun god.[579] They brought together with them a "sacred idol, a gilded image of the sun in anthropomorphic shape". Before the arrival of the Maga, it is said that the sun was venerated in India only in an aniconic form of a disk.[580] Carter has suggested that these Maga were Iranian priests from Sistan, who came to India in the third century CE, perhaps being expelled, according to one suggestion, through the actions of Kartīr.[581] If this is so, it is reasonable to assume that the statue that the Maga carried with them originally depicted an Iranian Mithra. Especially curious is the fact that this story credits Iranians with the introduction of the anthropomorphic statues into a previously aniconic Indian cult. It is also interesting to note that *Tārīkh-i Sīstān* mentions a temple of the sun (*khvarshīd*), distinct from a local fire-temple, which existed in Sistan by the time of the Muslim invasion.[582] This could well be a sanctuary dedicated specifically to Mithra.

---

576 Mukhtarov 1982: 14–20; Yakubov 1996: 38–42.
577 Yakubov 1996: 39.
578 Mukhtarov 1982: 16–17.
579 See Carter 1981: 80–82.
580 Carter 1981: 81.
581 Carter 1981: 86–87.
582 *TS* 93.

Al-Masʿūdī tells a story of another "temple of the Sun" built by king Kavus in Ferghana and destroyed by the Arabs.[583]

Returning to Sogdian art, the personification of the sun that the goddess Nana often holds in her raised hands together with that of the moon could allude to Mithra. The saddled, riderless horse, which frequently appears in Sogdian art in cultic scenes, is also sometimes understood as dedicated to Mithra.[584] However, this suggestion is primarily based on the evidence of Greek historians from the Achaemenian period, who often mention that horses were sacrificed by the Iranians to the Sun.[585] It appears that at least at one instance, on the so-called "Miho couch", this horse is likely to be a personification of the god Oxus.[586]

The image of the solar god riding a chariot eventually spread beyond the eastern fringes of the Iranian world. Three textiles discovered in the tombs in Dulan and Astana in Xinjiang depict a deity seated frontally on a quadriga drawn by winged horses, dated perhaps to the sixth-ninth centuries CE.[587] Compareti, who studied these textiles, suggested that they depict Mithra whose image originated from Sogdiana.[588] However, in Sogdiana almost all the possible images of Sogdian Mithra depict him seated on a throne with horses protome and these horses are not winged. Furthermore, on the only certain representation of the Sogdian Mithra—on the fragments of the wooden frieze from Panjikent VII/11—the horses are also wingless. The images with winged horses are more characteristic of Sasanian and Indian depictions of Mithra and Surya and, therefore, it is more plausible that the Dulan and Astana textiles were not produced in Sogdiana.

3. *Conclusions*

Despite possible earlier candidates it appears that the earliest definite image of Mithra is that of the Kushan Miiro. Like other Kushan deities, the iconography of Miiro was formed after the Graeco-Roman prototype; in this case Helios-Sol. Unfortunately the place and function of Miiro in the Kushan pantheon is not entirely clear.

The second representation of Mithra was created in Sasanian official art based on contemporary images of Sol on Roman provincial coins. Both images of the Sun god were created to serve royal ideology and it is significant that although belonging to a different period and region, they convey exactly the same message of divine investiture. The Sasanian Mithra was adopted by the Kushano-Sasanian king Ōhrmazd I, as a reverse design of his coins minted in Merv. Official Sasanian art also produced another type of Mithra with a unique attribute—the *barsom*—at Ṭāq-i Bustān.

The third type showing the enthroned Mithra is found on the coins of the Kushano-Sasanian king Ardašīr I and probably reflects an indigenous Bactrian development influenced by iconographic elements borrowed from Sasanian art.

At an uncertain date, a new type of Mithra as a driver of the solar chariot was introduced from the west into Sasanian art and eventually became the emblematic representation of the god in the Iranian world. The first appearance of the chariot of the solar god in the presumably Iranian milieu comes from the region of Bosporus in the first centuries CE. However, due to the complex ethno-cultural environment

---

583 Masʿūdī, vol. 2, 1379.

584 Marshak 2004: 28.

585 De Jong 1997: 306.

586 For further discussion of the riderless horse motif and the "Miho coach", see p. 129. In this context the veneration of Zoljanah, the white stallion of Imam Hoseyn among the Twelver Shi'ites, should be noted. Zoljanah—a white, riderless and saddled horse—plays an important role in the ceremonial processions of the month of Moharram and one account even connects him with the river Euphrates. On the representations of Zoljanah, see Frembgen 2012.

587 Compareti 2000.

588 Compareti 2000.

of this region, we cannot be certain that this image was indeed assimilated with Iranian Mithra. Later it is found on a number of Sasanian seals and its popularity perhaps should be sought in the fact that the astral chariot is probably the only divine image in Sasanian art which does not originate in official royal iconography. Under Sasanian influence, the solar charioteer also appeared in the eastern regions of the Empire. By the time these provinces were lost to the rising power of various nomadic states, this image of Mithra had already been absorbed by local artistic traditions and it was later reproduced in Bāmiān and in Sogdiana.

In at least three instances Mithra appears paired with Mao: on one type of Kushan coins,[589] on the reliquary of Kanishka and half a millenium later at Fondukistan. The fourth possible case is the astral spheres that Nana holds in her hands in Sogdian paintings. Interestingly, the partnership between Miiro and Mao does not accord with the norms recorded in the Avesta where it is Xwaršēd, and not Mithra, who corresponds to Māh.[590]

The rayed crown is the most characteristic and recognizable attribute of Mithra in Iranian art, in both the West and the East. However, on one type of Miiro on Kushan coins he has only an ordinary plain nimbus. Mithra was probably not depicted as an archer, or at least no such undisputable images of the god have survived. His most popular attributes and weapons in Eastern Iran are a spear and a sword, which emphasize the warlike aspect of the god also found in the Avesta. Mithra possesses the most diverse iconography among the Iranian gods. The study of his pictorial representations appears to confirm textual testimony as to the wide popularity of Mithra among Iranians.

14. *Mozdooano*

A deity labeled MOZΔOOANO appears on some rare gold coins of Kanishka. He is shown as a bearded man, closely resembling the Kushan king in his dress and appearance (pl. 14). Mozdooano wears the Kushan royal headgear tied with a diadem, is armed with a sword, holds a trident, and rides a two-headed horse. He is not known from any Zoroastrian text and is unique to Kushan Bactria.

1. *Western Iran*

Mozdooano does not appear to be found in Western Iran, neither in written nor material sources. It is worth mentioning, however, the intriguing suggestion that a deity *Mišdušiš* mentioned in the Persepolis Tablets may be related to Kushan Mozdooano.[591]

2. *Eastern Iran*

Mozdooano appears for the first time on the coinage of Kanishka. Before the discovery of the Rabatak inscription, the name Mozdooano was understood as "Mazdā the Victorious" and was thought to represent a manifestation of Ahura Mazdā,[592] or interpreted as a compound **mazda-wana-* "Winner of Wisdom", which was proposed to be a tribal god of the Kushans and patron of their royal family.[593] However, after the discovery of the Rabatak inscription where Mozdooano—spelled μοζδοο(α)νο—is mentioned in the tenth line in the fourth place, after Nana, Umma and Ahura Mazdā, it has become clear that Mozdooano and the supreme Zoroastrian god are in fact two separate deities.[594]

589 Göbl 1984 Mao-Miiro 1.
590 Humbach 1975b: 137.
591 Henkelman 2008: 373, n. 871.
592 E.g. Rosenfield 1967: 83; Mode 1991/1992: 187; Mode 1992: 478.
593 See the discussion of these etymologies in Sims-Williams 1997a: 336.
594 See p. 12–13.

Sims-Williams has proposed to derive μοζδοοανο from **miždwah* "generous, gracious" and therefore to translate the name of the Kushan deity as "the Gracious One".[595] This apparently links Mozdooano with the Indian Śiva whose name has a similar meaning ("kind, benevolent, auspicious").[596] However, the iconography of Mozdooano, besides a trident, is distinct from that of Oešo on the Kushan coins and therefore, as Sims-Williams himself cautiously concluded, the association with Śiva must remain speculative.[597] Nevertheless, nothing prevents us from considering the existence of two manifestations of Śiva; one that merged with Vayu creating the Kushan Oešo and another assuming the name of Mozdooano. Another attractive possibility is that Mozdooano is actually a Scythian ancestral god of the Kushans. Before the discovery of the Rabatak inscription, Helmut Humbach had already proposed that Mozdooano was "a sort of tribal god of the Kusanas, or a family god of their royal family".[598] A similar approach was recently adopted by Grenet, who suggested that Mozdooano was a deity inherited from the Scythian past of the Kushans whom they attempted to integrate into the Śivaite cult.[599]

The presumably intimate relationship between Mozdooano and the Kushan royal dynasty is apparently reflected not only in the important place the god occupies in the Rabatak divine list, but also in the striking similarity between the image of the god and that of the Kushan king himself. Mozdooano is not alone in his resemblance to the Kushan ruler. For instance, Iamšo also wears a similar royal headdress. However, Mozdooano is unique in that his facial features that mirror those of Kanishka and it appears almost certain that the image of Mozdooano was modeled on that of the king, although the latter is never shown mounted.[600]

One seal from Gandhāra depicts a standing deity with a Bactrian inscription that seems to identify him as Mozdooano (although seals usually carry the name of the owner) (fig. 91).[601] In his right hand he holds a long shafted weapon or a staff that is identified as a spear but could also be a trident. Ur Rahman and Falk believe that he has a knot on his head, although his image on the Kushan coins suggests that this might be a royal headdress. His left hand rests on the hilt of a sword. Above it there is an unidentifiable object. However, this iconography closely resembles that of another Kushan god—Maaseno.

Mozdooano may in fact be a deified ancestor of the Kushan dynasty, perhaps assimilated with one of the personalities of the Indian Śiva after the Kushans came to rule lands with considerable Indian population and became subject to profound Hindu religious influence. A cult of deified ancestors is attested among Scythians, Parthians and other Iranian nomads and it is only logical to assume that some of its reflections were still preserved by the Kushans in the period of their Imperial glory. Another detail possibly related to the Scythian origin of Mozdooano is the fact that he is the only Kushan deity shown mounted on a horse. One must only call to mind the predominance of equestrian figures on the coins of Indo-Scythian and Indo-Parthian rulers to strengthen the link between Mozdooano and nomadic culture.

The most curious iconographic feature of Mozdooano is undoubtedly his double-headed mount. This distinctive element was considered by some scholars to hold a key to the identity and the functions of the god. A connection to the dual nature of the god Vayu, the *way ī weh* "Vayu the better" and *way ī wattar*

---

595 Sims-Williams 1997a.

596 Sims-Williams 1997a: 338. This epithet is especially characteristic of Vedic Rudra, an early form of Śiva. See Wright 1997.

597 Sims-Williams 1997a: 338.

598 Humbach 1975b: 139.

599 Grenet 2012b: 17–18.

600 However, see the Gandhāran seal depicting a ruler on horseback: Callieri 1997: no. 7.17. It closely resembles Kushan royal representations and the images of Mozdooano, but has a crenellated crown not attested for the Kushan kings. Such crowns with three crenellations are typical of the Sasanians and therefore this seal probably depicts one of the local princes who ruled Gandhāra after the Sasanian conquest of the Kushan Bactrian territories.

601 Ur Rahman and Falk 2012: no. 07.01.03.

"Vayu the worse", which is found in Middle Persian Zoroastrian literature[602] hardly seems probable[603] as is the allusion to the Indian two-headed cow, Aditi.[604] Gnoli has further suggested that the double-headed mount could reflect the dual nature of Mozdooano as the deity of the "Rudra/Śiva type".[605] Markus Mode proposed to identify the Sogdian god seated on the throne supported by the foreparts of horses as Mozdooano.[606] I believe that this Sogdian god may rather represent Oxus.[607] No deity named Mozdooano is known in Sogdiana and the two-headed mount is still very different from the two horses serving as decorative support for the throne. It appears that this attribute should be viewed as reflecting a mythological tradition (perhaps Scythian or local Bactrian) regarding Mozdooano, which is regrettably a complete mystery to us, as is in fact the entire assemblage of beliefs, legends, practices and rituals connected to this enigmatic deity.

3. *Conclusions*

The god Mozdooano is unique to the Kushan royal pantheon of Kanishka and is not known from any other place or culture. His image was not based on that of any Greek or Roman divinity but was modeled on the Kushan king himself including his physiognomy. It is therefore plausible that Mozdooano was a Scythian tribal god of the Kushans or a deified ancestor of the ruling dynasty. Another, less likely, possibility is that he was a local Bactrian god, not attested among other Iranian people (as is the case with another Bactrian god—Zūn). The worship of Mozdooano probably ceased with the fall of the Kushans, as there is no evidence for his veneration in Bactria after the Rabatak inscription.

15. *Nana*

There are probably more studies dedicated to the iconography of Nana/Nanaia—the great goddess of Eastern Iran—than to any other Iranian deity.[608] Her origins and the exact etymology of her name are shrouded in the mists of history. Nana appears for the first time in Sumer in the royal pantheon of the Ur III period (2112–2004 BCE) and some specialists believe that her worship was imported from outside the Sumerian area, perhaps from Elam, since her name is possibly derived from the Elamite language.[609] Cuneiform sources indicate that Nana was not a manifestation of Inanna/Ištar and was probably distinct from her.[610] However, like Ištar, she was a goddess of love and possessed some of the traits of a warrior goddess.[611] In addition, Nana was considered to be a daughter of the Moon god Sin, but the fact that she was a Moon-goddess herself is not evident from Mesopotamian literary sources.[612]

In modern scholarship, Nana is often identified with other Iranian goddesses—most notably Anāhitā and Spəntā Ārmaiti—although this assumption is not borne out by the sources.[613] It appears that these

---

602 Sims-Williams 1997a: 338.
603 See the criticism in Gnoli 2009: 146–149.
604 Duchesne-Guillemin 1966: 104.
605 Gnoli 2009: 149.
606 Mode 1991/1992: 187; Mode 1992: 478.
607 See p. 130.
608 To mention just several important studies: D'yakonova and Smirnova 1967; Mukherjee 1969; Azarpay 1976b; Tanabe 1995b; Potts 2001; Ambos 2003; Ghose 2006.
609 Westenholz 1997: 58–60.
610 Westenholz 1997: 80; Potts 2001: 23. However, see Ambos 2003: 232, who writes that in the Old Babylonian texts Nana was equated with Ištar, although the two goddesses could also be worshipped separately.
611 Ambos 2003: 233.
612 Ambos 2003: 234.
613 See the discussion with references in Tanabe 1995a: 210–212. For the identification with Spəntā Ārmaiti see e.g. Azarpay 1981: 137–139. The only indirect evidence, which does not appear compelling, is the image of Anāhitā on the coin of the Kushano-Sasanian king Ōhrmazd II.

theories mainly result from a need felt by some scholars to explain why no certain images of the "central" Zoroastrian female deities Spəntā Ārmaiti and Anāhitā were known from Eastern Iran, where originally non-Iranian Nana became the prominent deity in the predominantly Iranian pantheons of the Bactrians and Sogdians. This problem is purely artificial and derives mainly from a desire to adjust the material data to fit the textual Zoroastrian tradition. Approached without this preconception in mind, both the written and archaeological materials provide no clear evidence for the assimilation of Nana with any Iranian goddess(es).

1. *Western Iran*

The cult of Nana is widely attested in literary and epigraphic sources and in the iconography of Mesopotamia, Syria and probably also in the Caucasus. It is therefore useful to provide a brief overview of some of the evidence from the periphery of Western Iran in order to achieve a better understanding of subsequent developments in the cult of Nana in the Iranian world itself.

Before the Hellenistic period, the only definite image of Nana is found on the *kudduru* of the Babylonian king Melišipak (1186–1172 BCE). Nana, shown enthroned, does not have any specific attribute, but wears a high headdress and the legs of her throne are shaped in the form of lion's paws.[614] During the Parthian period Nana enjoyed considerable popularity in Mesopotamia and there are a number of her depictions originating from cities such as Ashur and Hatra. On the famous pythos fragment from Ashur, a statue of Nana is shown placed on a flat throne and surrounded by worshippers and adorants.[615] The goddess is identified by an inscription, and is called "Our Lady" (Aramaic *mārtan*). She does not possess any specific attribute, but wears a curious headdress consisting of a flat base with a disk and her garments are decorated with crescent moons. This imagery led to the suggestion that she is shown here in the role of a moon goddess.[616] Another inscribed image of Nana dated to the middle of the second century CE is the statue of the goddess from Hatra holding a staff and wearing a high tiara.[617] Her worship and visual representations are also well attested in Palmyra, where Nana was identified with Greek Artemis,[618] and in Dura-Europos.[619]

Numerous literary and epigraphic sources attest to the central place occupied by Nana in the pantheon of Susa, Elymais.[620] From the time of the Parthian king Mithridates II (c. 110 BCE) and his successors Arsaces Theopator Euergetes and Phraates III (71/0–58/7 BCE) the city coins of Susa depict a figure wearing a crenellated/radiate crown, armed with a sword and holding a spear/bow or a bust wearing a radiate crown.[621] This figure is usually interpreted as Nana, modeled on the Greek Artemis.[622] However, these coins are not labeled and even the sex of the figure cannot definitely be established. From a purely iconographic point of view, the radiate bust could also represent Mithra in his characteristic crown. We also know from Graeco-Roman coins that the principal deity of a city does not necessarily dominate the city's coinage. It is noteworthy that a figure holding a spear/scepter and wearing a similar radiate crown appears on the Tang-i Sarvak II (NE side) rock-relief located in Elymais and dated to the second century CE.[623] Based on Susian coins, some have identified this image as that

614 Ambos 2003: 234, Fig. 1.
615 Ambos 2003: 238–240.
616 Ambos 2003: 241.
617 Ambos 2003: 240–242.
618 Kaizer 2002: 94–96, 106.
619 See Ambos 2003: 244–248.
620 See the references in Ambos 2003: 248–250.
621 Ambos 2003: Figs. 12–13, 14.
622 Ambos 2003: 250–251.
623 Kawami 1987: 89.

of the goddess Nana. However, it was recently and convincingly demonstrated that this figure has a moustache and is most probably male.[624]

A fragmentary marble relief found in Susa may be of paramount importance for evidence of the diffusion of the iconography of Nana.[625] It shows the goddess seated frontally on a lion marching to the right. The fragment is probably dated between the end of the first century CE and the beginning of the second century CE.[626] This demonstrates that a second type of Nana, completely different from the Artemis-type that appears on coins (if it is indeed Nana), also existed in Susa. This type is very close to the image of Nana on a lion depicted on Kushan coins.[627] The significance of this Susian relief lies in the fact that this is probably the earliest depiction of Nana with a lion in the West, which may only slightly postdate the image of Nana in the East or perhaps even be its contemporary.

Nana is commonly held to have acquired her lion companion from Ištar,[628] although, as we have already seen, a lion is not found together with the goddess before the Parthian/Kushan period. This development could perhaps be attributed to the Hellenistic period and may have been stimulated by the diffusion of the cult of Cybele.[629] In Mesopotamia Nana continued to be venerated into Late Antiquity and her name is mentioned on a Mandaic incantation bowl from Nippur.[630] A glazed terracotta rhyton from the same site provisionally dated to the late Parthian or early Sasanian period may depict the goddess as may another similar rhyton in the British Museum.[631] There is literary evidence that Nana was worshipped in the Sasanian court. In one Syriac source we read that king Šāpūr II ordered a convert to Christianity to venerate Nanaia, "the great goddess of the world".[632] Despite this evidence and her numerous visual representations from Mesopotamia, not a single image of Nana has come down to us from Western Iran.

Fabrizio Sinisi has proposed to interpret one variant of Tyche (wearing a *kalathos*) portrayed on Parthian coins, as the image of the goddess Nana. He rejects the Greek interpretation of her image, arguing that the Parthians "would have had no reason to picture a Greek deity" and that they may have understood Tyche "as the visual rendering of a deity from their own religious tradition".[633] The first statement alone is quite problematic and doubtful, and regarding the second, we do not really know what "their own religious tradition" was to begin with. There is no reason to think that by the time the Parthians came to rule Seleucia and other Greek *polei* of Mesopotamia, Greek deities had not become an integral part of the religious life of the Parthian elite and it is not certain that the Olympian gods necessarily required *interpretatio iranica* in each and every case. Tyche on the Parthian coins has no attributes of Nana as she is known from Eastern Iran (a difficulty acknowledged by Sinisi himself);[634] but more significantly also from the Parthian West. Most notably, there are no similarities between the Parthian Tyche and Nana as she appears on a jar shard from Ashur and the statue from Hatra[635] where the goddess is identified by the inscription, and on the coins of Susa (if they indeed depict Nana). Therefore, the Tyche on Parthian coins probably represents what it looks like at first glance—the prosperity and the fortune of *polis* embodied in the image of the Hellenistic Tyche.

---

624 Haerinck 2003.
625 Invernizzi 2010.
626 Invernizzi 2010: 31.
627 See below.
628 Azarpay 1976b: 539.
629 Ghose 2006: 99.
630 Westenholz 1997: 79.
631 See Carter 2010: 144–145.
632 See p. 27.
633 Sinisi 2008: 242–243.
634 Sinisi 2008: 244.
635 Ambos 2003: 238–240, Fig. 2.

2. *Eastern Iran*

It is usually thought that the cult of Nana penetrated Eastern Iran in the Hellenistic period.[636] However, since images of a goddess with a lion already appear in the BMAC, it has been suggested that the worship of Nana was already introduced to Central Asia by the end of the third millennium BCE from Elam.[637] The problem with this suggestion lies in the large chronological gap that falls between the Bronze Age goddess and the first images of Nana on a lion. A lion is the animal perhaps most commonly associated with the divine in many human cultures and it is entirely plausible that the "memory" and ancient tradition of a cult of a goddess on a lion in Central Asia facilitated the spread of the cult of Nana.

Although we lack direct material confirmation, it is likely that the worship of Nana was brought to Bactria during the Achaemenian period when almost the entire sedentary Iranian world was incorporated into a single political structure, allowing the free movement and circulation of ideas and cultural influences. As a province of the Achaemenian Empire, and perhaps also due to its special importance to the Persian kings, Bactria was subject to a strong Mesopotamian influence. This is evident from the architecture of some Bactrian temples and other edifices constructed in the Hellenistic period according to Mesopotamian building traditions. From fourth century BCE Aramaic documents from Bactria we know that the Mesopotamian god Bel was worshipped in Bactria in the Achaemenian period.[638] Furthermore, according to Sims-Williams the name of the goddess Nana (Bactrian ναναα) was borrowed into the Bactrian language from Old Persian in the Achaemenian period.[639] It is therefore plausible that the cult of Nana reached Eastern Iran under the Achaemenian kings. The introduction and reception of the cult of the goddess could well be part of this still poorly understood process of exceptional influence of Mesopotamian culture on Achaemenian Bactria.

Two silver plates depicting the goddess Cybele standing in a chariot drawn by lions were discovered in Bactrian Hellenistic temples—the "Temple with Indented Niches" at Ai Khanum and at the "Oxus Temple" at Takht-i Sangin[640]—suggesting that the cult of Cybele, or of other (local?) goddess(es) associated with her was widespread in Hellenistic Bactria. The most natural candidate for this local goddess would undoubtedly be Nana,[641] and it is therefore possible that the cult of Nana may have been practiced in both these temples. One might also mention the passage in the Syriac version of the *Alexander Romance* where the Macedonian conqueror is credited with the founding in Samarkand of a temple that was painted with gold, decorated with precious paintings, and dedicated to the goddess Rhea whom the Sogdians called Nani.[642] Rhea was strongly associated with Cybele. This description also corresponds to the interior of Sogdian temples adorned with beautiful paintings.

The earliest indisputable evidence for a cult of Nana in Central Asia comes from the coins issued by the Indo-Scythian rulers Sapadbizes and Agesiles (end of the first century BCE) that show on the reverse a standing lion with the inscription NANAIA (fig. 92). It is noteworthy that this first image of Nana is aniconic. The goddess is represented only by her zoomorphic attribute, the lion that precede the appearance of her anthropomorphic portrayals. The first human-shaped image of Nana (spelled NANA, NANAIA and NANAÞAO) appears on the coin of Vima Kadphises and would later become the most popular design on the reverses of the coins of Kanishka and the fourth most popular on the coinage of Huvishka. The image of Nana also continued to be used on the coins of Vasudeva. There are three main

636 Ambos 2003: 236.
637 Potts 2001: 27–30.
638 Naveh and Shaked 2012: C1:37.
639 Sims-Williams 2002: 227.
640 Francfort 1984: 93–105; Litvinskiy 2010: 226–230.
641 Carter 2005: 15; Carter 2008: 116, n. 76; Ghose 2006: 98.
642 Grenet 1995/1996b: 215–216.

iconographic types of Kushan Nana.[643] The most common type depicts her standing in profile, nimbate and wearing a diadem topped by a crescent (pl. 15). Her attributes are a staff terminating with a lion protome and a bowl. On one subtype, she also has a sword with a curved hilt attached to her belt. On some very rare copper coins, a figure is shown kneeling in front of her (fig. 93). The second type shows her sitting sideways on a lion (fig. 94). She wears a diadem with a crescent, has a nimbus surrounding her head, and holds a staff with a leonine protome. A particularly interesting variant of this type depicts her frontally, holding a scepter and a diadem in her hands and with a large crescent behind her back (fig. 95).[644] Finally, the third type shows her as an Artemis-like figure, standing in profile and holding a bow in her left hand while reaching with her right hand to pull an arrow out of a quiver on her back (fig. 96).[645] She is also nimbate and wears her distinctive diadem with a crescent. This type is very close to the image of Teiro on the coins of Huvishka.[646]

Nana is the most popular goddess on the coinage of this Kushan king, which corresponds to her primary position as the leader of the gods in the Rabatak inscription and the bestower of royal power. The assertion that Nana was the principal deity of Kanishka's pantheon was recently challenged by Gnoli, who argued that Nana was probably only "the deity to whom the Rabatak sanctuary was dedicated".[647] The Italian scholar has drawn a parallel with the position of Anāhitā in the West—whose temple at Eṣṭaḵr was a family sanctuary of the Sasanians, but she herself was never the head of the Sasanian pantheon. This is hardly convincing, since there is no certainty that the Rabatak sanctuary was dedicated to Nana[648]—it does not ensue from the inscription itself. Moreover, it seems that Kushan dynastic sanctuaries as a rule were not dedicated to a specific deity, but to numerous gods, protectors of the ruling dynasty.[649] Contrary to Gnoli, there are no sufficient grounds to doubt that Nana was the most important deity worshipped by Kanishka and the head of the royal dynastic pantheon of his time. This is confirmed by her place in the Rabatak inscription, the popularity of her image on coins and in personal names, and by the fact that Nana was also the most important goddess in neighboring Sogdiana and Chorasmia. It is unequivocally stated in the Rabatak inscription that Nana was the patron of the king and the source of his kingship. Curiously, the attribute most often associated with the investiture—a diadem—is held by Nana only on one unique coin of Kanishka III.[650] Usually the goddess herself wears a diadem topped by a crescent moon which indicates her astral connections and a lion or a staff with a lion protome that establishes her link with this animal. The type where she is depicted as Artemis the archer perhaps betrays influence from Susa, if the goddess with a bow depicted on its city coins is indeed Nana. Nana was also probably very popular with common people. One type of terracotta figurines depicting an enthroned female with a lunar crescent incorporated into her headdress possibly represents a vulgar image of the goddess in Kushan Bactria.[651] However, her most characteristic and recognizable attribute—the lion—is missing.

Images of Nana that closely resemble her representations on Kushan coins are also found on seals. One seal shows Nana facing right and holding a bowl and a scepter ending with a lion's protome (fig. 97).[652] She wears a diadem topped with a crescent. The seal carries a Sogdian inscription *nnyh-βntk*

643 For more detailed typology, see Göbl 1984: Nana 1–8, Nanaia 1, Nanašao 1–2.
644 Mukherjee 1969: Fig. 1 and 1A.
645 According to Carter 2008: 118, her iconography was adopted from Greek Artemis and Hecate.
646 See p. 149–150.
647 Gnoli 2009: 144–145.
648 Gnoli himself writes that it is only "probable".
649 Fussman 1998: 589.
650 Mukherjee 1969, Fig. 1 and 1A.
651 Abdullaev 2000; Abdullaev 2003. However, see Mkrtychev 2004: 351, who argues that the identification of these terracottas with Nana lacks argumentation.
652 Callieri 1997: U 7.21.

'wxsrδ, "Nanai-vandak (the son of) Aw-xsarth" or "Aw-xsarth (the son of) Nanai-vandak". It is strikingly similar to the most common image of Nana as depicted on the coins of Kanishka and therefore the seal may be dated to the second century CE. The second Kushan-era seal depicts a goddess seated on a prone lion who is turned to the left (fig. 98).[653] The goddess is shown in three-quarter view facing in the opposite direction and holding a short staff in her left hand. Her head is portrayed in full profile and is decorated with a crescent moon. On the left edge of the seal there is a Bactrian inscription giving the personal name of the owner.

After the fall of the Kushan Empire, Nana continued to be venerated in Eastern Iran. In the middle of the third century CE, when Bactria was subject to the rule of the Sasanian Kushanshahs a partially aniconic image of Nana appears on the coins of king Pērōz I. She is shown in the form of a female bust surmounted on an altar, very similar to the fire-altar used on the coins of the first Sasanian king Ardašīr I (fig. 99).[654] The bust is shown *en face*, is nimbate and has a crescent on top of its head. On both sides of the bust there are Bactrian inscriptions ΒΑΓΟ ΝΑΝΟ "The goddess Nana". Her identity here is beyond doubt thanks to the inscription. Nana can also be recognized by her characteristic attribute—a crescent moon—on top of her head.

The worship of Nana apparently survived in Bactria until the Muslim conquest, as is evident from the bronze plaque dated to the late seventh-eighth centuries CE that was purportedly found in the Laghman valley in Afghanistan. This small bronze plaque (8 × 5 inches) depicts a goddess seated *en face* on a lion facing left (fig. 100).[655] She wears a long robe and a crown decorated with tulips, a moon crescent, and a sun. The goddess holds a shallow cup in her right hand and clutches a plant stem in her left. Pots of flowers are depicted on both sides of the goddess and she has a crescent moon behind her back. What is exceptional in this particular representation is the strong association of Nana with vegetation. Not only her crown is decorated with tulips, but she also holds a plant stem and is flanked by flowerpots. It seems that in post-Kushan Bactria Nana acquired the characteristics of a nature/fertility goddess that are not found in her earlier Kushan representations or in later Sogdian ones, although any conclusions based on a single image are necessarily speculative. Another distinctive feature of this object is the crescent moon attached to the goddess's back in a manner similar to that of the Kushan Mao. In Mesopotamia Nana was connected with the moon god Sin and in Eastern Iran she usually has a crescent moon decorating her crown as a constant attribute in Bactrian, Sogdian and Chorasmian art.

Nana is the most representative example of the continuity between Kushan and Sogdian religious iconography. Despite inevitable transformations, the basic appearance and the main characteristics of Nana as an astral goddess on a lion were preserved during the period of political turmoil between the third and fifth centuries CE. The earliest Sogdian rendering of the goddess might be a frontal bust above the fire-altar that appears on the first copper coins struck in Bukhara (fig. 101).[656] It wears a round cap with ends folding up, which is decorated with a crescent and a sun. Braids of hair are shown on both sides. The figure wears a necklace and there are also two round groups of circles. These are depicted almost touching the altar's surface, but these undoubtedly show additional buckles of hair. This image is unquestionably borrowed from the coins of the Kushano-Sasanian king Pērōz I.[657] The crescent suggests that this could also be a depiction of Nana, but the round buckles of hair are a distinctively male headdress. This motif might therefore have been copied from Kushano-Sasanian coins, mixing the iconography of Nana and Bago Borzando.

653 Callieri 1997: U 7.23.
654 Carter 1985 Pl. 47, n. 4; Cribb 1990: no. 31.
655 Ghose 2005.
656 Naymark 1995.
657 See p. 121.

Another early possible image of Nana is found in the mural from Jartepa II Temple. This mural was painted on the northern wall of the cella of a Sogdian temple located between Samarkand and Panjikent.[658] The wall paintings are dated to the fourth or early fifth century CE and therefore constitute the earliest mural paintings yet discovered in Sogdiana. The composition of the Jartepa II mural consists of some nineteen figures arranged in two registers. The lower register shows hunting scenes. In the center of the upper register two figures are depicted seated on a throne supported by lion protomes (nos. 9 and 10) (fig. 102). These characters are male and female and in all probability represent a divine couple. The female figure (no. 10) to the right is wearing an orange robe and a white coat. The male figure seated beside her is dressed in an orange *kaftan* and trousers. The couple is flanked by figures of adorants. Grenet and Marshak reconstruct the diadems in the hands of figures nos. 14 and 15 and interpret this scene as a symbolic investiture by the gods.[659] It should be noted, however, that the scene with a deity investing a king with a diadem—so typical of Sasanian and Kushan art—is never attested in Sogdiana. The female figure seated together with her consort in the center of the upper register is most likely a goddess. Since the legs of the throne on which they are seated are formed in the shape of lion protomes, Grenet and Marshak proposed to identify her as Nana.[660] Unfortunately, due to the fragmentary state of the mural's preservation, it is not clear what attributes she has. A comparable composition of a couple on a large *takht* supported by lions is found on four Bactrian seals.[661] A male character is seated cross-legged and a female of somewhat larger proportions is depicted standing. In front of the *takht* a smaller kneeling figure extends a diadem towards the seated male.

As indicated by its coinage, Nana was apparently the principal deity of the city of Panjikent.[662] According to the Indus inscriptions, together with the river god Oxus she was also the deity most revered by Sogdian merchants.[663] Several Sogdian personal names contain the name of the goddess.[664] Statues of Nana were uncovered in Temple II in Panjikent, which was in all probability dedicated to the goddess. A huge figure of Nana was placed in front of the entrance to the sanctuary.[665] Small fragments of another painted clay sculpture were discovered on a bench to the south of the entrance in the western wall of room 13 in Temple II (X/13) in Panjikent (fig. 103).[666] The statue, originally four m. high, represented a goddess mounted on a standing lion. It is dated to the seventh or the first quarter of the eighth century CE. An additional sculpture of a goddess on a lion was found in a niche above the high podium attached to the southern wall in room 14 in Temple II at Panjikent (fig. 104).[667] Here, Nana is depicted seated not on a standing, but on a prone animal. The statue was flanked by painted figures of an armored male carrying a sword and a mace and a demon laying at his feet. It dates to the first quarter of the eighth century CE.

The temple has also yielded numerous murals depicting the goddess. An outline painting of Nana seated on a lion was discovered on the southern wall of room 14 in sector X (fig. 105).[668] Her figure was flanked by a male donor and a female figure. Four fragments of a complex cultic scene painted on a blue background were found in the fill belonging to paintings that were placed on the northern wall of the

658 Berdimuradov and Samibaev 2001.
659 Berdimuradov and Samibaev 2001: 59.
660 Berdimuradov and Samibaev 2001: 59.
661 Lerner and Sims-Williams 2011: D 1.1–D 7.
662 D'yakonova and Smirnova 1967.
663 Sims-Williams 1991: 177.
664 Lurje 2010: nos. 756, 757, 782, 786, 1462.
665 Shkoda 2009: 85.
666 Shkoda 2009: 78.
667 Shkoda 2009: 78.
668 Shkoda 2009: 75.

exterior courtyard in the temple (fig. 106).[669] In the center of the upper register a four-armed goddess is depicted seated on a lion. She wears a golden crown composed of almond-shaped elements and tied with a ribbon decorated with flowers. Her head is surrounded by a flaming nimbus and tongues of fire rise from her shoulders. From the preserved fragments it seems that Nana was portrayed holding a banner and the personifications of the Sun and the Moon. Two smaller female figures are shown beside her. They are nimbate, with shoulders aflame, carry spears and at least one of them wears armor.

Nana also appears on one of the most famous and complex wall paintings discovered in Panjikent—the so-called "Lamentation Scene"—which decorated the southern wall of the main hall of Temple II (fig. 107).[670] The subject of the painting is mourning over a deceased loved one, whose sex is difficult to establish. He or, more probably she, is lying under the doomed structure and surrounded by mourning attendants tearing out their hair in grief. Below, an additional group of people is shown cutting the lobes of their ears. To the left, three much larger figures are depicted, which probably represent only part of a larger procession, other participants of which were not preserved. The largest figure in this procession is a four-armed goddess whose head is surrounded by a rayed nimbus. With one hand, she appears to punch her own head as a display of mourning and desperation; another hand grasps an unidentifiable attribute. The other two arms are not preserved. Beside her, a smaller figure with a similarly rayed nimbus is depicted kneeling and planting in the ground an object resembling a torch. This mural is dated to the sixth century CE.

Images of Nana are also often found in private houses in Panjikent. For example, she occupies a central place in a painting depicting at least five divine figures found in room 2 in house XXVI in Panjikent (fig. 108).[671] Unfortunately, only fragments of the lower part of this painting were preserved, but they were sufficient to reconstruct a goddess on a prone lion flanked by four additional deities, two on each side. The first figure on the left is a warlike god striking a crouching demon with a spear. The second god is seated on a zoomorphic throne supported by rams. The throne was flanked by banners and the god itself had a sword attached to a belt. Unfortunately, all other details are lost. Only the end of the sword's scabbard and the bird's claw of his mount have survived from the god to the right of the goddess on a lion. The excavators have offered the reasonable suggestion that the god was riding a giant bird or a gryphon.[672] A bare foot set on mountainous terrain is all that is preserved from the last deity.

Another partially preserved large figure of Nana was uncovered on the southern wall of room 26 in house VI in Panjikent and depicts the goddess draped in blue and white garments (fig. 109).[673] The upper part of her head is damaged and only the floating ribbons, or perhaps parts of a veil attached to her headdress, can be clearly seen. The goddess has a nimbus surrounding her head and tongues of fire rise from her shoulders. In her outstretched hands, the goddess holds two disks. In the right hand, a blue disk with a feminine head framed by a crescent; and in the left, a golden disk with fragments of a badly damaged human figure.

Nana occupies the central place on one of the most complex religious paintings uncovered in Panjikent. It was excavated in 1977 in the niche of the northern wall of room 12 in house XXV (fig. 110).[674] The painting is divided into two main registers painted on a blue background. The composition is dominated by the towering figure of the four-armed Nana mounted on a marching lion. Her attributes have been reconstructed based on numerous parallels. In front of the goddess's face there is a small

669 Marshak, Raspopova, Shkoda 1999: 40–42; Shkoda 2009: 79.

670 For a detailed presentation and description, see D'yakonov 1954: 33–55. The most recent discussion of this mural is found in Grenet and Marshak 1998.

671 Marshak and Raspopova 2003: 47–49.

672 Marshak and Raspopova 2003: 48.

673 Belenitskiy 1959: 21–22. Belenitskiy 1973: 22.

674 Belenitskiy, Marshak, Raspopova and Isakov 1983: 197–204; Maršak and Raspopova 1991: 189.

kneeling figure holding a trumpet (?). Below him, there is a figure of a male god, seated on a throne supported by two dragons. He is beardless, but has a moustache, tongues of fire rise from his shoulders and he wears a headdress decorated with a figure of a dragon. The deity holds in his hands a long staff-like object, which was interpreted by Grenet and Marshak as an arrow.[675] Although the tip of this object is not preserved, the god holds the object in a manner different to the way in which a sword is usually held by the Sogdians. Its interpretation as an arrow is therefore possible. Beside the god, there is a small parasol. Behind the goddess on the lion, there are two additional human figures and an edifice with a lion standing in it. The composition in the lower register is framed by two standing figures holding banners. The left figure is beardless, wears a winged "Phrygian cap" tied with a diadem, and holds a small plate with a figure of a marching lion. The character on the right has a demonic physiognomy, a tousled beard, an animal ear and two goat-horns. The left figure faces another character seated on a throne supported by two human figures. He is nimbate, wears a winged crown and ribbons of his diadem are shown flying on both sides of his head. His attributes are a bowl, a sword and a jug attached to the throne. The center of the lower register is occupied by two buildings. The first is flanked by the two streams of smoke and is covered by scales. It is guarded by a lion and two characters painted in yellow that are seen inside—a large nimbate figure of a fully armored warrior carrying a mace and a sword, and wearing a winged crown, and a naked dwarfish character lying at his feet. The second building, flanked by two banners and adorned with jewelry and precious fabrics, is attended by two winged angel-like figures holding animal-headed maces. Windows and women can be seen inside the edifice. To the right, there is a portable altar with a kneeling figure of an adorant before it. The body of the altar carries an image of an armored deity standing in the niche. On the side wall, there are depictions of a dancing god with a trident and a skull at his feet and a cultic scene of three figures kneeling before a portable fire-altar.

In Ustrushana several paintings portray Nana involved in battle against demons. Her image as a four-handed goddess mounted on a lion is found in the lower of three registers of a mural which decorated the eastern wall of a "Small hall" in the palace of Bunjikat, the capital of this Sogdian principality (fig. 87).[676] The goddess faces right and wears finely decorated blue garments and an ornamental crown composed of crescent-like elements (pl. 16). In two raised hands she holds anthropomorphic representations of the Moon and Sun. In her third hand she holds a whip and with her fourth hand she makes a gesture of benefaction. The Sun is depicted as a golden disk with the bust of a beardless youth shown *en face*. Tongues of fire rise from his shoulders. The Moon is represented by a bust of an effeminate youth (perhaps a female?) wearing a complex ornamental crown mounted on a crescent. This bust also has tongues of fire rising from the shoulders. The upper register of the eastern wall of the "Small hall" at Bunjikat (fig. 111) shows a four-handed Nana mounted on a lion (fragments of the lion's mane and the leg of the goddess were preserved) portrayed in full frontal view (pl. 17).[677] Her crown, garments and jewelry correspond exactly to those of the four-handed goddess depicted in the lower register of the same painting. In her two hands, the goddess holds symbolic representations of the Sun and Moon and in the other two she holds a scepter, which has a finial in the form of a winged lion, and a standard topped by a golden bird. Her head is surrounded by a nimbus and tongues of fire rise from her shoulders.

In late Sogdian religious art Nana surpasses all other divinities in popularity. She has been found at almost every place where Sogdian paintings have been uncovered, notably at Panjikent and Ustrushana, once again bringing to mind the "temple of Nani" in Samarkand from the Syriac version of the *Alexander Romance*.[678] The visual representation of Nana became standardized and would have been easily recognized by all Sogdians. In late Sogdian art she is always depicted four-armed, seated on a prone

---

675 Grenet and Marshak 1998: 15.
676 Sokolovskiy 2009: 45–46.
677 Sokolovskiy 2009: 51.
678 See p. 28.

or marching lion, and holding personifications of the Sun and Moon. Nana was undoubtedly the most important divinity in the pan-Sogdian pantheon, although the veneration of Sogdian deities varied from one community to another. As the material from Panjikent clearly indicates, every family probably had its own patron god(s) or goddess(es).[679]

On one instance, in Ustrushana, Nana is portrayed holding a standard with a finial in the shape of a golden bird. This attribute is also attested with the image of the goddess on the ossuary from Khirmantepa. This ossuary was found in 1984 during earthworks conducted at the site of Khirmantepa, in the Kashka-darya region of Uzbekistan (southern Sogdiana). It is stamped on both long sides, with a scene of two four-handed figures placed under the arcade (fig. 112).[680] The left figure is a female, portrayed frontally, with her left leg tucked beneath.[681] She is nimbate and wears a tiara which widens at the top with a shawl attached to it, which falls to her shoulders. In her two right hands, she holds a scepter ending with the figure of a bird and a sun disk. In her two left hands, Nana holds a crescent and a short, massive object with a hilt—perhaps a mace or a short sword with an unusually wide blade. The second character is a male seated in the same pose. His head, however, is shown in profile, turned towards the goddess. His attributes are not as easily recognized. The god wears a helmet decorated with animal ears and chainmail. In his front hands he holds a narrow elongated object which was interpreted as a *tanbūr* (a variety of lute)[682] or as an arrow.[683] With his rear right hand, the god grasps a ring with a bird perched on it; and in his rear left hand, he holds a round object identified as a tambourine[684] or a shield.[685] Below, three musicians are depicted and this ossuary also features a figure of an "atlas" holding a column. The ossuary is dated to the sixth-seventh century CE.[686]

It is noteworthy that the Sogdian Nana does not have a single distinctive crown, but has several quite different types. This supports the general impression that crowns in Sogdian art (both of gods and mortals) were not personalized (as they were, for instance, for the early Sasanian kings and probably also for the gods depicted on their reliefs). In Sogdiana Nana is frequently depicted as accompanied by an armed male figure, who is probably to be identified as Tištrya. On the painting with the blue background from Temple II at Panjikent, Nana is attended by two warlike female personages. On one of the fragments of the wooden frieze discovered in the Sogdian palace of Kujruk-tobe in present day Southern Kazakhstan, Nana is depicted together with two small archer figures. This freeze, dated to the seventh or to the first half of the eighth century CE,[687] depicts deities from the Sogdian pantheon placed under an arcade.[688] Under the left arch on the first fragment, a goddess on a throne supported by gryphon protomes is depicted (fig. 113).[689] She wears a crenellated crown and in her left hand she holds a casket, perhaps an ossuary. The attribute in her right hand is difficult to identify. There seem to be three tongues of fire rising from her right shoulder. The right figure on the same fragment is a goddess seated on a throne supported by rams. She is shown almost frontally, with flying ribbons attached to her headdress. Her attributes are difficult to identify, but according to the excavator, Karl Bajpakov, she holds "a triangular object in the left hand and a scepter in the right".[690] The image of Nana

---

679 Maršak and Raspopova 1991: 192.
680 Lunina and Usmanova 1985.
681 Lunina and Usmanova 1985, interpret this pose as dancing, but numerous parallels in Sogdian art leave no doubt that the figures depicted with a leg tucked beneath are in fact shown seated on a carpet or enthroned.
682 Lunina and Usmanova 1985: 48, 50.
683 Grenet 1992: 47–48; Compareti 2008: 138.
684 Lunina and Usmanova 1985: 50.
685 Grenet 1992: 48.
686 Lunina and Usmanova 1985: 51.
687 Bajpakov and Grenet 1992: 48.
688 Bajpakov and Grenet 1992; Bajpakov 1998: 251–253.
689 Bajpakov 1998: 251, believes that the figure is male and interprets the zoomorphic throne supporters as "winged camels".
690 Bajpakov 1998: 251.

is carved on the second fragment (fig. 114). She is four-armed and flanked by two small archer figures whose significance is unclear. They might be connected with the alleged bellicose aspect of the goddess who is often shown battling against demons at the head of other divinities. It is also possible that the archers might specifically be associated with Tištrya-Tīr. In her raised hands, Nana holds two spheres, undoubtedly corresponding to the astral personifications. Only a small fragment of a hand holding a circular object is preserved from the deity to her right, but there is no doubt that it is the image of the same four-handed god depicted together with the goddess on the Khirmantepa ossuary.

In Sogdian art Nana is also represented by means of a large portable altar. This altar, the first and the tallest of three altars placed on a *takht* supported by a protomes of winged rams, is depicted on the mural in room 6/III in Panjikent.[691] The body of the altar is not preserved, but it is topped by a crenellated crown. In Sogdian and especially in Chorasmian art, a crenellated crown is the most common headdress of Nana.[692] Based on this, and on the fact that this altar probably represents the most important divinity in the local pantheon, it could an aniconic image of Nana.

The cult of Nana was not limited to the valleys of Zeravshan and Kashka-darya, but was also active in other regions of Eastern Iran. In Chorasmia her iconography and main attributes are almost identical to the way in which she is depicted in Sogdiana, suggesting that the functions of the Chorasmian Nana were close to those of the Sogdian goddess. Her images are mostly found on silver bowls. The first bowl, now in the British Museum, is dated to 658 CE by the Chorasmian inscription on its outer rim.[693] In a medallion in the middle of the bowl the four-armed goddess is seated on a prone lion in three-quarter view facing left (fig. 115). On her head, the goddess wears a high crown consisting of three crenellations and incorporating a crescent. In her two raised hands she holds a sun disk and a crescent moon and in her other hands she holds a short scepter and a bowl. In a recent article, Michele Minardi has showed that the goddess on this bowl exhibits numerous stylistic Byzantine influences and is probably to be dated to the end of the sixth century CE or to the first half of the seventh century CE.[694] A very similar bowl dated to the same year was found near the village of Bartym in the Perm region of Russia (fig. 116).[695] On another Chorasmian bowl discovered near the same village, Nana is depicted mounted on her lion companion (fig. 117).[696] Her crown and attributes correspond exactly to those on the first bowl, but the lion is shown marching to the left towards a small figure of a kneeling worshipper holding a cup in his hand. A further Chorasmian silver bowl, though of a cruder and linear style, is now in the State Hermitage Museum and dated to the 538 or 638 CE.[697] The medallion in the center of the bowl depicts a central frontal figure of the four-handed Nana (fig. 118). She wears a similar crenellated crown and has the same attributes as on other Chorasmian bowls, but the bowl is replaced by what seems to be a flower. Notable in his absence is the lion, the constant attribute of this goddess on other Chorasmian bowls and in Sogdian art. The image of Chorasmian Nana is possibly also found on two seal impressions from Teshik-Kala dated to the seventh-eighth centuries CE. They depict a four-armed figure in a frontal view wearing what may be a turreted crown.[698] These impressions are very close to the depiction

691 Shkoda 2009: 113–114.

692 See Minardi 2013: 127–131, who suggests that this element might have been borrowed from the iconography of the Eastern Roman Tyche.

693 Azarpay 1969: 186.

694 Minardi 2013.

695 Goldina, Pastushenko and Chernykh 2013: 885.

696 Azarpay 1969: 198–199; Goldina, Pastushenko and Chernykh 2013: 883–884, with further references to previous publications.

697 Azarpay 1969: 199–200.

698 D'yakonova and Smirnova 1967: Fig. 4.5–6.

of Nana on a Chorasmian bowl where the goddess is portrayed without a lion. However, they are not sharp enough for details to be distinguished.

Nana was apparently also worshiped in Parthiena. Four documents from the Parthian period discovered by Soviet archaeologists at the site of Old Nisa mention a "place of worship of praise of Nana" (*āyazan Nanēstāwakān*), but no image of the goddess has come to light from this region.[699] It was proposed that the sculpture of Artemis discovered in Old Nisa may have been called Nana by the Arsacids,[700] but this is impossible to prove.

The cult and images of the goddess on a lion spread further to the East, beyond the limits of the Iranian world. It infiltrated Gandhāra, the Indian peninsula,[701] Khotan, where an unmistakable image of Nana holding two disks of the Sun and Moon is found on the painted panel D. X. 3. recovered by Stein in the ruins of the Buddhist shrine (D. X.) at Dandan Uiliq (fig. 16),[702] and probably even reached as far as China.[703] Very similar representations of the "Khotanese Nana" are also found on three wooden plaques from the collection of the State Hermitage Museum.[704] Interestingly, one of them renders a goddess who is completely naked—a feature completely alien to Iranian art.[705] This may indicate that in this case the iconography of Nana was adopted to represent another, non-Iranian deity. The four-armed goddess continued to be depicted in Khotan up to the ninth-tenth centuries CE, as the drawing from Dunhuang currently housed in the *Bibliothèque nationale de France* demonstrates (fig. 54).

An image of four-armed Nana executed in the Sino-Sogdian style is also known from China. The goddess is depicted on a stone panel from the "Miho couch" accompanied by two female heavenly musicians (fig. 119).[706] The upper part of Nana's body is shown frontally, with four flying ribbons on both sides. In her two upper hands, the goddess holds two spheres—representations of the Sun and Moon. Beneath her are carved two heads of roaring lions, probably serving as the symbolic representation of her throne with lion's protomes. This Sino-Sogdian Nana wears a polos-like crown combined with a sphere surmounted by a trefoil.

3. *Conclusions*

Nana is an example of the incredible longevity of divine images in the Iranian world. Originally a Mesopotamian/Elamite goddess, she was probably imported to Bactria in the Achaemenian period, gradually gaining unusual popularity with the local population. Eventually Nana became the head of the Kushan, Sogdian and probably also of the Chorasmian pantheon and was transformed into "The Great Goddess" of Eastern Iran. In Mesopotamia Nana was connected with the moon god Sin and in Eastern Iran she has a crescent moon decorating her crown as a constant attribute in Bactrian, Sogdian and Chorasmian art. On two occasions—on a bronze plaque from Afghanistan, and on one Kushan coin—the crescent moon is also attached to the goddesses' back in a manner similar to the Kushan Mao. Eastern Iranian iconography and the Rabatak inscription point out that Nana was an astral goddess, perhaps closely associated with kingship and royal power.[707] Her personality in Sogdian religion also had a military aspect, since she is usually shown attended by a warlike lesser god(s) and often personally battles against demons.

---

699 Livshits 2008: 107.

700 Invernizzi 2001: 141.

701 See the discussion and examples in Ghose 2006: 100–103.

702 Stein 1907: 259–261.

703 See Carter 2008; who suggests that Nana might have contributed to the cult of the Chinese goddess Xiwangmu, Queen Mother of the West.

704 D'yakonova 1961: 259–260. Azarpay 1981: 138, writes that these are the representations of Saka Śśandrāmata, the equivalent of the Avestan Spəntā Ārmaiti. However, to my knowledge, there is no evidence supporting this identification.

705 D'yakonova 1961: 259.

706 Raspopova 2004: 50–51; Marshak 2004: 21; Grenet 2007: 469–470.

707 Tanabe 1995a: 209–210, also proposed to associate her with water and earth.

No images of Nana have been identified from the Iranian plateau, although numerous representations are known from the Western periphery in the Hellenistic and Parthian periods. Her earliest pictorial rendering is her zoomorphic companion—a lion—that appears on the coins of the Indo-Scythian rulers. The Kushans created her first anthropomorphic representations in the East, all of them incorporating a crescent moon and associated with a lion. In the Kushano-Sasanian era Nana continued to be venerated, appearing on the coins of Pērōz I. The worship of Nana seems to have penetrated Transoxiana from Bactria, perhaps in the first centuries CE (if not already in the Achaemenian period). Her visual representations are found at almost every site where Sogdian paintings have been uncovered. The Sogdians did not invent any new images of the goddess. Instead, they adopted the Kushan type of Nana seated on a lion with only slight "cosmetic" alterations, such as an additional pair of hands (an influence from Indian iconography), and two spherical personifications of the Sun and Moon, more vividly illustrating the astral aspect of the great goddess. In addition to her association with luminaries, the painting from Ustrushana showing Nana actively involved in a battle against demons probably indicates that in Sogdiana she acquired a warlike aspect not found in Bactria.

16. *Oxus/Vaxš*

Oxus (Bactrian Vaxš), the god of the river Amu Darya, was one of the most important and popular gods in Bactria, Sogdiana and Chorasmia. He is completely absent from the Avesta and Zoroastrian tradition and represents a layer of local Iranian cults and beliefs left outside the Zoroastrian scriptures and of which, therefore, very little is known.

1. *Western Iran*

Being the personification of the Amu Darya—the greatest river of Eastern Iran—Oxus was apparently unknown in the West where his veneration is not attested by any material or literary source.[708]

2. *Eastern Iran*

The worship of Oxus in Bactria is already attested in the Achaemenian period. Several personal names in the Aramaic documents from Bactria, which date to the fourth century BCE, contain the theophoric compound Vaxšu (Oxus).[709] It is also worth mentioning a finger ring from the Oxus Treasure, bearing the image of the winged bull and carrying an Aramaic inscription "Vaxšu".[710] The earliest representation of Oxus is probably a small bronze statuette depicting Marsyas, a river deity from Asia Minor (Phrygia), playing on a flute and surmounted on a votive stone altar of the Greek type, found in excavations of the Oxus Temple at Takht-i Sangin (modern Tajikistan) (pl. 18).[711] The altar carries a Greek inscription: *Εὐχὴν ἀνέθηκεν Ἀτροσωκης Ὀξωι* ('Atrosokes dedicated [his] vow to Oxus'). This may in fact be the earliest definite post-Achaemenian visual representation of any Iranian deity. Its complete adoption of the iconography of the Greek river god, Marsyas, is undoubtedly significant.[712] Moreover, this statue was presented to the temple by an individual with an Iranian name and with a dedication written in Greek

---

708 However, it is worth noting that the personal name "Oxus" appears on a gravestone from Mount Dindymus in Galatia, Asia Minor. See Mitchell 2007: 163.

709 For instance, Vaxšu-bandaka ("Slave or servant of the Oxus") and Vaxšu-data ("Created by the Oxus"). See Naveh and Shaked 2012: 59.

710 Dalton 1964: no. 105.

711 Litvinskiy, Vinogradov, Pichikjan 1985; Pichikyan 1991: 160–172. For the excavations reports, see final publications in Litvinskiy and Pichikyan 2000; Litvinskiy 2001b; Litvinskiy 2010.

712 However, see Francfort 2012: 121, who opposes this identification.

that uses the Greek name of the god. Interestingly, three additional Greek inscriptions uncovered at Takht-i Sangin in recent years also mention Oxus and were most probably dedicatory inscriptions ordered by individuals of Bactrian origin.[713]

In the Kushan period, a new and utterly different visual image of Oxus was created for the Kushan numismatic pantheon. The god Oaxšo (OAXÞO), portrayed on the unique gold coin of Huvishka (pl. 19), is absent from the Rabatak divine list.[714] He is shown in frontal view, turning his head in profile to the left. Oaxšo is bearded, with a nimbus surrounding his head and holding a staff (or perhaps a trident or spear) in his right hand and a large fish in his left. It has been proposed that the Kushan Oaxšo's visual representation was modeled on the image of Poseidon as he appears on coins of the Indo-Scythian king Maues (third quarter of the second century BCE).[715] It has also been suggested that an image of Triton carrying an oar and a large fish on seven plaques from the Saka graves at Tillya Tepe and on Indo-Greek coin of Hippostratos also represent Oxus.[716] On the Kushan coin, Oxus is shown holding a large fish, undoubtedly reinforcing his identity as a river god.

Henri-Paul Francfort has suggested that Oxus was, in fact, a female divinity—the principal deity of Central Asia in *la longue durée*.[717] Furthermore, the goddess Ardoxšo whose name was proposed to mean **Arda-Vakhshu* ("the righteous Oxus"), might be, according to the French scholar, the visual representation of Oxus.[718] Moreover, he has suggested that the goddess Cybele depicted on silver plates from the "Temple with Indented Niches" at Ai Khanum and the "Oxus Temple" from Takht-i Sangin are to be equated with the god Oxus—the principal deity of the two Bactrian temples.[719] However, the assumption that Oxus was considered to be female is not borne out by the available sources. The only two representations of Oxus—the statuette from Takht-i Sangin and the Kushan Oaxšo—are male. Moreover, it is highly improbable, not to say impossible, that the same deity would be represented twice on Kushan coins, under different names, assigned to different sexes and with different appearances. It is more plausible that Cybele would be identified in Bactria with Nana, the great Bactrian goddess with whom she shared her principal attribute—the lion.

To date, no definite images of Oxus have been identified in Sogdian art. This fact is surprising considering the undeniable popularity of the god among Sogdians, as attested by their personal names.[720] Pavel Lurje has suggested that *Xušūfayn*, a village in the vicinity of Samarkand, be interpreted as "The temple of Oxus" and it is therefore possible that a temple dedicated to the god existed in Sogdiana.[721] These considerations and the apparent importance of Oxus in Sogdian religion make it difficult to believe that his image did not exist among Sogdian art's rich repertoire of divine beings. There is some evidence to suggest that Oxus was worshipped in Sogdiana in zoomorphic form—that of a horse. A depiction of the veneration of a horse is found on the "Miho coach", a Sino-Sogdian funerary coach, now in the Miho Museum in Japan, dated to 570 CE.[722] The water stream and fishes depicted beneath its hooves have led to its interpretation as the river god Oxus.[723] It should be noted that the image of a riderless horse is well-known from Sogdiana itself and is found in different media, including paintings and ossuaries.[724]

---

713 See Ivantchik 2011.
714 Rosenfield 1967: 92, Pl. VIII, 155; Göbl 1984: Oaxšo 1.
715 Rosenfield 1967: 92.
716 Boardman 2012: 108, Figs. 8–9.
717 Francfort 2005/2006; Francfort 2012.
718 Francfort 2005/2006: 518–519. Francfort 2012: 130.
719 Francfort 2012.
720 Lurje 2010: nos. 219, 1355, 1356, 1364–1373.
721 Lurje 2004: 209.
722 Marshak 2004; Raspopova 2004.
723 This oral suggestion by Skjærvø was accepted by Marshak 2004: 20–21 and Grenet 2007: 470.
724 For a discussion of this motif in Sogdian art, see Riboud 2003.

The link between Oxus and the horse is also strengthened by an eighth century CE Chinese source that speaks of a temple located at the confluence of the Vakhsh and Panj rivers (very close to the location of the Oxus Temple at Takht-i Sangin) with a remarkable statue of a horse.[725] This may allude to the survival of local traditions of sanctity relating to the long-abandoned Oxus Temple site, preserving the cult of the god in the form of a horse. Moreover, at the entrance to the Oxus Temple itself, fragments of a colossal bronze statue (which could have been as tall as 5 m) were uncovered,[726] and recent excavations on the site indicate that the statue was probably four-footed.[727] Could these be the fragments of a giant statue of Oxus in the form of a horse? If Oxus was believed to manifest himself as a horse and given the visual appearance of a stallion, it is plausible to suggest that the Sogdian god on the throne supported by protomes of horses, who appears in Panjikent and is also the main protagonist of the paintings in the "Small Hall" at Bunjikat, Ustrushana, might be Oxus.[728] The god from the Doḵtar-e Nōšervān painting may also represent a Bactrian portrayal of Oxus. We know that Oxus was hugely popular in Bactria and especially in the region of Northern Afghanistan as attested by Bactrian legal documents from seventh and eighth centuries CE, where Oxus is addressed as βαγο οαχϸο βαγανο ϸαυο, "god Vaxš, the king of gods".[729] On one Bactrian seal he is called λωγο βαγο or ιωγο βαγο, that is, "the lord of the world" or "the one god".[730]

Interestingly, Oxus is not the only god in the Bactrian documents to bear the title "the king of gods". Another such god is Mithra, who is addressed as "Mihr-yazad the god of Ulishagan" (μιυροιαζαδο βαγο ολιραγαναγγο).[731] The title "king of gods" is also shared by a third, enigmatic deity called Kamird. The meaning of "Kamird", which could be an epithet rather than a name, is "head" or "chief".[732] It is therefore plausible that Kamird is simply an epithet of Oxus or Mithra. Moreover, the clerics or followers of Kamird mentioned in the same documents are known as *kēd*; and in Chinese sources this term is used to designate the worshipers of the god Zūn. Hence, it is likely, as Sims-Williams proposes, that Kamird should be identified with Zūn and that he was the god depicted on the Doḵtar-e Nōšervān painting.[733] Furthermore, it is possible that Zūn, whose etymology is not clear,[734] could be yet another title of Oxus or Mithra. The seventh century CE account of the Chinese pilgrim Xuanzang that attests to the great popularity of the god *Shu-na* (Zūn) also records a local legend connecting Zūn with the mountains, stating that he "arrived from afar".[735] Both these motifs appear inadequate for a local river god, but the connection with mountains aligns with the Avestan myth of Mithra who "surveys the whole material world" from Mount Harā. This motif is apparently depicted on one Sasanian seal from Eastern Iran.[736]

The title "king of gods" is given to more than one deity, indicating that, as in neighboring Sogdiana, each Bactrian city, community and even family tended to have a "patron" deity to whom they were particularly devoted.

---

725 Drège and Grenet 1987; Litvinskiy and Pichikyan 2000: 315–316.
726 Litvinskiy and Pichikyan 2000: 123.
727 Druzhinina and Inagaki 2008: 103–104.
728 See p. 111 ff.
729 Sims-Williams 2001/2005.
730 Lerner and Sims-Williams 2011: 56.
731 Sims-Williams 2007: 136–137. Ulishagan is probably modern Alishang in the Langhman Province in northeastern Afghanistan.
732 Sims-Williams 2000: 4.
733 Sims-Williams 1997b; Sims-Williams 2000: 4.
734 However, see Sims-Williams 2010: 66, for the suggestion that it derives from Zurwān.
735 Watters 1904: 126–127. Bosworth 1968: 35, suggested that the cult of Zūn might have been brought to Bactria by the Hephtalites.
736 See p. 108.

3. *Conclusions*

It is highly probable that the cult of Oxus predated the Achaemenian period and originated in remote prehistory, reflecting the local veneration of the life-giving water of the great Eastern Iranian river Amu Darya. He was perhaps already worshipped in the temples of BMAC in Gonur or Togolok, but in the absence of any written record from that era, this must be considered a speculation.

The earliest recorded image of Oxus is most probably that of a bronze statuette of Marsyas from the Oxus Temple dated from the Hellenistic period and of pure Greek iconography. A second image was crafted by the Kushans based on entirely different prototypes and iconographic conventions. Despite not being mentioned in the Rabatak inscription and probably suffering neglect by the Kushan rulers whose origin was far to the north of the great Central Asian river, Oxus was apparently able to retain his popularity in Bactria. Moreover, according to the Bactrian documents, he was honored as "the king of gods" as late as the time of the Arab conquest. If the assumption that Kamird and Zūn are both epithets referring to Oxus is correct, it would mean that Oxus-Zūn was the greatest god of Zāvulistān in Late Antiquity. The available evidence indicates that Oxus was also no less popular in Sogdiana. Assuming that the hypothesis linking Oxus with horse is correct, the Sogdian god on the throne supported by the foreparts of horses may be his visual manifestation in Sogdiana and in Doḵtar-e Nōšervān in Bactria.

17. *X*ʸ*arənah*

*X*ʸ*arənah* (MP. *xvarrah*, NP. فر, *far*(*r*), Scyth. *farn*) appears in the Avesta both as an abstract concept and as a *yazata* in Yt. 19, which is dedicated to it. There has been much controversy and debate over the exact meaning and etymology of the term *x*ʸ*arənah*. It was proposed to mean "fortune" in the sense of "good things, prosperity", to be derived from the Old Iranian word for "sun" and hence convey the idea of "luminosity", "shining",[737] or be a borrowing from the Scythian language with the original meaning "sovereignty, control", and then "abundance".[738] Whatever its etymology, the common and most fitting basic semantics of this word in the historical period appears to be "glory/fortune".[739]

Even when acting as a divinity, *x*ʸ*arənah* is abstract and is never described in the Avesta or in Pahlavi literature as taking anthropomorphic form. Its very name is always given in neuter form.[740] In these texts, *x*ʸ*arənah* is frequently directly or indirectly linked with fire, light and warmth. In the Avesta, *x*ʸ*arənah* also has strong connections with lakes and water and has been proposed that *x*ʸ*arənah* was originally an attribute of the deity Apąm Napāt who acts as its guardian.[741] The possession of *x*ʸ*arənah* necessarily required engagement in direct physical contact, as may be deduced from the myth of Yima and from the *Kār-nāmag ī Ardašīr ī Pābagān* where the *x*ʸ*arənah* in the form of a ram was described as being seated on the horse behind Ardašīr.[742]

Similar notions of "divine grace and fortune" existed among many ancient Eurasian people. Especially significant is the Mesopotamian conception of *melammu* found already in Sumerian mythology, which, like *x*ʸ*arənah*, also had connotations of brilliance and radiance.[743] Sumerian deities are said to

---

737 See the detailed overview and discussion by Gnoli 1999. Rastorgueva and Edelman 2007: 440–444, translate the Proto-Iranian **hu̯arnah-* as "brilliance, radiance". See also Boyce 1975b: 66–67.

738 Lubotsky 1998.

739 Gnoli 1999.

740 Boyce 1975b: 67. For a classic, in-depth study of *x*ʸ*arənah* in Iranian written sources, see Bailey 1971: 1–78.

741 Oettinger 2009.

742 *KAP* 4.11.16, 22–23. The *Shāh-nāma* supplies additional details regarding the appearance of this ram. He is sad to be of a purple color, winged, with a tail like that of a peacock and the head, ears and hooves of a horse. See *Shāh-nāma*, vol. 6, 155.

743 *Melammu* can be translated as "physical emanation or 'aura' surrounding its bearer": Winter 1994: 125. According to Emelianov 2010: 1112, the original meaning of the Sumerian word is "a bright garment of flame and light, covering the person

possess these luminous characteristics. For instance, it is written that goddess Inanna/Ištar "shines like daylight".[744] The *melammu* appears to have had a long and enduring presence in Mesopotamian mythology through the ages. In late Babylonian culture, that encountered by the Achaemenian Persians, divine light, radiating from the gods (most notably the Sun-god Shamash) continued to be "a basic characteristic" of the deities.[745] In the texts, both Mesopotamian gods and their statues are described as shining and emanating light.[746] Kings were also endowed with *melammu*. This idea appears for the first time in the Sumerian epics of Lugalbanda, in Gilgameš, and in the hymn of king Ur-Nammu of the Ur III Period (2047–2030 BCE) where we read that "Suen has selected Ur-Nammu in his heart, he is a charm-bearing king, whose radiance covers the country".[747]

Although gods and kings are described in texts as possessing *melammu*, only Ištar is ever depicted with a nimbus. This fact has led Irene Winter to suggest that the halo of the goddess is related not to the concept of *melammu*, but to Ištar's association with the Venus "star".[748]

1. *Western Iran*

From Zoroastrian literature, especially from the myth of Yima, one gains the impression that *x^varənah* was a concept of paramount importance for the legitimacy of Iranian kingship—the ultimate, necessary source of divine authority.[749] *X^varənah* (NP. *far*(*r*)) also occupies a similar place in the *Shāh-nāma* that often determines how ordinary Iranians and even some scholars (both consciously and unconsciously) perceive pre-Islamic Iran.[750] It is therefore unsurprising that art historians, archaeologists and historians have looked for and found *x^varənah* in numerous elements of ancient Iranian—and especially Sasanian—art. Visual representations of *x^varənah* have been recognized in dozens of real and fanciful renderings of animals, birds and plants, in various decorations (ribbons, jewelry, precious stones), in the Achaemenian figure in the winged ring, the nimbus, tongues of fire, royal diadem and elements of crowns, in wings and even in circular marks that appear on the faces of Parthian and Kushan kings on some of their coins.[751] And this is only a partial list![752] Indeed, anything connected with royal symbolism and seemingly conveying the idea of "glory", can, if in the Iranian context, be interpreted as representing *x^varənah*.

However, only three visual manifestations of *x^varənah* are explicitly described in the entire corpus of pre-Islamic Iranian literature:

(1) The Fire in the *Mihr Yašt*[753] and in the story of Zoroaster's birth in *Wizīdagīhā ī Zādspram*.[754]
(2) The *vārəγna* bird in the Avestan myth of Yima.[755]
(3) A wild ram (*warrag*) in *Kār-nāmag ī Ardašīr ī Pābagān*.[756]

---

dressed in it or endowed with it". See also the recent study by Aster 2012, who defines *melammu* in the second millennium BCE texts as "the covering, outer layer, or appearance of a person, being, or object, or the rays emanating from a being, which perceptibly demonstrate the irresistible or supreme power of that person, being or object" (p. 51).

744 Rochberg 2009: 49.

745 Rochberg 2009: 49.

746 Winter 1994: 124–125.

747 Emelianov 2010: 1117. For additional examples, see also Winter 1994: 126.

748 Winter 2012: 160.

749 See, for example, the classic study by Ehsan Yarshater, who writes that "the xvaranah is one of the most enduring concepts of Iranian tradition and figures prominently in the national history. No king could rule successfully without it.": Yarshater 1983: 345.

750 For the occurrences of *farr* in the *Shāh-nāma*, see Ghazanfari 2011: 130–138.

751 Tanabe 1988: 379.

752 See also Soudavar 2003 and Soudavar 2010.

753 Yt. 10.127. ed. and tr. by Gershevitch 1959: 136–137.

754 *WZ* 5. His mother already possessed a *x^varənah* in form of a blazing fire according to *Dk* 7.2.7.

755 Yt. 19.30–34.

756 *KAP* 4.11.16, 22–23.

No other objects or animals are ever directly associated with *x^v^arənah* by any pre-Islamic Iranian or non-Iranian text.[757]

Despite the fact that *x^v^arənah* seems to exist in most Iranian languages and is frequently attested as a compound in personal names, it is never found in Achaemenian royal inscriptions. It therefore does not seem to have played an important role in Achaemenian royal ideology.[758] Achaemenian kings exercised kingship due to their special relationship with their patron god, Ahura Mazdā, and this is constantly emphasized in royal inscriptions. This is not an Iranian, but a Mesopotamian idea.[759] The attempts to interpret the Achaemenian figure in the winged ring as *x^v^arənah* are untenable and not grounded in primary material.[760] Unfortunately, because of the paucity of sources, nothing definite can be said about the concept of *x^v^arənah* in the Hellenistic and Parthian periods.

X^v^arənah (MP *xvarrah*) appears for the first time in royal inscriptions and in epigraphy in the Sasanian period. At first, however, this evidence is inarticulate and problematic, allowing De Jong to argue that the popular "assumption that xvarrah was a central concept in Sasanian royal ideology is difficult to uphold".[761] Indeed, any reference to *xvarrah* is completely absent under the first six Sasanian kings. It appears for the first time in the Paikuli inscription of king Narseh who emphasizes that "glory and rulership had been given" to him[762] and claims that "the gods gave glory and rulership to the family of Sāsān".[763] The second reference to *xvarrah* is found in a short building inscription from Meshkin shahr (Eastern Azerbaijan) dated to the twenty-seventh year of Šāpūr II (236 CE).[764] In this inscription a man named Narseh writes that he completed the building of the castle "in the name of the gods for (?) the glory of the King of Kings (*xvarrah ī šāhān šāh*)". To the reign of Šāpūr II also belongs a Parthian inscription on a vessel found in Merv where *farn* appears in the meaning of "blessing", "fortune".[765] It seems that over the course of time the role and importance of *xvarrah* in Sasanian royal ideology was gradually, but steadily, increasing. Thus, Pērōz proclaims in the inscription on his seal that he is the one "who increased the glory (*xvarrah*) of the gods of the Ērān and Anērān".[766] An important milestone occurs during the reign of Xusrō II, when the legend *xvarrah* appears for the first time on the obverse of his coins followed by another type, which carries a longer formula—*xvarrah abzūd* ("whose xvarrah has increased").[767] This legend continued to be employed until the fall of the Sasanian dynasty.

757 However, there exists one additional description of *x^v^arənah* in *Dk* 816.13 where it is said that the *x^v^arənah* of the Kayānids was in the form of TYN' (*kayān xvarrah TYN' karb būd*). The reading of the Arameogramm TYN' as (*gil*), "clay" as well as the alternative *gar* "mountain", suggested by Kotwal 1984, does not seem to fit the context, since the necessary characteristic of *x^v^arənah* is its dynamism and mobility. Bailey 1971: xxxiii, proposed to read TYBA (*āhūg*), "gazelle" or TNYN' "sea monster", instead of TYN'. A "gazelle" seems the most appropriate manifestation of the *x^v^arənah*, but such a reading would require too much textual emendation. Regarding TNYN', according to Hintze 1999: 85 it is hard to imagine that *x^v^arənah* would assume a form of a monster. However, the narrative of this story rather seems to support this interpretation. This passage describes the unsuccessful attempt of Kay Us, urged on by the demons, to reach Heaven from the summit of mount Alborz, but his *x^v^arənah* assumes the form of TYN' and disappears. Therefore, the transformation of the *x^v^arənah* into a monster probably symbolizes the punishment of his *hubris* and the loss of his divine grace.

758 Gnoli 1974: 170–171; Gnoli 1989b: 96.

759 Gnoli 1980: 215–216.

760 See p. 47 ff.

761 De Jong 2004: 265. Although Gnoli is certainly right in his remark that the *xvarrah* was "an element peculiar to Sassanian propaganda". See Gnoli 1989b: 150–151, n. 26.

762 Paikuli 53, Humbach and Skjærvø 1983: 3.1., 52.

763 Paikuli 80, Humbach and Skjærvø 1983: 3.1., 65. For other occurrences of *xvarrah* in the Paikuli inscription, see Humbach and Skjærvø 1983: 3.2., 51.

764 Frye and Skjærvø 1996/1998.

765 "*Farn* came, (o) Burzwand, (you), whom so (= with fortune) let live (?) a thousand years". See Livshits and Nikitin 1991: 112–116.

766 See Panaino 2009a: 245, with references to previous publications of this seal.

767 Daryaee 1997; Gyselen 2000: 307.

As noted above, *x^varənah* (*farr*) occupies a place of central importance in the *Shāh-nāma*, being a necessary attribute of kingly grace bestowed on kings and great heroes.[768] Indeed, in the epic of Firdausī, *farr* is the ultimate source of legitimate kingship and a distinctive feature of the rightful Iranian king, which entitles him to rule. The *farr* in the *Shāh-nāma* is directly linked with light radiating from the body of the king.[769] Interestingly, in *Tārīkh-i Sīstān*, one of the earliest sources in the New Persian language, *farr* is described as the light above the ears of the king's horse.[770]

From the evidence surveyed above it is clear that *x^varənah* was not the central and necessary component of early Sasanian royal legitimacy that it is often presented to be, let alone in the Achaemenian and Parthian periods.[771] Attempts to recognize manifestations of *x^varənah* in the visual record during early periods or to attribute to it an important or even central place in royal ideology appear anachronistic. However, the increased significance of *x^varənah* in the later Sasanian period and its centrality to the royal ideology in the *Shāh-nāma* strongly suggest that a change occurred at some stage in Sasanian history. At this turning point, the Avestan concept of *x^varənah* was adopted by the Sasanians and elevated to a position of prime importance as the source of Iranian legitimate kingship. This shift was perhaps an outcome of a process which Daryaee has called a "Zoroastrianization of memory", and which resulted in the adoption of the "Kayānid ideology" by later Sasanian kings.[772] The growing influence of Zoroastrian clergy in the royal court and its deeper involvement in the management of the Empire seems to have led to a remodeling of the ideology of Sasanian kingship according to Avestan concepts. Rahim Shayegan has convincingly argued that the complex relations of the Sasanian Empire and its kings with the nomadic world to the East contributed to this shift and evoked mythical confrontations between the legendary Kayānid rulers and the Turanians, identified with the nomads.[773] Sasanian kings began claiming Kayānid lineage and presented themselves as the descendants of the mythical Avestan kings, the possessors of *xvarrah*. This is reflected in changes in the Sasanian royal titulature.[774] Under the king Yazdgerd II the standard formula on the coins *mazdēsn bay* [*name*] *šāhān šāh ērān kē čihr az yazdān* was replaced by a new title *kay* (Kayānid).

Anthroponyms containing *x^varənah* are widely attested in Old Persian, Parthian and Middle Persian. The notion of *x^varənah* as an abstract "divine glory" and probably also as the personified deity undoubtedly existed among Western Iranians during these periods, although it is impossible to ascertain to what extent these perceptions correspond to those in the Avesta. Western Iranian royal ideology was based on other principles of mainly Mesopotamian origin (with considerable Hellenistic and nomadic contributions) and Iranian kings did not regard it necessary or important to emphasize their possession of *x^varənah* in their inscriptions and monumental art. It is possible that under the early Sasanian kings the idea and concept of *x^varənah* were employed in a general sense, referring to abstract "glory". This situation had changed significantly by the time later Sasanian kings began to embrace the "Kayānid ideology" and employed *xvarrah* on their coins in the Avestan sense of the word. However, even in the late Sasanian period there is no compelling evidence that *x^varənah* (both as an abstraction and as a deity) was represented in visual art.

The most suitable candidates for this role in light of the written sources are probably a ram and a bird of prey—an eagle, a falcon or a hawk. These creatures, sometimes decorated with flying royal ribbons,

768 For the *farr* in the *Shāh-nāma* and the hero Rostam as its guardian, see Davidson 1994: 110–128.

769 For instance, the *farr* radiated from Feraydun as if he was the sun. See *Shāh-nāma*, vol. 1, 62, b. 110–111.

770 *TS* 35.

771 For instance, see Abkaʿi-Khavari 2000: 130 and Wiesehöfer 2010b: 136, who maintains that the Sasanian kings "derived their legitimacy" through *xvarrah* "already known to us from the Achaemenids and the Parthians".

772 Daryaee 2006b.

773 Shayegan 2013: 807–808.

774 On the evolution of Sasanian royal titles, see Shayegan 2003 and Shayegan 2013.

were often depicted on Sasanian seals.[775] They—and only they—are mentioned in Zoroastrian literature as manifestations of x^v*arənah*, although the possibility cannot be excluded that in the lost parts of the Avesta or in Middle Persian writings, x^v*arənah* may have also been symbolized by other animals found in the rich Sasanian bestiary. Taking into account that in the *Shāh-nāma farr* manifests itself as the light radiating from a king, it is possible that the nimbus could be the visual representation of x^v*arənah* in the art of the late Sasanians and perhaps also of other Iranian peoples. However, the automatic interpretation of a nimbus in any Iranian culture and period as the expression of x^v*arənah* appears unjustified.[776] In this context the story of the dream of Pābag from *Kār-nāmag ī Ardašīr ī Pābagān* may be revealing. In his dream Pābag sees that the sun shines from the head of Sāsān (*xwaršēd az sar ī sāsān be tābēd ud hamāg gēhān rōšnīh gīrēd*) betokening royal power.[777] It is significant that in this story, unlike in the *Shāh-nāma*, the light radiating from Sāsān is not called *xvarrah*, although the author was certainly familiar with this term, which is employed several times in the *Kār-nāmag*. Nevertheless, the imagery of this description is expressive enough and we cannot rule out that this text reflects a period when the nimbus was not yet directly linked with the manifestation of x^v*arənah*. It is quite possible that among various Iranian people in different historical periods, the nimbus could have had different meanings.

Another element often taken to represent x^v*arənah* in the art of the ancient Iranians are the tongues of fire rising from the shoulders of deities, kings and heroes.[778] This seemingly corresponds well to the Zoroastrian texts, where fire is one of the manifestations of x^v*arənah*. Tongues of fire appear for the first time on the coins of the Kushan king Vima Kadphises and later became an important attribute of the Kushan rulers and gods, even subsequently adopted for images of Buddha.[779] Burning shoulders are also frequent in Sogdian art, but they remain almost unknown in the art of Sasanian Iran. No Sasanian king except Balāš is ever depicted with shoulders aflame. If flames were indeed a visual expression of the idea of x^v*arənah*, one would expect this motif to have been exploited much more intensively by late Sasanian kings.

The diadem granted to the king by the deity on numerous Sasanian reliefs is also often regarded as the symbol of x^v*arənah*. Certainly, the diadem in the investiture scenes signifies the delegation of sacral kingship and the "divine mandate" to rule, which accords with perceptions of x^v*arənah* in Zoroastrian tradition and in the *Shāh-nāma*. However, in these sources neither a diadem nor a crown is ever associated with x^v*arənah*. Moreover, from the Paikuli inscription it is clear that the diadem and x^v*arənah* are not directly linked to each other.[780]

2. *Eastern Iran*

There are only three indisputable representations of x^v*arənah* in Iranian art, all originating from Eastern Iran—two from Bactria under the Kushan kings and the third from late Sogdian art. Only one is anthropomorphic—the Kushan Pharro (ΦΑΡΡΟ) who appears for the first time on the coins of Kanishka as a beardless youth, with his nimbate head turned to the right. Pharro wears a tunic, mantle, and a diadem with a small wing attached to its front. He holds a bowl in his right hand and a staff in his left.

---

775 For instance, see Bivar 1969: EP-ER (a ram), HG (a bird of prey). In a recent study, Grenet has proposed to interpret the figure of a standing man with a ram's head depicted on a Sasanian seal as the representation of x^v*arənah*, based on the *Kār-nāmag*. See Grenet 2013: 2004.

776 For instance, demons in Sogdian art also often have nimbi. I am inclined to think the observation of Grenet and Zhang Guangda 1996: 179; that "the nimbus is not so much a divine attribute as an indication of supernatural power, no matter whether good or bad" is probably correct.

777 *KAP* 1.8.

778 For instance, Herzfeld 1930: 29.

779 See Tsuchiya 1999/2000.

780 The only exception seems to be a Sogdian tale of Caesar and the thieves where "the diadem of *farn*" (*prn δyδym*) is mentioned. See p. 39.

Under Huvishka, Pharro continued to be represented, but several new types were added bringing the total number of iconographic variants to ten (figs. 120–124; pl. 20).[781] On three types (nos. 4, 5, 10) he has no mantle and on no. 9 he is armored. His attributes include a staff (nos. 1, 2, 4, 6, 8, 10), a caduceus (no. 3), a sword (nos. 2, 5, 6, 8, 10), a bowl (no. 1), fire (nos. 3, 4, 5), a diadem (nos. 7, 8) and a purse (no. 9). Eight types have a nimbus (nos. 1, 2, 4, 6, 7, 8, 9, 10), two have flames rising from both shoulders (nos. 5, 6). No. 3 stands on a round wheel-like object and nos. 2 and 3 make a gesture of benediction with the right hand. All types are inspired by Graeco-Roman examples and one (no. 3) may be specifically identified as following the imagery of Hermes, although it remains uncertain to what extent the iconographic similarities reflected the functional correspondence between the two gods.[782] Most of Pharro's attributes are not unique to him, but are also found in the possession of other Kushan deities. The only exception is the wing attached to his diadem, which was borrowed from Hermes. The purse is the only indication that Pharro was connected with fortune in the sense of fecundity, prosperity and wealth, which apparently accords well with the "Scythian" etymology of *x^v^arənah* proposed by Alexander Lubotsky. It should also be noted that Sims-Williams has recently put forward linguistic arguments in favor of a Scythian origin for the Kushan royal dynasty.[783] It is tempting to suggest that the material wealth, with which Pharro is iconographically associated, reflects the original Scythian meaning of *x^v^arənah* preserved by the Kushan ruling clan who traced its lineage to Central Asian nomads.

An additional type of Pharro is attested on a seal bearing a Kharoṣṭhī inscription, currently housed in the British Museum. The god depicted on this seal wears a diadem decorated with wings, holds a staff and purse and stands on two anthropomorphic busts.[784] It suggests that other variants of Pharro's iconography were created by alternative combinations from a "tool-kit of attributes", and it is different from those attested on coins that were also in circulation in the Kushan state. Carter has also proposed to interpret the image of a youthful god with a spear and flaming shoulders, which appears on a painted terracotta panel from northern Afghanistan, as Pharro (fig. 125).[785] This deity, attended by an adorant, is portrayed beardless, nimbate and with flames rising from his shoulders. He wears a red coat with long sleeves and a red crown made of oval elements topped by a crescent and a diadem. This god holds a spear in his right hand and grasps the hilt of a sword with his left hand. Although Pharro holds a staff instead of a spear on coins, taking into account the variety of types and the large number of associated attributes, the identification suggested by Carter is possible.[786]

It is significant that *x^v^arənah* is never mentioned in the Kushan royal inscriptions.[787] The Kushan kings were subjected to full deification (which already contradicts Avestan notions) and derived their legitimacy from other sources. Thus, Kanishka is said to have obtained kingship from "Nana and all the gods".[788] The popularity of Pharro in Kushan Bactria was probably high and was not limited to a certain religious confession. His image was even adopted by Kushan adherents of Buddhism. One Buddhist divine couple, whose sculptural representations are common in Gandhāran art, are often identified as Pharro and Ardoxšo. They are shown with symbols of fecundity such as a cornucopia and coins pouring from a purse.[789]

---

781 Nine, according to the typology of Carter 1986: 90–91, with one additional type.
782 On the equation of Pharro with Hermes, see Gnoli 1996b.
783 Sims-Williams 2002.
784 Callieri 1997 Cat. 7.1.
785 Carter 1997: 575–577. For other panels from this group, see p. 62–63 and p. 155–156.
786 Tigran Mkrtychev in his forthcoming study tends to identify this god as Kārrtikeya (personal communication). However, a cock, the principal attribute of Kārrtikeya, is missing.
787 Although Fussman 1998: 586, has proposed that Pharro is mentioned among the other gods in the Rabatak inscription, this translation seems unlikely. See Sims-Williams 2004/2008: 64.
788 Rabatak inscription, line 2.
789 Quagliotti 2003. Although she was also identified as the Indian goddess Śrī. See Fussman 1988.

An additional image that is traditionally interpreted as the visual representation of Pharro in the Buddhist context comes from the wall painting uncovered at the Bactrian monastery of Fayaztepa located within Old Termez, in the Surkhandarya region of modern Uzbekistan. The excavator, Lazar' Al'baum, maintained that it was built in the first century CE and functioned until the third century CE, when it was destroyed by the Sasanians.[790] However, Ciro Lo Muzio has recently produced convincing iconographic arguments for the dating of the Fayaztepa paintings to the fourth century CE.[791] On the eastern wall of the Fayaztepa temple, two figures were pictured walking towards Buddha, depicted on the southern wall (fig. 126). The first figure from the left is dressed in a yellow *kaftan* and is labeled by a Bactrian inscription "φαρο" placed above his head. However, φαρο may be a part of a theophoric name or of a longer inscription.[792] His right arm is bent and a pointed finger is directed towards Buddha in a gesture of adoration.[793] The northern wall is decorated with a group of figures in Kushan dress standing frontally. According to Al'baum, these depict the Kushan king Kanishka and various deities approaching as worshippers in the presence of Buddha.[794] On the eastern wall where "Pharro" is portrayed, the composition is different and might have originally depicted a procession of donors. However, the complete absence of any divine attributes and the very composition of the painting, undoubtedly representing a procession of donors, make the identification of the left figure as Pharro, improbable. Rather, he is more likely to be one of the donors.

Neither of the variants of Kushan Pharro were apparently continued in Kushano-Sasanian or Sogdian visual art.[795] If the image of the god of glory and fortune existed among Eastern Iranians after the fall of the Kushan Empire, it was probably different from the Kushan creation. Grenet has proposed to identify one of the enthroned divine figures in the Kushano-Sasanian painting at Ghulbiyan in the Faryab province in northwestern Afghanistan as Pharro.[796] These wall-paintings, discovered in a cave in 1978, probably represent a rare example of Kushano-Sasanian period art and are dated to the fourth-fifth centuries CE.[797] The preserved area of the painting (4.5 × 2 m.) depicts some sixteen figures painted on a red background (fig. 127). The far left part of the painting is occupied by a hunting scene and by a group of five adorants depicted in profile and headed by a larger figure, probably a local ruler (nos. 3–7). They are facing a group of enthroned figures portrayed frontally, who in all probability represent divinities (nos. 8, 9, 11, 14, 15). The first of these enthroned characters (no. 8) is nimbate and wears white and green clothes and a crown topped by a bird with outstretched wings. A round green object is pictured to the right of his head, perhaps representing an astral symbol. In his raised right hand the figure holds an arrow, but the object in his left hand is not preserved. His legs rest on a carpet covering an "aquarium" in which four fishes can be seen. Lee and Grenet note the outlines of three heads (perhaps of a man, a woman and a child) above the two fishes to the left, although it is impossible to identify them.[798] To his right there is a female figure (no. 9) draped in a green tunic with white cuffs and a veil, which covers her head. She holds a bowl in her left hand and makes a gesture with bended forefinger with her right hand. She turns in adoration toward another enthroned male figure to the right (no. 11) wearing white and red clothes whose attribute is a sword placed between his knees. Between them there is an image of a flying Nike (no. 10).

790 Al'baum 1990: 26.
791 Lo Muzio 2008/2012.
792 Lo Muzio 2008/2012: 193.
793 Al'baum 1990: 25.
794 Al'baum 1990: 26.
795 Although some notions that go back to the Kushan Pharro might have been preserved among the Sogdians. See below.
796 Grenet 1999.
797 Lee and Grenet 1998; Grenet 1999.
798 Lee and Grenet 1998: 79.

Further to the right and below, is another somewhat larger seated nimbate male figure (no. 14), wearing green and red, whose legs rest on a ram's head/skull. Behind him there are additional enthroned figures (nos. 15, 16a), who are unfortunately poorly preserved. A group of enthroned gods, a procession of two female and one male figures (nos. 12, 13, 16b), carrying small, portable fire-altars is shown below. It is significant that the figure of the principal adorant (ruler) (no. 7) is shown on a larger scale than the figure of the chief god (no. 8). We may assume that the Ghulbiyan painting depicts a scene of worship of a Kushano-Sasanian king and his retinue before the cultic statues of local deities. The suggestion that figure no. 14 be identified with Pharro is based on the presence of a ram's head on which the god rests his legs. A wild ram is the visual manifestation of *x^varənah* in the Sasanian text *Kār-nāmag ī Ardašīr ī Pābagān*, but it is impossible to be certain that an association between a wild ram and Pharro also existed in Bactria. The imagery of the god on the Kushan coins does not support this suggestion.

Primarily based on the same fragment from the *Kār-nāmag*, Boris Litvinskiy has argued that the ram was a manifestation of *x^varənah* among Central Asian Saka and Sarmatians.[799] Following him, numerous decorative images of rams found in Scythian art were also interpreted as personifications of *farn*.[800] It is certain that the notion of *x^varənah* existed among Scythians and Saka, since the names containing this theonym are common in Scythian onomastics.[801] However, there is no way of knowing whether *farn* indeed played any role in the royal ideology and religion of the Scythians and other Iranian nomads, since we possess no Scythian sources where the notion of *farn* could possibly have been manifested.[802] Although a ram, as was noted above, indeed could have acted as a visual manifestation of *x^varənah* in Sasanian art, it is problematic to interpret objects belonging to other people (albeit sharing common cultural heritage), different regions and historical periods based on the evidence of *Kār-Nāmag*, which is a product of Sasanian culture.

Grenet also attempted to identify a "god on camel" attested together with his female companion on several Sogdian paintings as a representation of *x^varənah* in Sogdian art. The mural from Panjikent (XXIV/2) depicts a divine couple seated on a zoomorphic throne with a protome of a camel on the left and a protome of a mountain ram on the right (fig. 128).[803] The painting is badly damaged and unfortunately very few details are clearly distinguishable. A painting from another house (Panjikent, XXIV/13) shows essentially the same scene as in Panjikent XXIV/2.[804] However, this painting is better preserved and more details of the divinities are visible, such as the nimbi behind the heads of the deities, the tongues of fire that rise from their shoulders and a bowl with a small figure of a camel that one of the figures holds in its hand (fig. 129). The same couple is found again on murals discovered in 1986 in house XXV located in the center of Panjikent.[805] All four walls of the main hall (room 28) were decorated with paintings executed between 690–720 CE.[806] On the southern wall, two huge figures of male and female deities were painted on a red background. Only the lower part of the painting is preserved, but numerous analogies have allowed the excavators to reconstruct a camel supporting the throne on the left side (of the male deity) and a protome of a mountain ram on the right (of the female) (fig. 130). The only attribute that is clearly distinguishable is a sword placed between the knees of the male god whose right leg tucked beneath. This pair of deities is also depicted on one of the first wall paintings discovered at the site of Afrosiab in 1965 (pl. 21). The mural with the divine couple was uncovered on the northern

799 Litvinskiy 1968.

800 Shaub 2004.

801 Litvinskiy 1968: 59–70.

802 The golden objects which fell from Heaven in the "Scythian genealogical myth" (Hdt. 4.5–6) are often taken to allude to *x^varənah*. For instance, see Litvinskiy 1968: 61.

803 Belenitskii and Marshak 1981: Fig. 7.

804 Belenitskii and Marshak 1981: Fig. 8.

805 Marshak and Raspopova 1990: 125.

806 Marshak and Raspopova 1990: 127.

wall of room IX.[807] The gods are portrayed seated under a red arch painted on a blue background. The male figure on the left turns his head backwards towards a female facing him. They wear red garments and white diadems and have a composite triple nimbus around their heads consisting of white, red, and yellow rings. There are traces of flames above the shoulders. In their right hands, they hold bowls with small standing animal figures. Although the lower part of the painting is missing, there is no doubt that the gods are sitting on a throne with camel and mountain ram protomes as on the examples from Panjikent.

Another painting showing the god on a camel was discovered in the Eastern Hall of the palace at Varakhsha, near modern Bukhara. It depicts a cultic scene involving three nimbate worshipers and a large altar.[808] On the leg of the altar there is an image of a male figure seated on a camel under an arch (fig. 131). His body is depicted frontally with his right leg tucked beneath. The god wears a crown consisting of three projecting elements and has a nimbus around his head, which is half-turned to the right. The camel on which the god is mounted faces left. According to Grenet, this "god on camel" could be a visual form given to *x^varənah* in Sogdian culture.[809] It is not impossible that in Sogdian religion *xᵛarənah* may have been perceived as a camel, but at present the state of our knowledge is such that no proof can be found for that.[810]

The only images in Sogdian art which certainly represent *farn* are fantastic flying creatures with the heads of lions, camels, horses or birds and with the bodies of fishes or dragons. They are depicted accompanying Rostam and other characters in paintings from Panjikent (fig. 132). A very similar creature was also often represented in Sasanian art where it is traditionally identified as *Sēnmurw* (Av. *mərəγō saēnō*), the mythological fabulous bird and the guardian of the heroes Zal and Rostam.[811] It is difficult to determine whether this identification is correct and whether the Sasanian "*Sēnmurw*" indeed portrays the same creature as the paintings from Panjikent. Both creatures were interpreted by scholars as the embodiment of *xᵛarənah*.[812] The connection of the Sogdian flying monsters with the notion of *xᵛarənah* has been unequivocally confirmed by the discovery of seventh century coins with a Sogdian countermark bearing an image of such a creature labeled by a Sogdian inscription *prn* (*farn*).[813] It is also important to note the variability of these flying hybrid monsters composed from parts of different animals, however, some conformity can be observed. In the Panjikent paintings of the "Rostam Circle" the creature that floats before Rostam always has the head of a lion, while other protagonists are depicted with different flying companions. This indicates that—probably in a similar way to Sasanian art—Sogdians could depict *xᵛarənah* in the shape of various creatures. However, each king, god or a hero seems to be associated with one particular creature that symbolized his personal *xᵛarənah*. Thereupon, one may cite the evidence of al-Bīrūnī who, while discussing the calendar and the feasts of the Persians, mentions a "Khurasan-xvarra" (خرسانخر)[814]—"the flying foxes", who personified the glory of the Kayānids.[815] This description appears especially fitting for the Sasanian "*Sēnmurw*".[816]

---

807 Al'baum 1975: 15–17.
808 Shishkin 1963: 158–162.
809 Grenet et al. 1993: 65; Grenet 1993: 156–159.
810 For a different view on the identification of this god see Marshak and Raspopova 1990: 141–145; Marshak 1999: 182.
811 See Schmidt 2002. For a discussion of the iconography of *Sēnmurw* and related problems, see Compareti 2006b; Compareti and Cristoforetti 2012; Cristoforetti and Scarcia forthcoming with references to previous literature. *Sēnmurw* appears for the first time at Ṭāq-i Bustān and Harper 2006: 73–74, believes that it developed under Western influences as apotropaic creature.
812 For instance, see Azarpay 1975a; Marshak 1998: 85; Marshak 1999: 182; Marshak 2002b: 37.
813 Nikitin and Roth 1995; Grenet 2002a: 219.
814 "The Eastern (heavenly) *farr*", according to Belenitskii and Marshak 1981: 73.
815 Bīrūnī 237.
816 Marshak 1999: 182.

However, the Sogdians probably also imagined *farn* in anthropomorphic form. A reflection of this notion is found in a Manichaean Sogdian tale about Caesar and the thieves.[817] The royal regalia in this story clearly act not as generic attributes of Sogdian *x*ᵛ*arənah*, but as a specific kingly *x*ᵛ*arənah* of Caesar. Gnoli's analysis of this fragment has pointed to the traits of *farn* as a trickster and psychopomp that draw him together with Hermes.[818] It is possible that they are echoes of the Kushan Pharro whose iconographic link with Hermes is beyond doubt.

3. *Conclusions*

Based on anthroponymic analysis, it seems certain that the notion of *x*ᵛ*arənah* was present among Iranians in all historical periods. However, evidence for the pivotal role of *x*ᵛ*arənah* in royal ideology dates only from late Sasanian times. One may safely conclude that no single, universally recognized visual symbol of *x*ᵛ*arənah* ever existed in the Iranian world. On the contrary, the available evidence suggests that a wide variety of visual images, both anthropomorphic and zoomorphic, could have been associated with *x*ᵛ*arənah* among different Iranian people in different periods.

To date, only one representation of *x*ᵛ*arənah* in human form has been definitely identified in the Iranian world—the Kushan Pharro depicted on coins and seals, whose iconography was inspired by Hermes. In addition, two non-anthropomorphic images were also employed in Eastern Iran to symbolize *x*ᵛ*arənah*—a bird perched on the hand of the Kushan Iamšo and the hybrid flying creatures in Sogdian art. In Kushan Bactria these two types of *x*ᵛ*arənah* seem to coexist (and two of them, Pharro and the bird of Iamšo, even within the same medium), reflecting the complex nature and different perceptions of *x*ᵛ*arənah*. It is possible that in Sasanian art the wild ram and the "*Sēnmurw*" may also have acted as visual representations of *x*ᵛ*arənah*. However, until additional, compelling evidence is obtained, these suggestions should be regarded as hypothetical.

18. *Rašnu*

Rašnu (MP. Rašn) is the Avestan *yazata* of judgment, whose very name means "judging, the one who judges",[819] or "the straightener".[820] In Zoroastrian tradition he is closely associated with Mithra and plays an important role in the Last Judgment of the soul.[821]

1. *Western Iran*

The appearance of Rašnu is not described in the Avesta, nor is he given any specific epithets shedding light on his visual image. However, the second "prince" with the balance in the vision of Kartīr is undoubtedly Rašnu[822] and it is significant that in the third century CE we find evidence for a fully developed notion of Rašnu (and other gods, mentioned in Kartīr's vision) as an anthropomorphic being. For the authors and editors of Zoroastrian Middle Persian literature, Rašn was also indisputably a human-shaped divinity. Together with Mihr, the good Wāy, Wahrām and Aštād he helps Wīrāz to cross the Činwad bridge. Wīrāz was even able to see Rašn, who holds a yellow golden balance in his hand.[823]

---

817 See p. 39.
818 Gnoli 1996a.
819 Gray 1929: 99–101; Boyce 1975b: 59.
820 Skjærvø 2011d: 16.
821 For references, see Gray 1929: 99–101.
822 See p. 11–12. Grenet 2003c: 21; Skjærvø 2011a.
823 See p. 32.

Although his name forms part of some personal names in the Achaemenian period,[824] no figural representations of Rašnu are known from this era. It is attested in several names in the Parthian Nisa documents[825] and also found at least twice in Middle Persian anthroponomastics,[826] but his Parthian and Sasanian images are equally unknown.

2. *Eastern Iran*

While absent from Bactrian nomenclature, Rašnu is known in Sogdiana from one personal name—*ršnδys* "(having) the appearance of Rašnu".[827] An individual named *Rašnδātak* ("created by Rašnu") is also attested in the ostracon from Kalaly-Gyr II in Chorasmia.[828] Two definite images of Rašnu are found on Sogdian ossuaries. The first comes from a fragment of a clay ossuary that probably originated in the vicinity of Samarkand, but is currently in Tashkent. It depicts a scene of the Judgment of the soul (fig. 133).[829] One figure wearing a crown with three crenellations is seated cross-legged in the left far side of the scene, holding a scale in his hand. He is approached by another figure also portrayed with a similar crown. In one hand, he holds what seems to be a small, portable altar and grasps the hand of the third figure, who unfortunately remains outside of the preserved fragment. The figure with a scale immediately evokes the description of Rašn from the *Ardā Wīrāz Nāmag* and from Kartīr's vision and constitutes a rare case when it is possible to match an image with a Zoroastrian text.[830] A more impressive representation of Rašnu is found on another Sogdian ossuary from Yumalaktepa, which depicts him in complete anthropomorphic form weighing the soul of the deceased on his scales.[831]

Central Asian toponymics suggest that a temple dedicated to Rašnu possibly existed in the vicinity of Samarkand. Smirnova has proposed that the original name of the Samarkand village of Rastivagn (**rst(y)βγn*) was **ršn[y]βγn*—"temple (of) Rašnu".[832] If this suggestion is sound, it is reasonable to assume that a statue of the god was housed in this sanctuary.

3. *Conclusions*

The popularity of Rašnu is widely attested in both Eastern and Western Iran by personal names and toponyms. Despite being perceived as an anthropomorphic god at least from the Sasanian period, no images of Rašnu are known from Western Iran. There are only two certain portrayals of Rašnu on Sogdian ossuaries from the environs of Samarkand and from Yumalaktepa. This scene, showing the Judgment of the soul, has remarkable textual parallels in Zoroastrian tradition.

19. *Scythian Anguipede Goddess*

An anguipede goddess, half-maiden, half-viper, features in Scythian genealogical mythology as a mother of the first Scythian man, born from Zeus or Heracles.[833] The goddess has distinctly chthonic characteris-

824 Mayrhofer 1973: nos. 8.1420–8.1422; Tavernier 2007: 542.
825 See Livshits 2004: 190.
826 Gignoux 1986: nos. 804, 805.
827 Lurje 2010: no. 1018.
828 Livshits 2004: 189–190.
829 Grenet 1986: 106–107; Grenet 2002b: 94.
830 See Grenet 1986: 106–107; Grenet 2002b: 94.
831 See p. 85.
832 Smirnova 1971: 93.
833 The main versions of the myth are found in Hdt 4.5; 4.8–10. Val. Flac. 6.48–59, Diod. Sic. 2.43 and in *Tabula Albana* IG XIV 1293 A 93–96. For the discussion, see e.g. Raevskiy 1977: 19–81; Bessonova 1983: 10–25; Ustinova 1999: 87–93; Ustinova 2005; Shaub 2007: 89–100.

tics—she is described as the daughter of the earth or of a local river-god and her dwelling is in a cave. She is usually identified with Apia from the Scythian pantheon recorded by Herodotus,[834] but this identification is far from certain.[835] Yulia Ustinova has suggested that the anguipede goddess is comparable to another Herodotian Scythian female deity—Argimpasa-Aphrodite[836]—emphasizing that the two goddesses remained distinct despite their close association and occasional "merging".[837] Mikhail Artamonov has argued that all female Scythian deities mentioned by Herodotus, Tabiti, Apia and Argimpasa gradually evolved from a single fertility goddess.[838] However, our knowledge of their origin is very limited. The snake-limbed goddess described by Herodotus in the Scythian genealogical myth is not named and is not linked by him with any Scythian goddess known to him. Scythians probably perceived her as their maternal ancestor, and although her local name cannot be established, her chthonic nature, underlined by all scholars, is beyond doubt.

1. *Western Iran*

Despite numerous infiltrations of nomads of Scythian origin and the considerable influences they undoubtedly exercised on the culture of the Iranian plateau, no clear traces of Scythian religious iconography have been identified in Western Iran. No comparable image of an anguipede goddess is known from Achaemenian, Parthian or Sasanian art.

2. *Eastern Iran*

A snake-limbed goddess is found on numerous objects of art uncovered from Scythian burials, as well as on those reflecting the visual culture of the Pontic Greek cities, with most representative objects coming from Tzymbalova mogila and Kul'-Oba kurgan.[839] The Tzymbalova mogila golden frentera originates from the kurgan in Zaporozh'e district in Ukraine.[840] The entire surface of this piece is occupied by a hybrid figure of a goddess with the upper part of a woman and three pairs of legs ending with the heads of snakes and gryphons and vegetal tendrils (pl. 22). Additional plant stems sprout from the *kalathos* on her head. The goddess depicted on the golden plaque from Kul'-Oba kurgan in Crimea has the upper part of the body of a female and two pairs of snake-shaped legs ending with the heads of snakes and gryphons (fig. 134).[841] An additional pair of tendrils terminating with the heads of horned lions rises from her shoulders. Distinctive features of this image are the small wings and bird's tail, placed below her waist between the snake-shaped limbs and a satyr's mask/a severed head that the goddess holds in her left hand.

Another image probably connected to the anguipede goddess is the tendril-limbed female deity who became widespread in Scythian art in the first centuries CE.[842] This winged, tendril-legged goddess wears a *kalathos* usually surrounded by abundant floral motifs. However, the nature of the connection between the snake- and tendril-legged goddesses remains unclear.

---

834 Hdt. 4.59.
835 See the discussion in Ustinova 1999: 91–93.
836 Ustinova 1999: 96–97.
837 Ustinova 1999: 122; Ustinova 2005: 78.
838 Artamonov 1961: 71. Shaub 2007: 80–123, adopts his conception and includes various female divine portrayals whose iconography and semantics are entirely distinct under the label "The Great Goddess".
839 Other objects with similar images are discussed and illustrated in Bessonova 1983: 93–98; Ustinova 1999: 94–99; Ustinova 2005: 66–70; Shaub 2007: 93, no. 13. Depictions of the anguipede goddess were also common outside immediate Scythian and Iranian cultural spheres—in the Balkans and Mediterranean. See Ustinova 1999: 99–107; Ustinova 2005: 70–74. However, they may have spread there from Scythia: Ustinova 2005: 76. See also Shaub 2007: 119, who proposes that her image originated in Anatolia.
840 Bessonova 1983: 93; Ustinova 1999: 94. An identical object was also discovered in kurgan Tolstaya mogila.
841 Bessonova 1983: 93; Ustinova 1999: 94.
842 Ustinova 2005: 68. Shaub 2007: 93, considers the snake- and the tendril-limbed goddesses to represent two variations of the iconography of the same deity.

It is significant that unlike Argimpasa—a second Scythian goddess known from the visual record[843]—the snake-limbed goddess is never shown in a cultic context or as part of a narrative scene, but appears in decorative and ornamental compositions only. An echo of the Scythian genealogical myth is also found in the legend of the origin of the local dynasty from Northern Pakistan recorded by a Buddhist Chinese pilgrim in the seventh century CE.[844] This legend was probably transmitted to Bactria and Gandhāra by the Saka nomads.

3. *Conclusions*

The Scythian anguipede goddess probably depicts the Scythian mythological maternal ancestor. Unfortunately, her name remains unknown and attempts to connect her with the Avestan or other Iranian pantheons have so far been unsuccessful. The Kushan and Indo-Scythian religious iconography that appears most fruitful for such parallels contains no comparable images.

Only one main type of image of anguipede goddess in known from Scythian art, although the tendril-limbed female deity may be an additional variation. The fact that the anguipede goddess is not mentioned in the list of Scythian deities by Herodotus, and that she was not represented in cultic scenes, probably indicates that she occupied a special place in Scythian religion. Perhaps the anguipede goddess was considered a remote, primordial power and was venerated through the mediation of other female deities.

20. *Šahrewar*

Šahrewar (Av. *xšaϑra vairiia*, "Desirable dominion/kingdom" or "well-deserved Command")[845] is one of the Aməša Spənta. In Zoroastrian textual tradition he is the guardian of the sky and of metal.[846]

1. *Western Iran*

The "god of good order" (εὐνομία) mentioned by Plutarch in the first-second centuries CE may be the earliest attestation of Šahrewar in historical sources.[847] However, to date no images of Šahrewar have been identified in Western Iran from any period.

2. *Eastern Iran*

The only definite visual representation of Šahrewar is the Kushan Šaoreoro (ÞAOPHOPO) attested on the gold coins of Huvishka. Göbl has divided the representations of Šaoreoro into four types.[848] The first shows the god facing right, wearing a Greek helmet, heavy body armor, and equipped with a sword and a shield (pl. 23). On the second type, the pose, helmet and armor are the same, but instead of the shield, he holds a sword and a plain nimbus encircles his head (fig. 135). The other three types do not have a nimbus. On the third type, Šaoreoro is portrayed facing left leaning on a long spear, but holding a round shield in his right hand (fig. 136). The fourth type almost mirrors the first, but the shield is placed behind the body rather than in front of it. Some scholars identify the unclear decoration on

843 See p. 86 ff.
844 Carter 1992.
845 Skjærvø 2011d: 14.
846 Gray 1929: 45–47; Boyce 1975b: 207–209.
847 Plut. *De Is. et Os.* 47. Discussion by De Jong 1997: 187.
848 Göbl 1984, Šaorēoro 1–3.

Šaoreoro's shield as *gorgoneon*.[849] Although Šaoreoro does not appear in the first Greek issue of Kanishka, his iconography of a heavily armored warrior is undoubtedly borrowed from Greek Ares as he appears on eastern Roman coinage.[850] Judging by his attributes, Šaoreoro appears to be the most "warlike" deity in the Kushan numismatic pantheon. This does not seem to correspond to his role in Zoroastrian written sources. Šaoreoro was not included in the Rabatak god's list and therefore his place in the Kushan royal pantheon remains obscure.

The subsequent fate of the Kushan Šaoreoro is equally unknown. He is not attested later in Bactria. It has been proposed that several Sogdian objects such as the Chilek plaque and some of the ossuary fragments from Biyanajman and Miankal carry images of Šahrewar.[851] While the possibility that the Chilek god is related to Šahrewar cannot be ruled out,[852] and it is even theoretically plausible taking into account the presidency of Šahrewar over metal, a domain of Hephaistos, this interpretation is not certain. His crown, like the crowns of most Sogdian divinities, does not provide any clues as to his identity and the sword is an attribute shared by many gods. The Chilek god holds what appears to be a shield with a *gorgoneon* emblem under his right arm, but there does not seem to be a clearly distinguishable *gorgoneon* on Kushan Šaoreoro's shield.[853] Furthermore, the *gorgoneon* appears on numerous Sogdian paintings as simply an ordinary piece of war equipment.[854] Moreover, there is an enormous chronological gap between the Chilek god and the Kushan Šaoreoro. Therefore, the identification of the Chilek god with Šahrewar is doubtful.

The figures on the Biyanajman and Miankal ossuaries identified by Grenet as Šahrewar, are according to my division, three different characters (nos. 6–8). Because of the presence of heavy body armor and a sword, figure no. 8 may be considered as a possible image of Šahrewar, although it remains speculative.

3. *Conclusions*

Based on his name it is expected that Šahrewar would be closely associated with royal power, ideology and thus frequently represented in official art. However, this was not the case. In fact, in Western Iran where vivid images of the Zoroastrian gods were put to service in royal Sasanian propaganda, Šahrewar was never given a concrete visual manifestation.

His only definite image, as well as two possible ones, originates from Eastern Iran. The iconography chosen for the Kushan Šaoreoro indicates that he was obviously considered a warlike deity and his functions were probably similar to those recorded in the Zoroastrian scriptures. One possible image of Šahrewar also exists in Sogdian art. If the figures on the Biyanajman and Miankal ossuaries indeed depict, at least partly, the Aməša Spənta, figure no. 8 could be a rendering of the Sogdian Šahrewar.

21. *Sraoša*

Sraoša, (MP. *Srōš*) is a prominent Avestan *yazata*, whose name means "obedience", "hearkening",[855] or "readiness to listen".[856] There are certain textual indications suggesting that Sraoša was perhaps an

---

849 For instance, Grenet forthcoming a.

850 Grenet forthcoming a.

851 For the Chilek plaque, see p. 92–93. For the Biyanajman and Miankal ossuaries, see p. 170. It is also worth mentioning several Sogdian terracotta plaques from Chaganian depicting a warrior standing under an arch and armed with a spear and a sword, who was suggested to represent Sogdian Šahrewar. See Ilyasov 1999.

852 This interpretation is preferred by Grenet et al. 1993: 59–60.

853 Contra other scholars, for instance, Grenet forthcoming a.

854 Marshak 1995/1996: 304.

855 Gray 1929: 106–109; Boyce 1975b: 60–62; Kreyenbroek 1985.

856 Skjærvø 2011d: 15.

Avestan creation rather than an ancient deity of the Indo-Iranian tradition.[857] The Zoroastrian scriptures associate Sraoša with prayer and stress his close links with Mithra and the goddess Aši. He also serves as a mediator between *mēnōg* and *gētīg* and often acts as the divine messenger.

1. *Western Iran*

Sraoša is not attested as part of personal names in the Achaemenian period, but he is found in a Greek papyrus from Hellenistic Egypt.[858] His name also appears in several anthroponyms on the Parthian ostraca from Nisa.[859] However, no representations of Sraoša are known in Western Iran from these periods. In addition, very few Sasanian personal names contain his name as a theophoric compound.[860] That Sraoša was perceived as anthropomorphic is clear from Zoroastrian literature, more specifically from the *Ardā Wīrāz Nāmag* where Sraoša together with Ādur accompanies Wīrāz through his journey to Heaven and Hell.[861]

Like many other Avestan deities, Sraoša rides a chariot drawn by "four white, radiant ... steeds".[862] However, in Zoroastrian literature he is most closely associated with a rooster as his favored bird.[863] The fact that Sraoša has survived in Islamic tradition as a cosmic cock, an angel rooster encountered by Muhammad during his ascension to Heavens,[864] testifies to the unusual endurance and longevity of the association of Sraoša with a cock. It is therefore reasonable to assume that if the image of Sraoša existed in Sasanian art it would have been associated with roosters. This is also suggested by a curious image found on a unique Sasanian seal, which depicts a juvenile, beardless head above two protomes of birds facing in opposite directions (fig. 137).[865] This is a conventional way of symbolically representing a divine chariot in Sasanian sigillography.[866] Although the wheels are missing, there can be no doubt that the seal shows a deity riding his chariot. The birds resemble most of all roosters, despite the unusual wings, which are however typical for all winged creatures on Sasanian seals, regardless of their type. I suggest that this image may be that of a chariot of Sraoša. There are numerous representations of roosters on seals from the Sasanian period. In the case of single roosters on Sasanian seals, an association with Sraoša is certainly possible, but it is important to keep in mind that when depicted alone they are devoid of any additional divine context like that provided by the symbolic divine chariot on the seal.

Besides Ahriman, Sraoša (NP. Surūsh) is the only pre-Islamic deity to appear in the *Shāh-nāma*. In Firdausī's epic poem, Surūsh acts as the divine messenger, an echo of one of his roles in Zoroastrian tradition. He is described as having a form "of a *pari* wearing a leopard skin" and is clearly anthropomorphic.[867]

2. *Eastern Iran*

In the Eastern Iranian world, we find further possible evidence for Sraoša's linkage with the rooster as well as several candidates for his anthropomorphic portrayal. Sraoša (Bac. σροþαρδο) occupies fifth place in the Rabatak god list.[868] However, no deity called Sroshard is known from the Kushan numismatic

857 Kreyenbroek 1985: 164.
858 Huyse 1990: no. 130.
859 For example, Diakonoff and Livshits 2001: nos. 2575:4; 1339:5.
860 Kreyenbroek 1985: 179.
861 See p. 32.
862 Y. 57.27.
863 See Kreyenbroek 1985: 118, who provides references to Middle Persian sources.
864 The motif of the cosmic cock in Islamic literature and art is discussed by Subtelny 2011.
865 Frye 1971: no. 68.
866 For other examples, see p. 103 ff.
867 See p. 44.
868 See p. 12–13.

pantheon. If Maaseno (Sk. Mahāsena) mentioned in the interlinear phrase in the Rabatak inscription is in fact the *interpretatio indica* of Srošard, then the deity of the same name on the coins of Huvishka is the Kushan representation of Sraoša, making this a unique case in which an Iranian divinity was represented under the name of his Indian counterpart on Kushan coins. Unlike most Kushan deities, the god Maaseno (MAACHNO) is depicted with both the body and the head in frontal view (pl. 24).[869] He wears a cloak over his shoulders and a nimbus surrounds his head. In his right hand, Maaseno holds a long staff surmounted by the figure of a cock and with his left hand he clasps the hilt of a sword. On the second type, Maaseno is shown standing within a sanctuary while smaller figures of deities named Skando-Kumaro and Bizago flank him on both sides and probably represent different forms of Maaseno (fig. 138).[870] The rooster perched on his staff also contributes to this identification. Additionally, a gold coin of Huvishka shows only Skando-Kumaro and Bizago (fig. 139).[871]

Like Mahāsena, Sraoša's personality has a pronounced warlike aspect, and his role as the vanquisher of demons is specifically emphasized in Zoroastrian literature.[872] Among his common epithets are "strong of arm" and "with mighty club".[873] In Middle Persian Zoroastrian literature Srōš is referred to as "the chief over the material world" (*pad gētīg sālār*)[874] and he is in charge of the "defense and protection of the creatures of the material world" (*pāsbānīh ud pānagīh ī gētīgān*).[875] It is possible that the Bactrian Srošard-Maaseno was even more bellicose. If the identification of Sraoša with Mahāsena is sound, an additional Kushan image of the god may be recognized in a seal originating from Gandhāra and depicting Mahāsena-Kārrtikeya wearing a breastplate and holding a long spear, and with a large cock facing him.[876]

It is noteworthy that Sraoša is also attested in one Bactrian name.[877] Sraoša was likewise known in other regions of Central Asia. Names containing the theonym Sraoša are found at Topraq-Qal'a, Chorasmia,[878] and in Sogdiana.[879] Furthermore, Sraoša is probably represented on the Sogdian ossuary fragment from the environs of Samarkand.[880] Although this ossuary is not inscribed, the imagery leaves no reasonable doubt that it depicts a scene from the Judgment of the soul in the afterlife as described in Zoroastrian texts. Therefore, the left figure with the scales would be the god Rašnu, while the one who leads the soul into Rašnu's presence is most probably Sraoša, who assists the soul in passing the Činwad bridge.[881] Grenet notes that the garments worn by Sraoša and Rašnu are not typical of Sogdian gods, but rather resemble those of priests.[882] Their crowns are also closer to those worn by divinities on Sasanian reliefs than to the headdresses of Sogdian deities, which are usually more elaborate and consist of several elements. Furthermore, Sraoša appears as a judge of souls only in Sasanian Middle Persian texts, but not in the Avesta.[883] It is therefore possible that the scene on this ossuary betrays Sasanian influences not only in the iconography but also in the theology underlying the whole scene.[884]

---

869 Rosenfield 1967: 79; Göbl 1984: Maasēno 1; Mann 2012: 129–135.
870 Göbl 1984: Maasēno 2; Mann 2012: 138–139.
871 Mann 2012: 135–138.
872 Gray 1929: 109. It is interesting to note that Mann 2001/2005, who discusses the formation of the iconography of Mahāsena in India, sees both the cock and the warlike appearance as borrowed from Sraoša. See also Mann 2012: 125–128.
873 Boyce 1975b: 61.
874 *IBd* 26.50.
875 *Dd* 27.6.
876 Callieri 1997: 7.2.
877 Sims-Williams 2010: no. 34.
878 Livshits 2004: 191.
879 Lurje 2010: nos. 61, 1092.
880 See p. 141.
881 *DMX* 2.114; Grenet 2002b: 94.
882 Grenet 2002b: 94.
883 Kreyenbroek 1985: 4.
884 However, see De Jong 2008/2012: 21, who ascribes Sraoša's transformation to the Achaemenian period, when both Pars

Just as statues of Srošard-Maaseno undoubtedly existed in Kushan Bactria, freestanding cultic sculptures of the god were also housed in Sogdian sanctuaries. Grenet has raised the possibility that a Sogdian image found on a painting from Panjikent (XXVI/3) is an image of Sraoša. The surviving fragments of the mural discovered in this room probably depict a large codex or a litter decorated with two divine figures and a golden statue probably carried in a procession (fig. 140).[885] The statue was not placed behind the codex/litter, but rather above, "rising" from it (fig. 141).[886] What seems certain, however, is that it represents a cultic image of a deity. A mace is shown in the god's right hand and his left hand probably holds an altar or a portable incense burner. According to the French scholar, the curious combination of an anthropomorphic statue with a book may be a literal illustration of the Avestan epithet of Sraoša, *tanu.mąϑra*: "whose body is the Sacred Word".[887] Another tentative image of the Sogdian Sraoša may be recognized in one of five deities in a badly preserved mural from Panjikent XXVI/2.[888] It is tempting to interpret the divine mount of the god portrayed to the right of Nana as a rooster—meaning its rider is likely Sraoša—but this is no more than conjecture. Furthermore, if the bird is a peacock its rider is probably Skanda, which, as we have seen, in Kushan art was also identified with Sraoša-Maaseno. Skanda was probably depicted riding on a peacock from the Gupta era.[889] A fragment of the image of Skanda mounted on a peacock is also found on the wall-paintings in Dilberjin in room 16 of the northeastern complex (fig. 142).[890] According to the excavators, it cannot be later than the fifth century CE.[891] This provides solid evidence for the diffusion of the Gupta iconography of Skanda to Bactria and Sogdiana, although it is not clear whether he was still assimilated with Sraoša in this period.

A god depicted on the ossuaries from Sivaz[892] may also represent Sogdian Sraoša,[893] but Grenet's proposal to identify him as Vohu Manah seems preferable.[894]

The discussion of possible Sogdian representations of Sraoša would not be complete without mention of several Sino-Sogdian tombs on which a curious design of two half-men, half-birds attending a fire-altar is depicted on walls, stone couches and sarcophagi (fig. 143).[895] The dated examples all belong to a short thirteen-year period between 579 and 592 CE.[896] They wear *padām* and are obviously performing the duties of a priest tending the fire. Similar "human-bird priests", but without the fire-altar, are also shown flanking the chariot of Mithra in the painting next to the head of the Small Buddha at Bāmiān[897] and probably also appear on fragments of two ossuaries discovered in Samarkand in 1999.[898] The avian portion of these priests is probably that of a rooster. In a passage in the *Vidēvdāt*, the rooster is presented in the role of a priest.[899] Therefore, scholars seeking to interpret these "human-bird priests" within

---

and Sogdiana were parts of a single political unity. However, evidence for any religious reforms or a deliberate policy of religious consolidation and unification attempted by the Achaemenian monarchs is lacking.

885 Codex according to de la Vaissière, Riboud and Grenet 2003: 134–136; a litter, according to Marshak and Raspopova 2003: 50–51.

886 Marshak and Raspopova 2003: 50.

887 de la Vaissière, Riboud and Grenet 2003: 134–136. This possibility is also discussed by Marshak and Raspopova 2003: 50–51.

888 See p. 123.

889 Mann 2012: 204.

890 Kruglikova 1979: 137–138.

891 Kruglikova 1979: 143.

892 See p. 84–85.

893 Marshak 1999: 185.

894 See p. 165.

895 Riboud 2007/2012. Previous studies of this motif include: Grenet, Riboud and Yang Junkai 2004: 275–276; Grenet 2007: 470–471; Berdimuradov and Bogomolov 2008.

896 Riboud 2007/2012: 2.

897 See p. 89.

898 Grenet 2003a: 40, Fig. 10; Riboud 2007/2012: Fig. 16.

899 Vd. 18.14.

Zoroastrian tradition have tended to identify them with Sraoša, following the oral suggestion made by Skjærvø.[900] In Sogdiana, representations of half-birds, half-women were found at Varakhsha and Panjikent, including on ossuaries.[901] Although they closely resemble Indian *kinnaras* and *kinnaris*, they seem to be related to harpies/sirens, who in Greek mythology accompanied souls on their journey to the underworld.[902] However, the "human-bird priests" on Sino-Sogdian tombs are always male, and this specific type may have originated in China.[903]

A similar composition, but featuring fully anthropomorphic priests and lacking the complete symmetry of the two Sino-Sogdian characters, are found on two Sogdian ossuaries from Molla Kurgan and Krasnorechesnkoe Gorodishche.[904] Penelope Riboud, who has recently analyzed the origin of the bird-priest composition, convincingly suggested that it was the result of an encounter between two funerary motifs: that of two birds found on Chinese tombs and that of Sogdian priests.[905] Based on this observation, it seems likely that these are not in fact divine images, but rather pictorial representations of Central Asian priests performing a funerary ritual merged with typically Chinese birds to fit the Chinese funerary settings. It is not improbable that the harpy-siren motif known in Sogdiana facilitated this fusion, which resulted in the creation of hybrid, Sino-Sogdian "bird-priests". However, if one insists on their divine interpretation, Sraoša should not be regarded as the only theoretical possibility. In his curious account of Zoroastrianism with Avestan echoes, the Syriac author Theodore bar Koni reports that Haoma "was a cock".[906] Furthermore, among the Avestan divinities it is Haoma who is most associated with the priesthood and is perceived as "the priest" *par excellence*.[907]

3. *Conclusions*

Aside from the Avesta, the first attestation of Sraoša's existence comes from the Parthian ostraca from Nisa. However, his earliest possible visual representation from Western Iran dates only from the Sasanian period. If the god riding a chariot drawn by roosters is indeed Sraoša, he would be only the third deity, together with Mithra and Māh, to be depicted as a charioteer in Sasanian art.

However, in the Eastern Iranian world, there are several possible candidates. The evidence of the Rabatak inscription unequivocally testifies that Sraoša was known in Bactria, where he was perhaps equated with the Indian Mahāsena and was depicted as the warrior-god with a cock on the coins of Huvishka. In Sogdiana, he is probably shown on the ossuary from Samarkand in his role as the guardian and guide of the souls of the righteous in the afterlife, but this particular image probably betrays Sasanian influence.

If all these images indeed portray Sraoša, it implies the existence of three completely different and independent iconographic types of the god in ancient Iranian art: 1) the Kushan warlike god with a cock; 2) the partly aniconic Sasanian charioteer; and 3) the fully anthropomorphic god on a Sogdian ossuary wearing a crenellated crown. This would make Sraoša one of very few deities to be depicted in Kushan, Sasanian and Sogdian art.

900 See Riboud 2007/2012: 6–10. Carter 2002: 266–267, identifies them as fravaši or possibly related to *x^varənah*.
901 For illustrations, see Berdimuradov and Bogomolov 2008: Figs. 3–4.
902 Lerner 1975: 167.
903 Grenet 2007: 470.
904 Grenet 1986: 104–105.
905 Riboud 2007/2012.
906 See p. 27.
907 Boyce 2003.

22. *Tištrya*

Tištrya (MP. *Tištar*) is one of the notable deities of the Zoroastrian pantheon, a god of the star Sirius.[908] He was probably already venerated by Indo-Iranians and perhaps even by Indo-Europeans.[909] In the Avesta, Tištrya is especially associated with water and rain;[910] and since he had also assimilated with the star Sirius, Tištrya was likened to an arrow.[911] Perhaps as early as the Achaemenian period, Tištrya was identified with Tīriya (Tīr), a deity of the planet Mercury of unclear origin, and with the Mesopotamian god of writing—Nabu.[912] Bernard has proposed that Nabu was first assimilated with Apollo in Hellenistic Mesopotamia and then with the Iranian Tīr in the Parthian period.[913]

1. *Western Iran*

We have solid evidence that in Mesopotamia and Armenia Tīr was identified with Greek Apollo, and his statues that stood in temples in Armenia, Seleucia on Tigris and other cities probably imitated the images of the son of Leto.[914] On the other hand, Apollo was usually equated with Iranian Mithra, a tendency well-attested in neighboring Commagene and elsewhere.[915] We know of at least two temples dedicated to Tīr—one in Seleucia on Tigris and another in Armenia. Ammianus Marcellinus tells us of a statue of Apollo captured by Romans in Seleucia on Tigris, which could perhaps be connected to the temple of Tīr mentioned in the inscription on the thigh of a statue of Heracles/Vərəθraγna from Mesene.[916]

No image associated with Tištrya/Tīr is known from Achaemenian, Parthian or Sasanian art from the Iranian plateau. Although the evidence cited above indicates that such temples and statues probably existed, at least under the Arsacids,[917] until such temples or statues or inscriptions mentioning them are discovered, there is no means of knowing this for certain.

2. *Eastern Iran*

The earliest attestation of Tīr in Eastern Iran comes from an inscription on a pottery flask from Chirik-rabat on the lower Syr-darya. It gives a personal name *Tīriβōδi* "incense of (god) Tīri" and is dated to the fourth to second centuries BCE.[918] However, the first visual representation of this god in the Iranian world is found on the unique gold coin of Huvishka (pl. 25).[919] The Kushan Teiro (TEIPO) is portrayed as a feminine figure facing right and draped in long garments. With his left hand, he clasps a large composite bow and with his right hand, he draws an arrow from a quiver on his back. Teiro wears a headdress resembling a small *kalathos*. His image apparently follows the iconography of Artemis, or perhaps that of Apollo, but it should be noted that Kushan Teiro is remarkably similar to one of the types of Nana on the Kushan coins. Teiro does not appear among the known examples of the first "Greek" minting of

---

908 See Panaino 2005 with references to previous studies.
909 Panaino 1995: 107.
910 Gray 1929: 115–116.
911 Panaino 2005.
912 Boyce 1982: 21–22; 204–206; Panaino 1995: 108.
913 Bernard 1990b: 57–62.
914 For the Armenian evidence, see p. 20.
915 Bernard 1990b: 52 with references.
916 See p. 11.
917 Several personal names in ostraca from Old Nisa were formed with Tīr. See, for example, Diakonoff and Livshits 2001: nos. 1646:2; 1060:5.
918 See Ivantchik and Lurje 2013.
919 Göbl 1984 Nana 2a; Bernard 1990b: 55; Grenet and Marshak 1998: 12.

Kanishka and it is therefore impossible to ascertain with what god of the Olympian pantheon he was identified in Bactria. It was certainly not Mithra, who in the Kushan pantheon was equated with Helios.

An additional image of Bactrian Tištrya was identified by Grenet in the Kushano-Sasanian painting at Ghulbiyan—the enthroned god who holds an arrow and has a fish-filled pond beneath his feet.[920] Since the figure interpreted by Grenet as Tištrya is the largest among the group of deities in this painting, he was probably also the most important deity depicted in the scene. If this god is indeed Tištrya (which seems the most cogent interpretation given the available evidence) his visual representation is remarkably different from the Kushan Teiro and from possible Sogdian images of the god. For Sogdians, Tištrya (Sog. *tyδr*) was one of the most popular gods judging by his occurrence in Sogdian personal names.[921] Grenet has proposed to identify him as the god who is at times shown accompanying the goddess Nana in Sogdian art.[922] It is to be noted that the same four-armed deity is also found on the wooden frieze from Kujruk-tobe palace.[923] The starting point for this hypothesis is the interpretation of the four-armed god from Khirmantepa ossuary as Tištrya/Tīr, because of the large arrow that the god holds in his hands (according to the French scholar).[924] His other attributes are a helmet decorated with animal ears, chainmail, a ring topped by a bird and a round object (a tambourine or most probably a shield). Grenet connects the decoration of his helmet to the Avestan zoomorphic incarnation of Tištrya, who assumes the form of a white stallion to fight Apaoša, the demon of drought;[925] and his body armor and shield are connected with his epithet *xwarāsān spāhbed*, "the general of the East" found in *Bundahišn*.[926]

Grenet and Marshak have also proposed to identify a god seated alongside a goddess (most probably Nana) on the earliest Sogdian painting from Jartepa II Temple, as Tištrya.[927] Unfortunately, the image of the god is very fragmentary and it is therefore impossible to determine what attributes he possessed. Another image of Tištrya was identified by Grenet and Marshak in a god wearing a dragon crown seated to the right of Nana on a painting from XXV/12 at Panjikent.[928] It is noteworthy that two other Panjikent paintings featuring Nana also depict a smaller masculine figure on the right side of the goddess. This figure is standing, not enthroned, has a sword and in one instance, a mace, and wears a different type of headdress. It is therefore unclear whether these three figures represent the same individual. If they are images of the same god it is unlikely that the figure from XXV/12 at Panjikent holds an arrow, as proposed by Grenet and Marshak, but that his attribute is a sword as on the other two representations. The main argument for his identification with Tištrya is therefore removed. Grenet and Marshak attempted to explain the union between Nana and Tištrya in light of the Graeco-Mesopotamian substrate of Sogdian religion.[929] In Mesopotamia, Nana was considered a consort of Nabu and since Nabu was syncretized with Apollo and Tištrya, his link with Nana was also maintained in Sogdiana. Despite the attractiveness of these identifications, they are based on a series of interconnected and unproven assumptions. It is not certain that the arrow is an attribute of the Sogdian Tištrya and that the god accompanying Nana indeed holds an arrow. Furthermore, the Kushan Teiro does not seem particularly close to Nana and the god from Ghulbiyan is not shown paired with the goddess either. However, if all the above mentioned figures are indeed images of Sogdian Tištrya, the iconography of this god in Sogdiana exhibits a truly

---

920 See p. 137–138. Lee and Grenet 1998: 79.
921 Lurje 2010: nos. 1004, 1277, 1278 (?), 1279, 1289, 1291, 1292, 1294.
922 Grenet and Marshak 1998: 10.
923 See p. 125–126.
924 For a description of the ossuary, see p. 125.
925 Yt. 8.6.20–22.
926 GBd 2.4. Grenet and Pinault 1997: 1058.
927 See p. 121–122.
928 Grenet and Marshak 1998: 15. For a detailed description of the painting, see p. 123–124.
929 Grenet and Marshak 1998: 15.

remarkable—even unparalleled—diversity. He was depicted four-armed and with the usual number of hands, seated on a carpet, or on a zoomorphic throne supported by winged dragons, wearing chain-mail and a helmet with animal ears or unprotected and wearing crown topped by a dragon. Only an arrow and his place to the left of Nana would be constant characteristics, albeit limited only to Sogdian art. The association of Tīr with Nana would also be a specifically Sogdian feature.

The veneration of Tīr also existed in Chorasmia, as attested by Chorasmian personal names containing this theonym.[930] However, while there are several representations of Nana on Chorasmian silver bowls, no image identifiable with Tīr has come to light.

3. *Conclusions*

Despite every reason to assume that Tištrya-Tīr was an important deity in Western Iran at least in the Parthian and Sasanian periods, visual representations and temples of Tištrya from this region are still completely unknown. The Kushan Teiro represents the only certain image of Tištrya-Tīr in pre-Islamic Iranian art. He was perhaps depicted as a juvenile archer because of his association with Greek Apollo, attested in the West. All other images discussed above are identified with Tištrya with varying degrees of probability. Especially curious is the Kushano-Sasanian "Tištrya" from Ghulbiyan. His iconography is completely different from that on the coin of Huvishka and probably represents a local variant in a region where Tištrya was a subject of special veneration.

The hypothesis advanced by Grenet and Marshak to identify a Sogdian Tištrya as the "consort" of Nana in Sogdian art appears attractive and is the best currently available. From his Sogdian iconography "Tištrya" appears to possess the traits and attributes of a warlike deity, acting as a sort of "guardian" of Nana. If all the characters from Sogdian art discussed above actually depict Tištrya it would indicate that this god enjoyed unusual popularity in the Sogdian pantheon, which apparently corresponds to the high number of Sogdian personal names containing Tištrya as a compound.

23. *Vanant*

Despite having his own Yašt (20), Vanant ("victorious, conqueror") is a minor god in the Avesta.[931] Unfortunately, the visual appearance of Vanant is not described in ancient Iranian written sources. In Middle Persian literature he is identified with the star Vega.

1. *Western Iran*

Because of her name and visual representation in Kushan art (see below), Vanant is often automatically associated with the Greek Nike. Numerous representations of Nike are known from Western Iran during the Hellenistic and Parthian periods. However, there are no indications that the image of the Greek goddess conceals Iranian Vanant. No sources allow this identification and no "deity of Victory" which could be interpreted as Vanant is ever mentioned in historical sources. Therefore, at present we are left with no convincing candidature for the visual image of Vanant from Western Iran.

2. *Eastern Iran*

Vanant (Bac. ΟΑΝΙΝΔΟ) appears for the first time on the coinage of the Kushan king Huvishka (pl. 26).[932] Oanindo is nimbate and is portrayed standing in full profile, holding a cornucopia or a staff/scepter,

---

930 Livshits 2004: 191; Ivantchik and Lurje 2013: 287.
931 Gray 1929: 166–167.
932 Rosenfield 1967: 91–92.

and offering a diadem. There are two basic types. On the first she is turned to the left, and on the second she is facing right.[933] Besides the wind god, Anemos, she is also the only winged deity in the Kushan numismatic pantheon. Despite being a male deity in the Avesta, the Kushan Oanindo is female and her iconography is undoubtedly derived from the Graeco-Roman Nike, who is curiously not found on the first Greek issue of Kanishka. It demonstrates that Oanindno, like the Avestan Vanant, was also primarily associated with victory and triumph. It is not entirely clear, however, whether the difference of sex reflects original differences between the Avesta and the Kushan pantheon, or whether this change should be ascribed to the influence of Nike.

Nike is already known from Eastern Iran on Graeco-Bactrian and Indo-Scythian coinage and she was often depicted on Roman coins contemporary with the Kushans.[934] The image of Nike was also frequent in early Kushan art. Most notable examples are the winged goddess crowning a prince with a wreath on the coins of Heraios, the statue of flying Nike from Khalchayan,[935] and a terracotta medallion from the same site depicting the enthroned king.[936] However, it is not clear whether she was already associated with Iranian Vanant at this point. Oanindo does not feature in the Rabatak divine list, but it is possible, albeit unlikely, that the temple at Surkh-Kotal was in fact dedicated to her.

The subsequent fate of Oanindo and her cult are unclear. An image of a floating Nike crowing a seated divinity with a wreath is found on Kushano-Sasanian paintings from Ghulbiyan,[937] although it is difficult to know whether this is a continuation of the Kushan Oanindo. Grenet has raised the possibility that the right charioteer on the painting of the epiphany of Mithra at Bāmiān could be Vanant.[938] However, although the character is winged, it holds a bow and arrow—attributes wholly alien to Kushan Oanindo and those that are not associated with Vanant in the Avesta.

Vanant was probably known in Sogdiana, as can be deduced from the name of the village *Wanandūn* in the vicinity of Bukhara.[939] However, identifying her image in Sogdian art poses significant obstacles. Images of Nike are found in Sogdian art, for example, in the hunting scene from the citadel of Panjikent,[940] but there are no indications that she was identified with Vanant. According to Marshak and Raspopova, the goddess on the mountain ram paired with a god on a camel in Panjikent art may be identified as Vanant (Čisti is put forward as another possibility).[941] Unfortunately, there is no solid evidence to confirm or refute this identification.

3. *Conclusions*

The only certain representation of Vanant in the visual record of the ancient Iranian world is the Kushan goddess Oanindo modeled after Nike. However, it is not known whether other images of Nike found in Western and Eastern Iran were also understood and interpreted as Vanant. Oanindo remains the only case when this identification is secure. Despite toponymic evidence, it is uncertain if the image of Vanat existed in Sogdian art.

---

933 Göbl 1984: Oanindo 1–2.
934 Rosenfield 1967: 91.
935 Pugachenkova 1971: 43–44.
936 Pugachenkova 1971: Fig. 54.
937 See p. 137–138.
938 Grenet 1993/1994: 91. For the painting of the Bāmiān Mithra, see p. 89.
939 Lurje 2004: 210.
940 Marshak 1996: 426–427, Fig. 1.
941 Marshak and Raspopova 1990: 145.

24. *Vāta*

Vāta (MP. *Wād*) "wind" is the wind deity in the Avestan pantheon.[942] *Vāta* is also used in the Avesta as the word for wind, often making it difficult to distinguish between the god and the natural phenomenon.[943] Vāta was probably an ancient Indo-Iranian deity since his figure and functions are similar both in the Avesta and in the Rig Veda. Vāta appears very close in personality and functions to another Avestan god—Vayu—but seems to possess a less complex nature than his atmospheric colleague.

1. *Western Iran*

Vāta is attested in two Old Persian names,[944] but was not represented in Western Iran and no possible images of the god are known.

2. *Eastern Iran*

The only certain portrayal of Vāta comes from Kushan coinage. Like many other Kushan deities, Vāta also had a Greek name (ANEMOC) on the first issue of Kanishka (fig. 144), before being renamed "Oado" (OAΔO). The reverses with his portrait continued to be produced under Huvishka (fig. 145). There are two main iconographic types. The first shows Oado running left, and on the second he is heading in the opposite direction.[945] On both types, Oado appears as a bearded male with floating hair and a large cape. This image derives from the Greek wind god Anemos who is depicted on the unique gold coin of Kanishka. However, unlike other Kushan gods whose iconography was virtually unaffected in this language change, Anemos lost his wings when he became Oado. Moreover, while the image of Anemos is found on the unique gold coin, Oado was "relegated" to bronze coinage.[946]

The iconography of Anemos-Oado has been convincingly demonstrated by Tanabe to be derived from Greek and Hellenistic images of the wind god.[947] Oado features in Bactrian personal names,[948] but his history following the Sasanian conquest of the Kushan lands is unknown. Two wind-genies with floating scarves that appear in the upper corners of the Mithra-painting at Bāmiān[949] can be identified as a continuation of the Kushan Oado, although they are not labeled.

Vāta is also possibly attested in one Sogdian personal name,[950] but no divinity in Sogdian art seems to possess the attributes and visual appearance suitable for the wind god.

3. *Conclusions*

The only image of the wind-god Vāta in the Iranian world seems to be that of the Kushan Oado. However, it is possible that in sixth century CE Bactria, the wind-god was represented as a flying genie holding floating scarves at Bāmiān. If this is indeed the image of Vāta, it would indicate a remarkable continuity of the Kushan type whose main attribute is a floating scarf.

---

942 Gray 1929: 167–168.
943 Boyce 1975b: 79.
944 Tavernier 2007: 543.
945 Göbl 1984: Oado 1–2; Tanabe 1990: Figs. 5–6.
946 Grenet forthcoming a, suggests that this could be due to the rising popularity of another "atmospheric" god, Oešo. However, it does not imply that the gods depicted on the more prestigious, but extremely rare, gold coins were necessarily more popular than those portrayed on bronze and copper coinage. In fact, the opposite could be the case, and deities chosen for the coins made of less prestigious metals, but which were in wide circulation, could have been viewed by the minting authorities as more important.
947 Tanabe 1990.
948 Sims-Williams 2010: no. 468.
949 See p. 89.
950 Lurje 2010: no. 1370.

25. *Vayu*

Vayu (MP. *Wāy*) is essentially a wind-god, but he was also associated with the life-breath of all the living beings and is described in the Avesta as a warlike, conqueror and ruthless deity.[951] In Sogdian, one of his names is "adorned with red" (*krm'yr py'tk*).[952] Other appellations conveying the notions of victory, power and warfare are also attested in both Avestan and Sogdian texts.[953]

1. *Western Iran*

There are no images of Vayu in Western Iran from the entire pre-Islamic period. The Persian veneration of natural phenomena, including the wind, is a popular *topos* among Greek and Latin authors.[954] It is not clear whether this can be taken as an evidence for the worship of Vayu. Neither he, nor any other atmospheric deity, is known from the Armenian and Georgian pantheons.

2. *Eastern Iran*

Vayu was undoubtedly known in Parthiena, since he is attested as a theophoric component in several names from Nisa.[955] The possible inclusion of Vayu in the Kushan and Sogdian pantheons has been the subject of much debate and controversy. During the excavations of Panjikent, Soviet archaeologists discovered a painting of a deity labeled *wyšprkr* (Wēšparkar) whose iconography was very close to the god known from the Kushan pantheon as Oešo (OHÞO). Oešo is the second most common god on Kushan coins and exhibits the most diverse iconography.[956] Oešo is the only god to be depicted on the coins of Vima Kadphises. He features alongside numerous other gods on the issues of Kanishka and Huvishka. He again becomes the exclusive deity on the reverse of Vasudeva's coins and shares the reverses of Kanishka II, Vasishka, Kanishka III and Vasudeva II with the goddess Ardoxšo.

This god, whose iconographic features and attributes are entirely those of Indian Śiva, is labeled οηþο starting from Kanishka. Joe Cribb has divided the images of Oešo on Kushan coinage into six main categories:

(1) without a bull, two armed, single headed (fig. 146).
(2) without a bull, two armed, three headed.
(3) with a bull, two armed, single headed.
(4) with a bull, two-or four armed, three headed (pl. 27).
(5) without a bull, four armed, single headed (pl. 28).
(6) without a bull, four-or six armed, three headed (fig. 147).

His attributes are numerous and include a trident-axe or simple trident (an obligatory attribute that appears on all types), a thunderbolt, a water pot, a lion skin, a lotus flower, an antelope, an elephant goad, a wheel and a club. On some types, Oešo has a nimbus (sometimes flaming) and wears a diadem.[957]

951 See Wikander 1941; Gray 1929: 169–171; Boyce 1975b: 79–82; Boyce 1993/1994: 35–37.
952 Panaino 2002b: 113.
953 Panaino 2002b: 113.
954 De Jong 1997: 29, 304, 413.
955 For instance, Diakonoff and Livshits 2001: nos. 593:10; 304:4.
956 His iconography was described and classified by Cribb 1997. To be supplemented with new types published in Bopearachchi 2008.
957 Cribb 1997.

In 1975 Helmut Humbach recognized *wyšprkr* as deriving from the Avestan epithet of Vayu—*vaiiuš uparō.kairiiō*, "Vayu, whose activity lies in the upper region" and suggested that οηþο represents Bactrian *wēš*, from the Avestan *vaiiuš*.[958] Therefore, both Kushan Oešo and Sogdian Wēšparkar are local variants of the same Iranian Vayu. Humbach's hypothesis was adopted by some scholars,[959] and criticized by others who preferred to identify Oešo with the Indian Śiva.[960] In fact, Oešo poses a serious dilemma. On the one hand, it is incontestable that "OEŠO, as any student of Indian iconography can tell you, is Śiva"[961] and it is true that "as far as iconography is concerned, Bactrian Vesh [Oešo] is undeniably Shiva himself and, judging by the attributes, there is no evidence of his connection with Iranian Vayu".[962] However, on the other hand, Indologists have failed to produce a convincing alternative "Śivaite" etymology for Oešo that would prove Humbach wrong.[963] Notable is the suggestion of Gail who attempted to link Oešo with *Bhūteśa*, one of the names of Śiva in Mathurā where the god was venerated as *Śiva Bhūteśvara*, "Lord of the demons".[964] This etymology has recently gained support from such prominent Iranists as Gnoli who also noted that "nothing excludes the possibility that οηþο was the name or epithet of a proto-Śiva figure characteristic of the Gandhāra region and deeply rooted in a complex and composite religious world that was essentially Indian ...".[965]

While the etymology of Oešo does not provide an unambiguous answer, Wēšparkar, I believe, supplies the necessary evidence. The fact that Sogdian *wyšprkr* reflects Avestan *vaiiuš uparō.kairiiō* has never been seriously doubted and his iconography is undeniably that of Śiva. Wēšparkar is also identified with Mahādeva (Śiva) in the Buddhist text *Vessantara Jātaka* 913–921.[966] Chinese sources also provide evidence for the linkage between Śiva and Wēšparkar.[967] Therefore, the association between Śiva and Vayu might be considered firmly established at least for the Sogdian pantheon. Although the possibility cannot be ruled out that the visual representation of Śiva was borrowed for Wēšparkar directly from Indian art whose influence on Sogdian art was indeed substantial, it is more reasonable to suppose that Śiva-Wēšparkar is in fact a continuation of the Kushan Oešo who was an exceptionally popular deity in Kushan and Kushano-Sasanian Bactria.

Oešo is completely absent from the Rabatak inscription, although it is not inconceivable that he was substituted by Mozdooano—another possible manifestation of Śiva in the Kushan pantheon who occupies fourth place in the Rabatak gods' list. The first images of Oešo on early issues of Vima Kadphises are aniconic and represent the god through his most recognizable symbols, a trident combined with an axe and a bull.[968] His anthropomorphic image was created during the reign of this king, perhaps incorporating features from the iconography of Poseidon, Zeus and Heracles.[969] Besides coins, images of Oešo are also recorded in other media, for instance on two painted terracotta panels in the Metropolitan Museum and in a private collection.[970] On one panel, a worshipper is shown whose upper part of the body is not preserved, but who holds in his right hand an object resembling a bowl (fig. 148).[971] In front of him stands a half-naked, three-headed, nimbate god. Only two of his three heads are preserved. The

958 Humbach 1975a: 402–408.
959 Tanabe 1991/1992; Boyce 1993/1994: 35–36; Carter 1995b; Cribb 1997; Grenet 2006/2010: 88–89.
960 Gail 1991/1992; Lo Muzio 1994/1995; Zeymal 1997; Gnoli 2009: 146–149.
961 Carter 1995b: 143.
962 Marshak 1995/1996: 305.
963 See references to some of these suggested etymologies in Gnoli 2009: 149, ns. 50, 51.
964 Gail 1991/1992.
965 Gnoli 2009: 148.
966 Wendtland 2009: 120–121.
967 See p. 39.
968 Cribb 1997: A1, C1.
969 Giuliano 2004: 59.
970 For other panels from this group, see p. 62–63 and p. 136.
971 Carter 1997: 577.

central head is that of a young man with a thin moustache and a third eye. The left head belongs to a bearded man in a white cap. Oešo has four arms, but only two attributes are clearly recognizable—a trident and a vessel. On the second panel, in contrast with the other from this group, the worshipper is shown on the right side while Oešo occupies the position on the left edge (fig. 149).[972] The deity also holds a trident and a vessel in his right hands (the left are missing), and is tricephalic. The central head is similar to that from the first panel, but the other heads are different. The head on the right side wears a red cap and belongs to a child or a young girl. The left head is beardless but it seems to depict a mature male. Both these representations correspond to type VI of Cribb's typology.[973]

After the Sasanian conquest of Kushanshahr Oešo not only continued to be used by the Kushano-Sasanians, but in fact became the most popular reverse type on their coins. However, he was now labeled by the Bactrian inscription βορζοανδο ιαζαδο, which is a borrowing from MP. *Burzāwand yazad*,[974] meaning "the exalted god" or "the god who possesses the heights". The reasons for this change are not clear. Alongside the standard Kushan reverse type of a standing Oešo with the bull Nandī on the coins of the Kushano-Sasanian Pērōz I,[975] the other type of this king shows a male frontal bust on top of the altar with the Bactrian inscription ΒΑΓΟ ΒΟΡΖΑΝΔΟ (fig. 150).[976] His fiery hair stands on end and two large locks of hair rest on his shoulders. A silver drachm of Ōhrmazd I minted in Merv shows a king performing a libation on a small altar set before the enthroned statue of the same god now identified not by Bactrian, but by a Middle Persian inscription as *Burzāwand yazad* (fig. 151).[977] The god is portrayed seated on a throne very similar to that of the goddess on a coin of Ōhrmazd II and the significance of the composition is clearly the same—a king worshipping before the enthroned statue of a deity. *Burzāwand yazad* is beardless and a fiery nimbus surrounds his head. In his left hand he holds a spear, while with his right hand he offers a royal crown tied with a diadem to the king.

Such statues were undoubtedly housed in Bactrian temples, although we lack archaeological confirmation. The only possible sculptural representation of Oešo is the life-size statue excavated by the Soviet-Afghan mission in the main room of sanctuary X in Dilberjin. Unfortunately, it is known only from a brief description in a single, not easily accessible publication, and four small photos of inadequate quality (fig. 152).[978] The statue depicts a nude (although it is possible that garments were painted but did not survive) male figure seated frontally on a throne placed on a podium in front of the entrance. The head is missing, but there are traces of locks of hair falling on his shoulders. The figure wears two necklaces and a palmette pendant. His right hand was not preserved and his left hand is lowered. The statue was accompanied by two other statues placed to the left of the lower seats—a female figure on the far left, and an additional figure of whom only small fragments have survived placed between them. The only god in the Kushano-Sasanian pantheon who is shown partially naked, with such a hairstyle and with necklaces is Oešo/βαγο βορζανδο on the coin of the Kushano-Sasanian king Pērōz I. The statue might therefore depicted this very god, who, according to numismatic evidence, was one of the most important deities of Kushano-Sasanina Bactria. It is furthermore tempting to speculate that his missing right hand might have grasped a trident and his left hand originally held one of the attributes of Oešo known from coins.

Interestingly, the deity Apąm Napāt in the Avesta has the epithet *bərəzant*, "The High One", derived from the same root (in Middle Persian he is called *burz yazad*). Moreover, Wēšparkar from Pan-

972 Carter 1997: 581.
973 Cribb 1997: VI.
974 Sims-Williams 2002: 232.
975 Grenet 2006/2010: Fig. 11.
976 Carter 1985: Pl. 50, no. 37; Cribb 1990: no. 32.
977 Cribb 1990: no. 59, no. 23, is the reduced copper version of the same reverse design.
978 Kruglikova 1982: 169.

jikent XXII/1 is probably shown in the presence of Apąm Napāt, providing additional material for speculation of a close association between these two divinities.

Two significant changes were introduced to the new types of Kushano-Sasanian Oešo. He is shown offering a diadem or a crown, and a trident—his obligatory attribute on all Kushan types—is replaced by a spear. It is noteworthy that according to the Avesta, the main attribute/weapon of Vayu is a spear. His epithets include "the sharp-speared one" (*tižiiaršta*), "the wide-speared one" (*pərəϑuuarəšta*) and "the one with a brandished lance" (*vaēžiiaršta*).[979] It is tempting to connect this change of attribute with the influence of the Avestan concept of Vayu, as a part of conjectured Sasanian attempts to bring the Śiva-like Oešo nearer to the Avestan god.

Contrary to Kushan Oešo whose iconography is purely Śivaite, the Sogdian Wēšparkar possibly shows signs of proximity to the functions of the Avestan Vayu. The left of Wēšparkar's three heads blows a horn—an attribute alien to Śiva, but fully appropriate for the wind god.[980] However, it could also be a war-horn, which might rather reflect a militant side of the god. Wēšparkar is one of only two gods in Sogdian art who are identified by an inscription.[981] He is also probably depicted on the leg of a large altar from a mural at Panjikent III/6.[982] In Ustrushana, Wēšparkar is portrayed in the center of the lower register of the eastern wall of a "Small hall", as a mounted three-headed and four-handed deity engaged in a battle against demons (fig. 153).[983] The central head is significantly larger than the other two and all three wear a crescent-shaped crown. The god is armored and equipped with a bow, a spear and a short dagger attached to his belt.

His second representation is found in the upper register, to the left of the four-handed Nana (pl. 29).[984] Wēšparkar is armored, has a moustache, a nimbus and a crown decorated with a crescent. His head is slightly turned towards the goddess. With one of his right hands, the god grasps a trident. Unfortunately, his other attributes are not preserved.

We should also add a seal from Kafir-Kala depicting a three-headed figure with a trident, which is undoubtedly Wēšparkar.[985] A representation of Wēšparkar is also found on panel D. X. 3. from the Buddhist shrine (D. X.) at Dandan Uiliq at Khotan (fig. 16) where the god appears together with the other Sogdian gods, Nana and Āδβāγ.[986] Further to the east, Wēšparkar is depicted on the right panel of the eastern side of the Sino-Sogdian funerary bed of Wirkak (579 CE) (fig. 162).[987] Here, the god assumes the iconography of Śiva Maheśvara (albeit with some variations, for instance he has one head instead of his usual three). His supremacy over the scene of the ascent of the souls to Heaven is remarkable. Although according to Zoroastrian scriptures Vayu indeed assists the souls in their crossing of the Činwad bridge, he is only one of several divine "assistants" (Mihr, Rašn, Wahrām and Aštād). However, in the most detailed Iranian account of the journey to Heaven, the *Ardā Wīrāz Nāmag*, Vohu Manah clearly occupies a place of greater importance than Vayu.[988] Therefore, the depiction of Vayu-Wēšparkar as presiding over the Činwad bridge crossing possibly reflects either a personal preference for Wirkak and his wife or a specifically Sogdian variant of religious beliefs connected with the afterlife which differ in this aspect from canonical Zoroastrian literature. The latter suggestion is also supported by the Chinese

979 Panaino 2002b: 83–84.
980 Grenet 2006/2010: 92.
981 Airyaman being the second.
982 Belenitskii and Marshak 1981: 30–31.
983 Sokolovskiy 2009: 49–50.
984 Sokolovskiy 2009: 51–52.
985 Compareti 2013: 128–131, Fig. 1.
986 Stein 1907: 259–261.
987 Grenet, Riboud and Yang Junkai 2004: 281–282, Fig. 3.
988 See p. 32.

chronicle *Liangjing xinji* which attests to the existence among Sogdians of a temple of a Wēšparkar-Śiva Maheśvara, referred to as a "Heavenly god".[989]

The presence of Vayu in the Sogdian pantheon is also attested by a single personal name (*Wēšδāt*, "Given by Vayu") from one document from Mount Muγ.[990] Vayu was also known in Chorasmia as is evident from an anthroponym formed with *vayu* from Topraq-Qal'a documents.[991] Although no reliable data exist for the cult of Vayu among Scythians, Vasiliy Abaev has equated Ossetian *wæjug* "giant" with OIr. **vayuka-*; and the Scythian god Οἰτόσυρος reported by Herodotus with OIr. **vayuka-sura*, suggesting that Vayu was venerated among Scythians as the god of death.[992] Be that as it may, no divine image in Scythian art can be convincingly associated with Vayu.

3. *Conclusions*

All visual representations of Vayu are confined to the Eastern Iranian world and appear to have originated from numerous and diverse types of Kushan Oešo. It is perhaps best to approach Oešo as a syncretistic deity fusing elements of Śiva with Iranian Vayu, although in the absence of any written evidence describing the traits and qualities of Oešo it is not clear which characteristics of Vayu, as he is known from Zoroastrianism, Oešo possessed. The cult of Śiva in the lands conquered by the Kushans was deeply rooted and influential.[993] Furthermore, it is likely that in the religious worldview of the Iranian population of the Kushan Empire the position of Vayu was far more elevated and significant than just being "another Kushan wind god".[994] He was possibly considered a powerful god, a Lord of Life and Death and, as such, was believed to stand close in his functions to Śiva. Judging by the extraordinary popularity of Oešo on Kushan coins, one is inclined to think that he was one of the most important deities in Bactria, although his enigmatic absence from the Rabatak list of gods presents a problem that can hardly be resolved on the basis of our current data.

Sasanian rule in Bactria saw the introduction of a number of changes to the image of Oešo. Some of them perhaps reflect an attempt to adjust his cult to more "Zoroastrian" perceptions of Vayu. The popularity of Oešo had seemingly even increased and there is no evidence for him being "challenged" by the principal Sasanian god—Ahura Mazdā—as there are no signs of his very existence in the Kushano-Sasanian pantheon. Anāhitā was perhaps the only divinity imported from Western Iran. Along with the continuation of the standing type of Kushan Oešo and his bull, a new type appeared, sometimes represented enthroned in fully anthropomorphic shape, and sometimes reduced to a torso and called in Bactrian and Middle Persian "the exalted god". He has a flaming nimbus and a spear and offers the king a diadem or a crown.

Among all these Kushan and Kushano-Sasanian representations, only one iconographic type of three-headed Oešo was probably continued in Sogdiana (where this god was called Wēšparkar). There are indications that also in the Sogdian pantheon, Vayu occupied a more important place than that reserved for him in Zoroastrian literature. His personality undoubtedly included a dominant warlike aspect, since in Ustrushana Wēšparkar is depicted as a rider combating demons and he possibly also played an important role assisting the souls of the just in their journey to heaven. Future investigation of his possible links with Apąm Napāt could prove illuminating and yield interesting results.

---

989 See p. 39.
990 Lurje 2010: no. 1385.
991 Livshits 2004: 191.
992 Abaev 1960.
993 See Fussman 1991.
994 As the title of the important article by Tanabe 1991/1992 proclaims.

26. *Vərəϑraγna*

Vərəθraγna (MP. *Wahrām*) is the Old Iranian god of war and victory whose personality preserves traces of Indo-Iranian and Indo-European mythology.[995] He occupies a prominent place in the Avesta, as a mighty warrior-god whose very name means "smiting of resistance". Vərəθraγna holds a peculiar record among Avestan deities for his number of incarnations—ten overall; among them can be found nearly all major animals appearing in Iranian art. This provides a vast field for speculation. Moreover, since Vərəθraγna is a god of war and victory, any divine figure that has a weapon or armor may also be interpreted as Vərəθraγna.

1. *Western Iran*

Vərəθraγna is not attested at all in the Achaemenian period as a theophoric compound in personal names and there are no assured visual representations in the artistic record of this era. His position and very existence in Achaemenian Iran is therefore questionable. The earliest attestation of Vərəθraγna in the west, beyond the borders of the Iranian world, is in Commagene in the first century BCE where his image is entirely that of Heracles (fig. 163).[996] Heracles was probably the most popular and widely represented Greek deity in the Iranian world.[997] The relief from Commagene and the statue of Heracles from Mesene[998] provide unquestionable examples of his identification with Iranian Vərəθraγna. On the other hand, in the Iranian world itself the situation seems to be somewhat different. Heracles appears under his own name on Kushan coins, distinct from Vərəθraγna (Orlagno) even after the so-called "Reform of Kanishka",[999] clearly demonstrating that images of Heracles originating from the Iranian world should not automatically be associated with Vərəθraγna.[1000]

Numerous images of Heracles have come down to us from the Parthian Empire, but few of them originate from the Iranian plateau. The only certain representation of Heracles-Vərəθraγna is the abovementioned bronze statue from Mesene. In pre-Christian Armenia ruled by the offshoot line of the Arsacid dynasty, Heracles was also associated with Vahagn (Vərəθraγna) and his statues—probably modeled on Anatolian and Greek images—were set up in temples.[1001] No descriptions of the statues of Vahagn have survived, but it is reasonable to assume that his iconographic type closely followed that of a purely Greek Heracles as he appears on the coins of some Artaxiad kings—naked, and holding a club and a lion skin.[1002] However, it is interesting to note the unusual association of the Armenian Vahagn with fire. In a fragment of an ancient Armenian hymn preserved by Movsēs Xorenac'i, Vahagn is described as a fiery red-headed boy.[1003]

With the ascent of the Sasanian dynasty, there are numerous indications that Vərəθraγna did in fact maintain his widespread popularity. The first and the fourth "princes" of Kartīr's vision might be Vərəθraγna.[1004] If so, it indicates that Vərəθraγna was considered and imagined as a fully anthropomorphic god in third century CE Sasanian Iran. However, no definite visual representations of the god of Victory have been found in Sasanian art. One of the small figures placed between the king and the god on

995 Benveniste and Renou 1934; Gnoli 1989c.
996 See Boyce and Grenet 1990: 323–324 with references.
997 See Jamzadeh 1989; Boyce and Grenet 1991: 62–65; Carter 1995a; De Jong 2003a. On the cult of Heracles in Eastern Iran, see also Pugachenkova 1977.
998 See p. 11.
999 See below.
1000 Carter 1995a, provides the most complete list of Heracles imagery from the Hellenistic East.
1001 See p. 20.
1002 Russell 1987: 84.
1003 See p. 21–22.
1004 Skjærvø 2011a. For his vision, see p. 11–12.

the relief of Ardašīr I at Naqš-e Rağab is usually recognized as that of Heracles assimilated here with the Iranian Vərəθraγna.[1005] Due to the relief's poor preservation, the attributes of this figure are not clearly distinguishable and it is impossible to be sure that this is indeed the image of the Greek god. This figure looks remarkably similar to a figure that appears on the reverse of coins belonging to the mid-second CE ruler of Pars who was recently identified as Pakorus III.[1006] This reverse design is unprecedented among the coinage of Hellenistic and Parthian Pars. It shows a naked, bareheaded figure with a roundly-cut beard, holding a club-like object in his right hand.[1007] If this character is the same as that on the relief of Narseh, it provides strong support for the divine nature of the latter. However, if the figure on the Naqš-e Rağab relief is indeed a deity, it is difficult to find a satisfactory explanation for his inferior size compared to Ahura Mazdā, the king and even to his retinue. There are no examples of inner height hierarchy between different deities found on Sasanian rock-reliefs—gods are always depicted as the same size. On the other hand, the second small figure is shown in a pose of adoration toward him. Because of this ambiguity, these two characters still defy any convincing interpretation.

It is noteworthy that the half-sized figures placed between the main protagonists are also found in Sogdian art. In Panjikent VI/41 (the "Rostam Room") in one of the scenes of the third, upper register, a small figure of a female harpist is placed between two heroes and the "king".[1008] Marshak has interpreted this as the "fame" of the heroes.[1009] I believe that the central position of these small characters between the god and king is not accidental. Could they be a sort of "mediator" between human and divine, between *gētīg* and *mēnōg*?

Additional images proposed to represent Vərəθraγna in Sasanian monumental art, include two figures wearing chainmail from the column capitals at Ṭāq-i Bustān and an armored horseman from the lower register of the large grotto at the same site.[1010] It is unlikely that the figure of the heavily armored horseman from the relief of the grotto at Ṭāq-i Bustān represents Vərəθraγna or, in fact, any deity. Although one may agree that Ṭāq-i Bustān is indeed an exceptional monument,[1011] all known representations of deities in Sasanian monumental art are connected with scenes of royal investiture. Moreover, gods in Sasanian art are always depicted in royal attire and have royal attributes.[1012] The Ṭāq-i Bustān horseman is completely different from these images, but is almost identical to the equestrian figures on bullae of some high-ranking Sasanian generals.[1013] The Ṭāq-i Bustān horseman is even depicted turned to the right—precisely as the horsemen on the seals are always shown. The only difference seems to be the nimbus of the Ṭāq-i Bustān warrior[1014] and he may therefore depict someone higher than the generals, but not of divine nature—probably a Sasanian king himself. If the king who commissioned the monument of Ṭāq-i Bustān is Xusrō II, his desire to show himself as a victorious warrior fits perfectly the historical context of his rule—an epic struggle with the Byzantium Empire.

The Sasanian column capitals with figural representations were gathered from different locations, but clearly form a single typological group. Six of them are currently placed in a park adjacent to the Ṭāq-i Bustān monument, one is at Čehel Sotun Palace in Isfahan and the last is at Irān-e bāstān Museum

1005 Hinz 1969: 123–124; Ghirshman 1975: 125; Vanden Berghe 1988: 1522; de Waele 1989: 817; Boyce and Grenet 1991: 63, n. 61; Levit-Tawil 1992: 192; Carter 1995a: 129. For a description of the relief, see p. 51.

1006 See Rezakhani 2010.

1007 See the excellent images in Rezakhani 2010.

1008 Marshak 2002b: Figs. 25–26.

1009 Marshak 2002b: 57.

1010 This was already proposed by von Gall 1990: 100 and recently reformulated by Compareti 2006a.

1011 Compareti 2006a: 166.

1012 Marshak 1998: 86.

1013 See Gyselen 2001.

1014 This is also noted by Compareti 2006a: 168.

in Tehran (figs. 154–161).[1015] All of them are carved with the similar motif of various deities extending a diadem. On the opposite side, the capitals are decorated with the representation of a Sasanian king stretching his arm (for the diadem), or with a floral ornament. There can be little doubt that these figures represent deities, since they are depicted in the "canonical" Sasanian scene of investiture. If we reject the identification of the Ṭāq-i Bustān horseman as Vərəθraγna, the only argument left in favor of the interpretation of two of the figures on these capitals (nos. 1 and 4) as the god of Victory is the fact that they wear chainmail. Indeed, given the presumable popularity of Vərəθraγna in the Sasanian period and his position of importance in the Zoroastrian pantheon, he is the most likely candidate for the "god wearing armor", but this identification is by no means certain. One can also envisage other deities from the Zoroastrian pantheon being armored, for instance Šahrewar.

Evidence for the representations of Vərəθraγna in Sasanian minor art, seals and coins is also ambiguous. Choksy identified one of three busts which appear on the obverse of the coins of Wahrām II as Vərəθraγna. According to him, Vərəθraγna is a youth wearing a horse, eagle, or boar-headed bonnet.[1016] As has already been noted, the identification of Vərəθraγna based on his animal Avestan incarnations is highly problematic,[1017] although the fact that on some types he is offering a diadem to the royal couple seems to suggest his divine nature. Furthermore, Gyselen, drawing on parallels with Roman coinage depicting an emperor, empress and the crown prince, has suggested that the coins of Wahrām II actually follow this model and portray a similar assemblage: a king, a queen and a crown prince.[1018] This alternative suggestion seems preferable.

2. *Eastern Iran*

The earliest evidence for the existence of Vərəθraγna in Eastern Iran is found in personal names from Old Nisa.[1019] The paucity of historical sources makes it impossible to establish whether Vərəθraγna was worshipped in other regions before making his first definite appearance on the Kushan coins. Vərəθraγna, Bactrian Orlagno (ΟΡΛΑΓΝΟ) is portrayed on the reverses of several golden coins of Kanishka (pl. 30).[1020] He is depicted standing, facing right, and dressed in the Kushan noble costume. In his left hand he holds a spear and his right hand rests on the hooked hilt of the sword, probably shaped in the form of a bird's head. Orlagno's head is surrounded by a nimbus and he wears a headdress surmounted by a bird of prey. He clearly exhibits an iconographical type completely independent from Heracles or any other Graeco-Roman deity and is an original Kushan creation based on the image of the Kushan prince with some alterations, such as the eagle headdress. Its earlier prototypes are unknown as are its descendants.

The bird-helmet of Orlagno is usually taken to allude to one of the Avestan incarnations of Vərəθraγna.[1021] However, as pointed out by Carter, this headdress probably originates among the Central Asian nomads and is attested in Chorasmia and among the Scythians.[1022] Judging by Bactrian onomastics, the popularity of Orlagno does not appear to be very high; his name is attested as a theophoric compound in only one name.[1023] Interestingly, Orlagno is the only Iranian deity from Kanishka's coinage that does not continue on the coins of Huvishka.

1015 Compareti 2006a.
1016 Choksy 1989: 134.
1017 See p. 176.
1018 Gyselen 2010b: 203.
1019 For instance, Diakonoff and Livshits 2001: nos. 151:4; 1520:6.
1020 See Rosenfield 1967: 95–96; Göbl 1984: 63/8.
1021 For instance, Grenet 1993: 152.
1022 Carter 1995a: 125. For a discussion of the symbolism of Iranian headdresses, see p. 178.
1023 Sims-Williams 2010: no. 195.

There is one uncertain attestation of Vərəθraγna—Sogdian Wašagn (*wšγn*)—in Sogdian personal names.[1024] In Sogdian art no definite image of Vərəθraγna has yet been identified, but several candidates have been proposed. Since the camel is one of the incarnations of the Avestan Vərəθraγna, Shishkin and later Marshak proposed to identify the Sogdian god associated with a camel as Vərəθraγna.[1025] This god on a camel is usually depicted together with a female goddess whose attribute is a mountain ram, although sometimes he is also shown alone.[1026] His image is found not only in monumental art such as wall-paintings, but also on tokens and terracotta.[1027] Numerous appearances of the "camel-god" in Sogdian art indicate the unusual popularity that he enjoyed among the Sogdians. However, as with the coins of Wahrām II, the animal attribute alone cannot suffice for identification, especially as it relies on the unproven assumption that a camel was also an attribute of the Sogdian Wašagn. Even leaving aside the methodological issues involved in using the Avesta, there is another divinity in the Zoroastrian holy hymns who also assumes the shape of a camel—Dahmān Āfrīn.[1028]

Grenet has also proposed to recognize Vərəθraγna in the image of a four-handed god from the Khirmantepa ossuary.[1029] His identification was generally based on the warlike appearance of the god. Even if he holds a shield and an arrow, as the French scholar maintains contra Lunina and Usmanova, this does not necessarily imply his identification with Vərəθraγna. After all, the Kushan Orlagno—the only definitely established image of Vərəθraγna—has different attributes and definitely does not possess the most warlike appearance among the Kushan gods. In a recent article, Grenet has changed his mind and has proposed to interpret the god from the Khirmantepa ossuary as Tīr-Tištrya.[1030] If the main attribute of the god on this ossuary is indeed an arrow, the identification as Tīr-Tištrya seems possible. An additional, hypothetical Sogdian Vərəθraγna was recognized in a wall painting which decorated the portico of Temple I at Panjikent, depicting a charioteer riding a chariot drawn by wild boars.[1031] Once again we face the problem of identifying a Sogdian god according to its Avestan animal incarnation. An image of a four-handed armored warrior from the wall painting recently found in Panjikent was interpreted as Vərəθraγna by the Tajik archaeologists.[1032] The warrior holds two swords and a mace and has human hands and a skull decorating his helmet. However, this character is in all probability a demon, as was convincingly demonstrated by Marshak.[1033]

3. *Conclusion*

In Commagene and Mesopotamia—the Western periphery of the Iranian world—Vərəθraγna assumed the appearance of the Greek Heracles. Based on this evidence, it is logical to suppose that at least some of the numerous images of Heracles that circulated in the Iranian world in the Hellenistic and Parthian periods were also assimilated with Vərəθraγna. The Kushan Orlagno unequivocally demonstrates that this assimilation was probably limited to Western Iran, while in the East Heracles and Vərəθraγna were considered separate gods. Given the important place that Vərəθraγna presumably enjoyed in Sasanian Iran, it is difficult to understand his absence from official Sasanian art.

1024 Lurje 2010: no. 1347.

1025 Shishkin 1963: 203; Marshak and Raspopova 1990: 141–145; Marshak 1999: 182. According to an alternative suggestion by Grenet, this god should be identified as *x*ᵛ*arənah*, Grenet et al. 1993: 65; Grenet 1993: 156–159.

1026 See p. 138–139 ff.

1027 These are reproduced in Shkoda 2009: Fig. 124.

1028 See Boyce 1993a.

1029 Grenet 1992: 48; Grenet et al. 1993: 62. For the Khirmantepa ossuary, see p. 125.

1030 Grenet and Marshak 1998: 10; Grenet 2006/2010: 94.

1031 Marshak 1999: 182.

1032 Karimova and Kurbanov 2008.

1033 Karimova and Kurbanov 2008: 185. Marshak 2009: 11, calls him "a king of demons".

The only certain image of Vərəθraγna is Orlagno—an original Kushan creation, not copied from any Graeco-Roman deity. Like the majority of gods found on Kanishka's and Huvishka's coins, Orlagno had no continuation in Kushano-Sasanian Bactria or Sogdiana. If representations of Vərəθraγna actually existed in the rich Sogdian iconography, we are still unable to identify it.

27. *Vohu Manah*

Vohu Manah (MP. *Wahman*, "Good Thought") is one of the six Aməša Spənta. He appears in the Avesta both as an abstract idea and as a concrete divine being—the protector and patron of animals and especially of cattle.[1034] The Avesta does not inform us of his physical appearance, but he is described as seated on a golden throne welcoming the souls of the righteous to Paradise.[1035]

1. *Western Iran*

Like all the Aməša Spənta Vohu Manah is not mentioned in the Achaemenian period and his representations are unknown. In the Parthian era, Vohu Manah is seemingly referred to for the first time as the "god of benevolence" (εὔνοια) mentioned by Plutarch.[1036] Moreover, the existence of a wooden cultic statue of Vohu Manah in Cappadocia documented by Strabo for the same period indicates that the abstract Aməša Spənta could also have been represented anthropomorphically.[1037] Unfortunately, Strabo does not describe the statue in more detail and no material examples of the imagery of Vohu Manah have come down to us either from Western Iran or from its immediate periphery.

Middle Persian literature contains three references to the visual form of Vohu Manah. Two of them are among the most detailed descriptions of the anthropomorphic appearance of a Zoroastrian divinity in the entire Zoroastrian written tradition. In *Dēnkard* and in *Wizīdagīhā ī Zādspram* Vohu Manah is said to be "in a form of a man" (*pad mard ēwēnag*), and he has a "height of three spears of a man". He is handsome, shining and radiant, and dressed in silken clothing. His hair is said to be "divided, like what is divided is a sign of duality". In *Ardā Wīrāz Nāmag* Vohu Manah sits on a golden throne and greets the righteous Wīrāz by taking hold of his hand.[1038] The third "prince" from Kartīr's vision is probably also Vohu Manah, since he sits on a golden throne.[1039] It is interesting to note that in his hand this "prince" holds an object called **čayēn/čiyēn* that turns into a bottomless well full of evil creatures. Perhaps this unusual transformation can be understood as a manifestation of Vohu Manah's duality, manifested by his "dual" hairstyle described in the *Wizīdagīhā ī Zādspram*. If the third "prince" from Kartīr's vision is indeed Vohu Manah, it provides us with safely dated evidence that in the third century CE, he was perceived as a completely anthropomorphic being, although we do not possess any of his representations in Sasanian art.

2. *Eastern Iran*

Although Vohu Manah is attested in personal names from the Nisa ostraca,[1040] his earliest possible visual representation in Eastern Iran is that of the god known from the Kushan coins of both Kanishka and

---

1034 See Narten 1989; Gignoux 1989.
1035 See p. 14. Boyce and Grenet 1991: 333, n, 121; write that Vohu Manah leads the souls "on into the presence of Ahura Mazdā himself, who is unquestionably also enthroned".
1036 Plut. *De Is. et Os.* 47. See the discussion by De Jong 1997: 185–186.
1037 See p. 17.
1038 See p. 32.
1039 See p. 11–12.
1040 For instance, Diakonoff and Livshits 2001: no. 264:4.

Huvishka as Manaobago (ΜΑΝΑΟΒΑΓΟ) (pl. 31).[1041] He appears seated on a throne with curved legs terminating with lion's paws of the type also found on some issues of Vima Kadphises.[1042] The lower part of his body and his torso are shown frontally, while his head and four arms are turned to the right. Manaobago wears a loose dress and a Bactrian variant of the Greek "Boeotian" helmet, which was apparently the most popular type in Graeco-Bactria.[1043] In his middle hands he holds a wheel and a ring, a plough in his upper hand and a purse tied with a flying ribbon in his lower hand.[1044] Based on his name, Manaobago is traditionally identified with Vohu Manah. His name consists of two compounds, one of which is *manah*, but instead of *vohu*, there is *baga-* ("god") and thus the name of the Kushan deity could be translated as "The God Thought". However, Humbach has argued against the identification of Manaobago with Vohu Manah and has compared Manaobago with Vedic *Mánasas Páti* ("Lord of Thought")—a deity of dreams who was connected with the moon.[1045]

A Bactrian inscription on a Roman silver plate recently published by Sims-Williams states that it was donated to the temple of Manaobago: "this *plate was acquired for the god Mana (*μαναο βαγο*) by Sen-gul, the son of Friy-gul, the satrap. And(?) … from the vineyard and from the …, of the year forty-three, this (is) the *income belonging to the god Mana".[1046]

Even for diverse Kushan imagery, the iconography of Manaobago is exceptionally eclectic and is unique in several respects. He is the only deity portrayed seated—a striking parallel with textual descriptions of Vohu Manah—and the only one to wear a helmet modeled after the helmets of Graeco-Bactrian rulers, although the significance of this last element is not clear. Manaobago is four-armed, reflecting an Indian influence and two of his four attributes, a plough and a wheel, are probably borrowed from the Hindu gods Krishna and Balarāma.[1047] The crescent moon rising from the shoulders of Manaobago is also found in images of the moon god Māh, who is, according to the Avestan texts, one of Vohu Manah's assistants, and in two representations of the goddess Nana.

The iconography of Manaobago poses many questions with few ready answers. Does the helmet allude to a warlike aspect of the deity? Why was Manaobago, judging by his name an Iranian deity, depicted four-armed like the Hindu gods and given their attributes? Unlike in Sogdian iconography, Kushan gods were not usually depicted with Indian attributes and with abnormal numbers of hands. Turning to the Avesta is not particularly helpful in answering these questions[1048] and unlocking the complex iconography and identity of Manaobago, clearly demonstrating how little is known about the Kushan religion and religious iconography. It is impossible to establish whether Manaobago reflects a Kushan variation of Vohu Manah, or perhaps another deity coming from the same Indo-Iranian background whose name also included a component *manah*. From a linguistic point of view, the identification of Manaobago with Vohu Manah is not certain, as pointed out by Humbach, and the German scholar's proposal connecting the Kushan god to the Vedic *Mánasas Páti* should not be ruled out.

The case of Manaobago highlights the problems inherent in dealing with Iranian religious iconography. It clearly demonstrates the limits and ambiguity involved when comparing the iconography and the Avestan texts whose relevance to most Iranian cultures in most historical periods is obscure, or at best debatable. With no accompanying legend unequivocally identifying this bizarre four-handed, helmeted Kushan deity, no one would ever think of connecting it to the Avestan Vohu Manah. Manaobago

---

1041 Rosenfield 1967: 79–80; Göbl 1984: Manaobago 1–2.
1042 Cribb 1997: 37.
1043 Nikonorov 1997: 48. On Boeotian helmets, see Litvinskiy 2001a: 351–355.
1044 Cribb 1997: 37. According to Grenet forthcoming a, Manaobago holds an "untied ribbon diadem".
1045 Humbach 1975b: 138–139.
1046 Sims-Williams 2009/2013: 192–195.
1047 Grenet forthcoming a.
1048 See Grenet forthcoming a.

is not mentioned in the Rabatak inscription and therefore his place in the divine hierarchy of Kushan Bactria is impossible to determine. His image remains unique to Kushan coins and is not encountered afterwards in Eastern Iran.

It appears that Vohu Manah was known in Sogdiana, as several Sogdian names contain the compound *xym'n*—a Sogdian form of his name.[1049] Identifying his possible visual representations in Sogdiana, however, proves to be a perplexing task. Three possible images of Vohu Manah have been suggested. As part of his theory that the figures on the ossuaries of Biyanajman and Miankal correspond to the Aməša Spənta, figure no. 1 on these ossuries was interpreted by Grenet as the representation of Vohu Manah.[1050] The second candidate is the seated figure on the extreme right from the Sivaz and Yumalaktepa ossuaries.[1051] The identification with Vohu Manah was proposed by Grenet, mostly based on the so-called "Vohu Manah" figure from the ossuaries of Biyanajman and Miankal.[1052] Both figures are characterized by the same gesture of two raised fingers and it is probable that they also share a second attribute, a ladle for libations. Unfortunately, the upper part of the head of the Sivaz figure is not preserved, making it impossible to determine which type of crown the figure originally wore. On the other hand, Marshak, based on the account of *Ardā Wīrāz Nāmag*, proposed to identify the figure with Rašnu or Sraoša and identified the lefthand god on the same ossuary as Ātar.[1053]

The interpretation of the scene depicted on the Sivaz ossuaries as the journey of a soul (identified as a naked bended figure) to Paradise,[1054] seemingly supports the idea that Vohu Manah—whose task is to greet the souls of the righteous in Paradise—is one of the figures shown on the ossuary. However, the (golden) throne, the most distinctive attribute of Vohu Manah that characterizes him both in the Avesta and in Middle Persian literature, is missing here. On the more detailed version of this scene from the Yumalaktepa ossuaries that feature Rašn, the figure purportedly identified with Vohu Manah is portrayed without any attribute. On both the ossuries of Sivaz and Yumalaktepa, the gods make a gesture with a raised finger. In this context, one should recall that in Kartīr's vision, the last "prince" points a finger at Kartīr's *hangirb* and smiles (§ 34).

We may assume that Vohu Manah was also known in Chorasmia, as follows from the personal name *Wahumanδāt* ("created by Vohu Manah") attested in documents from the palace of Topraq-Qal'a.[1055]

3. *Conclusions*

Both the textual and material records from Western Iran provide compelling evidence that Vohu Manah was conceived there as possessing an anthropomorphic shape, and it seems that he was occasionally thus represented. However, his images, as well as those of other Aməša Spənta, are completely absent from the Iranian plateau. If Manaobago and the figures from the Sogdian ossuaries are indeed renderings of Vohu Manah, they reflect two independent, completely unrelated iconographic types, which were created separately in Kushan and Sogdian art. This radical difference in iconography may also reflect entirely different perceptions of Vohu Manah in Kushan and Sogdian religion, which also differed from his Middle Persian descriptions.

1049 Lurje 2010: nos. 4, 35, 311, 635, 1440.

1050 Grenet 1987a: 50–51. For a detailed discussion of the figures on this group of ossuaries, see p. 170.

1051 See p. 84–85.

1052 Grenet et al. 1993: 61–62; Grenet 2009: 107–108.

1053 Marshak 1999: 185.

1054 Additional evidence for this interpretation was recently supplied by Grenet, who recognized a depiction of the *sedra* (Zoroastrian funerary ritual) as part of the scene. See Grenet 2009: 107–108.

1055 Livshits 2004: 191.

29. *Yima*

Yima (Av. *yima xšaēta*,[1056] MP. *Jam/Jamšēd*) is one of the most complex figures in Iranian mythology. In the period of Indo-Iranian unity he seems to have been primarily regarded as the First Man and the "civilizing hero".[1057] In the Avesta, Yima is the king of Paradise, ruling over humankind during the Golden Age.[1058]

1. *Western Iran*

To date, no image of Yima has been identified in Western Iran. He was known as early as the Achaemenian period, since his name is found as a compound in several personal names from Persepolis.[1059] However, contrary to Kushan religion,[1060] Yima was not deified in Western Iran. This concurs with what we know of Yima's position in Zoroastrian tradition where he was never ascribed a divine status.

Boyce believed that "pre-Zoroastrian" Yima was the god of the underworld and proposed to identify him with Herodotus' "god under the earth" to whom Xerxes performed sacrifices.[1061] This underworld god has so far defied any conclusive interpretation and several other candidates have been suggested. Gnoli has opted for Aŋra Mainyu[1062] while Martin Schwartz has recently argued that this divinity was part of the old Median, "pre-Zoroastrian" pantheon.[1063] To these proposals another speculative suggestion can be added. The only deity in Iranian mythology with a pronounced chthonic aspect is Rapithwin. He was believed to rule over summer months and then retreat under the earth at the beginning of winter to reappear on the vernal equinox.[1064] A festival connected with Rapithwin is described in the Avesta and his cult could have been practiced by some Iranians at a very early date.[1065] Therefore, if Herodotus' account is indeed credible, it is possible that this underground god may be identified with Rapithwin, rather than with Yima or any other deity whose chthonic connections are not immediately grounded in written sources.[1066]

2. *Eastern Iran*

A single clear visual representation of Yima is found on the unique coin of the Kushan king Huvishka, where Yima is labeled IAMÞO. Iamšo is depicted in full profile facing to the right (fig. 164). Of all the divinities shown on Kushan coins, Yima resembles the Kushan king most closely.[1067] He is armored and wears a typical Kushan costume and a high conical tiara with a diadem, the ribbons of which can be seen falling down his back. This headdress is unique to Iamšo and closely resembles that of king Huvishka himself. Iamšo appears to have a short beard and is armed with a spear and a sword, hilt of which is shaped in the typical Kushan form of a bird's head. On his right outstretched hand a bird-of-prey is perched.

1056 No explanation of his epithet is accepted by all specialists. It seems to have had a solar meaning, perhaps referring to the color of the sun. See Skjærvø 2008.
1057 Shaked 1987: 239. See also Kellens 1984 and the recent comprehensive treatment of Yima's figure in Iranian mythology by Skjærvø 2008.
1058 Yt. 19.33.
1059 Mayerhofer 1973: nos. 8.1792–8.1795; Tavernier 2007: 543.
1060 See below.
1061 Hdt., 7.114. Boyce 1975b: 83, 94, 109.
1062 Gnoli 1980: 151, n. 164; Gnoli 1989a: 921.
1063 Schwartz 2005: 149.
1064 See Boyce 1968a; Krasnowolska 1998: 101–103.
1065 Boyce 1968a: 215.
1066 However, see below for the possible Sogdian representation of Yima as the guardian of Hell.
1067 Grenet 1984: 253–254.

The Bactrian form of his name probably derives from OIr **yama-xšāwan* "Yima the King".[1068] Unlike in Zoroastrian tradition, in Kushan religion, Yima was undoubtedly considered a god, as only divinities are shown on the reverse of Kushan coins.[1069] His divine status among the Bactrian population is also evident from numerous Bactrian names with the theophoric component ιαμþο.[1070] The fact that Yima was probably considered divine in other Iranian cults and religions also finds indirect confirmation in the veneration of the god Imrā among the Nuristani people.[1071] The functions and position of Yima in the Kushan pantheon are anything but clear. His attributes associate him with warfare and royal power, and more specifically with divine favor and royal legitimacy, which is represented by a *x^varənah* in the form of a bird (although the moment captured by the artisan seems to be, in fact, that of the departure of the *x^varənah*).[1072]

Although Yima was undoubtedly also known in Sogdiana where some anthroponyms contain his name,[1073] it is impossible to establish whether he was a hero, a mythical ruler as in the Avesta or whether he possessed a divine status as in Kushan Bactria. It is possible that visual representations of Yima also existed in Sogdian art. Grenet has convincingly demonstrated that the figure depicted as a guardian of Hell on a wall-painting from Panjikent XXV/12 served as a prototype for a specific iconographic type of the warlike Buddhist deity Vaiśravaṇa.[1074] According to the French scholar, his Iranian counterpart would be Yima.[1075] This proposal, although well-argued, should remain hypothetical at present, until more data on the Sogdian pantheon and religious iconography are accumulated, which will hopefully provide conclusive proof for this identification.

3. *Conclusions*

To date only one certain representation of Yima in pre-Islamic Iranian art has been identified—the Kushan Iamšo. Deified by the Kushans, his representation was probably modeled on that of a Kushan prince. Iamšo's iconography is one of the most striking examples of correspondence between a divine image and the Avestan texts. It demonstrates beyond any doubts that despite being deified, some of the Kushan mythological stories connected with the figure of Yima were similar to those recorded in the Avesta.

30. *Unidentified Deities*

This study has confirmed the identification (with varying degrees of probability) of the visual representations of twenty-one gods and goddesses known from the Avesta. However, the iconography of many other deities mentioned in Zoroastrian texts, if indeed it ever existed, remains unknown. Two indicative examples are that of Spəntā Ārmaiti and Haoma who were certainly understood as possessing a human form, but whose images have not yet been found in the artistic record and were perhaps never produced.

1068 Grenet 1984: 254–255; Grenet 2012a: 85. *Þo* is probably a form of *Þao*, "king, ruler". See Sims-Williams 1997/1998: 196–197. However, see Humbach 2002: 69, n. 3, who thinks that *Iamšo* is a short form of **Iamšēdo*.

1069 Grenet 1993: 153. However see Gnoli 1989a, who argues that Yima was not a god in the Kushan pantheon.

1070 Sims-Williams 2010: nos. 167–172

1071 See Fussman 2012.

1072 See the interesting suggestion by Grenet 2012a: 87–88, who connects it with royal falconry.

1073 Lurje 2010: no. 1488 and probably also no. 1489.

1074 Grenet 1995/1996a. For the Panjikent XXV/12 wall painting, see p. 123–124.

1075 Grenet 1995/1996a: 283.

Spəntā Ārmaiti, one of the Aməša Spənta and guardian of the earth[1076] is described several times in Middle Persian literature as a young girl in shining garments and golden girdle, sitting alongside Ahura Mazdā and embracing him.[1077] She was known in Western Iran as early as the Achaemenian period, since her name was recently identified in an Elamite tablet from Persepolis.[1078] Written sources and onomastics also attest to her existence in Armenia[1079] and probably also in Bactria[1080] and Sogdiana.[1081] The language of the Khotanese Saka preserves the word *śśandrāmata*, indicating that the cult of Spəntā Ārmaiti as the "bounteous, devoted Earth" may in fact go back to the Indo-Iranian pantheon.[1082] Scholars have tended to identify Spəntā Ārmaiti with Nana, Anāhitā and other female deities venerated in the Iranian world and to recognize her in various female images.[1083] However no concrete evidence has ever been supplied and the goddess must be considered as yet unrepresented in the Iranian world.

Haoma—the personification of the ritual *haoma* plant—is also clearly anthropomorphic in the Avesta and is said to have the form of a most handsome man.[1084] Anthropomorphic perceptions of Haoma are also reflected in the story of Afrāsiāb's hiding in the cave in the *Shāh-nāma*. Haoma is attested in six Achaemenian proper names.[1085] Despite his apparent anthropomorphism no pictorial representations of him have been recognized in Iranian iconography. I have suggested that the Sogdian "bird-priest" might be an image of Haoma, but the evidence for this is indirect and speculative.[1086]

The sum of deities venerated by Iranian people was undoubtedly much higher than that included in the Avestan pantheon. We have discussed visual representations of at least five deities not attested in the Avesta. Examination of Iranian personal names reveals the existence of additional otherwise unknown deities, seemingly outside of Zoroastrian tradition. Sogdian anthroponymics, for instance, attest to the existence of divine beings called *Rēw*,[1087] *Rām*,[1088] *Āpox*,[1089] *xšwm*,[1090] *Wanēpat* (a name probably meaning "Lord of the forests"),[1091] *Avyāmanand*,[1092] and others. It is entirely possible that one or more of these divine names may be matched with some of the Sogdian representations discussed below, but unfortunately we are not yet in a position to establish such a connection.

1. *Nimbate Gods on the Persepolis Tablets*

Several seal impressions from Persepolis depict divinities surrounded by a rayed nimbus. The first of these seals belonged, according to the description, to Irtashduna, the wife of Darius I. The impression shows a hero battling two winged monsters and a floral element (fig. 165).[1093] Floating above the latter, a figure in the triple ring may be seen, surrounded by rays which end in stars. The figure seems to be

1076 See Boyce 1987b.
1077 See p. 32 and p. 34–35.
1078 Razmjou 2001.
1079 On the Armenian Sandarmet, see Russell 1987: 323–361.
1080 In two personal names. See Sims-Williams 2010: nos. 30, 450.
1081 In one personal name. See Lurje 2010: no. 128 and probably in the name of the village *Aspandizā* in the district of Samarkand. According to Smirnova 1971: 95–96, its original name was **'sp'ntrmtδyz'*, "the citadel (of) Aspan[darmat]".
1082 Bailey 1967; Boyce 1975b: 207.
1083 For references to studies where Spəntā Ārmaiti was associated with Nana and Anāhitā, see Tanabe 1995a: 210.
1084 See p. 15. On Haoma see Boyce 2003.
1085 Tavernier 2007: 541.
1086 See p. 148.
1087 Lurje 2010: no. 281.
1088 Lurje 2010: nos. 998–1004.
1089 Lurje 2010: no. 24.
1090 Lurje 2010: nos. 212, 1356.
1091 Sims-Williams 1991: 177.
1092 Sims-Williams 1991: 177.
1093 Garrison pre-publication: 40.

beardless and wears a conical headdress with a knot on top. Garrison thinks that it is probably female, but it is difficult to be certain based on the drawing of the seal. The second seal depicts a bearded deity with a raised hand, whose upper body is surrounded by a notched nimbus (fig. 166).[1094] He wears a long robe and a tiara and is flanked by winged genies holding a bucket and raising their hands in gestures of adoration. The third seal shows a partly preserved figure of undistinguishable sex encircled by a rayed nimbus, raising his hand in a gesture of benefaction towards a facing worshipper.[1095] An altar or a spade-like symbol of the Babylonian god Nabu is placed between them.

It is plausible that these are pictorial representations of the various gods of the "Persepolitan pantheon" mentioned in the Persepolis tablets.[1096] These deities of Iranian and Elamite origin might have indeed been understood as "Persian" gods by the population of Pars, as shown by Wouter Henkelman.[1097] However as far as the iconography is concerned, it is typically Mesopotamian and does not demonstrate any specific Iranian traits. Although these deities were probably part of Persian religious life in Persepolis and its environs area, it is impossible to establish whether any of these gods were in fact of Iranian origin.

2. *A God Mounted on a Dragon*

This seal impression was excavated at the site of Erkurgan, ancient Nakhshab, near modern Karshi in Uzbekistan (fig. 167).[1098] It portrays a rider mounted on a fantastic dragon-like beast with two huge claws instead of hooves. The dragon-rider holds a whip in his extended right hand and faces a standing figure wearing a long dress, perhaps a female, that holds a bowl in one hand and grasps the reins of a dragon with the other. The rider either has long hair or part of a headdress falling down his back. A seven-pointed star and a crescent are depicted to his left. The sealing was found in layers dated to the third century CE.[1099]

The excavator, Rustam Suleymanov, has identified the rider on this seal as the ruler of Nakhshab and the woman as a goddess. According to Suleymanov, the scene represents a ritual of sacred marriage.[1100] Suleymanov draws appropriate parallels with the Scythian goddess, who is frequently depicted holding a vessel and in the presence of an equestrian.[1101] However, the seal impression from Erkurgan exhibits considerable differences both in general conception and in its detail. The Erkurgan rider is mounted on a fantastic, dragon-like creature, and not on a horse. This mount alone appears sufficient to identify him not as a mortal, but as a divine personage. The composition itself also unequivocally subordinates the female figure to that of the dragon-rider.[1102] It is instructive that in Scythian art, the goddess occupies the center and is usually enthroned (she is never shown standing), while the woman from Erkurgan is depicted standing to one side. She does not simply hold the vessel, as on the Scythian examples, but clearly offers it to the rider. Therefore, it is safe to assume that this seal impression depicts a scene of adoration of an unknown local deity, riding a dragon. The similarity of the rider's hairstyle with that of the ruler of Nakhshab as depicted on coins does not prevent this interpretation, as the image of the divine was usually modeled on that of the king.

1094 Garrison pre-publication: 40.
1095 Garrison pre-publication: 40.
1096 See the comprehensive study by Henkelman 2008.
1097 Henkelman 2008.
1098 Abdullaev, Rtveladze and Shishkina 1991: no. 289; Suleymanov 2000: 285–288.
1099 Suleymanov 2000: 285.
1100 Suleymanov 2000: 285–286.
1101 See p. 86.
1102 Abdullaev 1996: 58, interprets the figure with a bowl as a "priest".

3. *A Four-Armed Goddess on a Dragon*

The four-armed goddess seated on the back of a fantastic dragon-like beast is one of the most colorful and impressive divine images from Panjikent, but it has also proved to be one of the most difficult to identify. It was discovered in room 5–6 of the Temple II complex (pl. 32).[1103]

The goddess is portrayed frontally with her left leg tucked beneath. Her head is missing, but traces of a nimbus and ribbons, which were probably part of the diadem worn over the crown, are evident. Tongues of fire rise from her shoulders. The goddess is dressed in garments richly decorated with jewelry and gold. She holds a flagstaff in one hand and the other grasps the flap of her dress. Two additional hands are not preserved. She was probably covered with a baldachin. Facing the goddess on both sides are six partly preserved figures of adorants, three on each side.[1104]

Her only preserved attribute—a flagstaff—is not indicative, but the dragon on which the goddess is mounted appears to be a unique feature. It was equated with *makara*—a sea-monster—that serves as the *vāhana* of several Indian deities, most notably of Ganga—a personification of the river Ganges—and therefore the Panjikent goddess has been suggested to represent a similar personification of the local river Zeravshan.[1105] Furthermore, additional subjects of paintings from Temple II attest to the importance of the theme of water in this particular sanctuary.[1106] However, like the other Indian elements, *makara* could have been reinterpreted by the Sogdians and assigned to a deity not necessarily related to water. Another appealing suggestion was provided by Carter, who connected the goddess with the Scytho-Saka river goddess from the Scythian genealogical legend that was allegedly popular in Gandhāra and also found its way into the Sogdian pantheon.[1107] Might she indeed be a reflection of the Scythian Anguipede goddess? Until new evidence comes to light, these two proposals must remain hypothetical.

4. *The "Grain God"*

The image of this deity is found in the middle register of the northern wall in room 28 in Panjikent XXV which depicts a scene of grain crop distribution.[1108] On the left, an enthroned figure of an elderly bearded man is painted larger than the others (fig. 168). He is dressed in a *kaftan* and wears a white pointed cap decorated with a wreath of leaves. The figure has long hair and his head is surrounded with a nimbus. Tongues of fire rise above his shoulders and two ribbons flutter over them. His attributes, including the nimbus, flames, royal ribbons and his superior size, suggest that he is a deity. He is clearly associated with agriculture and fecundity. Based on the ethnographic material, the excavators proposed to identify this god as a "Grandfather Tiller", a character from contemporary Tajik folklore who acts as a patron of agriculture.[1109] It is plausible that this god depicts a Sogdian divinity of agriculture, whose later reminiscences are found in the Tajik "Grandfather Tiller".

5. *Ossuaries from Biyanajman and Miankal*

The interpretation of the figures decorating these two groups of closely related ossuaries poses one of the most complex problems in Sogdian iconography. The ossuries were discovered in 1908 at Biyanajman near Kattakurgan,[1110] and during the 1970s and early 1980s in the region of Miankal located between

1103 Belenitskiy 1973: 13–14.
1104 Belenitskiy 1973: 13, Fig. 2.
1105 Belenitskiy 1973: 45; Shkoda 2009: 75, Fig. 115.
1106 Shkoda 2009: 105–106.
1107 Carter 1992: 75.
1108 Marshak and Raspopova 1990: 153–154.
1109 Marshak and Raspopova 1990: 155.
1110 Published in Kastal'skiy 1909; Kalmykov 1909 and studied by Borisov 1940 and Staviskiy 1961.

Samarkand and Kattakurgan in modern Uzbekistan.[1111] Most of them carry very similar stamped decorations and are executed in a roughly similar style, which has determined their study as a unified complex probably characteristic to the region.[1112] The ossuaries are usually dated based on their style and iconography to the sixth-seventh centuries CE.[1113] Marshak has also pointed out that the ceramics associated with the ossuaries excavated at Ishtikhan (Miankal) are not earlier than the second half of the seventh century CE.[1114] Therefore, the date for the whole complex of these ossuaries can probably be corrected to the seventh and perhaps even the beginning of the eighth century CE.

The most common type of design on these ossuaries shows a group of crowned male and female figures holding various attributes and standing or sitting under arches forming an arcade. On the ossuary from Ishtikhan the heads of the figures are surrounded by toothed nimbi. With one exception (no. 7), all of them are of the same size and without any visible iconographic hierarchy. Although all these figures clearly form one typological group and some of their attributes, the shape of crowns, and their facial features are very similar, very few of them are in fact identical. Therefore, their division into different characters depends mostly on the approach taken by the scholar in question. According to the "maximalist stance" assumed by Pugachenkova, who identified no less than thirteen figures, different crowns or attributes represent different figures.[1115] Grenet adopted a "minimalist approach" and reduced them to six—three males and three females—interpreting differences as mere "variations" of the same character.[1116]

I propose that in fact eight distinct characters can be identified:

1) A female figure wearing a crown consisting of a palmette-like half-oval element flanked by rosettes. According to some scholars, she holds a mortar and pestle in one hand and an object resembling a forked rod in the other.[1117] Pugachenkova proposed to interpret it as tongs used to provide a flaming material for the fire, while according to Grenet this is a stylized depiction of the *haoma* plant. Marshak states that she holds an "upright sprout" and "something like a reed".[1118] Her headdress consists of three elements probably representing a stylized crenellated crown. She is found on two ossuaries from Ishtikhan (Iš-1, Iš-2) (figs. 169–172), on the ossuary from Durmentepe (Dr) (figs. 173–174) and on three ossuaries from Biyanajman (Bn-1, Bn-2, Bn-4) (figs. 175–178). On all fragments the figure has the same attributes and a crown with only slight stylistic variations.
2) A male figure with a short round beard.[1119] His crown is formed by two large crenellations terminating with three small disks and crescents. In all four variations of this figure (Iš-1, Dr, Iš-2, Bn-1) his hand rests on an object best described as a "small shovel". On Iš-1 and Bn-1 his other hand (right and left respectively) is raised in a two fingered benedictory gesture. In Dr and Iš-2 his left hand supports a small plate with two different objects; one resembling an animal (Dr) and probably a crown (Iš-2).[1120] According to Grenet, this animal is most probably a swine, a boar,[1121] or a hedgehog.[1122] On Iš-1 and Iš-2 there is also a kind of coat slipped over his shoulders and on Bn-1 the elbow of his right

1111 Pugatchenkova 1985.
1112 See Yakubov 1987; Grenet 1987a; Marshak 1995/1996.
1113 Grenet 1986: 99.
1114 Marshak 1995/1996: n. 1.
1115 Pugatchenkova 1985 and Pugachenkova 1987.
1116 Grenet 1986: 110.
1117 Grenet 1986: 113; Grenet 1987a: 45.
1118 Marshak 1995/1996: 302.
1119 Grenet 1987a: 45–46.
1120 A winged crown with solar symbols, according to Abdullaev and Berdimuradov 1991: 74.
1121 Grenet 1986: 113.
1122 Personal communication.

hand rests on an additional attribute—a sword ending with a serpent's head. On Iš-2, the figure is nimbate as are all other figures on this specific ossuary.

3) A beardless male figure is attested five times on Iš-1, Dr, Bn-2, Bn-4, Bn-5 (fig. 179). On Dr he has a moustache. On all variants the character wears a winged crown incorporating an element resembling a lyre and his attributes are a fire-altar and a shovel, lifted up or placed on the ground.[1123]
4) A female figure wearing a turreted crown and holding a cornucopia is found on five fragments, Iš-1, Iš-2, Dr, Bn-2, Bn-5.[1124] The cornucopia on Iš-2 is often erroneously identified as a plant with sprouts. Her representation on Iš-1 is exceptional for an additional attribute, most probably a diadem, that she holds in her right hand.
5) A female figure is depicted twice on Iš-1 and Bn-1.[1125] On Bn-1 her attributes are a large key and a casket with a triangular cover resembling a certain group of Sogdian ossuaries. On Iš-1 only the left hand of the figure with a key is preserved.
6) A male figure with a long beard is found on Iš-70 (fig. 180) and Bn-1. They wear different crowns, but have similar attributes. In one hand, they hold a plate with several objects that are difficult to identify, and the other hand leans on a sword (on Bn-1 the hilt ends with a serpent's head). The objects on the plate perhaps represent a crown (Iš-1) and mountains, clouds or wind (Bn-1).
7) A bearded male figure wearing a winged crown with an astral symbol in the center is found only on Bn-2. He sits on a carpet with his left leg tucked beneath. In his right hand, he holds a short axe and his left hand rests on the straight hilt of a sword. There is a semi-oval object attached to his left shoulder. Pugachenkova has proposed that this could be a quiver with arrows,[1126] however, these are probably tongues of fire rising from the man's shoulders. The fact that the flame on the altar which holds a figure to the right (no. 3) is rendered in a completely different manner may simply suggest that the artisan who copied this composition from another source did not understand this detail. According to Grenet, this figure is a variation of no. 6. However, his pose is entirely different, as he is the only figure depicted seated and the only one to have flames rising from his shoulders. He has also a unique attribute, an axe. It therefore seems that he should be regarded as a distinct character.
8) A male figure whose head and left hand are missing appears once on Iš-1. Because his right hand rests on the hilt of a sword, he could have been taken as a variant of no. 6, but he has a distinctive attribute—scale armor—and may therefore represent a different personage.

The composition of figures of deities standing under arches is attested as early as the first-second centuries CE on Buddhist reliquaries, long before its appearance in Sogdiana.[1127] Figures placed under arches supported by pillars are characteristic of the early phase of Gandhāran art in the Peshawar region and Taxila.[1128] Specialists of Gandhāran art consider this motif to be a Western, Parthian influence.[1129] Deities standing under arcades are also found on Byzantine caskets and it was proposed that the Sogdians borrowed this "archade composition" from Byzantine art, changing the attributes of the characters to fit their own gods.[1130] The composition in which arcades of equal dimensions are based on the columns is found only on ossuaries. Such arcades are not known from Sogdian architecture.

1123 Grenet 1986: 113–114; Grenet 1987a: 46.
1124 Grenet 1986: 114; Grenet 1987a: 46–47.
1125 Grenet 1986: 114; Grenet 1987a: 47.
1126 Pugachenkova 1996: 43.
1127 Walter 2009: 187–189.
1128 Brancaccio 2006: 220.
1129 Brancaccio 2006: 220.
1130 Mkrtychev and Naimark 1991: 65.

Therefore, the origin of this composition is not Sogdian.[1131] Arcade depictions were widespread in late Roman and early Byzantine art and it seems certain that it was adopted from the decoration on Western sarcophagi. However, the immediate origin of this composition on Sogdian ossuaries is to be sought in the Buddhist art of Gandhāra.[1132]

Interpretation of the characters on these ossuaries is undoubtedly complicated by the fact that their iconography differs considerably from the majority of known Sogdian divine representations on wall-paintings and was perhaps even created especially for them.[1133] An instructive case is that of the ossuary from Khirmantepa where the goddess Nana is depicted without her animal, a lion that almost always accompanies her on wall-paintings.[1134] This indicates that we should also expect unusual variations in the iconography of other gods on ossuaries. It is also possible that the Biyanajman and Miankal ossuaries reproduce a specifically local iconography. They might constitute a phenomenon limited to a clearly defined region, as no ossuaries of the same group have been discovered in other regions of Sogdiana. Furthermore, the murals of this region (Kashka-darya basin, Shahr-i Sabz and Erkurgan) are unfortunately almost unknown.

As one of the first known examples of Sogdian artistic expression, these ossuaries have been discussed numerous times by various scholars. Borisov has suggested that the figures on the Biyanajman and Miankal ossuaries are personifications of Water, Earth, Fire and Air.[1135] This is also accepted in principle by Marshak.[1136] The most reasoned and coherent theory explaining the figures on the Biyanajman and Miankal ossuaries was put forward by Grenet, who argued that this group represent the six Aməša Spənta participating in the *frašegird*—the final renovation and transfiguration before the resurrection.[1137] His hypothesis, however, was never fully accepted by the other notable specialists of Sogdian art—Pugachenkova, Marshak and Abdullaev.[1138]

The decorations on these ossuaries are almost unanimously connected by scholars with notions of the afterlife. However, similar compositions of divine figures under arches or in medallions are also found on other Sogdian objects that clearly have no funeral connotations, such as the wooden friezes from Panjikent and from Kujruk-tobe and on the fragment of an incense burner from Jartepa II (although, as already mentioned, arches supported by columns are attested only on ossuaries).[1139] Even if we adhere to the idea that the figures on the Biyanajman and Miankal ossuaries are linked with the afterlife, *frašegird* does not have to be the only interpretation. Sogdian ideas on the afterlife undoubtedly departed from Zoroastrian ones and the best illustration for this fact is the presence of the goddess Nana, who clearly has no place in Zoroastrian eschatology, on at least one Sogdian ossuary.

It seems that the unusual iconography of the Biyanajman and Miankal ossuaries favors Grenet's suggestion, since pictorial representations of the Aməša Spənta have not yet been identified in Sogdian monumental art. However, I believe that there are more than six characters, and if some of them are indeed Aməša Spənta, they are certainly not depicted alone. Furthermore, in my opinion, even the group of four personifications of Water, Earth, Fire and Air, identified by Borisov, is not so readily recognized. No. 3 could indeed be Fire, although it should be noted that a portable fire-altar is the attribute of a number of Kushan and Sogdian deities. Female character no. 1 may be the personification of plants, but she may equally well be a pictorial representation of Haoma. Figure no. 2 may indeed be Vohu Manah,

1131 Naymark 1988: 282.
1132 Naymark 1988: 284.
1133 Marshak 1995/1996: 300.
1134 See p. 125.
1135 Borisov 1940.
1136 Marshak 1995/1996: 301.
1137 Grenet 1986; Grenet 1987a.
1138 Abdullaev and Berdimuradov 1991: 74; Marshak 1995/1996; Pugachenkova 1996.
1139 See p. 110, pp. 125–126 and p. 101.

as suggested by Grenet, since he is close to the figure from the Sivaz ossuary,[1140] although this argument is of course, circular. No. 4 holds a cornucopia and may be identified with the Sogdian Aši assuming this distinctive attribute of the Kushan Ardoxšo was continued in Sogdiana. The casket that figure no. 5 holds is not necessarily a miniature ossuary. In fact, it could be a chest to be opened by the key that she holds in her left hand.[1141] This character is identified by Grenet as Spandarmad.[1142] If the attribute that figure no. 6 holds on a plate is indeed a stylized wind, he could be Vāta.

Character no. 7 is distinguished from the others, since he is not standing, but is seated on a carpet. Lazar' Rempel proposed to combine him with another ossuary fragment depicting a piece of a carpet and one side of a throne supported by the foreparts of a horse.[1143] The folds of the garments indeed seem to fit each other on the two fragments, but the two parts of the sword clearly do not combine in a straight line and therefore these two fragments probably do not belong together.[1144] However, there is no doubt that this god is seated on a zoomorphic throne. As to his identity, Grenet identified him as Šahrewar,[1145] Marshak as Saošyant,[1146] and Pugachenkova has proposed Yima.[1147] Without knowing what animals supported his throne it is difficult to make any secure suggestions, but the axe is found together with royal images in Sogdian and Bactrian art. Finally, figure no. 8 is armored and therefore is most probably a warlike deity, but the poor preservation of the garment does not allow any further enquiry.

In conclusion, there seem to be at least eight different characters represented on these ossuaries and indeed future finds may reveal additional characters. I believe that these figures represent images of gods from the Sogdian pantheon (of whom Aməša Spənta were obviously a part) that the deceased would meet in Paradise. It is possible that they reproduce actual statues that stood in Sogdian temples. Unfortunately, present attempts to individually identify them must remain, for the most part, hypothetical.

6. *The Ossuary from Xantepa*

This ossuary was discovered during earthworks near the city of Shahr-i Sabz, in the Kashka-darya region of Uzbekistan.[1148] It is dated between the sixth-eight centuries CE. The scene stamped on the long side of the ossuary depicts a male figure with a moustache seated on a carpeted throne with lions protomes (fig. 181). His body is shown frontally and his head in profile turned to the left. He sits in a typical Sogdian pose with one leg tucked up beneath. The upper part of his head is badly stamped and there is no means of knowing which type of headdress he originally wore. His open right palm, turned upwards, supports a fire-altar and in his left hand he holds a long rod with a horizontal crossbar, terminating in a spherical object. This figure is flanked by two musicians.

The lion, a principal attribute of Nana, is not attested with any other deity in Sogdian art. A fire-altar is found with character no. 3 on the Biyanajman and Miankal ossuaries who is, however, beardless, while the god on this ossuary has a moustache. Grenet deliberated between Aša Vahišta, Ātar and the personification of the *x*ᵛ*arənah*.[1149] However, in the absence of other parallels and additional evidence, no convincing identification for the Xantepa god can be proposed.

1140 See p. 84–85.
1141 However the proposal that this is the representation of a key used to open a *naos* is possible. See Grenet 1986: 127.
1142 Grenet 1986: 126–128.
1143 Pugachenkova 1996: Fig. 2.
1144 This observation was made by Grenet (personal communication).
1145 Grenet 1986: 123–124.
1146 Marshak 1995/1996: Fig. 10.
1147 Pugachenkova 1996: 50.
1148 Grenet et al. 1993: 55–59.
1149 Grenet et al. 1993: 62–65.

CHAPTER 4

INTANGIBLE SPIRITS: IRANIAN ANICONISM[1]

In studies dedicated to cultic iconography and aniconism in the Ancient Near East, the Iranian world is noticeable by its absence. Research has tended to focus exclusively on Mesopotamian, Israelite, Syrian, Anatolian, Aegean, Greek, Roman and Egyptian examples, while Iranian material remains outside of the general discussion. This situation has come about because the subject of aniconism has never been treated systematically by Iranists themselves.

In his influential book, *No Graven Image? Israelite Aniconism in its Ancient Near Eastern Context*, T.D.N. Mettinger defines aniconism as "cults where there is no iconic representation of the deity (anthropomorphic or theriomorphic) serving as the dominant or central cultic symbol ...".[2] Furthermore, he makes an important distinction between what he calls "material aniconism" and "empty-space aniconism"—aniconic symbolism or sacred emptiness, respectively—both of which replace a figural representation of the deity.[3] In a recent article, Mettinger has also observed that the distinction between iconic and aniconic refers only to material symbols, while "the *mental* notions of deity nurtured by the worshipers may well be anthropomorphic, even if the cult object is aniconic".[4] Examples of both "material aniconism" and "empty-space aniconism", as defined by Mettinger, are undoubtedly found in the Iranian world together with examples that fall into the categories of "semi-aniconism" and "elemental aniconism".

From the very beginning, the religious art of the Iranian people, in particular those of western Iran, has demonstrated significant aniconic trends, especially when compared with the evidence from some contemporary Near Eastern cultures. It is generally claimed that the roots of Iranian aniconism are evident in the earliest written sources describing Indo-Iranian cultic practices and religious rites.[5] Indeed, the Avesta and the Rig Veda, the sacred scriptures of Zoroastrianism and Hinduism and our earliest literary sources on Indo-Iranian religion, make no mention of either idols or cultic statues; furthermore, they provide no detailed anthropomorphic descriptions of the deities of the Indo-Iranian pantheon. The aniconism of the Persians is also a well-known *topos* in Greek and Latin sources, which make up the major part of the available literary evidence.

1. *"Material Aniconism"*

The most famous manifestation of "material aniconism" among the Iranians is the worship of a warrior-god in the form of a sword thrust into the ground, as reported by Herodotus.[6] Adoration of a sword among the Alans, who were the successors of the Scythians and the Sarmatians in the Pontic steppes, is described by Ammianus Marcellinus.[7]

---

1 Parts of this text have already appeared in Shenkar 2008/2012.

2 Mettinger 1995: 19.

3 Mettinger 1995: 19.

4 Mettinger 2006: 275.

5 In Louis Gray's words describing Avestan religion: "This Iranism was so primitive that like Vedism it had not even developed beyond the aniconic stage in the representation of its divinities": Gray 1913/1914: 38.

6 See p. 16.

7 See p. 16

An *akinakes* dated to the fifth century BCE, found thrust into the artificial fill between two kurgans at Nosaki in modern day Ukraine, has been interpreted as the sanctuary and idol of Ares as described by Herodotus.[8] Finds of weapons (spears, axes, daggers and swords) thrust into the ground are also attested in a number of Scythian burial sites.[9] The unique stele excavated at the Scythian settlement of Ust' Al'minsk in Crimea might be further evidence for this cult in the material culture.[10] The stele, dated to the second century CE, is approximately three m. high and bears an image of a sword (fig. 182).[11] It is possible that this is the same non-figural representation of the Scythian god of war that is mentioned in the writings of classical authors.[12]

In the context of "material aniconism", we might also mention the sole piece of evidence for the worship of standing stones or *maṣṣebot* in Elymais—a region closely related to Iran throughout history. A relief carved on stone at Tang-i Sarvak and probably dated to the beginning of the third century CE, shows a local king worshiping before a standing stone decorated with ribbons (fig. 183).[13] This practice, apparently alien to the Iranian world, was probably introduced to Elymais by Semitic peoples to the west. However, it never gained wide popularity and acceptance among Iranians and is not attested on the Iranian plateau.[14]

2. *Zoomorphic Symbols*

Many Avestan deities have animal incarnations. For that reason, it has become commonplace for scholars to consider various animals appearing in Iranian art as allusions to deities or as their zoomorphic representation.[15] However, none of these animals, which are especially abundant in Sasanian art, are ever identified by an inscription, and none ever appear in clear cultic contexts. As De Jong has rightly put it, when these animals can be explained as Avestan zoomorphic manifestations, they are readily interpreted as such, but when there is no appropriate Avestan explanation, they remain "just animals" and require no further interpretation.[16] Thus, a bird of prey is usually seen as a *vārayna* bird, a wild boar is conventionally Vərəθrayna (although Sasanian kings are often portrayed killing them in depictions of the royal hunt on silver plates), and a horse is Mithra, Tištrya or even Vərəθrayna, depending on the context and the predilection of the interpreter.[17]

---

8 Boltrik 1978; Ol'khovskiy 1991: 133. On the "altars of Ares", see also Bessonova 1984: 5–7.

9 Ol'khovskiy 1991: 110.

10 Vysotskaya 1984.

11 Vysotskaya 1984: 135.

12 Nevertheless, the worship of a sword can hardly be considered specifically Iranian, and it is not attested in any Iranian source. It could potentially be a holdover from an ancient heritage going back to Indo-European unity or borrowed from autochthonous pre-Indo-European people. The revering of a sword as an icon of the divine was practiced by Indo-European Thracians, Illyrians and some Germanic tribes as well as non-Indo-European people such as Turks and Huns: Maenchen-Helfen 1973: 278–280; Bessonova 1983: 49. The origin of this cult is difficult to determine. However, it is worth noting that already in early Sumer, divine weapons belonging to the gods were not merely a symbolic representation of the anthropomorphic deity, but were considered independent deities in their own right.

13 Vanden Berghe and Schippmann 1985: 76–79.

14 On the cult of *maṣṣebot* and Western Semitic aniconism, see Patrich 1990; Mettinger 1995; Mettinger 2006: 284–289; Gaifman 2008. Further comparison with Western Semitic material might prove rewarding and illuminating. However, it will require a separate study.

15 This is characteristic, for instance, of works of the prominent Soviet scholar Vladimir Lukonin: Lukonin 1977: 159–160; Lukonin 1987: 102; Trever and Lukonin 1987: 56, 91; Loukonine and Ivanov 2003: 26. For an example of a recent study that connects animals with Zoroastrian deities, see Compareti 2009/2010.

16 De Jong 2009: 37.

17 It is worth noting that Boyce 1975b: 63, n. 276 already pointed out that "it is hardly justifiable to regard every poetic simile or heraldic badge with the boar as referring to this god [Vərəθrayna]". Tištrya also shares with Vərəθrayna his other two visual manifestations—a bull and a young man.

However, the Sasanian bestiary is much broader, and includes lions, bears, elephants, zebus, roosters, scorpions, deer and many more. Not only are some of these animals not explained as Zoroastrian symbols; they are, in fact, *xrafstra*—a special category of creatures, the creations of the Evil Spirit. It is plausible that, in some cases, these beasts and birds could indeed be symbolic representations of Iranian gods. Moreover, this practice could be seen as going back to ancient Mesopotamia. Of the forty divine symbols that replaced the anthropomorphic images of deities in Mesopotamia listed by Green, fifteen represent real and fantastic beasts and an additional four are staves ending with animal heads.[18] However, the interpretation of animals in Iranian art as symbolic representations of deities appears justified in only a few cases and should be limited to a specific cultural sphere. For instance, a ram decorated with ribbons could indeed represent *x^{v}arənah* in Sasanian art, based on the evidence from *Kār-nāmag ī Ardašīr ī Pābagān*.[19] Another case is that of the earliest image of the goddess Nana in the Eastern Iranian world. On the coins issued by the Indo-Scythian rulers Sapadbizes and Agesiles (end of the first century BCE), she is represented only by her animal, a lion, which is identified by the inscription NANAIA.

It is worth noting that the first images of the god Oešo on the early issues of the Kushan king Vima Kadphises are aniconic and represent the god by his most recognizable symbols, a trident combined with an axe and a bull.[20] This anthropomorphic image was created during Vima Kadphises's reign, most likely by incorporating features taken from the iconography of Poseidon, Zeus and Heracles. It is possible that a bull already depicted on a group of coins of Kujula Kadphises represents Oešo.[21]

In most cases, the animal symbols may possibly be connected with totemism. The Parthians, a dynasty of originally nomadic origin, introduced many elements of Eurasian steppe culture—such as costume, and social and military organization—to the Iranian plateau, and the Sasanians inherited many of these features from their Parthian predecessors.[22] In Sasanian visual art we find certain elements from the nomadic Eurasian world, such as *tamga* signs, adopted as emblems of clans and ranks and equestrian investiture. The conquest of the lands of the former Kushan Empire and constant interaction with successive nomadic confederations of Chionites, Kidarites, and Hephtalites undoubtedly also contributed to the absorption of cultural elements characteristic of the Eurasian nomads in Sasanian Iran.[23]

The Sasanian bestiary could therefore also have been influenced by steppe culture and art and might even have been distantly related to the famous Scythian "animal style". The interpretation of this phenomenon in Scythian art is highly problematic and controversial. Scholarly opinions range from totemic, magical notions connected with the hunt to representations of the Scythian gods (the latter is itself obviously based on the Avesta).[24] Raevskiy regarded them as symbols of Scythian divinities rather than their representations.[25] Either the totemic or the symbolic interpretations seem most preferable, since Herodotus, in his Scythian *logos*, did not mention any connection between animals and the gods of the Scythians, as he did, for example, in Egypt.[26]

---

18 Green 1995: Fig. 1 and Tab. 1.
19 *KAP* 4.11.16, 22–23.
20 Cribb 1997: I.A1.
21 Cribb 1997: 26.
22 For an important evaluation of Parthian steppe background and heritage, see Olbrycht 2003.
23 On this period, see Grenet 2002a.
24 Even a cursory outline of the literature dedicated to this subject is impossible. See the useful survey in Raevskiy 1977: 4–7 and Perevodchikova 1994.
25 Raevskiy 1978: 69–70.
26 Raevskiy 1978: 68; Schiltz 1994: 51.

In this context, it is worth mentioning that the *Shāh-nāma* describes the banners of heroes as decorated with different beasts: elephants, lions, wolves, wild boars.[27] It is likely that these are reflections of Eurasian nomad totemism rather than references to Iranian deities.

3. *Sasanian Royal Crowns*

The crowns of the Sasanian kings are yet another category of object frequently taken to allude to Zoroastrian deities.[28] Beginning with Ardašīr I, and perhaps already with his direct predecessors, every Sasanian king employed a distinctive, specially designed, elaborate crown or a number of crowns, which often serve as a sort of "identifier". However, from the fifth-sixth century CE the royal crowns become stereotyped and lose their individuality.[29]

Associations of various elements on Sasanian royal crowns with Zoroastrian gods and concepts are found in various studies and are usually taken as obvious and self-evident. For instance, the wings decorating the crowns of several Sasanian kings are usually interpreted as a symbol of Vərəθraγna.[30] However, no known written source makes an explicit connection between the crown and the divine. It is only in rare cases like that of the rayed crown of Wahrām I that we can state with some confidence that it indeed refers to Mithra since we have unquestionable iconographic and epigraphic evidence that this type of crown was specific to Mithra.[31] In other cases, like association of plants and the arcade of Narseh with Anāhitā, these are necessarily speculations as all the evidence we possess is indirect. It is often claimed that the animal heads incorporated in some royal crowns allude to specific gods[32] and that these represent the symbols of the eponymous deity of the king. The example that is usually given is that of Wahrām II whose crown is decorated with wings, an expression of the king's personal devotion to Vərəθraγna, a deity whose name Wahrām II carried.[33]

In my opinion, this approach is too simplistic. Little attention is paid to the fact that no less than six Sasanian kings were named Wahrām and only two of them, Wahrām II and Wahrām IV, wore a winged crown while others chose different types. Moreover, the only king who has the entire bird-of-prey incorporated into his crown is Ōhrmazd II, whose name has nothing to do with Vərəθraγna. This suggests that the individual designs of Sasanian crowns were determined according to other guiding principles and considerations.

The headdress topped by an image of a bird or an animal and incorporating various faunal elements is common among Scythians and other Iranian Eurasian nomads. The felt headdresses of the Pazyrik culture (sixth-third centuries BCE) capped by a bird and decorated with animals might be an early prototype of Sasanian animal headdresses.[34] They are obviously connected to the "animal style" phenomenon mentioned above. It is my contention that zoomorphic elements in Sasanian crowns were inspired by the headdresses of eastern Iranian nomads. The channel of transmission was probably via Bactria, where the Sasanians were involved in intense interaction and cultural exchange with Kushans,

---

27 Pugachenkova 1999: 207–208.

28 For example, see Lukonin 1969: 96, 155; Göbl 1971; Göbl 1983: 325; Choksy 1988: 42–43; Choksy 1989; Peck 1993; Tanabe 1993: 60; Curtis 2008: 138. Also accepted in principle by Schindel 2013: 829.

29 Harper 2006: 20. On the identification, typology and evolution of the Sasanian royal crowns, see Herzfeld 1939; Erdmann 1951; Göbl 1971; Peck 1993 and Schindel 2013: 829–830.

30 See, e.g., the most recent excellent survey of the Sasanian coinage, Schindel 2013: 829–830.

31 Gyselen connects it with the cult of Sol Invictus in Rome that flourished in this period. See Gyselen 2010b: 193.

32 E.g. Grenet 1995: 110. For a recent discussion of animal headdresses among ancient Iranians, see also Lerner 2009: 219–224, who interprets them as symbols of Iranian deities.

33 Curtis 2008: 140; Gyselen 2010b: 195.

34 See Polos'mak 2004: 143–163, Figs. 104–105.

Chionite, Kidarite and Hephtalite nomads. It seems that the animal-headed *kulāf* worn by various dignitaries and princes in Sasanian art should also be viewed in this light.[35]

4. *"Empty-Space Aniconism"*

An empty chariot drawn by white horses that seems to have played a prominent role in Achaemenian royal military processions may be the most significant piece of evidence regarding Iranian "empty-space aniconism" preserved in the classical sources.[36] Such aniconic representations of deities, apparently residing invisibly in a sacred empty chariot, have Urartian and Mesopotamian parallels. In Mesopotamia, many gods such as Anu, Bel, Ea, Enlil, Marduk and others, are mentioned in the texts as owning chariots.[37] In Assyria, chariots bearing statues of Aššur and Ištar were drawn by white horses in religious processions. There is also textual evidence for chariots being treated as deities in certain, albeit limited, circumstances.[38] A divine, empty chariot without any cult image is depicted on the Lachish relief and empty chariots and carts as divine objects are also attested in Urartu.[39]

5. *"Elemental Aniconism"*

Perhaps the most celebrated and frequently remarked upon stereotype regarding Iranian cults is that of the worship of fire. As noted above, the veneration of fire probably has its roots in the remote Indo-Iranian past.[40] From the Achaemenian period, if not earlier, fire functioned as a visual manifestation of the divine. Achaemenian kings can be seen worshipping in front of the stepped fire-altar at Naqš-e Rostam and similar altars are indeed attested in the archaeological record—the most famous being the two monumental plinths in the Sacred Precinct at Pasargadae.[41]

After the Achaemenians, fire-altars appear on the coins of the *frataraka* rulers of Pars and their successor, Ardašīr I, the founder of the Sasanian dynasty.[42] On most coin types of Ardašīr I, the altar is depicted in combination with lion legs (fig. 184), which should perhaps be interpreted as a joint image of the fire-altar and divine throne, thus emphasizing the fire-altar as the seat of an invisible, aniconic divinity.[43] In this regard it is also worth mentioning the fire-altar supported by three camels depicted in the center of a ritual scene carved on the tympanum of the entrance door of the Sino-Sogdian tomb of An Jia (579 CE) (fig. 185). It is likely that this unusual camel-base is nothing more than a typical Sogdian zoomorphic divine throne, the standard attribute of Sogdian gods.

In the fourth century CE a bust was added to the fire-altar on the reverse of Sasanian and Kushano-Sasanian coins.[44] It is shown both *en face* and in profile and a similar bust also appears on two Sasanian seals. While the identity of the Sasanian bust on the fire-altar is controversial, the Kushano-Sasanian bust portrays Nana and Oešo.

---

35 See a recent study of this headdress by Gyselen 2005/2009.
36 See Calmeyer 1974; De Jong 2010a: 547–548.
37 Porter 2009: 172.
38 Porter 2009: 173–174.
39 Ornan 2005a: 86. See Seidl 1994: 118, who thinks that it could be a symbol of principal Urartan god, Haldi.
40 Boyce 1989.
41 On fire-altars, see Yamamoto 1979; Yamamoto 1981; Houtkamp 1991 and Garrison 1999, with references to previous literature.
42 Yamamoto 1979: Pl. 53–55.
43 Alram and Gyselen 2003: Type I(1)/2(1)-VIII. For the discussion of this motif, see Harper 1979 and also Schindel 2013: 834–834.
44 See p. 90 ff.

Besides fire, other elements such as water, the sun and moon, earth, wind and sky were considered important manifestations of deities or even divine beings in their own right. The *topos* that Persians took the natural elements to be the only possible incarnation of their various gods is found in many classical accounts and fully accords with the available Iranian sources. This phenomenon adds another aniconic category that could perhaps be labeled "elemental aniconism".

The worship of elements and celestial bodies and even the deification and anthropomorphization of natural entities such as rivers and mountains is also attested in Mesopotamia.[45] It is possible that Iranian aniconism and anthropomorphism owed much to its Mesopotamian heritage. Indeed, Iranian avoidance of deities in human form was probably determined not only by an "aniconic nomadic heritage", but also by the incorporation of cultic practices and ideas originating in first millennium BCE Mesopotamia: the substitution of human-shaped portrayals of deities by non-anthropomorphic symbols. Non-anthropomorphic portrayals are known in Mesopotamian iconography as early as the late fourth millennium BCE, but a strong tendency to avoid anthropomorphic images of deities becomes more evident from the second half of the second millennium, reaching its peak in the first half of the first millennium BCE. It was especially predominant in Babylonia from the seventh to the fifth centuries BCE and in Assyria during the last century of the Neo-Assyrian Empire.[46] In ancient Mesopotamia, deities were commonly perceived to have human form and were represented anthropomorphically.[47] It is, however, important to note that the two principal gods of the Mesopotamian pantheon, Anu and Enlil, were never portrayed in human form.[48] This avoidance of pictorial representation is difficult to explain, but as Tallay Ornan puts it:

> … such an absence may indicate an inherent difficulty for Mesopotamians to giving concrete form through visual images to the conceptual image of a human-shaped god … while deities were conceived of as personified entities, they were not always thus represented.[49]

On the reasons behind the replacement of cultic images with non-figural representation, Ornan concludes that:

> … the reasons for the transformation of the cult image into a non-anthropomorphic icon are highly conjectural, since the ancient records are not explicit about this issue. Thus we can only speculate that it was the awesome sacred status of Mesopotamian deities, or perhaps their sublime splendor, which prevented their visual representations from being viewed by humans.[50]

It is important to note that Iranians maintained close contact with Assyrians and Babylonians for at least five hundred years before the founding of the Achaemenian Empire and their relations with the Elamites have recently been described in terms of "Irano-Elamite acculturation".[51] Moreover, the latest study by Henkelman has convincingly demonstrated that the religion of Pars in the period recorded by the *Persepolis Foundation Archive* was essentially an amalgam of heterogeneous Elamite and Iranian cults.[52]

Among the "semi-aniconic" representations in Sasanian art, aside from the abovementioned bust on the fire-altar, we may also point to symbolic representations of the divine chariots of Mithra, Māh and other unidentified deities on Sasanian seals and sealings.

---

45 Ornan 2009: 97–98; Porter 2009: 156–169.
46 See in-depth studies by Ornan 2005a and Ornan 2009.
47 Ornan 2005a: 41; Ornan 2009: 93.
48 Ornan 2005a: 46; Ornan 2009: 93–94.
49 Ornan 2009: 94.
50 Ornan 2009: 147.
51 Henkelman 2008.
52 Henkelman 2008: 58–59.

CHAPTER 5

GRAVEN IMAGES: IRANIAN ANTHROPOMORPHISM

1. *Cultic Statuary, "Idols" and "Idol-Temples"*

1. *Western Iran*

At the beginning of the twentieth century the American Iranist A.V.W. Jackson confidently stated that "the Persians from the earliest antiquity had no idols in the sense of representations of the godhead set up as objects of worship",[1] and that "throughout the history of the religion of Irān, idolatry played no part".[2] Almost a century later, Boris Marshak, a prominent Central Asian archaeologist, agreed that "ancient Iran had neither cult statuary nor an iconographical tradition of its own".[3]

Indeed, the excavated Median and Achaemenian sanctuaries have not produced any evidence for the employment of cultic statues. However, the Babylonian priest Berossus, writing in Greek in the Hellenistic period, credited Artaxerxes II with the introduction of statues of Anāhitā into several temples in the cities of the Empire.[4] The Roman historian Curtius Rufus also mentions a chariot in a royal Achaemenian procession, adorned with statues of Nin and Bel and divine statues in Persepolis destroyed by Alexander of Macedon.[5] Despite Berossus' claims, cultic sculpture is not found in Iran before the Macedonian conquest. This comes as no surprise, since only a few examples of freestanding sculpture are known from Achaemenian art.[6] Moreover, to date, no closed temples that could house such statues and serve as the "House of God" have been uncovered in Achaemenian Western Iran.[7] Anthropomorphic cultic statuary was seemingly never part of the royal Achaemenian cult, although the gods themselves were perceived by the Persian kings as anthropomorphic beings.[8] Herodotus concluded that the Persians did not think of their gods in human form because they tended not to erect anthropomorphic statues. Interestingly, the Greek historian Hecataios of Abdera says of Moses in his *Aegyptiaca*:

> He [Moses] had no images whatsoever of the gods made for them, being of the opinion that God is not in human form rather the Heaven that surrounds the earth is alone divine and rules the universe.[9]

The Greeks were mistaken about the anthropormorphic status of the Jewish God, and used a similar rationale to draw similarly mistaken conclusions about Persian deities.

Although there is no reason to think that the Hellenistic period was marked by a profound change in cult practices, in this period the first archaeological evidence appears for the existence of cultic statues set within temples whose plans were taken from the repertoire of Oriental architectural types.[10] In addition to the examples discussed in Chapter 3, we should also note the as yet unpublished fragments of

---

1 Jackson 1914: 274.
2 Jackson 1915: 151.
3 Marshak 2002c: 8.
4 See p. 16.
5 See p. 16–17.
6 The statue of Darius I originally made in Egypt and found in Susa. See Root 1979: 68–72; Ladynin 2011, and fragments of two or three statues from the same site: Root 1979: 110–114.
7 See Shenkar 2007: 173–179; Shenkar 2011: 117.
8 See also the brief discussion of Iranian anthropomorphism by Duchesne-Guillemin 2002 in a short entry in the *EIr*.
9 Diod. Sic. 40.3.4 (tr. *LCL*).
10 See Shenkar 2011.

a marble statue uncovered by Iranian archaeologists in recent excavations in the "Frataraka Temple" in Persepolis.[11] There is a complex debate, however, as to whether these statues represent Greek or Iranian deities, or perhaps both.

Nevertheless, it is clear that the depiction of deities in human form in the Iranian world existed from the Achaemenian period onwards. The iconographic repertoire of Achaemenian imperial art is rich in human-shaped and theriomorphic representations and, in that sense, may indeed be labeled as a successor to Mesopotamian and Elamite artistic traditions.[12] At least some of the anthropomorphic deities portrayed on seals and tablets from the *Persepolis Fortification Archive* may indeed represent cultic statues,[13] which possibly existed in the sanctuaries in the Pars region—essentially an amalgam of heterogeneous Elamite and Iranian cults.[14] Although compared to Eastern Iran very few sanctuaries have been excavated and studied in the West, on the basis of our current archaeological data the only case where traces of a cultic statue have been found is in the "Frataraka Temple" at Persepolis from the Hellenistic period. The clear absence of closed temples in any of the Achaemenian centers of Western Iran[15] speaks for itself that the royal cult, to which the kings were personally devoted, was not characterized by a pronounced image-orientated ritual and was conducted under the open sky. This does not necessarily mean that they did not sponsor and participate in cults that included anthropomorphic cultic imagery and did not attend sanctuaries originally belonging to non-Iranian religious traditions, which housed such statues.

In the Parthian period, Strabo describes a religious procession in which the image of the god Ōmanos was carried by Magi in Cappadocia.[16] Unsurprisingly, the practice of bearing a cultic image of a deity in processions is also known in Mesopotamia. Human-shaped images were kept inside temples and they would be revealed to common people on special occasions, once or twice a year.[17] It is, however, important to note that when Mesopotamian deities were exhibited outside the temples during the year, their images were usually represented by a non-anthropomorphic icon.[18] In addition, although sculpture finds become more numerous in the Parthian period, only a handful can be shown to represent deities.[19] We know that the statue of Heracles-Vərəθraγna from Mesene was set up in the temple of Apollo–Tīr in Seleucia of Tigris.[20] The soldiers of Lucius Verus captured in 164 CE a statue of Comaean Apollo from the same city,[21] and Flavius Josephus alludes to the domestic idols venerated by a "Parthian" wife of Anilaeus.[22] However, these data relate to predominantly Graeco-Semitic Mesopotamia and evidence for such cults on the Iranian plateau is almost entirely absent.

The Parthian coins depict numerous anthropomorphic images of Greek gods and often show kings interacting with them. It is possible that they were in fact modeled on cultic statues, which existed not only in Mesopotamian temples but also on the Iranian plateau, but any archaeological evidence as to their existence is yet to appear. According to Boyce "it is presumably largely due to Zoroastrian iconoclasm in the Sasanian period that no such cult statues survive in Iran itself".[23]

---

11 Callieri 2007: 61–62.

12 See Garrison 2000 and especially his forthcoming study of Achaemenian divine iconography: Garrison pre-publication.

13 Garrison 2000: 143, n. 64. The seal from Gorgippia (see p. 68) might also portray a cultic statue of Ištar.

14 Henkelman 2008: 58, 336–337.

15 However, it is possible that the monumental building, which is currently being excavated by the Italo-Iranian team at Tol-e Ājori on the Persepolis plain, might be a temple. See Chaverdi, Callieri and Gondet 2013. One must, nevertheless, wait to see if the final results of the excavation provide convincing data for the religious function of the building.

16 See p. 17.

17 van der Toorn 1997: 233; Ornan 2005a: 114.

18 Ornan 2009: 142–143.

19 A general discussion of Parthian sculpture is found in Colledge 1977; Colledge 1986; Kawami 1987; Mathiesen 1993.

20 See p. 11.

21 See p. 18.

22 See p. 17

23 Boyce and Grenet 1991: 66, n. 71.

The existence of a militant iconoclasm in the Sasanian period was postulated by Boyce in a groundbreaking article published in 1975,[24] and has since been accepted by scholars almost without reservation. I have argued in detail elsewhere that no iconoclastic movement ever existed within Sasanian Zoroastrianism.[25] The attacks against "idols" and "idolatry" in Middle Persian literature should be viewed in the context of discourse against idolatry common to monotheistic religions and as a response to Christian and Manichaean missionary activities. "Idol-worship" (*uzdēs-parastīh*), like "demon worship" (*dēwēzagīh*), *ag-dēn* and *duš-dēn* ("bad/evil religion"), *an-ēr* (non-Iranian), *dēwēsn* (demon-worshipper), *jādūg* (sorcerer) and *ahlomoγ* (heretic/apostate), appear to be polemical terms that lack substance and definition and could be applied to any religious tradition deemed alien by the Zoroastrian priesthood.[26] They were intended mostly for "Zoroastrian self-definition *per negationem*", through the idea of what is excluded.[27]

The Sasanians did not develop any prohibition against anthropomorphic representations of gods, and in the surviving Zoroastrian literature and inscriptions there is no evidence of either theological disputes over idols or a deliberate eradication of them by the Persian kings. The destruction of the statues in Armenia after its conquest by Ardašīr I, as well as his acts of extinguishing fires from the fire-temples,[28] should be understood as efforts towards centralization and unification of the cult by suppressing *any* public religious activities—sacred fires and cultic statues alike—associated with the previous dynasties and rulers that had been overthrown by the founder of the Sasanian Empire.[29] The seizure of huge amounts of money assembled in these sanctuaries in formerly Parthian domains would have been a strong secondary motivation.[30]

The Sasanian cult was aniconic, probably following a tradition sustained in the region of Pars from the Achaemenian period, and Sasanian temples were free of figural imagery.[31] However, Sasanian culture was not iconoclastic. In fact, Sasanian kings were responsible for the creation of the first fully anthropomorphic images of Iranian gods in Western Iran and ordered images of their representations receiving diadems from the hands of Ahura Mazdā in human form. Alongside the aniconic cult, sculptural depictions in the round were clearly part of public and private spaces in Sasanian Iran[32] and historical and archaeological evidence clearly demonstrates that Sasanian visual culture was anything

24 Boyce 1975.

25 See Shenkar forthcoming a.

26 However, unlike all other terms, *uzdēs-parastīh* is not found in the Avestan texts. I have suggested that is a calque of the Greek Christian term εἰδωλολατρεία which was adopted in the Sasanian period to counter Christian polemics. See the detailed discussion in Shenkar forthcoming a.

27 De Jong 2003c: 22.

28 See p. 21 and Boyce 1968: 47.

29 See also De Jong 2006: 234–235.

30 De Jong 2006: 232–233.

31 Although they contained anthropomorphic and zoomorphic representations, which are reported by Byzantine sources (see p. 28–29) and attested by the archaeological finds. The German team that conducted the excavations of Taḵt-e Solaymān uncovered fragments of anthropomorphic and zoomorphic stucco reliefs in the fill under the floors of the last Sasanian phase of the temple. See Kröger 1982: 141–148. Furthermore, if the interpretation of the large complex at the northern limits of Bīšāpūr as a fire-temple is sound, it means that the famous mosaics with Dionysiac scenes in fact decorated the fire-temple. See Callieri 2009: 54; Callieri 2011.

32 Notable examples are the colossus of Šāpūr I in the cave near Bīšāpūr and the statue of Šāpūr I that once stood at the main intersection of the same city. Statues are also mentioned by Muslim authors in the accounts of booty taken by Arabs in Iranian cities (see p. 40). The enclosure walls of the *Palais B* at Bīšāpūr were decorated with blocks bearing reliefs of charging equestrians and standing figures. See Bier 2009. Both the public and private Sasnaian edifices reveal a wealth of figural stucco decorations. See Kröger 1982 (especially 248–255), who assembled and studied stucco fragments from several Sasanian sites. In additions, see also material from the manor house at Hājīābād: Azarnoush 1994; and the recently excavated Sasanian complex at Bandiān in northern Khurāsān: Rahbar 1998; Rahbar 2004; Rahbar 2007; Rahbar 2011; Gignoux 2008.

but iconoclastic. However, images of gods in Sasanian culture were limited to rock-reliefs, coins and seals, and seem to have been excluded from the urban landscape, temples and palatial complexes.

In Middle Persian literature, the common term for the "idol-temple" is *uzdēszār*. It has also been suggested that Iranian temples containing cultic imagery, which were in this way distinct from aniconic fire-temples, were labeled by terms derived from OIr. **bagina*—"(place) belonging to god".[33] Words deriving from *bagina* are attested in Imperial Aramaic (*bagina*), Armenian (*bagin*), Georgian (*bagini*), Bactrian (**βaγən*), Sogdian (*vaγn* (*βγn-*)), Parthian (*bagin*) and Middle Persian (*bašn*).

It is certain that Armenian, Bactrian, Sogdian and perhaps also Parthian *baginas* contained cultic images. However, translating them as "idol-temples" is misleading and carries negative connotations that are only appropriate within the context of the Pahlavi books, as they speak of a category of "idolatry" that only makes any sense from a hostile, monotheistic perspective. It is only for the outside observer, who considers himself anti-idolic and negatively predisposed towards images, that the sanctuaries of the Armenians, Bactrians and Sogdians would be considered "idol-temples". For the Armenians, Bactrians, and Sogdians themselves, this term in their own languages probably meant nothing more than simply "temple".[34] The Middle Persian *bašn* is attested only twice in Manichaean polemical texts and in the geographical treatise *Šahrestānīhā ī Ērānšahr*.[35] Since both relate to the Eastern Iranian world, we might assume that in Middle Persian, *bašn* might have been used as a specific reference to Sogdian—and perhaps also to Bactrian—temples, which were certainly viewed by the Sasanians as essentially different from their own fire-temples.

2. *Eastern Iran*

The tradition of anthropomorphic religious iconography in Eastern Iran goes back to the BMAC (Bactria-Margiana Archaeological Complex), also known as the Oxus Civilization, which covered a large region in Central Asia before the arrival of the Indo-Iranians.[36] However, the local Iranian cults that existed in Eastern Iran before and immediately after the Achaemenian conquest are virtually unknown. It is only in the Hellenistic period that the two Bactrian temples at Ai Khanum and Takht-i Sangin provide the first direct archaeological evidence for cultic statues, found *in situ*.

The Kushan kings and the Sogdian rulers in what is today Afghanistan, Northern Pakistan and parts of Uzbekistan and Tajikistan should be credited with the final anthropomorphization of most Iranian deities. Of the twenty-six divinities depicted on Kushan coins in full anthropomorphic shape, at least seventeen have a definite Iranian background. It is to this period, or slightly earlier, before the rise of the Kushan dynasty as the region's dominant force forging an empire out of the various principalities ruled by the nomadic clans, that the creation of the first anthropomorphic images of Buddha and Śiva (and other Indian deities) are also usually dated.[37] The Kushan dynasty kept alive Graeco-Bactrian sculptural traditions and blended them with Indian motifs to create a body of fully anthropomorphic art.[38] Fragments of numerous statues made of unbaked clay have been found in the palace/temple of Khalchayan[39] and from the Rabatak inscription we know that Kushan sanctuaries housed statues of gods and of rulers. Kushan dynastic art seemingly absorbed both the rich artistic heritage of Hellenistic Bactria as well as the influence of contemporary Roman art, thus determining the appearance

33 Boyce 1975: 99; Boyce 1982: 227; Grenet 1988.
34 For a detailed discussion, see Shenkar: forthcoming a.
35 See p. 38 and *SE* 7.
36 For a recent excellent survey of the Oxus Civilization, see Francfort 2005. For the religious iconography and pantheon, see pages 281–285.
37 Giuliano 2004. For the genesis of figural representations of Buddha and Buddhist aniconism, see also Seckel 2004.
38 The basic studies of Kushan art are still Rosenfield 1967; Pugachenkova 1979.
39 Pugachenkova 1966; Pugachenkova 1971.

of Iranian gods and goddesses in human form. The Sogdians went even further in combining Hellenistic and Kushan legacies with Sasanian and Indian influences, creating the Iranian world's most complete series of divine personages.

The Kushan temples at Surkh-Kotal and Rabatak undoubtedly housed cultic statues of gods. This is confirmed not only by the inscriptions, but also by the rectangular niches on the top of the Surkh-Kotal platform that contained clay, painted sculptures, a few small fragments of which were discovered by the French expedition. The painted panels from the Metropolitan Museum probably represent worshippers before cultic statues.[40] Golden statuettes of Nana, Mao and Mithra are reported to been recently discovered in Peshawar among a huge hoard of gold coins from the early Kushan period. Unfortunately, these statuettes disappeared shortly after their discovery, before they were even photographed.[41] While we have very limited information on the rituals performed in Bactrian Kushan sanctuaries, there is no reason to doubt that the cultic statues of the gods played an important, perhaps even central part in it, as in the Iranian temples from the Hellenistic period and in Sogdian sanctuaries.

Although no inscriptions and temples have been uncovered in Bactria from the Kushano-Sasanian era, Kushano-Sasanian iconography depicts numerous scenes of kings worshipping before image(s) of the god(s) that most probably represent cultic statue(s). It is clear that the pictorial data provides no evidence of "iconoclasm" following the Sasanian occupation of Bactria. Veneration of images not only continued under the Sasanian viceroys, but it presumably flourished. Statues for new western deities, like Anāhitā, were manufactured and their veneration was shown on coins.[42]

The thematic repertoire of Sogdian art is exceptionally rich in anthropomorphic representations. As suggested most interestingly by Marshak, Sogdian religious iconography developed due to competition with Buddhism and Manichaeism, whose devotees employed religious art in their propaganda.[43] A wealth of statues, part of Sogdian visual culture, is attested numerous times in written sources and by archaeological finds, and Sogdian temple cults were clearly centered around these figures,[44] as deduced both from written sources and from archaeology. Medieval accounts of the Muslim conquest of Transoxiana contain numerous references to idols captured in Sogdian sanctuaries.[45] It is especially noteworthy that Muslim authors, as a rule, do not distinguish between idol- and fire-worship in Sogdiana, which for them were clearly part of the same cult. The two temples in Panjikent—the best studied Sogdian sacred buildings—housed numerous sculptures and statues of deities, confirming that their central ritual was the kindling of fire before images of the gods.[46] In addition to the examples discussed in Chapter 3, one may also note that the niches in the western walls of the main halls of Panjikent temples housed clay statues of the gods that unfortunately were not preserved. A large bronze ear of a statue of an animal was found in Temple I, probably belonging to the zoomorphic throne of a huge statue.[47]

Sogdian idols were completely anthropomorphic and, as the statue from the Surkh mountains, were often made of wood.[48] The three heads found in a large storage jar hidden under the floor of the "Large Hall" at the Sogdian fortress of Chilhujra in Ustrushana form another interesting example.[49] These heads are almost life size with only slight differences between them. The storage jar and the heads show traces of intense burning. All three heads belong to males and exhibit distinct individual features. The first

40 See p. 63, p. 136 and pp. 155–156.
41 Bopearachchi 2008: 5.
42 See p. 75–76.
43 Marshak 1999: 177.
44 Shkoda 1989: 86. See a recent study of the rituals in Sogdian cult based on the Panjikent temples in Shkoda 2009: 98–121.
45 See pp. 40–42
46 Shkoda 2009: 124.
47 Shkoda 2009: 87–88.
48 See p. 112.
49 Pulatov 1975: 90–93, 96–100.

head is the best preserved among the three (fig. 186). It shows a man with almond-shaped eyes and carefully modeled facial features. His hair was probably tied with a diadem. On the back, there is a "T" shaped projection allowing it to be attached to something, probably to a body, which was carved independently.[50] The second head is slightly larger and more damaged (fig. 187). The main part of the face, especially on the left side, is missing or burned, but the hair is relatively well preserved. The figure wore some sort of headdress, perhaps a crown.[51] Finally, the third head was reassembled from small fragments of burned wood (fig. 188). Its extremely poor state of preservation does not allow any facial features to be distinguished. It probably also had a tall headdress.[52] Unfortunately, the Chilhujra heads are too effaced and lack any characteristic features that would allow identification. However, the idol from the Surkh Mountains that was not only uniquely preserved in its entirety, but also discovered together with accompanying objects and elements of its decorations and dress, is also not readily associated with any known Sogdian god.

It is certain that the statues from Panjikent, and probably also those of Chilhujra and of the Surkh mountains, stood as cultic images in Sogdian sanctuaries. And at least some of the fragments of statues uncovered at the temple at Erkurgan may also represent statues of deities.[53]

The group of four figures on the southern wall of the Afrosiab paintings standing within the building toward which a procession is directed, has also been identified as depicting the statues of gods.[54] However, only the lower parts of these characters are preserved and the interpretation of the building itself as a cultic site is conjectural. Furthermore, these figures are of normal size, while in Sogdian art, divine images are always distinguished by their superior dimensions. Wall paintings are undoubtedly the most productive source for the study of Sogdian religion and for the iconography of deities in the Sogdian pantheon. In Central Asia, monumental paintings, including representations of cultic scenes of the veneration of deities probably evolved first in Bactria in the Kushan and Kushano-Sasanian periods. In the fifth-sixth centuries CE the Bactrian artistic tradition gave impulse to this development in Sogdian art.[55] The region's Hellenistic artistic legacy, perhaps also partly through Bactrian mediation, was equally significant.[56] Sogdian murals have been uncovered in four main locations, Panjikent, Afrosiab (Samarkand), Varakhsha and Bunjikat (Ustrushana). Sogdian paintings of the fifth century CE are very close to the Kushan and Kushano-Sasanian art of Bactria. In the Kushano-Sasanian and the Hephtalite periods, elements of Sasanian iconography also entered Sogdian art.[57]

Indian influence likewise played an important role in the formation of Sogdian art. The Indian elements seem to have been borrowed not from the Kushan tradition, but directly from the art of northwestern India in the fifth-sixth centuries CE.[58] The main influx of foreign influences on Sogdian art can probably be attributed to the sixth century CE, followed by a period in which the iconographical canon stabilized in the seventh-eight centuries CE, when new borrowings appear to dwindle.[59] It is to this period that most of the examples of Sogdian paintings discussed in this book (and especially those from Panjikent) belong.

---

50 Pulatov 1975: 90–92.
51 Pulatov 1975: 92–93.
52 Pulatov 1975: 93.
53 See Suleymanov 2000: 110–111.
54 Compareti 2009a: 196.
55 Marshak 1983: 53.
56 The principal studies of Sogdian art and religious iconography, are that of Belenitskiy 1954; Belenitskiy 1973; Azarpay 1975a; Azarpay 1975b; Belenitskiy and Marshak 1976; Belenitskiy and Marshak 1981; Maršak and Raspopova 1991; Marshak 1987; Marshak 1989; Mode 1991/1992; Marshak 1999; Marshak 2002b; Marshak 2009.
57 See Marshak 1983: 53.
58 Marshak 1983: 53; Marshak 1989: 118. See also recent articles by Grenet 2006/2010 and Compareti 2009b.
59 Marshak 1999: 177.

Eleven idols uncovered *in situ* at the manor house at Kayragach, Ferghana represent an instance of cultic statues used in the domestic, private cult (fig. 189).[60] They were found in three adjacent rooms that probably served as a private sanctuary. One of these rooms contained a pedestal on which the idols were placed. Four statues were actually found nearby, overthrown from the pedestal when the building was destroyed. Another idol was discovered just to the north of the sanctuary, bringing their total number to twelve.[61] The idols are made of alabaster and clay and all belong to the same type. They have disproportionally large heads and almond-shaped eyes, but they also demonstrate some individual features. The largest idol is 66.9 cm high.[62] They are dated by the excavator to the end of the fourth-sixth century CE. Unfortunately, almost nothing is known about the religious beliefs of Late Antique Ferghana, but the inhabitants of Kayragach, who were most probably Iranians, clearly employed idols as part of their everyday cultic routine. Isolated finds of similar "domestic" idols have also been made in other regions of Central Asia.[63] Brykina connects the Kayragach idols with an ancestral cult,[64] which may well be the truth. In any case, these idols demonstrate nothing that would suggest their association with any known Iranian deity.

Numerous anthropomorphic statues have also been discovered in other areas of Eastern Iran, for example at Topraq-Qal'a at Chorasmia, but unfortunately none of them can be identified as an image of a deity with any degree of certainty.[65] The remains of mural art have been found at several sites in Chorasmia, but figural images were discovered only at Kalaly-gyr II (a horse and a rider), Koi-krylgan-kala (a human figure), and Kazakly-yatkan (animals and human processions, portraits of Chorasmian kings) and none of them portray a deity.[66]

When Herodotus visited the Scythians in the fifth century BCE, he observed that with the exception of Ares, who was visualized as *akinakes*, the Scythians did not make images of their gods. However, several dozen of schematic human-shaped stone statues have been found in the Scythian domains.[67] They are usually dated to the sixth-fifth centuries BCE, thus predating any other anthropomorphic image in Scythian art.[68] These statues are generally believed to be of a funereal character, and, according to Raevskiy, they might represent both Targitaius (the mythical ancestor of the Scythians) and the Scythian kings (who as the descendants of Targitaius were held to be his personifications).[69] The explicit anthropomorphization of Scythian art probably began around the time of Herodotus' visit and the majority of the human-shaped representations of Scythian deities are not dated earlier than the second half of the fourth century BCE.[70] The influence of Greek art might have played a significant role here,[71] but the basic conception of at least some Scythian gods as anthropomorphic beings was probably present from the very beginning.[72] However, it is important to note that the principal Scythian gods,

60 Brykina 1982.

61 Brykina 1982: 89–90.

62 Brykina 1982: 90–94.

63 See Brykina 1982: 94–103. See also Kruglikova 1988, who discusses four idols found during the excavations of the gate fortifications at Dilberjin.

64 Brykina 1982: 104–113.

65 Rapoport 1994.

66 See Kidd et. al. 2004/2008. For a study of the techniques employed in Central Asian murals, see Kossolapov and Marshak 1999. For a general survey of the Central Asian paintings, see also Antonini 2003.

67 Raevskiy 1983.

68 Raevskiy 1983: 43.

69 Raevskiy 1983: 52, 57.

70 Bessonova 1983: 81; Schiltz 1994: 51; Rusyayeva 2007: 97

71 However, anthropomorphic imagery was present in Scythian art before the Greeks. See Schiltz 1994 10–11; Ustinova 1999: 21. There are, however, very few images of gods independent of Greek iconography, and given its anepigraphic character, the interpretation of Scythian divine iconography is highly problematic and unclear.

72 Artamonov 1961: 82; Raevskiy 1977: 178; Raevskiy 1978: 68–69.

Tabiti-Hestia and Papaeus-Zeus, were probably never depicted in human shape.[73] The appearance of anthropomorphic iconography among Sarmatians may be dated as late as the second-first centuries BCE.[74]

Finally, two finds of female wooden statues associated with the Alans are known from the region between Volga and Don rivers. One such statue was discovered in a kurgan burial.[75]

2. *Anthropomorphic Mental Notions of the Divine*

After surveying the artistic evidence, we will now turn to the Iranian written sources. The Avesta and the corpus of Zoroastrian Middle Persian literature preserve clear indications of tensions between the initial Iranian anthropomorphic perception of the divine and its aniconic representations. This tension is expressed in two important parallel notions, two modes of being found in the Zoroastrian scriptures—*mēnōg* and *gētīg*.[76] *Gētīg* stands for "the material, earthly (world), that which can be apprehended through the senses" while *mēnōg* is best described as "that which is non-material, non-sensual, intelligible, incorporeal and unperceived by the senses".[77] The principal distinction is usually made between the visible and material characteristics of *gētīg* and the invisible and non-material ones of *mēnōg*.[78] A possible allusion to the existence of the concept of the invisible plane inhabited by incorporeal entities among Iranians is found in Diogenes Laertius, who quotes Sotion's evidence that the Magi "… say that the air is filled with shapes that enter the eyes of the sharp-sighted through a stream caused by evaporation".[79] Only persons of extraordinary qualities, such as Zoroaster and his patron king Vištaspa, are quoted as seeing *mēnōg*. Curiously, new-born children are also said to be capable of it.[80] Ahura Mazdā is called the "*mēnōg* of *mēnōg*", possessing the highest degree of "invisibility", and even the *mēnōg* beings—including the other deities themselves—are incapable of seeing him, just as the inhabitants of *gētīg* are usually unable to see *mēnōg* creatures.[81]

A hierarchy existed between other divine beings too. Thus in the *Sīh-rōzag* we find a passage stating that:

> Wahman ud Māh ud Gōšurwan har 3 gōspand-tōhmag hēnd; Wahman mēnōg ī a-wēnāg ud a-grftār, Māh mēnōg ī wēnāg ud a-griftār, Gōšurwan wēnāg ud griftār.
>
> Wahman, Māh and Gōšurwan are all three of the seed of cattle; Wahman is an invisible and intangible spirit, Māh a visible and intangible spirit, Gōšurwan visible and tangible.[82]

In a passage from the Avesta (preserved only in the Middle Persian work *Šāyast ne Šāyast*) Ahura Mazdā is described as having a fully anthropomorphic appearance.[83] Unequivocal allusions to the anthropomorphic shape of Ahura Mazdā and the Aməša Spənta are also found in Middle Persian literature. The *Sīh-rōzag* states that "the likeness of Ohrmazd in the *gētīg* is the righteous men" (*hangōšīdag ī Ohrmazd*

---

73 The male figure in the eagle headdress from the finial from Lysaya Gora is usually identified as a unique image of Papaeus. See Bessonova 1983: 41–42; Schiltz 1994: 182, Fig. 133. However, naked and ithyphallic images are not found in Iranian divine iconography and therefore it is hardly possible that it depicts an Iranian deity. Perhaps it should rather be understood as a depiction of a priest-shaman (?).

74 Yatsenko 1992: 192.

75 Yatsenko 1992: 104.

76 Shaked 1971; Shaked 2001.

77 Shaked 1971: 60.

78 Shaked 1971: 63.

79 Diog. Laert. 1.7.

80 Shaked 1971: 61–62.

81 Shaked 1971: 77–78.

82 *Sr* 12.

83 See p. 33.

pad gētīg mard ī ahlaw).[84] In the *Pahlavi Rivāyat Accompanying the Dādestān ī Dēnīg*, Ohrmazd and Spandarmad are described as an affectionate, embracing couple.[85] In the *Dādestān ī Dēnīg* itself, we find the notion that it is possible to see Ohrmazd in *mēnōg* "through wisdom and the power of similitude".[86] In the *Pahlavi Rivāyat Accompanying the Dādestān ī Dēnīg* and in a passage by the Muslim author al-Jayhānī quoted by al-Shahrastānī, Ohrmazd is said to have created the world out of his body.[87]

Mardānfarrox ī Ohrmazddādān, the author of the polemical and theological essay *Škand Gumānīg Wizār*, argues that the god is necessarily incorporeal and possess no *čihr* ("form").[88] The creator must exist only in *mēnōg*, but not in *gētīg*. A passage from chapter 14 that is concerned with a polemic against Judaism provides a good illustration of this concept. Mardānfarrox, relying on the authority of Jewish scripture, relates that the Jewish god

> … sits on a throne which four angels carry on their wings which from its weight a fiery river flows out. Now when he is spiritual and not corporeal, what is the reason those four pitiful ones painfully bear that heavy burden?[89]

What is evident from these texts, and from several other places in Pahlavi literature, is that gods were essentially perceived as having human form in *mēnōg*, but their manifestations in the visible world, *gētīg*, usually assumed symbolic, metaphoric, elemental and aniconic shape. The idea that deities do not have an anthropomorphic representation in the physical plane, which is visible to ordinary people, may have been one of the main theoretical concepts behind the Iranian inclination to represent their gods in aniconic form. It is also clear that human-shaped images existed during certain periods in some Iranian religions, but there is usually no way of knowing whether this reflects nuances in cult or even religious belief.

In light of these observations, the Sasanian reliefs pose an interesting problem, as they depict not only kings, but also dignitaries and courtiers seeing and even interacting with the divine. This seemingly indicates, once again, that the notions and concepts developed by priests in theological treatises were not universally shared by society and were not unquestionably relevant in the matters of royal ideology and propaganda, just as the very scene of investiture depicted on the reliefs is nonexistent in Zoroastrian literary tradition.

3. *Conclusions*

The cultic practices attested among Pre-Islamic Iranians were very diverse, encompassing both "material" and "empty-space" aniconism, alongside the most frequent and common practice of "elemental aniconism". Any conception of aniconism as a "primitive" and "ancient" form of worship that preceded figural representation can be laid to rest. It is clear that in most cultures, cultic statues coexisted with non-figural symbols, and aniconism was simply "another way to visualize the divine".[90]

Iranian deities were essentially perceived as anthropomorphic. Iranian gods were always viewed as possessing a human form in *mēnōg*, but were not always represented in this way in *gētīg* in certain regions and periods. For instance, although the Sasanian cult was probably predominantly aniconic (but not iconoclastic), the Kushan and Sogdian cults included cultic images. At this stage of research,

---

84 *Sr* 1.
85 See p. 34–35.
86 See p. 34.
87 See p. 35 and p. 43–44.
88 *ŠGW* 5.46, ed. and tr. by de de Menasce 1945: 67.
89 *ŠGW* 14.34–35, tr. by Thrope 2012: 93–94.
90 Mylonopoulos 2010: 10. See also Gaifman 2008.

it seems likely that aniconic trends were present among Iranians from the very beginning, reflecting their nomadic origins, ideology and religious beliefs, but that these trends were also inspired by similar developments in Mesopotamia, Elam and Urartu. The influence that these civilizations have had on the formation of Iranian culture has long been acknowledged,[91] but the tremendous extent of this influence is only now starting to be fully appreciated.

91 See especially Gnoli 1974; Gnoli 1988; Panaino 2000.

CHAPTER 6

CONCLUSIONS

The foremost outcome of this study is the identification (or confirmation of already proposed identifications) of the anthropomorphic pictorial representations of twenty-eight Iranian deities. As there is no need to repeat here the conclusions reached for the development of the iconography of each deity, we will now turn to general observations that emerge from the material assembled and discussed above.

For Achaemenian art, only one Iranian divine representation, that of Ahura Mazdā as the figure in the winged ring, was recognized. No other human-shaped image has been shown beyond doubt to portray an Iranian deity. The sole image of an Iranian god associated with the art of the Parthian Empire, is that of the statue of Heracles from Mesene, which was, however, produced in Mesopotamia. From the Hellenistic period, only the statuette of the god Oxus as Marsyas on the votive altar from Takht-i Sangin can be identified as an image of an Iranian deity.

Kushan art has produced no less than eighteen assured images of Iranian deities as well as two that are more doubtful: Ahura Mazdā, Aši, Arštāt, Ātar, Drvāspā, Māh, Mithra, Mozdooano, Nana, Oxus/Vakhsh, X^{v}arənah, Šahrewar, Sraoša, (?), Tištrya/Tīr, Vanant, Vāta, Vayu, Vərəθraγna, Vohu Manah (?), Yima. Sasanian art contains five certain and several possible divine images: Ahura Mazdā, Anāhitā, Aŋra Mainyu, Ātar (?), Māh, Mithra, Sraoša (?), Vərəθraγna (?). In Sogdian art, images of six deities and a further seven possible ones are found: Airyaman, Anāhitā (?), Apąm Napāt, Ātar (?), Daēnā (?), Drvāspā (?), Māh, Mithra, Nana, Oxus/Vakhsh (?), Rašnu, Sraoša (?), Tištrya/Tīr (?), Vayu. Kushano-Sasanian art has representations of four Iranian divinities: Anāhitā, Mithra, Nana and Vayu. Finally, in post Kushano-Sasanian Bactria we have recognized the visual images of two gods and one that is doubtful: Mithra, Māh, Oxus/Vakhsh (?). In Chorasmia, only the portrayal of Nana, the great goddess of Eastern Iran, was identified.

From this list alone it is immediately evident that the Eastern Iranian iconography was much richer than that of Western Iran. Curiously, the only deity to appear in Western Iran, but not in Eastern Iran, is Aŋra Mainyu. Pre-Islamic Iranian divine iconography was clearly not a homogenous assemblage in terms of characteristic style and recognizable iconographic conceptions and cannot be compared to other religious traditions; Egyptian iconography, for instance. This is readily explicable, since Sasanians, Sogdians and Kushans by no means possessed the same pantheon and their artistic language developed under varying conditions, in different periods and geographical environments. We are, in fact, dealing with independent or semi-independent pantheons and cultural traditions sharing the same background and with very complex interconnections between them. They shared an assortment of deities originating from the common Proto-Iranian pantheon, but the iconographical data indicates that more often than not, these gods developed in different directions and had different functions, personalities and even different gender. The only deity visually represented among Sasanians, Kushans, and Sogdians was Mithra (and perhaps also Sraoša). Furthermore, according to the iconographic data, Mithra was one of the most frequently reproduced deities in the Iranian world. Interestingly, in Eastern Iran, the chief deity always appears to be female; Hestia-Tabiti of the Scythians, Nana in Bactria, Sogdiana and Chorasmia.

Among more than one hundred divine representations, encompassing most of the currently known Iranian divine iconography, only six have been identified as having parallel descriptions in the

Zoroastrian canon.[1] These are: Anāhitā on the coin of coins of Ōhrmazd I;[2] Apąm Napāt from the Panjikent painting;[3] Mithra rising from the mountain;[4] the chariot of Mithra Bāmiān;[5] Rašnu on the Sogdian ossuaries[6] and the Kushan Iamšo.[7] It is instructive that five of them originate from Eastern Iran and only one example is taken from Sasanian art. This substantiates the veracity of De Jong's observations cited in the Introduction,[8] supporting his other statement that:

> not a single item of the iconography on these [Sasanian] reliefs has been convincingly interpreted as being based on Avestan imagery. The same is true of Sasanian silver-work and of an astounding number of Sasanian seals, which bear all sorts of images.[9]

It can therefore be considered an established fact that even the art of the Sasanian Empire, from which the religious tradition of modern Zoroastrianism directly evolved, drew upon sources other than the Avesta and the materials later assembled in Middle Persian literature. Above all, these sources drew on Mesopotamian imagery with additional Graeco-Roman influences as well as elements coming from Eurasian nomads (either inherited from the Parthians, or acquired through direct contact).

Borrowing was by no means uni-directional. One example of an Iranian contribution is a plain nimbus that appears for the first time with the gods on the coins of Kanishka and would eventually become one of the most recognized attributes of the divine in Eurasia, penetrating the iconography of many religions including Christianity, Hinduism, Buddhism and Islam. Huvishka was the first to incorporate the nimbus in his portrait; and subsequently this element was also frequently associated with royalty in Sasanian Iran and in the Roman and Byzantine Empires. In addition to the nimbus, the divine status of Iranian gods was usually graphically conveyed by means of their focal place in the composition, superior size, enthroned pose, animal attributes (often *pars pro toto*), attributes of royalty and astral and elemental symbolism, such as the crescent moon and flames rising from the shoulders. The ultimate Mesopotamian origin of the nimbus (but not the plain nimbus), crescent and flaming shoulders has been noted by Ernst Herzfeld, who attempted to explain their puzzling presence in Bactria by commenting that they are "the old Oriental, the Sumerian way of adding divine attributes to figures, and we must suppose that Graeco-Bactrian art has here revived a feature long forgotten in the West".[10]

Herzfeld, however, preferred not to linger the question of how and why this feature was revived, how this "Mesopotamian" tradition reached Bactria and where it was kept for all those years to be rejuvenated in a region, far removed from the centers of Mesopotamian civilization. It now seems that features of Mesopotamian culture were constantly and strongly present in the cultural landscape of Bactria as early as the Achaemenian period.[11] Although, elements of Mesopotamian-inspired divine iconography are not found in the Graeco-Bactrian period, its influence in Bactria remained appreciable.[12] This we learn from the extraordinarily diverse pantheon of Kanishka and Huvishka who infused it with the region's Hellenistic legacy and dominant Roman influences to create their outstanding galleria of divine

---

1 Although we should possibly also add Drvāspā from Panjikent and Daēnā on a Kushano-Sasanian (?) seal. See p. 97 and p. 94–95.
2 See p. 69.
3 See p. 82.
4 See p. 108.
5 See p. 89.
6 See p. 141.
7 See p. 166.
8 See p. 6.
9 De Jong 2009: 37.
10 Herzfeld 1930: 29.
11 For example, the evidence for the cult of Bel. See p. 61–62.
12 However, a "Mesopotamian type" of Graeco-Bactrian temples was modeled after Mesopotamian prototypes. See Shenkar 2011.

pictorial representations. Furthermore, it was contact with Mesopotamian divine imagery that probably provided the originally aniconic Iranians with the initial impulse for the visual anthropomorphization of their gods. Starting from the Achaemenians, the echoes of this impact of Mesopotamian religious iconography are traceable in Kushan, Sasanian, and even Sogdian iconography. However, as we have seen, not only anthropomorphism, but also the Iranian inclination towards aniconism, was probably influenced by the developments in the first millennium Babylonian cult.

The representation of the divine in the ancient Iranian world was generally modeled on that of royalty, probably exploiting the ideological base of divine agency of kingship that appears to be common to most Iranians. The royal insignia, crown and/or diadem became the essential accessories of an Iranian divinity. This observation especially holds true for Sasanian and Sogdian art where deities are almost always pictured crowned and in royal attire. The parallelism between the king and the god in Sasanian art, expressed through similar dimensions, pose, garments and attributes is exceptional in the art of ancient Iranians and is not found in other periods. The very anthropomorphic image of Ahura Mazdā was created by the first Sasanian monarch in order to augment his own exceptional status and to liken himself to a deity.

In the Hellenistic period, the iconocentric Greek cult, which became the cult of the ruling elites in many regions of the Iranian world, undoubtedly contributed to the visual anthropomorphization of Iranian gods and to the expansion of anthropomorphic imagery in Iran. It is in this period that the first evidence of cultic statuary appears in the archaeological record. Despite preferences for aniconic representations of deities, especially in Western Iran, it seems that the perception of the divine among ancient Iranian people was anthropomorphic from the very beginning. Textual evidence confirming this observation is found already in the Avesta, and appears in an elaborated form in Middle Persian literature, reflected in the notions of *mēnōg* and *gētīg*. While the deities of the Zoroastrian texts possess a fully anthropomorphic shape in *mēnōg*, and could be seen by the chosen ones, in *gētīg* their representations often assumed symbolic or aniconic form.

There is a sharp distinction in the nature of the cult between Western and Eastern Iran. The Achaemenian and Sasanian cults were aniconic, but not iconoclastic. The Persian dynasties adopted anthropomorphic representations of the divine for their official and proclamatory uses, but their sanctuaries and sacred precincts were free from statues of the divine in human form. As for the elusive Parthians, the only solid evidence we possess—the statue of Heracles in Mesene—indicates that at least in Mesopotamia, free-standing sculptures of the Iranian deities identified with the Olympian gods were erected in temples. Unfortunately, the situation on the ethnically and culturally different Iranian plateau is completely unknown.

Following the collapse of Greek rule, it appears that cultic iconography in Eastern Iran developed in a remarkably different manner. Eastern Iranian people, like the Kushans and the Sogdians, not only made unprecedented use (by Western Iranian standards) of portrayals of their gods in human form, but also venerated their man-made representations in temples. This cultic dissimilarity between Eastern and Western Iran may be explained in terms of different intrinsic developments in Proto-Iranian religion, as it contained ideas and elements with both aniconic and iconic potential. Human-shaped representations of the divine are found already in the BMAC in the second millennium, but they were probably not continued by eastern Iranians. Diffusionists will draw attention to the exceptionally strong Hellenistic influence in Eastern Iran, as distinct from Western Iranian regions, especially Pars with its well-known tradition of preserving the Achaemenian, Persian legacy well into the Parthian and Sasanian periods. Aniconic worship was probably part of that heritage. It is interesting that the first representations of the principal Bactrian gods, Nana and Oešo, were also aniconic, perhaps reflecting the predominantly aniconic religious culture of the nomadic newcomers. However, under Kanishka, a complete anthropomorphism became the guiding principle of Bactrian religious iconography. Iranian anthropomorphic divine imagery therefore initially emerged from contact with Mesopotamian civilization, and most divine attributes and visual conventions used in Iranian iconography in fact go back to ancient Mesopotamia. These conventions were reformulated and given a new impulse, dispersion and cultic role under the influence of Greek and Roman iconography. In the particular case of Sogdian art, the influx of Indian divine iconography constitutes yet another important layer.

Representations of anthropomorphic divine images of Iranian deities assembled in this book are intended to serve any future enquiry into the sphere of pre-Islamic Iranian iconography. Many particular problems with the iconography of specific deities still remain unsolved, as are several important issues related to the religious and cultural history of the pre-Islamic Iranian world, which are poorly understood and require further in-depth investigation. For instance, the presence of strong Mesopotamian influences in Achamenian Bactria is yet to be explained satisfactorily. With critical use of Zoroastrian written sources, awareness of their extreme complicity, and their careful and conditional appliance to cultures other than late Sasanian, it is hoped that further research will be able to offer new solutions to these questions. Treating the various Iranian cultures as independent entities within one pre-Islamic Iranian cultural space, and exploring the multifaceted relations between the particular and the general appears to be the most attractive and sound approach.

It is my hope that this research has succeeded in demonstrating the importance and the immense potential of iconography for the history of Iranian religions, and that it has contributed to our understanding of the fascinating artistic and intellectual world of the Iranian people that were, and still are, major actors on the Eurasian stage.

APPENDIX

IRANIAN DYNASTIES[1]

Teispids

Cyrus the Great (550–530 BCE)
Cambyses (530–522 BCE)
Bardya (522 BCE)

Achaemenians

Darius I (522–486 BCE)
Xerxes I (486–465 BCE)
Artaxerxes I (465–424 BCE)
Xerxes II (424–423 BCE)
Darius II (423–405 BCE)
Artaxerxes II (405–359 BCE)
Artaxerxes III (359–338 BCE)
Artaxerxes IV/Arses (338–336 BCE)
Darius III (336–330 BCE)

Arsacids

Arsaces (c. 238–211 BCE)
Phraates I (c. 177–171 BCE)
Mithridates I (c. 171–138 BCE)
Phraates II (c. 138–237 BCE)
Artabanus I (c. 127–124 BCE)
Mithridates II (c. 123–191 BCE)
Gotarzes I (c. 91–87 BCE)
Orodes I (c. 90–80 BCE)
Mithridates III (c. 57–54 BCE)
Orodes II (c. 57–38 BCE)
Phraates IV (c. 38–2 BCE)
Phraataces/Phraates V (c. 2 BCE–4 CE)
Tiridates (c. 29–27 BCE)
Vonones I (c. 8–12 CE)
Artabanus II (c. 10–38 CE)
Vardanes (c. 39–45 CE)
Gotarzes II (c. 40–51 CE)
Vonones II (c. 51 CE)
Vologases I (c. 51–78 CE)
Artabanus III (c. 80–90 CE)
Pacorus II (c. 78–105 CE)
Vologases III (c. 105–107 CE)
Osroes I (c. 109–129 CE)
Parthamaspates (c. 116 CE)
Mithridates IV (c. 140 CE)
Vologases IV (c. 147–191 CE)
Vologases V (c. 191–208 CE)
Vologases VI (c. 208–228 CE)
Artabanus IV (c. 216–234/4 CE)

Sasanians

Ardašīr I (223/4–241 CE)
Šāpūr I (c. 240–272/3 CE)
Ohrmazd I (272/3 CE)
Wahrām I (273–276 CE)
Wahrām II (276–293 CE)
Wahrām III (293 CE)
Narseh (293–303 CE)
Ohrmazd II (303–309 CE)

---

[1] Adopted with some changes from Errington and Curtis 2007, and Bopearachchi 2013: 133.

Šāpūr II (309–379 CE)
Ardašīr II (379–383 CE)
Šāpūr III (383–388 CE)
Wahrām IV (388–399 CE)
Yazdegerd I (399–420 CE)
Wahrām V (420–438 CE)
Yazdegerd II (439–457 CE)
Ohrmazd III (457–459 CE)
Pērōz (457/9–484 CE)
Balāš (484–488 CE)
Kavād I (484, 488–496, 499–531 CE)
Jāmāsp (497–499 CE)
Xusrō I (531–579 CE)
Ohrmazd IV (579–590 CE)
Wahrām VI (590–591 CE)
Bištam (591/2–597 CE)
Ohrmazd V (593 CE)
Xusrō II (590, 591–628 CE)
Kavād II (628 CE)
Ardašīr III (628–630 CE)
Xusrō III (629 CE)
Bōrān (630–631 CE)
Āzarmīgdūxt (631 CE)
Ohrmazd VI (?) (631/2 CE)
Yazdegerd III (632–651 CE)

Kushans

Kujula Kadphises (c. 40–90/95 CE)
Vima Takto (c. 90–95 or 95–100 CE)
"Soter Megas" (c. 92/97–110 CE)
Vima Kadphises (c. 100/105–127 CE)
Kanishka I (c. 127–150 CE)
Huvishka (c. 150–190 CE)
Vasudeva I (190–227 CE)
Kanishka II (c. 227–246 CE)
Vasishka (c. 246–267 CE)
Kanishka III (c. 267–280 CE)
Vasudeva II (c. 280–320 CE)
Shaka (c. 320–326 CE).

Kushano-Sasanians

Ardašīr I–II (c. 258–271 CE)
Pērōz I (c. 271–310 CE)
Ohrmazd I (c. 310–325 CE)
Ohrmazd II (c. 325–334 CE)
Pērōz II (c. 334–360 CE)
Wahrām (c. 360–395)

BIBLIOGRAPHY

Abaev, V.I. 1960. "Dokhristianskaya religiya alanov [The Pre-Christian Religion of the Alans]", *Trudy XXV mezhdunarodnogo kongressa vostokovedov* [*Proceedings of the 25th International Congress of Orientalists*], Moscow, 11–15.

———. 1962. "Kul't semi bogov u skifov [The Cult of Seven Gods among Scythians]", in *Drevniy Mir. Akademiku V.V. Struve* [*Ancient World. Academician V.V. Struve Festschrift*], 445–451.

———. 1984. "Avestica", *Orientalia J. Duchesne-Guillemin Emerito Oblata*, (*AI* 23), Leiden, 29–35.

Abdullaev, K. 1994. "Recenziya na: [Review of:] History of Zoroastrianism. Vol. III. Zoroastrianism under Macedonian and Roman Rule, by Mary Boyce and Frantz Grenet with Contribution by Roger Beck, Leiden, 1991", *VDI* 3, 239–245.

———. 1996. "Ellinisticheskaya traditsiya Sogda i Baktrii [The Hellenistic Tradition of Sogdiana and Bactria]", *IMKU* 27, 52–61.

———. 2000. "K attribuzii tronnykh izobrazheniy v Kushanskoy koroplastike [On the Identification of the Enthroned Figures in Kushan Coroplastic Art]", *VDI* 2, 18–30.

———. 2003. "Nana in Bactrian Art", *SRAA* 9, 15–39.

———. 2005. "Les motifs dionysiaques dans l'art de la Bactriane et de la Sogdiane", in Bopearachchi, O. and Boussac, M.-F. (eds.), *Afghanistan ancien carrefour entre l'est et l'ouest*, Turnhout, 227–259.

Abdullaev, K. and Berdimuradov, A.E. 1991. "Novyy pamyatnik sogdiyskogo iskusstva [A New Monument of Sogdian Art]", *VDI* 3, 64–76.

Abdullaev, K.A., Rtveladze, E.V. and Shishkina, G.V. 1991. *Culture and Art of Ancient Uzbekistan: Exhibition Catalogue*, 2 vols, Moscow.

Abka'i-Khavari, M. 2000. *Das Bild des Könings in der Sasanidenzeit*, Hildersheim.

Akhundov, D.A. 1986. *Arkhitektura drevnego i rannesrednevekovogo Azerbaydzhana* [*The Architecture of Ancient and Early Medieval Azerbaijan*], Baku.

Al'baum, L.I. 1975. *Zhivopis' Afrasiaba* [*The Paintings of Afrasiab*], Tashkent.

———. 1990. "Zhivopis' svyatilishcha Fayaztepa [The Paintings of the Fayaztepa Sanctuary]", in Pugachenkova, G.A. (ed.), *Kul'tura Srednego Vostoka: izobrazitel'noe i prikladnoe iskusstvo* [*The Culture of Central Asia: Paintings and the Applied Arts*], Tashkent, 18–28.

Alemany, A. 2000. *Sources on the Alans: A Critical Compilation*, Leiden.

Alram, M. 2004. "The History of the Silk Road as Reflected in Coins", *Parthica* 6, 47–69.

———. 2008. "Early Sasanian Coinage", in Curtis, V.S. and Stewart, S.R.A. (eds.), *The Sasanian Era* (*The Idea of Iran* 3), London and New York, 17–30.

Alram, M. and Gyselen, R. 2003. *Sylloge Nummorum Sasanidarum, Band 1: Ardashir I. – Shapur I.*, Wien.

Alram, M., Blet-Lemarquand, M. and Skjærvø, P.O. 2007. "Shapur, King of Kings of Iranians and Non-Iranians", in Gyselen, R. (ed.), *Des Indo-Grecs aux Sassanides: données pour l'histoire et la géographie historique* (*Res Orientalis* 17), Bures-sur-Yvette, 11–40.

Álvarez-Mon, J. 2010. *The Arjān Tomb. At the Crossroads of the Elamite and the Persian Empires*, (*AI* 49), Leuven.

Ambos, C. 2003. "Nanaja—eine ikonographische Studie zur Darstellung einer altorientalischen Göttin in hellenistisch-parthischer Zeit", *Zeitschrift für Assyriologie* 93/2, 231–272.

Andrés Toledo, M.Á. 2013. "The Dog(s) of the Zoroastrian Afterlife", in Pirart, É. ed., *Le sort des Gâthâs et autres études iraniennes in memoriam Jacques Duchesne-Guillemin*, Leuven, 13–25.

Antonini, C.S. 2003. *Da Alessandro Magno all'Islam. La pittura dell'Asia Centrale*, Roma.

Arevshatyan, S.S. 2008. (ed. and tr.), *Eznik Kokhbazi. Oproverzhenie sekt* [*Eznik Koghbac'i, Refutation of the Sects*], Erevan.

Artamonov, M.I. 1961. "Antropomorfnye bozhestva v religii skifov [Anthropomorphic Deities in the Scythian Religion]", *AGE* 2, 57–88.

Aster, S.Z. 2012. *The Unbeatable Light: Melammu and Its Biblical Parallels*, Münster.

Azarnouche, S. 2013. (ed. and tr.), *Husraw i Kawādān ud rēdag-ē. Khosrow fils de Kawād et un page*, Paris.

Azarnoush, M. 1994. *The Sasanian Manor House at Hājīābād, Iran*, Firenze.

Azarpay, G. 1969. "Nine Inscribed Choresmian Bowls", *Artibus Asiae* 31/2–3, 185–203.

———. 1972. "Crowns and Some Royal Insignia in Early Iran," *IA* 9, 108–115.

———. 1975a. "Some Iranian Iconographic Formulae in Sogdian Painting", *IA* 11, 168–178.

———. 1975b. "Iranian Divinities in Sogdian Painting", *Monumentum H.S. Nyberg*, (*AI 4*), Leiden, 19–29.

———. 1976a. "The Allegory of *Dēn* in Persian Art", *Artibus Asiae 38/1*, 37–49.

———. 1976b. "Nanā, the Sumero-Akkadian Goddess of Transoxania", *JAOS 96 /4*, 536–542.

———. 1981. "The Pictorial Epic in Oriental Art", in Azarpay, G. (ed.), *Sogdian Painting. The Pictorial Epic in Oriental Art*, Berkeley—Los Angeles—London, 79–205.

———. 1995. "A Jataka Tale on a Sasanian Silver Plate", *BAI 9*, 99–127.

———. 1997. "The Sasanian Complex at Bandian: Palace or Dynastic Shrine", *BAI 11*, 193–197.

———. 2000. "Sasanian Art Beyond the Persian World", in Curtis, J. (ed.), *Mesopotamia and Iran in the Parthian and Sasanian Periods: Rejection and Revival c. 238 BC–AD 652*, London, 67–76.

———. 2011. "Imagery of the Sogdian Dēn", in Gyselen, R. and Jullien, C. (eds.), *Florilège offert à Philippe Gignoux pour son 80e anniversaire*, Paris, 53–97.

Back, M. 1978. *Die sassanidischen Staatsinschriften*, (*AI 19*), Tehran and Liège.

Bailey, H.W. 1967. "Saka śśandrāmata", in *Festschrift für Wilhelm Eilers*, Wiesbaden, 136–143.

———. 1971. *Zoroastrian Problems in the Ninth-Century Books*, Oxford.

Bajpakov, K.M. 1998. "Medieval Towns in South Kazakhstan and Semireč'e", *Rivista degli Studii Orientali 72*, 245–263.

Bajpakov, K.M. and Grenet, F. 1992. "Nouvelles données sur la culture sogdienne dans les villes médiévales du Kazakhstan", *SI 21*, 33–45.

Bakhos, C. and Shayegan, M.R. 2010. (eds.), *The Talmud in Its Iranian Context*, Tübingen.

Barkova, L.L. 2009. "Novye issledovaniya importnykh tkaney iz Bol'shikh Altayskikh Kurganov [New Research on Imported Textiles from the Big Altai Kurgans]", *SGE 67*, 5–21.

Barthold, W. 1968. *Turkestan Down to the Mongol Invasion*, London.

Basirov, O. 2001. "Evolution of the Zoroastrian Iconography and Temple Cults", *ANES 38*, 160–177.

Bedjan, P. 1890/1897. *Acta Martyrum et Sanctorum*, 7 vols., Paris.

Belenitskiy, A.M. 1954. "Voprosy ideologii i kul'tov Sogda po materialam Pyandzhikentskikh khramov [The Ideology and the Cults of Sogdiana according to the Material from the Temples of Panjikent]", in Yakubovskiy, A.Yu. (ed.), *Zhivopis' drevnego Pyandzhikenta [The Paintings of Ancient Panjikent]*, Moscow.

———. 1959. "Novye pamyatniki iskusstva drevnego Pyandzhikenta [New Monuments of Art from Ancient Panjikent]", in Belenitskiy, A.M. and Piotrovskiy, B.B. (eds.), *Skul'ptura i zhivopis' drevnego Pyandzhikenta [The Sculpture and the Art of Ancient Panjikent]*, Moscow, 11–87.

———. 1973. *Monumental'noe iskusstvo Pendzhikenta [The Monumental Art of Panjikent]*, Moscow.

———. 1976. "Otchet o raskopkakh na gorodishche drevnego Pendzhikenta v 1972 g. [Panjikent 1972, Excavations Report]", *ART 12*, 85–102.

Belenitskiy, A.M. and Marshak, B.I. 1976. "Cherty mirovozreniya sogdiytsev VII–VIII vv. v iskusstve Pendzhikenta [Features of the Worldview of the Sogdians in the 7th–8th c. CE According to the Art of Panjikent]", in *Istoriya i kul'tura narodov Sredney Azii, drevnost' i srednie veka [The History and Culture of People of Central Asia, Antiquity and the Middle Ages]*, Moscow, 75–89.

———. 1981. "The Paintings of Sogdiana", in Azarpay, G. (ed.), *Sogdian Painting. The Pictorial Epic in Oriental Art*, Berkeley—Los Angeles—London, 11–79.

Belenitskiy, A.M., Marshak, B.I, Raspopova, V.I. and Isakov, A.I. 1983. "Raskopki drevnego Pendzhikenta v 1977 godu [The Excavations of Ancient Panjikent in 1977]", *ART 17*, 187–210.

Benveniste, É. 1929. *The Persian Religion According to the Chief Greek Texts*, Paris.

———. 1932/1933. "Le témoignage de Théodore bar Kônay sur le Zoroastrisme", *Le Monde Oriental 26–27*, 170–215.

Benveniste, É. and Renou, L. 1934. *Vṛtra et Vṛϑragna. Étude de mythologie indo-iranienne*, Paris.

Berdimuradov, A. and Samibaev, M. 2001. "Une nouvelle peinture murale sogdienne dans le temple de Džartepa II (Avec les notes additionnelles par F. Grenet et B. Marshak)", *SI 30*, 45–66.

Berdimuradov, A.E. and Bogomolov, G.I. 2008. "Obraz pritsecheloveka na rel'efakh pogrebal'nykh sooruzheniy sogdiytsev v Severnom Kitae [The Bird-Human Image on Sogdian Burial Reliefs in Northern China]", *IMKU 36*, 171–189.

Berdimuradov, A.E., Bogomolov, G.I., Daeppen, M. and Khushvaktov, N. 2012. "A New Discovery of Stamped Ossuaries near Shahr-i Sabz (Uzbekistan)", *BAI 23*, 137–143.

Bernard, P. 1969. "Quatrième campagne de fouilles d' Aï Khanoum (Bactriane)", *CRAI*, 315–355.

———. 1970. "Campagne de fouilles 1969 à Aï Khanoum en Afghanistan", *CRAI*, 301–349.

———. 1971. "La campagne de fouilles de 1970 à Aï Khanoum (Afghanistan)", *CRAI*, 385–455.

———. 1974. "Fouilles d' Aï Khanoum (Afghanistan) campagnes de 1972 et 1973", *CRAI*, 280–309.

———. 1989. "Āy Ḵānom", *EIr 3*, 124–126.

———. 1990a. "L' Architecture religieuse de l' Asie centrale a l'époque hellenistique", *Akten des XIII internationalen Kongresses fur klassische Archäologie*, Berlin, 51–59.

———. 1990b. "Vicissitudes au gré de l'histoire d'une statue en bronze d'Héraclès entre Séleucie du Tigre et la Mésène", *Journal des savants*, 3–68.
———. 2008. "The Greek Colony at Aï Khanoum and Hellenism in Central Asia", in Hiebert, F. and Cambon, P. (eds.), *Afghanistan, Hidden Treasures from National Museum, Kabul*, Washington, 81–106.
———. 2009. "La découverte et la fouille du site hellénistique d'Aï Khanoum en Afghanistan: comment elles se sont faites", *Parthica 11*, 33–57.
Berndt-Ersoz, S. 2006. *Phrygian Rock-Cut Shrines, Structure, Function and Cult Practice: A Study of Structure, Function, and Cult Practice*, Leiden.
Bessonova, S.S. 1983. *Religioznye predstavleniya skifov [The Religious Views of the Scythians]*, Kiev.
———. 1984. "O kul'te oruzhiya u skifov [On the Cult of Weapons Among Scythians]", in *Vooruzhenie skifov i sarmatov [The Arms of Scythians and Sarmatians]*, Kiev, 3–22.
Bidez, J. and Cumont, F. 1938. *Les mages hellénisés: Zoroastre, Ostanès et Hystaspe d'après la tradition grecque*, 2 vols., Paris.
Bier, L. 1983. "A Sculptured Building Block from Istakhr", *AMI 16*, 307–317.
———. 2009. "*Palais B* at Bishapur and its Sasanian Reliefs", in Gyselen, R. (ed.), *Sources pour l'histoire et la géographie du monde iranien (224–710) (Res Orientales 18)*, Bures-sur-Yvette, 11–41.
Bivar, A.D.H. 1969. *Catalogue of the Western Asiatic Seals in the British Museum. Stamp Seals II: The Sasanian Dynasty*, London.
———. 1998. *The Personalities of Mithra in Archaeology and Literature*, New York.
Brancaccio, P. 2006. "Gateways to the Buddha: Figures under Arches in Early Gandhāran Art", in Brancaccio, P. and Behrendt, K. (eds.), *Gandhāran Buddhism: Archaeology, Art, Texts*, Vancouver, 210–225.
Briant, P. 2002. *From Cyrus to Alexander. A History of the Persian Empire*, Winona Lake.
Brunner, C.J. 1979. "Sasanian Seals in the Moore Collection. Motive and Meaning in Some Popular Subjects", *MMJ 14*, 33–50.
Brykina, G.A. 1982. *Yugo-zapadnaya Fergana v pervoy polovine I tysyacheletiya nashey ery [The Southwestern Ferghana in the First Half of the 1st c. CE]*, Moscow.
Brykina, G.A. and Gorbunova N.G. 1999. "Fergana" in Brykina, G.A. (ed.), *Srenyaya Aziya v rannem Srednevekov'e [Central Asia in Early Mediaeval Period]*, Moscow, 93–114.
Black, J., Green, A. 1992. *Gods, Demons and Symbols of Ancient Mesopotamia*, London.
Boardman, J. 1970. *Greek Gems and Finger Rings*, London.
———. 2000. *Persia and the West. An Archaeological Investigation of the Genesis of Achaemenian Art*, London.
———. 2012. "Tillya Tepe: Echoes of Greece and China", in Aruz, J. and Valtz Fino, E. (eds.), *Afghanistan: Forging Civilizations along the Silk Road*, New York, 102–112.
Boltrik, Yu.V. 1978. "Svyatilishche Areya v urochishche Nosaki [The Sanctuary of Ares in the Nosaki Hole]", *Arkheologicheskie issledovaniya na Ukraine v 1976–1977 gg [Archaeological Research in Ukraine in 1976–1977]*, Uzhgorod.
Bopearachchi, O. 1991. *Monnaies gréco-bactriennes et indo-grecques. Catalogue raisonné*, Paris.
———. 2008. "Les premiers souverains kouchans: chronologie et iconographie monétaire", *Journal des savants*, 3–57.
———. 2012. "Chronology of the Early Kushans: New Evidence", in Jayaswal, V. (ed.), *Glory of the Kushans: Recent Discoveries and Interpretations*, New Delhi, 123–137.
Borisov, A.Ya. 1940. "K istolkovaniyu izobrazheniy na biyanajmanskikh ossuariyakh (VI–VII vv.) [To the Interpretation of Images on Biya-najman Ossuaries (6–7 c. CE.)]", *TOVGE 2*, 25–49.
Bosworth, C.E. 1968. *Sīstān Under the Arabs, From the Islamic Conquest to the Rise of the Ṣaffārids (30–250/651–864)*, Rome.
———. 2002. "Zūn", *EI2 11*, 571.
———. 2008. "The Appearance and Establishment of Islam in Afghanistan", in de la Vassière, É. (ed.), *Islamisation de l'Asie centrale*, Paris, 97–115.
Boyce, M. 1968a. "Rapithwin, Nō Rūz, and the Feast of Sade," in Heesterman, J.C., Schokken, G.H. and Subramoniam, V.I. (eds.), *Pratidānam: Indian, Iranian and Indo-European Studies Presented to Franciscus Bernardus Jacobus Kuiper on his Sixtieth Birthday*, The Hague and Paris, 201–215.
———. 1968b. *The Letter of Tansar*, Roma.
———. 1975a. "Iconoclasm among the Zoroastrians", in Neusner, J. (ed.), *Christianity, Judaism and Other Greco-Roman Cults: Studies for Morton Smith at Sixty*, Leiden, 93–111.
———. 1975b. *A History of Zoroastrianism, vol. 1: The Early Period*, Leiden.
———. 1981. "Varuna the Baga", in *Monumentum Georg Morgenstierne (AI 1)*, Leiden, 59–74.
———. 1982. *A History of Zoroastrianism, vol. 2: Under the Achaemenians*, Leiden.

———. 1984. *Textual Sources for the Study of Zoroastrianism*, Chicago.
———. 1985a. "Ahura Mazdā", *EIr 1*, 684–687.
———. 1985b. "Airyaman", *EIr 1*, 694–695.
———. 1987a. "Apąm Napāt", *EIr 2*, 148–150.
———. 1987b. "Armaiti", *EIr 2*, 413–415.
———. 1989. "Ātaš", *EIr 3*, 1–5.
———. 1993a. "Dahm Yazd", *EIr 6*, 556–557.
———. 1993b. "Corpse", *EIr 6*, 279–286.
———. 1993/1994. "Great Vayu and Greater Varuna", *BAI 7*, 35–41.
———. 2001. "Mithra the King and Varuna the Master", in Schmidt M.G. and Bisang, W. (eds.), *Philologica et Linguistica: Historia, Pluralitas, Universitas. Festschrift für Helmut Humbach zum 80. Geburtstag am 4. Dezember 2001*, Trier, 239–256.
———. 2002. "Fravaši", *EIr 10*, 195–199.
———. 2003. "Haoma ii. The Rituals", *EIr 11*, 662–667.
Boyce, M. and Grenet, F. 1991. *A History of Zoroastrianism, vol. 3: Zoroastrianism under Macedonian and Roman Rule*, Leiden.
Bracey, R. 2012. "Policy, Patronage, and the Shrinking Pantheon of the Kushans", in Jayaswal, V. (ed.), *Glory of the Kushans: Recent Discoveries and Interpretations*, New Delhi, 197–218.
Brock, S.P. 2009. *The History of the Holy Mar Ma'in. With a Guide to the Persian Martyr Acts*, Piscataway NJ.
Brosius, M. 2010a. "The Royal Audience Scene Reconsidered", in Curtis, J. and Simpson, J. (eds.), *The World of Achaemenid Persia. History, Art and Society in Iran and in Ancient Near East*, London, 141–153.
———. 2010b. "Women. i In Pre-Islamic Persia", *EIr, Online Edition*, March 15, 2010, available at http://www.iranicaonline.org/articles/women-i.
Callieri, P. 1990. "On the Diffusion of Mithra Images in Sasanian Iran. New Evidence from a Seal in the British Museum", *EW 40*, 79–99.
———. 1997. *Seals and Sealings from the North-West of the Indian Subcontinent and Afghanistan (4th Century BC–11th Century AD): Local, Indian, Sasanian, Graeco-Persian, Sogdian, Roman*, Naples.
———. 2002. "Regalità, guerra e fecondità: interpretazione iconografica della glittica del Nord-Ovest del subcontinente indiano in età Kusàna", in Antonini, C.S., Alfieri, B.M. and Santoro, A. (eds.), *Oriente e Occidente. Convegno in ricordo di Mario Bussagli*, Roma, 53–65.
———. 2003. "At the Roots of the Sasanian Royal Imagery: The Persepolis Graffiti", in Compareti, M., Raffetta, P. and Scarcia, G. (eds.), *Ērān ud Anērān: Studies presented to Boris Ilich Marshak on the Occasion of His 70th Birthday, Transoxiana Webfestschrift Series I.* http://www.transoxiana.org/Eran/
———. 2006. "Water in the Art and Architecture of the Sasanians", in Panaino, A. and Piras, A. (eds.), *Proceedings of the 5th Conference of the Societas Iranologica Europœa Held in Ravenna, 6–11 October 2003*, vol. 1, Milano, 339–351.
———. 2007. *L'archéologie du Fars à l'époque achéménide: quatre leçons au Collège de France, 8, 15, 22 et 29 mars 2007*, (*Persika 11*), Paris.
———. 2009. "Bishapur: The Palace and the Town", in Gignoux, P., Jullien, C., and Jullien, F. (eds.), *Trésors d'Orient: mélanges offerts à Rika Gyselen*, Paris, 51–67.
Calmeyer, P. 1974. "Zur Genese altiranischer Motive II. Der leere Wagen", *AMI 7*, 49–79.
———. 1975. "The Subject of the Achaemenid Tomb Reliefs", in *Proceedings of the 3rd Annual Symposium on Archaeological Research in Iran. 23rd October-1st November*, Tehran, 233–242.
———. 1977. "Vom Reisehut zur Kaiserkrone: B. Stand der archäologischen Forschung zu den iranischen Kronen", *AMI 10*, 168–191.
———. 1979. "Fortuna—Tyche—Khvarnah," *JDAI 94*, 347–365.
———. 1983. "Simvol Khaldi [The Symbol of Haldi]", *Drevniy Vostok 4*, 179–190.
———. 1993. "Crown I. In the Median and Achaemenid Periods", *EIr 6*, 407–408.
———. 1994. "Babylonische und assyrische Elemente in der achaimenidischen Kunst", in Sancisi-Weerdenburg, H., Kuhrt, A. and Root, M. (eds.), *Continuity and Change* (*Achaemenid History 8*), Leiden, 131–147.
Calmeyer-Seidl, U. 1999. "Eine Triumphstele Darius' I. aus Babylon", in Renger, J. (ed.), *Babylon: Focus mespotamischer Geschichte, Wiege früher Gelehrsamkeit, Mythos in der Moderne*, Saarbrücken, 297–306.
Canepa, M.P. 2009. *The Two Eyes of the Earth. Art and Ritual of Kingship Between Rome and Sasanian Iran*, Berkeley—Los Angeles—London.
———. 2010. "Technologies of Memory in Early Sasanian Iran", *AJA 114 /4*, 563–597.
Cantera, A. 2012. "Preface", in Cantera, A. (ed.), *The Transmission of the Avesta*, Wiesbaden, VII–XIX.
———. 2013. "Talking with God: The Zoroastrian *ham.parsti* or Intercalation Ceremonies", *JA 131.1*, 85–138.
Carter, M.L. 1981. "Mithra on the Lotus", *Monumentum Georg Morgenstierne* (*AI 1*), Leiden, 74–99.

———. 1985. "A Numismatic Reconstruction of Kushano-Sasanian History", *The American Numismatic Society Museum Notes 30*, 215–281.
———. 1986. "Trifunctional Pharro", *SI 15*, 89–98.
———. 1990. "Early Sasanian and Kushano-Sasanian Coinage from Merv", *BAI 4*, 11–17.
———. 1992. "A Scythian Royal Legend from Ancient Uḍḍiyāna", *BAI 6*, 67–79.
———. 1995a. "Aspects of the Imagery of Verethragna: The Kushan Empire and Buddhist Central Asia", in Fragner, B.G. et al. (ed.), *Proceeding of the Second European Conference of Iranian Studies*, Rome, 119–141.
———. 1995b. "OEŠO or Śiva", *BAI 9*, 143–159.
———. 1997. "Preliminary Notes on Four Painted Terracotta Panels", in Allchin, R. and Allchin, B. (eds.), *South Asian Archaeology 1995*, vol. 2, New Delhi and Calcutta, 573–588.
———. 1999/2000. "A Note on Sarapis-like Bust in the Necklace of a Gandhāran Bodhisattva Sculpture in the Norton Simon Musem", *SRAA 6*, 9–19.
———. 2002. "Notes on Two Chinese Stone Funerary Bed Bases with Zoroastrian Symbolism", in Huyse, Ph. (ed.), *Iran: questions et connaissance. Actes du IVe Congrès européen des études iraniennes, Paris, 6–10 septembre 1999*, vol. 1, Paris, 263–287.
———. 2005. "A Silver Statuette from the Oxus Treasure: Aspects of Indo-Iranian Solar Symbolism", in Daneshvari, A. and Gluck, J. (eds.), *A Survey of Persian Art. From the Prehistoric Times to the Present*, vol. 17, Costa Mesa, 1–35.
———. 2006. "Kaniska's Bactrian Pantheon in the Rabatak Inscription", in Panaino, A. and Piras, A. (eds.), *Proceedings of the 5th Conference of the Societas Iranologica Europœa Held in Ravenna, 6–11 October 2003, vol. 1*, Milano, 351–359.
———. 2008. "China and Mysterious Occident: the Queen Mother of the West and Nanā", *RSO 79*, 97–131.
———. 2010. "Nanā with Crescent in Kuṣāṇa Numismatic Imagery", in Franco, E. and Zin, M. (eds.), *From Turfan to Ajanta. Festschrift for Dieter Schlingloff on the Occasion of his Eightieth Birthday*, vol. I, 141–151.
Cazzoli, S. and Cereti, C.G. 2005. "Sealings from Kafir Kala: Preliminary Report", *ACSS 11/1–2*, 133–165.
Cereti, C.G. 1995. *The Zand ī Wahman Yasn: A Zoroastrian Apocalypse*, Roma.
———. 2001. *La letteratura Pahlavi*, Milano.
Chaumont, M.L. 1958. "Le culte de Anāhitā à Stakhr et les premiers Sassanides", *Revue de l'Histoire des Religions 153*, 154–175.
———. 1965. "Le culte de la Anāhitā (Anahit) dans la religion des monarques d'Iran et d'Armenia au Ier siècle de notre ère", *JA 253*, 167–183.
———. 1979. "A propos de la chute de Hatra et du couronnement de Shapur Ier", *AAASH 27*, 207–237.
———. 1985. "Anāhīd iii. The Cult and Its Diffusion", *EIr 1*, 1009–1011.
Chaverdi, A.A., Callieri, P. and Gondet, S. 2013. "Tol-e Ājori, a New Monumental Building in Pārsa: Preliminary Cross Interpretations from Recent Surveys and Excavations Works around Persepolis (2005–2012)", *Arta 2013*.
Choksy, J.K. 1988. "Sacral Kingship in Sasanian Iran", *BAI 2*, 35–52.
———. 1989. "A Sāsānian Monarch, His Queen, Crown Prince and Deities: The Coinage of Wahram II", *AJN 1*, 117–137.
———. 1990. "Gesture in Ancient Iran and Central Asia II: Proskinesis and the Bent Forefinger", *BAI 4*, 201–209.
———. 2002. "In Reverence for Deities and Submission to Kings: A Few Gestures in Ancient Near Eastern Societies", *IA 37*, 7–29.
Chunakova, O.M. 1987. *Kniga deyaniy Ardashira, syna Papaka* [*The Book of Deeds of Ardashir, son of Papak*], Moscow.
———. 1991. *Izvedat' dorogi i puti pravednykh. Pekhleviyskie nazidatel'nye texty* [*Come to Know the Paths of Righteous. The Pahlavi Didactic Texts*], Moscow.
———. 1997. *Zoroastriyskie teksty* [*The Zoroastrian Texts*], Moscow.
———. 2001. *Pekhleviyskaya Bozhestvennaya Komediya. Kniga o Pravednom Viraze (Arda Viraz Namag i drugie teksty)* [*The Pahlavi Divina Comedia. The Book of the Righteous Wiraz (Arda Viraz Namag and Other Texts)*], Moscow.
Chuvin, P. 1999. ed. *Les arts de l'Asie Centrale*, Paris.
Colledge, M.A.R. 1977. *Parthian Art*, London.
———. 1986. *The Parthian Period*, Leiden.
Collon, D. 2001. *Catalogue of the Western Asiatic Seals in the British Museum, vol. 5: Neo-Assyrian and Neo-Babylonian Periods*, London.
Compareti, M. 2000. "Iranian Divinities in the Decoration of Some Dulan and Astana Silks", *Annali di Ca' Foscari 39*, 331–369.
———. 2006a. "Iconographical Notes on Some Recent Studies on Sasanian Religious Art (with an additional note on an Ilkhanid monument, by Rudy Favaro)", *Annali di Ca' Foscari 45/3*, 163–201.

———. 2006b. "The So-Called Senmurv in Iranian Art: A Reconsideration of an Old Theory", in Borbone, P.G., Mengozzi, A., and Tosco, M. (eds.), *Loquentes linguis: Studi linguistici e orientali in onore di Fabrizio A. Pennacchietti*, Wiesbaden, 185–200.
———. 2007. "The Eight Pointed Rosette: A Possible Important Emblem in Sasanian Heraldry", *Parthica 9*, 205–231.
———. 2008. "The Painting of the 'Hunter King' at Karkak", *Annali di Ca' Foscari 47/3*, 131–151.
———. 2009a. "Remarks on the Sogdian Religious Iconography in 7th Century Samarkand", in Pande, A. (ed.), *The Art of Central Asia and the Indian Subcontinent in Cross-Cultural Perspective*, New Delhi, 194–201.
———. 2009b. "The Indian Iconography of the Sogdian Divinities and the Role of Buddhism and Hinduism in its Transmission", *Annali dell'Istituto Orientale di Napoli 69*, 175–210.
———. 2009/2010. "'Holy Animals' of Mazdeism in Iranian Arts: Ram, Eagle and Dog", *NIB 9/1–2*, 27–43.
———. 2013. "Two Seal Impressions from Kāfer Qal'a (Samarkand) and the Representations of Iranian Divinities", *JPS 6*, 127–142.
Compareti, M. and Cristoferetti, S. 2012. "Il fumo iranico della pipa di Perm", in *Mvlta & Varia. Studi offerti a Maria Ferraccioli e Gianfranco Giraudo, Milano, Biblion Edizioni srl*, vol. I, 239–250.
Cornelius, I. 1989. "The Lion in the Art of the Ancient Near East: A Study of Selected Motifs", *JNSL 15*, 53–87.
Cribb, J. 1990. "Numismatic Evidence for Kushano-Sasanian Chronology", *SI 19*, 151–195.
———. 1997. "Shiva Images on Kushan and Kushano-Sasanian Coins", in Tanabe, K., Cribb, J. and Wang, H. (eds.), *Studies in Silk Road Coins and Culture. Papers in Honour of Professor Ikuo Hirayama on his 65th Birthday*, Kamakura, 11–67.
———. 2007. "Money as a Marker of Cultural Continuity and Change in Central Asia", in Cribb, J. and Herrmann, G. (eds.), *After Alexander, Central Asia before Islam, (PBA 133)*, 333–375.
Cristoferetti S. and Scarcia G. forthcoming. "Talking about Sīmurġ and Ṭāq-i Bustān with Boris I. Marshak. (On the so-called Sīmurġ)", in *Proceedings of the International Conference held in St. Petersburg, St. Petersburg, November 16–17–18, 2008*.
Curtis, V.S. 1998. "The Parthian Costume and Headdress", in Wiesehöfer, J. (ed.), *Das Partherreich und seine Zeugnisse: Beiträge des internationalen Colloquiums, Eutin, (27.–30. Juni 1996)*, Stuttgart, 61–75.
———. 2004. "Investiture ii. The Parthian Period", *EIr, Online Edition*, 15 December 2004, available at http://www.iranica.com/articles/investiture.
———. 2007. "Religious Iconography on Ancient Iranian Coins", in Cribb, J. and Herrmann, G. (eds.), *After Alexander. Central Asia before Islam (PBA 133)*, 413–434.
———. 2008. "Royal and Religious Symbols on Early Sasanian Coins", in Kennet, D. and Luft, P. (eds.), *Current Research in Sasanian Archaeology, Art and History*, Oxford, 137–147.
———. 2010. "The Frataraka Coins of Persis: Bridging the Gap between Achaemenid and Sasanian Persia", in Curtis, J. and Simpson, J. (eds.), *The World of Achaemenid Persia. History, Art and Society in Iran and in Ancient Near East*, London, 379–397.
Dalton, O.M. 1964. *The Treasure of the Oxus*, London.
Dandamaev, M.A. 1997. "Assyrian Traditions during Achaemenid Times", in Parpola, S. and Whiting, R.M. (eds.), *Assyria 1995. Proceedings of the 10th Anniversary Symposium of the Neo-Assyrian Text Corpus Project Helsinki, September 7–11, 1995*, Helsinki, 41–48.
Dandamaev, M.A. and Lukonin, V.G. 2004. *The Culture and Social Institutions of Ancient Iran*, Cambridge.
Daryaee, T. 1997. "Religio-Political Propaganda on the Coinage of Khusro II", *AJN 9*, 41–54.
———. 2002. *Šahrestānīhā ī Ērānšahr. A Middle Persian Text on Late Antique Geography, Epic and History*, Costa Mesa.
———. 2006a. "Sasanians and Their Ancestors", in Panaino, A. and Piras, A. (eds.), *Proceedings of the 5th Conference of the Societas Iranologica Europœa Held in Ravenna, 6–11 October 2003*, vol. 1, Milano, 387–395.
———. 2006b. "The Construction of the Past in Late Antique Persia", *Historia 55*, 493–503.
———. 2008. "Kingship in Early Sasanian Iran", in Curtis, V.S. and Stewart, S.R.A. (eds.), *The Sasanian Era (The Idea of Iran 3)*, London and New York, 60–70.
———. 2012. (ed.), *The Oxford Handbook of Iranian History*, Oxford.
Davidson, O.M. 1994. *Poet and Hero in the Persian Book of Kings*, Ithaca and London.
Davis, D. 2006. *Ferdowsi, Shahnameh: The Persian Book of Kings*, New York.
Delehaye, H. 1907. *Les versions grecques des actes des martyrs persans sous Sapor II. Textes grecs et traductions, (Patrologia Orientalis 2/4)*, Paris, 401–560.
Diakonoff, I.M. and Livshits, V.A. 2001. *Parthian Economic Documents from Nisa, Texts I*, London.
Dietrich, M. and Loretz, O. 1992. *'Jahwe und seine Aschera': Anthropomorfisches Kultbild in Mesopotamien, Ugarit und Israel. Das biblische Bilderverbot*, Münster.

Dirven, L. 2009. "My Lord With His Dogs. Continuity and Change in the Cult of Nergal in Parthian Mesopotamia", in Greisiger, L., Rammelt, C. and Tubach, J. (eds.), *Edessa in hellenistisch-römischer Zeit: Religion, Kultur und Politik zwischen Ost und West*, Würzburg, 47–68.

———. 2011. "Religious Frontiers in the Syrian-Mesopotamian Desert", in Heckster, O. and Kaizer, T. (eds.), *Frontiers in the Roman World. Proceedings of the Ninth Workshop of the International Network Impact of Empire (Durham, 16–19 April 2009)*, Leiden, 157–175.

Downey, S. 1988. *Mesopotamian Religious Architecture: Alexander through the Parthians*, Princeton.

Drège, J.-P. and Grenet, F. 1987. "Un temple de l'Oxus près de Takht-i Sangin, d'après un témoignage chinois du VIIIe siècle", *SI 16/1*, 117–121.

Drijvers, J.W. 1999. "Ammianus Marcellinus' Image of Arsaces and Early Parthian History", in Drijvers, J.W. and Hunt, E.D. (eds.), *The Late Roman World and its Historian: Interpreting Ammianus Marcellinus*, London and New York, 193–206.

Druzhinina, A. and Inagaki, Kh. 2008. "Obshchie rezul'taty arkheologicheskikh issledovaniy na gorodishche Takht-i Sangin v 2007 g. [General Results of the Archaeological Excavations at Takht-i Sangin in 2007]", *ART 33*, 101–137.

Duchesne-Guillemin, J. 1966. *Symbols and Values in Zoroastrianism: Their Survival and Renewal*, New York.

———. 1972. "A la rechèrche d'un art mazdéen", *International Congress of Iranian Art and Archaeology V*, Tehran, 265–272.

———. 1974. "Art and Religion under the Sasanians", in Gignoux, Ph. and Taffazoli, A. (eds.), *Memorial Jean de Menasce*, Louvain, 147–168.

———. 1978. "Iran and Greece in Commagene", in Duchesne-Guillemin, J. (ed.), *Études Mithriaques (AI 17)*, Leiden, 187–199.

———. 1985. "Ahriman", *EIr 1*, 670–673.

———. 2002. "Anthropomorphism", *EIr, Online Edition*, 20 July, 2002, available at http://www.iranicaonline.org/articles/anthropomorphism.

Durkin-Meisterernst, D. 2004. *Dictionary of Manichaean Middle Persian and Parthian*, Turnhout.

Dvurechenskaya, N. 2005. "Izuchenie terrakotovoy plastiki Sredney Azii. Drevnost' i rannee srednevekov'e (arkheologicheskiy aspekt)", [The Study of Central Asian Terracottas. Antiquity and Late Antiquity (The Archaeological Aspect)], *PIFK 15*.

D'yakonov, M.M. 1954. "Rospisi Pyandzhikenta i zhivopis' Sredney Azii [The Murals of Panjikent and the Paintings of Central Asia]", *Zhivopis' drevnego Pyandzhikenta [The Paintings of Ancient Panjikent]*, Moscow, 83–159.

D'yakonov, I.M. 1983. "K voprosu o simvole Khaldi [On the Question of the Symbol of Haldi]", *Drevniy Vostok 4*, 190–195.

D'yakonova, N.V. 1961. "Materialy po kul'tovoy ikonografii Tsentral'noy Azii domusul'manskogo perioda [Materials on the Cultic Iconography of Central Asia in the Pre-Islamic Period]", *TGE 5*, 257–272.

D'yakonova, N.V. and Smirnova, O.I. 1967. "K voprosu o kul'te Nany (Anakhity) v Sogdiane [On the Cult of Nana (Anāhitā) in Sogdiana]", *SA 1*, 139–175.

Eichler, S. 1984. *Götter, Genien und Mischwesen in der urartäischen Kunst*, Berlin.

Elizarenkova, T.Ja. 1999. *Rigveda*, vol. 1, Moscow.

Elman, Y. 2007. "Middle Persian Culture and Babylonian Sages: Accommodation and Resistance in the Shaping of Rabbinic Legal Tradition", in Fonrobert, Ch.E. and Jaffe, M.S. (eds.), *The Cambridge Companion to Talmudic Literature*, Cambridge, 165–198.

Emelianov, V.V. 2010. "On the Early History of *melammu*", *Language in the Ancient Near East. Proceedings of the 53e Rencontre assyriologique internationale*, Eisenbrauns, 1109–1119.

Erdmann, K. 1951. "Die Entwicklung der sasanidischen Krone," *Ars Islamica 15/16*, 87–123.

Errington, E. 2002. "Numismatic Evidence for Dating the 'Kaniṣka Reliquary'", *SRAA 8*, 101–121.

Errington, E. and Cribb, J. 1992. *The Crossroads of Asia: Transformation in Image and Symbol*, Cambridge.

Errington, E. and Curtis, J. 2007. (eds.), *From Persepolis to the Punjub. Exploring Ancient Iran, Afghanistan and Pakistan*, London.

Ettinghausen, R. 1972. *From Byzantium to Sasanian Iran and the Islamic World*, Leiden.

Feldman, M.H. 2007. "Darius I and the Heroes of Akkad: Affect and Agency in the Bisitun Relief", in Cheng, J. and Feldman, M.H. (eds.), *Ancient Near Eastern Art in Context: Studies in Honor of Irene J. Winter by Her Students*, Leiden and Boston, 265–295.

Finn, J. 2011. "Gods, Kings, Men: Trilingual Insrciptions and Symbolic Visualizations in the Achaemenid Empire", *Ars Orientalis 41*, 219–275.

Francfort H.-P. 1984. "Le sanctuaire du temple à niches indentées. 2. Les trouvailles", *Fouilles d'Aï Khanoum 3, (MDAFA 27)*, Paris.

———. 2005. "La civilisation de l'Oxus et les Indo-Iraniens", *Āryas, Aryens et Iraniens en Asie Centrale*, Paris, 253–329.

———. 2005/2006. "Archéologie de l'Asie intérieure de l'Âge du Bronze à l'Âge du Fer", *EPHE IV*[3], *Livret-annuaire 21*, 511–520.
———. 2012. "Ai Khanoum 'Temple with Indented Niches' and Takht-i Sangin 'Oxus Temple' in Historical Cultural Perspective: Outline of a Hypothesis About the Cults", *Parthica 12*, 109–137.
Frembgen, J.W. 2012. "The Horse of Imam Hoseyn: Notes on the Iconography of Shi'i Devotional Posters from Pakistan and India", in Khosronejad, P. (ed.), *The Art and Material Culture of Iranian Shi'ism: Iconography and Religious Devotion in Shi'i Islam*, London and New York, 179–195.
Frye, R.N. 1954. *The History of Bukhara by Narshaki*, Cambridge.
———. 1971. *Sasanian Seals in the Collection of Mohsen Foroughi*, London.
———. 1972. "Gestures of Deference to Royalty in Ancient Iran", *IA 9*, 102–108.
———. 1978. "Mithra in Iranian Archaeology", *Études Mithriaques* (*AI 17*), Leiden, 205–211.
———. 1984. *The History of Ancient Iran*, München.
Frye, R.N. and Skjærvø, P.O. 1996/1998. "The Middle Persian Inscription from Meshkinshahr", *BAI 10*, 53–63.
Fukai, S. and Horiuchi, K. 1972. *Taq-i Bustan*, vol. 2, Tokyo.
Fussman, G. 1983. *Surkh Kotal. Tempel der Kuschan-Zeit in Baktrien*, München.
———. 1988. "Une statuette gandharienne de la déesse Śrī", *AIUO 48/1*, 1–9.
———. 1991. "Une effigie en laiton de Śiva au Gandhara", *JA 279*, 137–174.
———. 1998. "L'inscription de Rabatak et l'origine de l'ère śaka", *JA 286*, 571–651.
———. 2012. "Qu'y a-t-il dans un nom: Imrā au Nouristan", in Azarnouche, S. and Redard, C. (eds.), *Yama/Yima, Variations indo-iraniennes sur la geste mythique*, Paris, 67–83.
Gaifman, M. 2008. "The Aniconic Image of the Roman Near East", in Kaizer, T. (ed.), *The Variety of Local Religious Life in the Near East in the Hellenistic and Roman Periods*, Leiden, 37–72.
———. 2010. "Aniconism and the Notion of the 'Primitive' in Greek Antiquity", in Mylonopoulos, J. (ed.), *Divine Images and Human Imaginations in Ancient Greece and Rome*, Leiden, 63–87.
Gariboldi, A. 2004. "Astral Symbology on Iranian Coinage", *EW 54*, 31–55.
Gero, S. 1981. *Barṣauma of Nisibis and Persian Christianity in the Fifth Century*, Leuven.
Gagošidze, J. 1992. "The Temples at Dedoplis Mindori", *EW 42*, 27–48.
Gail, A.J. 1991/1992. "OHÞO = Bhūteśa: Śiva as Lord of the Demons in the Kuṣāṇa Realm", *SRAA 2*, 43–51.
Garrison, M.B. 1999. "Fire Altars", *EIr 9*, 613–619.
———. 2000. "Achaemenid Iconography as Evidenced by Glyptic Art, Subject Matter, Social Function, Audience and Diffusion", in Uehlinger, C. (ed.), *Images as Media. Sources for the Cultural History of the Near East and the Eastern Mediterranean (1st Millennium BCE)*, Göttingen, 115–165.
———. 2011. "By the Favour of Ahuramazdā: Kingship and the Divine in the Early Achaemenid Period", in Iossif, P.P., Chankowski, A.S., and Lorber, C.C. (eds.), *More than Men, Less than Gods: Studies on Royal Cult and Imperial Worship*, Leuven—Paris—Walpole, MA, 15–105.
———. pre-publication. "Visual Representations of the Divine and Numinous in Early Achaemenid Iran: Old Problems, New Directions", *Iconography of Deities and Demons in the Ancient Near East: Electronic Pre-Publication.* http://www.religionswissenschaft.uzh.ch/idd/prepublications/e_idd_iran.pdf.
Garsoïan, N.G. 1985. *Armenia Between Byzantium and the Sasanians*, London.
———. 1989. (ed. and tr.), *The Epic Histories Attributed to P'awstos Buzand*, Cambridge.
Gershevitch, I. 1959. *The Avestan Hymn to Mithra*, Cambridge.
Ghazanfari, K. 2011. *Perceptions of Zoroastrian Realities in the Shahnameh: Zoroaster, Beliefs, Rituals*, Berlin.
Ghirshman, R. 1948. "Etudes iraniennes II: Un ossuaire *en pierre sculptée*", *Artibus Asiae 11*, 292–310.
———. 1954. *Iran from the Earliest Times to the Islamic Conquest*, Harmondsworth.
———. 1962. *Iran. Parthians and Sassanians*, London.
———. 1964. *Persia from the Origins to Alexander the Great*, London.
———. 1970. "Une coupe sasanide à 'scène d'investiture'", in Boyce, M. and Gershevitch, I. (eds.), *W.B. Henning Memorial Volume*, London, 175–180.
———. 1975. "Les scènes d'investiture royale dans l'art rupestre des sassanides et leur origine", *Syria 52*, 119–130.
Ghose, M. 2005. "A Rare Image of the Goddess Nanā from Afghanistan", in Bopearachchi, O. and Boussac, M.-F. (eds.), *Afghanistan ancien carrefour entre l'est et l'ouest*, Turnhout, 259–271.
———. 2006. "Nana: The 'Original' Goddess on the Lion", *JIAAA 1*, 97–113.
Gignoux, Ph. 1978. *Catalogue des sceaux, camées, et bulles sasanides de la Bibliothèque Nationale et du Musée du Louvre. II: Les sceaux et bulles inscrits*, Paris.
———. 1979. "Problèmes de distinction et de priorité des sources", in Harmatta, J. (ed.), *Prolegomena to the Sources on the History of Pre-Islamic Central Asia*, Budapest, 137–141.
———. 1986. *Noms propres sassanides en moyen-perse épigraphique*, Wien.

———. 1989. "Bahman ii. In the Pahlavi Texts", *EIr* 3, 488.
———. 1991. *Les quatre inscriptions du mage Kirdīr. Textes et concordances*, Paris.
———. 1998. "Sāsān ou le dieu protecteur", in Sims-Williams, N. (ed.), *Proceedings of the Third European Conference of Iranian Studies*, Wiesbaden, 1–9.
———. 2005. "A propos de l'anthroponymie religieuse d'époque sassanide", in Weber, D. (ed.), *Languages of Iran: Past and Present. Iranian Studies in Memoriam David Neil MacKenzie*, Weisbaden, 35–42.
———. 2008. "La site de Bandiān revisité", *SI* 37, 163–174.
———. 2009. "Syriac Language ii. Syriac Writings on Pre-Islamic Iran", *EIr*, *Online Edition*, 20 July, 2009, available at http://www.iranica.com/articles/syriac-language-ii-syriac-writings-on-pre-islamic-iran.
Gignoux, Ph. and Gyselen, R. 1982. *Sceaux sasanides de diverses collections privées*, Leuven.
———. 1987. *Bulles et sceaux sassanides de diverses collections*, Paris.
———. 1989. "Sceaux de femmes à l'époque sassanide", *Archaeologia Iranica et Orientalis. Miscellanea in Honorem Louis Vanden Berghe*, Gent, 877–896.
Gignoux, Ph. and Tafazzoli, A. 1993. (ed. and tr.), *Anthologie de Zādspram*, Paris.
Gnoli, G. 1974. "Politique religieuse et conception de la royauté sous les Achéménides", *Commémoration Cyrus. Hommage universel* 2 (*AI* 2), Téhéran and Liège, 117–190.
———. 1980. *Zoroaster's Time and Homeland*, Naples.
———. 1987. "Aštād", *EIr* 2, 826.
———. 1988. "Babylonia ii. Babylonian Influences on Iran", *EIr* 3, 334–336.
———. 1989a. "On Kushan and Avestan Yima", in de Meyer, L. and Haerinck, E. (eds.), *Archaeologia Iranica et Orientalis. Miscellanea in honorem Louis Vanden Berghe*, Gent, 919–928.
———. 1989b. *The Idea of Iran: An Essay on its Origin*, Rome.
———. 1989c. "Bahrām (1) i. In Old and Middle Iranian texts", *EIr* 3, 510–513.
———. 1993/1994. "A Sasanian Iconography of the Dēn", *BAI* 7, 79–87.
———. 1996a. "Farn als Hermes in einer soghdischen Erzählung", in Emmerick, R.E. et al. (ed.), *Turfan, Khotan und Dunhuang: Vorträge der Tagung "Annemarie v. Gabain und die Turfan-forschung," veranstaltet von der Berlin-Brandenburgischen Akademie der Wissenschaften in Berlin (9.-12.12.1994)*, Berlin, 95–100.
———. 1996b. "Note Kuṣāṇa: a proposita di una recente interpretazione di Pharro", *La Persia e l'Asia Centrale da Alessandro al X secolo*, Rome, 685–705.
———. 1999. "Farr(ah)", *EIr* 9, 312–319.
———. 2006. "Indo-Iranian Religion", *EIr* 13, 97–100.
———. 2009. "Some Notes upon the Religious Significance of the Rabatak Inscription", in Sundermann, W., Hintze, A. and De Blois, F. (eds.), *Exegisti monumenta. Festschrift in Honour of Nicholas Sims-Williams*, Wiesbaden, 141–161.
Göbl, R. 1960. "Investitur im sasanidischen Iran und ihre numismatische Bezeugung", *WZKM* 56, 36–51.
———. 1971. *Sasanian Numismatics*, Braunschweig.
———. 1973. *Der Sasanidische Siegelkanon*, Braunschweig.
———. 1983. "Sasanian Coins", in Yarshater, E. (ed.), *The Cambridge History of Iran. vol. 3(1): The Seleucid, Parthian and Sasanian Periods*, Cambridge, 322–343.
———. 1984. *System und Chronologie der Münzprägung des Kušanreiches*, Vienna.
———. 1999. "The Rabatak Inscription and the Date of Kanishka", in Alram, M. and Klimburg-Salter, D.E. (eds.), *Coins, Art, and Chronology: Essays on the pre-Islamic History of the Indo-Iranian Borderlands*, Wien, 151–177.
Godard, A. 1965. *The Art of Iran*, New York.
Goldina, R.D., Pastushenko, I. Ju. and Chernykh, E.M. 2013. "The Nevolino Culture in the Context of the 7th-century East-West Trade: the Finds from Bartym", in Zuckerman, C. (ed.), *Constructing the Seventh Century*, Paris, 865–930.
Goldman, B. 1988. "The Celestial Chariot East and West", *BAI* 2, 87–107.
———. 1991/1992. "Women's Robes: The Achaemenid Era", *BAI* 5, 83–107.
Grantovskiy, E.A. 1998. *Iran i irantsy do akhemenidov* [*Iran and the Iranians before the Achaemenians*], Moscow.
———. 2007. *Rannyaya istoiya iranskikh plemen Peredney Azii* [*The Early History of the Iranian Tribes in the Near East*] (2nd ed.), Moscow.
Gray, L.H. 1913/1914. "Zoroastrian and Other Ethnic Religious Material in the Acta Sanctorum", *JMEOS* 1–2, 37–55.
———. 1929. *The Foundations of the Iranian Religions*, Bombay.
Green, A. 1995. "Ancient Mesopotamian Religious Iconography", in Sasson, J.M. (ed.), *Civilization of the Ancient Near East*, vol. 3, New York, 1837–1855.
Greenwood, T. 2008. "Sasanian Reflections in Armenian Sources", *e-Sasanika* 5. http://www.humanities.uci.edu/sasanika/pdf/e-sasanika5-Greenwood.pdf

Grenet, F. 1984. "Notes sur le panthéon iranien des Kouchans," *SI 13*, 253–262.

———. 1986. "L'art zoroastrien en Sogdiane", *Mesopotamia 21*, 97–131.

———. 1987a. "Interpretatsiya dekora ossuariev iz Biyanajmana i Miankalya [Interpretation of the Decoration of the Ossuaries from Biyanajman and Miankal]", in *Gorodskaya kul'tura Baktrii-Tokharistana i Sogda: Antichnost', Rannee Srednevekov'e [The Urban Culture of Baktria-Tokharistan and Sogd: Antiquity and Late Antiquity]*, Tashkent, 42–54.

———. 1987b. "L'Athéna de Dil'berdzin", in Bernard, P. and Grenet, F. (eds.), *Cultes et monuments religieux dans l'Asie Centrale préislamique*, Paris, 41–45.

———. 1988. "Bagina", *EIr* 3, 15–16.

———. 1991. "Mithra au temple principal d'Aï Khanoum?", in Bernard, P. and Grenet, F. (eds.), *Histoire et cultes de l'Asie centrale preislamique*, Paris, 147–151.

———. 1992. "Note additionnelle sur les panneaux mythologiques du palais de Kujruk-tobe (Keder)", *SI 21*, 46–49.

———. 1993. "Znanie yashtov Avesty v Sogde i Baktrii po dannym ikonografii [The Knowledge of the Yašts of the Avesta in Sogdiana and Bactria According to the Iconography]", *VDI 4*, 149–161.

———. et al. 1993. "Trois nouveaux documents d'iconographie religieuse sogdienne", *SI 22*, 49–69.

———. 1993/1994. "Bāmiyān and the *Mihr Yašt*", *BAI 7*, 87–94.

———. 1995. "Mithra et les planètes dans l'Hindukush central: essai d'interprétation de la peinture de Dokhtar-i Nôshirvân", in Gyselen, R. (ed.), *Au carrefour des Religions: Mélanges offerts à Philippe Gignoux (Res Orientales 7)*, 105–119.

———. 1995/1996a. "Vaiśravaṇa in Sogdiana. About the Origins of Bishamon-ten", *SRAA 4*, 277–299.

———. 1995/1996b. "I) Étude de documents sogdiens; II) Documents sur le zoroastrisme en Asie centrale", *AEPHE 105*, 213–217.

———. 1996. "Crise et sortie de crise en Bactriane-Sogdiane aux IVe–Ve siècles: de l'héritage antique à l'adoption de modèles sassanides", *La Persia e l'Asia Centrale da Alessandro al X secolo*, Rome, 367–391.

———. 1999. "La peinture sassanide de Ghulbiyan (Afghanistan)", *Dossiers d'Archeologie 243*, 66–67.

———. 1999/2000. "I) La perception du zoroastrisme d'Asie centrale par les cultures étrangères; II) Étude de textes sogdiens", *AEPHE 108*, 175–180.

———. 2001/2002. "I) Lecture commentée du Kârnâmag î Ardakhshêr î Pâbagân (suite et fin). II) Le panthéon zoroastrien de la Sogdiane (suite et fin)", *AEPHE 110*, 207–211.

———. 2002a. "Regional Interaction in Central Asia and Northwest India in the Kidarite and Hephthalite periods", in Sims-Williams, N. (ed.), *Indo-Iranian Languages and People*, (*PBA 116*), 203–224.

———. 2002b. "Zoroastrian Themes on Early Medieval Sogdian Ossuaries", in Godrej, P.J. and Mistree, F.P. (eds.), *A Zoroastrian Tapestry*, Middletown, 90–98.

———. 2003a. "Mithra, dieu iranien: nouvelles données", *Topoi 11*, 35–59.

———. 2003b. *La Geste d'Ardashir fils de Pâbag*, Paris.

———. 2003c. "Pour une nouvelle visite à la 'vision de Kerdīr'", *Studia Asiatica 1–2*, 5–27.

———. 2005. "An Archaeologist's Approach to Avestan Geography", in Curtis, V.S. and Stewart, S. (eds.), *The Birth of Persian Empire, (The Idea of Iran 3)*, London and New York.

———. 2006. "Mithra ii. Iconography in Iran and Central Asia", *EIr, Online Edition*, 15 August 2006, available at http://www.iranica.com/articles/mithra-2-iconography-in-iran-and-central-asia.

———. 2006/2010. "Iranian Gods in Hindu Garb. The Zoroastrian Pantheon of the Bactrians and Sogdians, Second—Eighth Centuries", *BAI 20*, 87–101.

———. 2007. "Religious Diversity Among Sogdian Merchants in Sixth-Century China: Zoroastrianism, Buddhism, Manichaeism, and Hinduism", *Comparative Studies of South Asia, Africa and the Middle East 27/2*, 463–478.

———. 2009. "Le rituel funéraire zoroastrien du sedra dans l'imagerie sogdienne", in Gignoux, P., Jullien, C., and Jullien, F. (eds.), *Trésors d'Orient. Mélanges offerts à Rika Gyselen*, Paris, 103–113.

———. 2010. "Cosa sappiamo dei pellegrinaggi nel mondo iraniano preislamico?", in Balbeo, A. and Piano, S. (eds.), *La bisaccia del pellegrino: fra evocazione e memoria*, Torino, 167–183.

———. 2008/2012. "Mary Boyce's Legacy for the Archaeologists", *BAI 22*, 29–47.

———. 2012a. "Yima en Bactriane et en Sogdiane: nouveaux documents", in Azarnouche, S. and Redard, C. (eds.), *Yama/Yima, Variations indo-iraniennes sur la geste mythique*, Paris, 83–95.

———. 2012b. "The Nomadic Element in the Kushan Empire (1st–3rd century AD)", *JCES 3*, 1–22.

———. 2013. "Some Hitherto Unrecognized Mythological Figures on Sasanian Seals: Proposed Identifications", in Tokhtasev, S. and Lurje, P. (eds.), *Commentationes Iranicae. Vladimiro f. Aaron Livschits nonagenario donum natalicium*, Saint Petersburg, pp. 201–211.

———. forthcoming a. "Zoroastrianism among the Kushans", in Boyce, M. and De Jong, A. (eds.), *A History of Zoroastrianism, vol. IV: Parthian Zoroastrianism*, Leiden.

———. forthcoming b. "Le panthéon iranien illustré des Sogdiens: système ou bricolage?", *Colloque franco-japonais, Interactions et translations culturelles en Eurasie. Traditions narratives et figuratives* (12–13 décembre 2002).
Grenet, F. and Azarnouche, S. 2007/2012. "Where are the Sogdian Magi?", *BAI* 21, 159–179.
Grenet, F. and Zhang Guangda. 1996. "The Last Refuge of the Sogdian Religion: Dunhuang in the Ninth and Tenth Centuries", *BAI* 10, 175–187.
Grenet, F. and Khasanov, M. 2009. "The Ossuary from Sangyr-tepe (Southern Sogdiana): Evidence of the Chionite Invasions", *JIAAA* 4, 69–81.
Grenet, F. and Marshak, B.I. 1998. "Le mythe de Nana dans l'art de la Sogdiane", *Arts Asiatiques* 53, 5–18.
Grenet, F. and Pinault, G.-J. 1997. "Contacts des traditions astrologiques de l'Inde et de l'Iran d'après une peinture des collections de Turfan", *CRAI*, 1003–1061.
Grenet, F., Riboud, P. and Yang Junkai. 2004. "Zoroastrian Scenes on a Newly Discovered Sogdian Tomb in Xi'an, Northern China", *SI* 33, 273–284.
Grenet, F., Lee, J., Martinez, Ph. and Ory, F. 2007. "The Sasanian Relief at Rag-i Bibi (Northern Afghanistan)", in Cribb, J. and Herrmann, G. (eds.), *After Alexander, Central Asia before Islam*, (*PBA* 133), 257–261.
Gubaev, A. 1971. "Sasanidskie bully iz zamka Ak-Depe (predvaritel'naya publikatsiya) [The Sasanian Bullae from Fortress Ak-Depe (Preliminary Publication)]", *EV* 20, 46–50.
Gubaev, A.G., Loginov, S.D., and Nikitin, A.B. 1996. "Sasanian Bullae from the Excavations of Ak-Depe by the Station of Artyk", *Iran* 34, 55–61.
Giuliano, L. 2004. "Studies in Early Śaiva Iconography: (I) The Origin of the triśula Some Related Problems", *SRAA* 10, 51–97.
Gvelesiani, M. 2008. "The Notion of Iranian *x^{v}arənah* in Post-Achaemenid Georgian Kingship", *JPS* 1, 174–182.
Gyselen, R. 1990. "Note de glyptique sassanide. Quelques éléments d'iconographie religieuse", in Vallat, F. (ed.), *Contribution à l'histoire de l'Iran. Mélanges offerts à Jean Perrot*, Paris, 253–269.
———. 1993. *Catalogue des sceaux, camées et bulles sassanides de la Bibliothèque Nationale et du Musée du Louvre. I. Collection générale*, Paris.
———. 1995a. "Les Sceaux des Mages de l'Iran Sassanide", in Gyselen, R. (ed.), *Au Carrefour des Religions. Mélanges offerts à Philippe Gignoux*, Bures-sur-Yvette, 121–151.
———. 1995b. "Une scène de banquet rituel dans la glyptique sassanide", in Fragner, B.G. et al. (ed.), *Proceeding of the Second European Conference of Iranian Studies*, Rome, 245–255.
———. 2000. "Un dieu nimbé de flammes d'époque sassanide", *IA* 35, 291–314.
———. 2001. *The Four Generals of the Sasanian Empire: Some Sigillographic Evidence*, Rome.
———. 2003. "Les grands Feux de l'empire sassanide: quelques témoignages sigillographiques", in Cereti, C.G., Maggi, M., and Provasi, E. (eds.), *Religious Themes and Texts of Pre-Islamic Iran and Central Asia: Studies in Honour of Professor Gherardo Gnoli on the Occasion of his 65th Birthday on 6th December 2002*, Wiesbaden, 131–138.
———. 2004. "New Evidence for Sasanian Numismatics: The Collection of Ahmad Saeedi", *Contributions à l'histoire et la géographie historique de l'empire sassanide* (*Res Orientales XVI*), Bures-sur Yvette, 49–140.
———. 2007. *Sasanian Seals and Sealings in the A. Saeedi Collection* (*AI* 44), Louvain.
———. 2005/2009. "Vahrām III (293) and the Rock Relief of Naqsh-i Rustam II: A Contribution to the Iconography of Sasanian Crown Princes in the Third Century", *BAI* 19, 29–37.
———. 2010a. "Romans and Sasanians in the Third Century: Propaganda Warfare and Ambiguous Imagery", in Börm, H. and Wiesehöfer, J. (eds.), *Commutatio et Contentio. Studies in the Late Roman, Sasanian, and Early Islamic Near East in Memory of Zeev Rubin*, Düsseldorf, 71–89.
———. 2010b. "Les Wahramides (273–293 A.D.): quelques aspects de leur langage monétaire", *SI* 39, 185–223.
———. 2010c. "'Umayyad' Zāvulistān and Arachosia: Copper Coinage and the Sasanian Monetary Heritage", in Alram, M. et al. (eds.), *Coins, Art and Chronology II. The First Millenium C.E. in the Indo-Iranian Borderlands*, Wien, 219–245.
Hackin, J. 1959. "La monastère bouddhique de Fondukistan (fouilles de J. Carl, 1937)," *MDAFA* 8, 48–59.
Haerinck, E. 2003. "Again on Tang-i Sarvak II, NE-Side. Goddesses Do Not Have Moustaches and Do Not Wear Trousers", *IA* 38, 221–246.
Haerinck, E. and Overlaet, B. 2008. "Altar Shrines and Fire Altars: Architectural Representations on Frataraka Coinage", *IA* 43, 207–233.
Hämeen-Anttila, J. 2006. *The Last Pagans of Iraq: Ibn Wahshiyya And His Nabatean Agriculture*, Leuven.
Hannestad, L. and Potts, D. 1990. "Temple Architecture in the Seleucid Kingdom", in Bilde, P. (ed.), *Religion and Religious Practice in the Seleucid Kingdom*, Aarhus, 91–124.
Harper, P.O. 1971. "Sources of Certain Female Representations in Sasanian Art," in *Atti del convegno internazionale sul tema: La Persia nel Medioevo*, Rome, 503–515.

———. 1978. *The Royal Hunter. Art of the Sasanian Empire*, New York.
———. 1979. "Thrones and Enthronement Scenes in Sasanian Art", *Iran 17*, 49–64.
———. 1983. "Sasanian Silver", in Yarshater, E. (ed.), *The Cambridge History of Iran. vol. 3(2): The Seleucid, Parthian and Sasanian Periods*, Cambridge, 1113–1130.
———. 1999. "Geographical Location and Significant Imagery: Taq-i Bostan", in Alram, M. and Klimburg-Salter, D.E. (eds.), *Coins, Art, and Chronology: Essays on the pre-Islamic History of the Indo-Iranian Borderlands*, Wien, 315–321.
———. 2006. *In Search of a Cultural Identity: Monuments and Artifacts of the Sasanian Near East, 3rd to 7th Century A.D.*, New York.
Hawting, G.R. 1999. *The Idea of Idolatry and the Emergence of Islam*, Cambridge.
Henkelman, W.F.M. 1995/1996. "The Royal Achaemenid Crown", *AMI 28*, 275–295.
———. 2003. "An Elamite Memorial: the *šumar* of Cambyses and Hystaspes", in Henkelman, W.F.M. and Kuhrt, A. (eds.), *Essays in Memory of Heleen Sancisi-Weerdenburg*, Leiden, 101–173.
———. 2008. *The Other Gods who are: Studies in Elamite-Iranian Acculturation Based on the Persepolis Fortification Texts*, Leiden.
———. 2011. "Parnakka's Feast: *šip* in Pārsa and Elam", in Álvarez-Mon, J. and Garrison, M.B. (eds.), *Elam and Persia*, Winona Lake, 89–167.
Henning, W.B. 1945. "Sogdian Tales", *BSOAS 11/3*, 445–487.
———. 1968. "Ein persischer Titel im Altaramäischen", *Memoriam Paul Kahle*, Berlin, 138–145.
Herman, G. 2005. "Ahasuerus the Former Stable-Master of Belshazzar, and the Wicked Alexander of Macedon: Two Parallels between the Babylonian Talmud and Persian Sources," *AJSReview 29/2*, 283–298.
———. 2006. "Iranian Epic Motifs in Josephus' Antiquities (XVIII, 314–370)", *JJS 57/2*, 245–269.
———. 2012. *A Prince Without a Kingdom. The Exilarch in the Sasanian Era*, Tübingen.
———. forthcoming. "'Like a Slave Before his Master' A Persian Gesture of Deference in Sasanian Jewish and Christian Sources", *Proceedings of the Aram Twenty Eighth International Conference on 'Zoroastrianism in the Levant', which was held at The Oriental Institute, the University of Oxford, 5–7 July 2010, Aram.*
Herrmann, G. 1977. *Naqsh-i Rustam 5 and 8, Sasanian Reliefs Attributed to Hormuzd II and Narseh, (Iranische Denkmäler 8)*, Berlin.
———. 1981. *The Sasanian Rock Reliefs at Bishapur: Part 2, (Iranische Denkmäler 10)*, Berlin.
———. 1983. *The Sasanian Rock Reliefs at Bishapur: Part 3, (Iranische Denkmäler 11)*, Berlin.
———. 1996. "Dārāb (2). iii. Rock Reliefs", *EIr 7*, 7.
Herrmann, G. and Curtis, V.S. 2002. "Sasanian Rock Reliefs", *EIr, Online Edition*, 20 July 2002, available at http://www.iranica.com/articles/sasanian-rock-reliefs.
Herzfeld, E. 1930. *Kushano-Sasanian Coins*, Calcutta.
———. 1939. "Khusraus II Krone: Al tādj al-kabīr. Die Kronen der sasanidischen Könige", *AMI 9*, 101–159.
Hespel, R. and Draguet, R. 1982. *Théodore bar Koni. Livre des scolies (recension de Séert)*, 2 vols, Louvain.
Hintze, A. 1998. "The Migrations of the Indo-Iranians and the Iranian Sound-Change *s* ⟩ *h*", in Meid, W. (ed.), *Sprache und Kultur der Indogermanen. Akten der X. Fachtagung der Indogermanischen Gesellschaft, Innsbruck, 22.-28. September 1996*, Innsbruck, 139–153.
———. 1999. "The Saviour and the Dragon in Iranian and Jewish/Christian Eschatology", in Shaked, S. and Netzer, A. (eds.), *IJ 4*, Jerusalem, 72–91.
———. 2009. "Avestan Literature", in Emmerick, R.E. and Macuch, M. (eds.), *The Literature of Pre-Islamic Iran (A History of Persian Literature 17)*, London and New York, 1–72.
———. 2012. "On the Prophetic and Priestly Authority of Zarathustra", in Choksy, J.K. and Dubeansky. J. (eds.), *Gift to a Magus. Indo-Iranian Studies Honoring Firoze Kotwal*, New York, 43–59.
Hinz, W. 1969. *Altiranische Funde und Forschungen*, Berlin.
Hoffmann, G. 1880. *Auszüge aus syrischen Akten persischer Märtyrer*, Leipzig.
Hollard, D. 2010. "Julien et Mithrā sur le relief de Tāq-e-Bostān", in Gyselen, R. (ed.), *Sources for the History of Sasanian and Post-Sasanian Iran, (Res Orientalis 19)*, Bures-sur-Yvette, 147–165.
Holloway, S.W. 2002. *Aššur is King! Aššur is King!*, Leiden.
Horn, P. 1893. *Grundriss der neupersischen Etymologie*, Strassburg.
Houtkamp, J. 1991. "Some Remarks on the Fire Altars of the Achaemenid Period", in Kellens, J. (ed.), *La religion iranienne à l'époque achéménide*, Gent, 23–49.
Huff, D. 2004. "Archaeological Evidence of Zoroastrian Funerary Practices", in Stausberg, M. (ed.), *Zoroastrian Rituals in Context*, Leiden and Boston, 593–631.
———. 2008. "Formation and Ideology of the Sasanian State in the Context of Archaeological Evidence", in Curtis, V.S. and Stewart, S.R.A. (eds.), *The Sasanian Era (The Idea of Iran 3)*, London and New York, 31–59.

Hultgård, A. 1993. "Trône de Dieu et trône des justes dans les traditions de l'Iran ancient", in Philonenko, M. (ed.), *Le Trône de Dieu*, Tübingen, 1–18.
Humbach, H. 1975a. "Vayu, Śiva und der Spiritus Vivens im Ostiranischen Synkretismus", in *Monumentum H.S. Nyberg, vol. 1 (AI 4)*, Teheran and Liège, 397–408.
———. 1975b. "Mithra in the Kuṣāṇa Period", in Hinnels, J. (ed.), *Mithraic Studies*, vol. 1, Manchester, 135–142.
———. 2002. "Yama/Yima/Jamšēd, King of Paradise of the Iranians", *JSAI 26*, 68–77.
Humbach, H. and Skjærvø, P.O. 1983. *The Sasanian Inscription of Paikuli. Parts 3.1 and 3.2, Restored Text and Translation*, Wiesbaden.
Humbach, H. and Faiss, K. 2012. *Herodotus's Scythians and Ptolemy's Central Asia: Semasiological and Onomasiological Studies*, Wiesbaden.
Huyse, Ph. 1990. *Iranische Namen in den griechischen Dokumenten Ägyptens*, Wien.
———. 2006. "Die sasanidische Königstitulatur: Eine Gegenüberstellung der Quellen", in Wiesehöfer, J. and Huyse, Ph. (eds.), *Ērān ud Anērān: Studien zu den Beziehungen zwischen dem Sasanidenreich und der Mittelmeerwelt*, München, 181–203.
———. 2009. "Inscriptional Literature in Old and Middle Iranian Languages", in Emmerick, R.E. and Macuch, M. (eds.), *The Literature of Pre-Islamic Iran (A History of Persian Literature 17)*, London and New York, 72–116.
Ilyasov, D.Ya. 1999. "Shakhrevar v Chaganiane [Shahrewar in Chaganian]", *Izuchenie kul'turnogo naslediya Vostoka [The Study of the Cutural Heritage of the Orient]*, Saint Petersburg, 141–142.
Ingholt, H., Seyrig, H. and Caquot, A. 1955. *Receuil des tessères de Palmyre*, Paris.
Invernizzi, A. 2001. "Arsacid Dynastic Art", *Parthica 3*, 133–157.
———. 2005. "Representations of Gods in Parthian Nisa", *Parthica 7*, 71–80.
———. 2010. "A Goddess on the Lion from Susa", *PIFK 1*, 28–35.
Ivantchik, A. 2011. "Novye grecheskie nadpisi iz Takhti Sangina i problema vozniknoveniya baktriyskoy pis'mennosti [New Greek Inscriptions from Takht-i Sangin and the Problem of the Origin of the Bactrian Script]", *VDI 4*, 110–131.
Ivantchik, A.I. and Lurje, P.B. 2013. "Dve nadpisi iz Chirik-rabata [Two Inscriptions from Chirik-rabat]", in Tokhtasev, S. and Lurje, P. (eds.), *Commentationes Iranicae. Vladimiro f. Aaron Livschits nonagenario donum natalicium*, Saint Petersburg, pp. 286–295.
Jaafari-Dehaghi, M. 1998. *Dādestān ī dēnīg, Part I*, Paris.
Jackson, A.V.W. 1914. "Allusions in Pahlavi Literature to the Abomination of Idol-worship" in Modi, J.J. (ed.), *Sir Jamsetjee Jejeebhoy Madressa Jubilee Vol. 1*, Bombay, 274–285.
———. 1915. "Images and Idols (Persian)", *The Encyclopaedia of Religion and Ethics*, vol. 7, 151–155.
Jacobs, B. 1987. "Das Chvarnah. Zum Stand der Forschung", *MDOG 119*, 215–248.
———. 1991. "Der Sonnengott im Pantheon der Achämeniden", in Kellens, J. (ed.), *La religion iranienne à l'époque achéménide*, Gent, 49–80.
———. 2000. "Die Religionspolitik des Antiochus I. von Kommagene", in Wagner, J. (ed.), *Gottkönige am Euphrat*, Mainz, 45–49.
———. 2001. "Kultbilder und Gottesvorstellung bei den Persern. Zu Herodot, Historiae 1.131 und Clemens Alexandrinus, Protrepticus 5.65.3", in Bakır T. (ed.), *Achaemenid Anatolia. Proceedings of the First International Symposium on Anatolia in the Achaemenid Period, Bandırma 15–18 August 1997*, Leiden, 83–90.
Jamasp-Asana, J.D.M. 1992. *Pahlavi Texts (Transcription, Translation)*, Tehran.
Jamzadeh, P. 1982. "The Winged Ring with Human Bust in Achaemenid Art as a Dynastic Symbol", *IA 17*, 91–99.
———. 1989. "Bahrām (1) ii. Representation in Iranian Art", *EIr 3*, 513–514.
Jolivet, J. and Monnot, G. 1993. *Shahrastani. Livre des religions et des sects*, vol. 2, Leuven.
De Jong, A. 1995. "Khvarenah", in van der Toorn, K., Becking, B. and van der Horst, P.W. (eds.), *Dictionary of Deities and Demons in the Bible*, Leiden, 903–908.
———. 1997. *Traditions of the Magi: Zoroastrianism in Greek and Latin Literature*, Leiden.
———. 2003a. "Heracles", *EIr, Online Edition*, 15 December 2003, available at http://www.iranicaonline.org/articles/heracles-gk.
———. 2003b. "Women and Ritual in Medieval Zoroastrianism", in Cereti, C.G. and Vajifdar, F. (eds.), *Ātaš-e Dorun. The Fire Within. Jamshid Soroush Soroushian Memorial Volume*, Vol. 2, 148–161.
———. 2003c. "Zoroastrian Self-Definition in Contact with Other Faiths", *IJ 5*, 17–27.
———. 2004. "Sub specie maiestatis: Reflections on Sasanian Court Rituals", in Stausberg, M. (ed.), *Zoroastrian Rituals in Context*, Leiden and Boston, 345–365.
———. 2005. "The Contribution of the Magi", in Curtis, V.S. and Stewart, S. (eds.), *The Birth of Persian Empire, (The Idea of Iran 3)*, London and New York, 85–100.

———. 2006. "One Nation under God? The Early Sasanians as Guardians and Destroyers of Holy Sites", in Kratz, R.G. and Spieckermann, H. (eds.), *Götterbilder, Gottesbilder, Weltbilder. Polytheismus und Monotheismus in der Welt der Antike*, vol. 1, Tübingen, 223–241.
———. 2009. "The Culture of Writing and the Use of the Avesta in Sasanian Iran", in Pirart, É. and Tremblay, X. (eds.), *Zarathushtra entre l'Inde et l'Iran: études indo-iraniennes et indo-européennes offertes à Jean Kellens à l'occasion de son 65e anniversaire*, Wiesbaden, 27–42.
———. 2010a. "Religion at the Achaemenid Court", in Jacobs, B. and Rollinger, R. (eds.), *Der Achämenidenhof*, Wiesbaden, 533–559.
———. 2010b. "Ahura Mazdā the Creator", in Curtis, J. and Simpson, J. (eds.), *The World of Achaemenid Persia. History, Art and Society in Iran and in Ancient Near East*, London, 85–91.
———. 2008/2012. "Regional Variation in Zoroastrianism: The Case of the Parthians", *BAI 22*, 17–29.
Jullien, C. 2008. "Martyrs, Christian", *EIr, Online Edition*, December 15, 2008, available at http://www.iranica.com/articles/martyrs-christian
Kaim, B. 2009. "Investiture of Mithra. Towards a New Interpretation of So Called Investiture Scenes in Parthian and Sasanian Art", *IA 44*, 403–415.
Kaizer, T. 2002. *The Religous Life of Palmyra*, Stuttgart.
Kalmykov, A.D. 1909. "Otkrytie V.N. Kastal'skogo 'Biyanajmanskie ossuarii' [The Discovery of V.N. Kastal'skiy 'Biyanajman Ossuaries'", *PTKLA 13*.
Kalmin, R. 2006a. "The Formation and Character of the Babylonian Talmud", in Katz, S. (ed.), *The Cambridge History of Judaism, vol. 4, The Late Roman-Rabbinic Period*, Cambridge, 840–876.
———. 2006b. *Jewish Babylonia between Persia and Roman Palestine*, Oxford.
———. 2008. "Idolatry in Late Antique Babylonia: The Evidence of the Babylonian Talmud", in Eliav, Y.Z., Friedland, E.A. and Herbert, S. (eds.), *The Sculptural Environment of the Roman Near East: Reflections on Culture, Ideology, and Power*, Leuven, 629–659.
———. 2010. "Talmudic Attitudes Toward Dream Interpreters: Preliminary Thoughts on their Iranian Cultural Context", in Bakhos, C. and Shayegan, M.R. (eds.), *The Talmud in Its Iranian Context*, Tübingen, 83–100.
Karimova, G.R. and Kurbanov, Sh.F. 2008. "Mural Painting from Panjikent (to the Problem of Symbols and Cults)", *BMM 8*, 185–216.
Kastal'skiy, B.N. 1909. "Biyanajmanskie ossuarii [The Ossuaries from Biyanajman]", *PTKLA 13*.
Kawami, T.S. 1987. *Monumental Art of the Parthian Period in Iran*, (*AI 26*), Leiden.
Keel, O. and Uehlinger, C. 1998. *Gods, Goddesses and Images of God in Ancient Israel*, Philadelphia.
Kekelidze, K. 1936. "Itrujani", *TSUS 1*, 266–270.
Kellens, J. 1984. "Yima, magicien entre les dieux et les homes", *Orientalia J. Duchesne-Guillemin emerito oblate*, (*AI 23*), Leiden, 267–281.
———. 1996. "Drvāspā", *EIr 7*, 565.
———. 1998. "Considérations sur l'histoire de l'Avesta", *JA 286/2*, 451–519.
———. 2002. "L'idéologie religieuse des inscriptions achéménides", *JA 290*, 417–464.
———. 2002/2003. "Le problème avec Anāhitā", *Orientalia Suecana 51/52*, 317–327.
———. 2013. "Les Achéménides et l'Avesta", *Séptimo centenario de los estudios orientales en Salamanca*, Salamanca, 551–559.
Khakimov, A. 2004. ed. *Masterpieces of the Samarkand Museum*, Tashkent.
Khaleghi-Motlagh J. 1988/2008. *Abu'l-Qasem Ferdowsi. The Shahnameh* (*The Book of Kings*), Vols. 1–8, New York.
Kidd, F., et al. 2004/2008. "Ancient Chorasmian Mural Art", *BAI 18*, 69–97.
Kiperwasser, R. forthcoming. "The Encounter Between the Iranian Myth and Rabbinic Mythmakers in the Babylonian Talmud", in Gabbay, U. and Secunda, Sh. (eds.), *Encounters by the Rivers of Babylon: Scholarly Conversations between Jews, Iranians, and Babylonians*, Tübingen.
Kiperwasser, R. and Shapira D.Y. 2008. "Irano-Talmudica I: The Three-Legged Ass and *Ridyā* In B. Ta 'Anith: Some Observations About Mythic Hydrology In the Babylonian Talmud and In Ancient Iran", *AJS Review 32/1*, 101–116.
———. 2012. "Irano-Talmudica II: Leviathan, Behemoth and the "Domestication" of Iranian Mythological Creatures in Eschatological Narratives of the Babylonian Talmud", in Fine, S. and Secunda, Sh. (eds.), *Shoshannat Yaakov: Jewish and Iranian Studies in Honor of Yaakov Elman*, Leiden and Boston, 203–237.
———. forthcoming. "Irano-Talmudica III: Interwoven: Between Bestiarium Iranicum to Bestiarium Rabbinicum, Between Avestan and Pslams, Bundahishn and Babylonian Talmud", in Rubanovich, J. (ed.), *Orality and Textuality in the Iranian World: Patterns of Interaction across the Centuries*, Leiden.
Kipiani, G. 2004. "Achaemenian Heritage in Ancient Georgian Architecture", *ANES 41*, 167–191.
Klimburg-Salter, D. 1993. "Dokhtar-i-Noshirwan (Nigar) Reconsidered", *Muqarnas 10*, 355–368.

Klimkeit, H.-J. 2001. "The Question of Image Worship in Manichaeism", in Sedov, A.V. (ed.), *Drevnie Tsivilizatsii Evrazii: Istoriya i Kul'tura [Ancient Civilizations of Eurasia: History and Culture]*, Moscow, 219–227.

Knauss, F.S. 2005. "Caucasus", in Boucharlat, R. and Briant, P. (eds.), *L'Archéologie de l'empire achéménide: nouvelles recherches*, Paris, 197–217.

Knauss, F.S. 2006. "Ancient Persia and the Caucassus", *IA 41*, 79–118.

Koch, H. 1995. "Theology and Worship in Elam and Achaemenid Iran", in Sasson, J.M. (ed.), *Civilizations of the Ancient Near East*, vol. 3, New York, 1950–1969.

Korol'kova, E.F. 2006. *Vlastiteli stepey [The Rulers of the Steppes]*, Saint-Petersburg.

Koshelenko, G.A. and Gaibov, V.A. 2010a. "Numizmaticheskie dannye po probleme tsarskogo kul'ta v Parfii [Numismatic Data on the Royal Cult in Parthia]", *VDI 3*, 169–179.

———. 2010b. "Novye postupleniya v numizmaticheskuyu kollektsiyu Gosudarstvennogo istoricheskogo muzeya [New Acquisitions of the Numismatic Collection of the State Historical Museum]", *VDI 1*, 190–195.

Kossolapov, A.J. and Marshak, B.I. 1999. *Stennaya zhivopis' Sredney i Tsentral'noy Azii [Murals Along the Silk Road]*, Saint-Petersburg.

Kotwal, F.M. 1969. *The Supplementary Texts to the Šāyest nē-šāyest*, Copenhagen.

———. 1984. "Review of Kaikhusroo M. JamaspAsa (ed. and tr.), Aogəmadaēcā: A Zoroastrian Liturgy", *Indo-Iranian Journal 27*, 163–166.

Kramers, J.H. and Wiet, G. 1964. *Ibn Ḥauqal. Configuration de la terre (Kitab surat al-ard)*, Beyrouth and Paris.

Krasnowolska, A. 1998. *Some Key Figures of Iranian Calendar Mythology: Winter and Spring*, Kraków.

Krauss, S. 1940. *Persia and Rome in Talmud and Midrashim*, (in Hebrew), Jerusalem.

Kreyenbroek, Ph.G. 1985. *Sraoša in the Zoroastrian Tradition*, Leiden.

———. 2008/2012. "On the Construction of Zoroastrianism in Western Iran", *BAI 22*, 47–57.

Kröger, J. 1982. *Sasanidischer Stuckdekor. Ein Beitrag zum Reliefdekor aus Stuck in sasanidischer und frühislamischer Zeit*, Mainz.

Kruglikova, I.T. 1976. "Nastennye rospisi Dil'berdzhina [The Wall Paintings of Dilberjin]", *Drevnyaya Baktriya: materialy Sovetsko-Afganskoy ekspeditsii 1969–1973 gg, t. 1 [Ancient Bactria: Excavations of Soviet-Afghan Expedition 1969–1973, vol. 1]*, Moscow, 87–111.

———. 1977. "Idoly iz Dil'berdzhina [Idols from Dilberjin]", *Istoriya i kul'tura antichnogo mira [The History and Culture of the Ancient World]*, Moscow, 86–91.

———. 1979. "Nastennye rospisi v pomeshchenii 16 severo-vostochnogo kul'tovogo kompleksa Dil'berdzhina [Wall Paintings in the 16th South-East Cultic Complex at Dilberdjin]", *Drevnyaya Baktriya: materialy Sovetsko-Afganskoy ekspeditsii 1969–1973 gg, t. 2 [Ancient Bactria: Excavations of Soviet-Afghan Expedition 1969–1973, vol. 2]*, Moscow, 120–145.

———. 1982. "Dil'berdzhin—kushanskiy gorod v severnom Afganistane [Dilberjin—the Kushan City in Northern Afghanistan]", *Arkheologiya Starogo i Novogo Sveta [The Archaeology of Old and New Worlds]*, Moscow, 153–176.

Kuhrt, E. 2010. "Achaemenid Images of Royalty and Empire", in Lanfranchi, G.B. and Rollinger, R. (eds.), *Concepts of Kingship in Antiquity*, Padova, 87–107.

Kuz'mina, E.E. 2002. *Mifologiya i iskusstvo skifov i baktriytsev [Mythology and Art of Scythians and Bactrians]*, Moscow.

Ladynin, I.A. 2011. "Statuya Dariya I iz Suz: k interpretazii pamyatnika v svete religiozno-ideologicheskikh predstavleniy Egipta i Perednego Vostoka [The Statue of Darius I from Susa: an Essay of Interpretation in the Light of Egyptian and Near Eastern Religious and Ideological Notions]", *VDI*, 3–28.

Lazard, G., Grenet, F. and De Lamberterie, Ch. 1984. "Notes Bactriennes", *SI 13*, 199–233.

Lecoq, P. 1984. "Un problème de religion achémenide: Ahura Mazda ou Xvarnah?", *Orientalia J. Duchesne-Guillemin Emerito Oblata (AI 23)*, Leiden, 301–326.

———. 1997. *Les inscriptions de la Perse achéménide*, Paris.

Lee, J. and Grenet, F. 1998. "New Light on the Sasanid Painting at Ghulbiyan, Faryab Province, Afghanistan", *South Asian Studies 14*, 75–85.

Lemaire, A. 2003. "Les pierres et inscriptions araméennes d'Arebsun, nouvel examen", in Shaked, S. and Netzer, A. (eds.), *IJ 5*, 138–165.

Lerner, J.A. 1975. "A Note on Sasanian Harpies", *Iran 13*, 166–171.

———. 2009. "Animal Headdresses on the Sealings of the Bactrian Documents", in Sundermann, W., Hintze, A. and de Blois, F. (eds.), *Exegisti monumenta: Festschrift in Honour of Nicholas Sims-Williams (Iranica 17)*, Wiesbaden, 371–386.

———. 2010. "An Achaemenid Cylinder Seal of a Woman Enthroned", in Curtis, J. and Simpson, J. (eds.), *The World of Achaemenid Persia. History, Art and Society in Iran and in Ancient Near East*, London, 153–165.

Lerner, J.A. and Sims-Williams, N. 2011. *Seals, Sealings and Tokens from Bactria to Gandhara (4th to 8th century CE)*, Vienna.
Lerner, K.B. 2004. *The Wellspring of Georgian Historiography: The Early Medieval Historical Chronicle, the Conversion of K'art'li and the Life of St. Nino*, London.
Levit-Tawil, D. 1992. "The Sasanian Rock Relief at Darabgird—A Re-Evaluation", *JNES 51/3*, 161–180.
Lewis, T.J. 1998. "Divine Images: Aniconism in Ancient Israel", *JAOS 118*, 36–53.
Litvinskiy, B.A. 1968. *Kangyuysko-sarmatskiy farn* [*The Kangju-Sarmatian Farn*], Dushanbe.
———. 2001a. *Khram Oksa v Baktrii, tom 2, Baktriyskoe vooruzhenie v drevnevostochnom i grecheskom kontekste* [*The Temple of the Oxus in Bactria, vol. 2, The Bactrian Arms and Armor in the Near Eastern and Greek Context*], Moscow.
———. 2001b. "Fondoqestān", *EIr 10*, 78–79.
———. 2010. *Khram Oksa v Baktrii, tom 3, iskusstvo, khudozhestvennoe remeslo, muzykal'nye instrumenty* [*The Temple of Oxus in Bactria, vol. 3, Art, Fine Art, Musical Instruments*], Moscow, 2010.
Litvinskiy, B.A. and Pichikyan, I.R. 2000. *Ellinisticheskiy khram Oksa v Baktrii* [*The Hellenistic Temple of the Oxus in Bactria*], Moscow.
Litvinskiy, B.A., Vinogradov, Yu.G. and Pichikyan, I.R. 1985. "Votiv Atrosoka iz khrama Oksa v Severnoy Baktrii [Offering of Atrosokes from the Temple of Oxus in Northern Bactria]", *VDI 4*, 84–110.
Livshits, V.A. 2004. "Nadpisi i dokumenty [Inscriptions and Documents]", in Vainberg, B.I. (ed.), *Kalaly-Gyr II. Kul'tovyy tsentr v drevnem Khorezme IV–II vv. do n.e.* [*Kalali-Gir II. The Cultic Center in Acient Chorasmia 4th–2nd centuries BCE*], Moscow, 188–213.
———. 2008. "Parfyanskie khozyaystvennye dokumenty na ostrakakh iz Nisy [The Parthian Documents on Ostraca from Nisa]", *TGE 39*, 105–110.
———. 2010. "Sogdiyskie 'Starye pis'ma' (II, IV, V). Vstuplenie, perevod i primechaniya V.A. Livshitsa [The Sogdian 'Ancient Letters' (II, IV, V). Introduction, Translation and Notes by V.A. Livshits", *VDI 3*, 238–244.
Livshits, V.A. and Nikitin, A.B. 1991. "The Parthian Epigraphic Remains from Göbekli-depe and Some Other Parthian Inscriptions", in Emmerick, R.E. and Weber, D. (eds.), *Corolla Iranica: Papers in Honour of Prof. Dr. David Neil MacKenzie on the Occasion of his 65th Birthday on April 8th, 1991*, 109–127.
Lo Muzio, C. 1994/1995. "OHÞO: A Sovereign God", *SRAA 4*, 161–175.
———. 2008/2012. "Remarks on the Paintings from the Buddhist Monastery of Fayaz Tepe (Southern Uzbekistan)", *BAI 22*, 189–207.
Lordkipanidze, O. 2001. "Introduction to the History of Caucassian Iberia and its Culture of the Achaemenid and Post-Achaemenid Periods", *AMI 32*, 3–19.
Loth, A.-M. 2003. *Védisme et hindouisme, images du divin et des dieux*, Paris.
Loukonine, V. and Ivanov, A. 2003. *Persian Art*, London.
Lubotsky, A. 1998. "Avestan *x^varənah-*: the Etymology and Concept", in Meid, W. (ed.), *Sprache und Kultur. Akten der X. Fachtagung der Indogermanischen Gesellschaft Innsbruck, 22.-28. September 1996*, Innsbruck, 479–488.
Lukonin, V.G. 1969. *Kul'tura sasanidskogo Irana* [*The Culture of Sasanian Iran*], Moscow.
———. 1971. "Po povodu bull iz Ak-Depe [On the Bullae from Ak-Depe]", *EV 20*, 50–53.
———. 1977. *Iskusstvo drevnego Irana* [*The Art of Ancient Iran*], Moscow.
———. 1987. *Drevniy i rannesrednevekovyy Iran* [*The Ancient and Early Medieval Iran*], Moscow.
Lukonin, V.G and Borisov, A.Ya. 1963. *Sasanidskie gemmy* [*Sasanian Gemstones*], Leningrad.
Lunina, S.B. and Usmanova, Z.I. 1985. "Unikal'nyy ossuariy iz Kashkadar'i", *ONU 3*, 46–51.
Lurje, P.B. 2004. *Istoriko-lingvisticheskiy analiz sogdiyskoy toponimii* [*Historico-linguistic Analysis of Sogdian Toponimy*], Unpublished PhD Dissertation, Saint-Petersburg.
———. 2010. *Personal Names in Sogdian Texts*, Wien.
Luschey, H. 1968. "Studien zu dem Darius-Relief von Bisutun", *AMI 1*, 63–94.
———. 1987. "Ardašīr I ii. Rock Reliefs", *EIr 2*, 377–380.
Mac Dowall, D.W. 1975. "The Role of Mithra among the Deities of the Kuṣāṇa Coinage", in Hinnels, J. (ed.), *Mithraic Studies I*, Manchester, 142–150.
———. 2007. "Coinage from Iran to Gandhāra—with Special References to Divinities as Coins Types", in Srinivasan, D.M. (ed.), *On the Cusp of an Era. Art in Pre-Kuṣaṇa World*, Leiden, 233–267.
Macuch, M. 1981. *Das sasanidische Rechtsbuch. Mātakdān i hazār dātistān* (Teil II), Wiesbaden.
Maenchen-Helfen, O.J. 1973. *The World of the Huns*, Berkley.
Malandra, W. 2013. "What's in a Name?", in Choksy, J.K. and Dubeansky. J. (eds.), *Gift to a Magus. Indo-Iranian Studies Honoring Firoze Kotwal*, New York, 105–103.
Malek, M. 2002. "The Sasanian king Husro II and Anāhitā", *NIB 2/1*, 23–45.

Mann, R. 2001/2005. "Parthian and Hellenistic Influences on the Development of Skanda's Cult in North India: Evidence from Kuṣaṇa-Era Art and Coins", *BAI* 15, 111–129.
———. 2012. *The Rise of Mahāsena. The Transformation of Skanda-Kārttikeya in North India from the Kuṣāṇa to Gupta Empires*, Leiden.
Marr, N.Ya. 1902. "Bogi yazycheskoy Gruzii po drevne-gruzinskim istochnikam [The Gods of Pagan Georgia according to the Ancient Georgian Sources]", *Zapiski vostochnogo otdeleniya Imperatorskago russkago arheologicheskago obshchestva 14/2–3 [Proceedings of the Oriental Section of the Russian Imperial Archaeological Society]*, 1–30.
Marshak, B.I. 1983. "Monumental'naya zhivopis' Sogda i Tokharistana v rannem srednevekov'e [The Monumental Paintings of Soghd and Tokharistan in the Early Medieval Period]", in Litvinskiy, B.A. et al. (ed.), *Baktriya-Tokharistan na drevnem i srednevekovom Vostoke [Bactria-Tokharistan in the Ancient and the Medieval Orient]*, Moscow, 53–55.
———. 1987. "Iskusstvo Sogda [The Art of Sogd]", in Pyotrovskiy B., Bongard-Levin, G. (eds.), *Tsentral'naya Aziya: Novye pamyatniki pis'mennosti i iskusstva [Central Asia: New Monuments of Epigraphy and Art]*, Minsk.
———. 1989. "Bogi, demony i geroi pendzhikentskoy zhivopisi [Gods, Demons, and Heroes in the Paintings of Panjikent]", in *Itogi rabot arheologicheskikh ekspeditsiy Gosudarstvennogo Ermitazha: Sbornik nauchnykh trudov [Proceedings of State Hermitage Archaeological Expeditions]*, Leningrad, 115–127.
———. 1990. "Les fouilles de Pendjikent", *CRAI*, 286–313.
———. 1995/1996. "On the Iconography of Ossuaries from Biya-Naiman", *SRAA* 4, 299–321.
———. 1996. "New Discoveries in Pendjikent and a Problem of Comparative Study of Sasanian and Sogdian Art", *La Persia e l'Asia Centrale da Alessandro al X secolo*, Rome, 425–439.
———. 1998. "The Decoration of Some Late Sasanian Silver Vessels and its Subject-Matter", in Curtis, V.S., Hillenbrand, R., and Rogers, J.M. (eds.), *The Art and Archaeology of Ancient Persia. New Light on the Parthian and Sasanian Empires*, London, 84–93.
———. 1999. "Sogd V–VIII vv. Ideologiya po pamyatnikam iskusstva [Sogdiana in the 5th–8th c. Ideology according to the Monuments of Art]", in Brykina, G.A. (ed.), *Srenyaya Aziya v rannem Srednevekov'e [Central Asia in Early Medieval Period]*, Moscow, 175–192.
———. 2000. "The Ceilings of the Varakhsha Palace", *Parthica* 2, 153–171.
———. 2001. "La thématique sogdienne dans l'art de la Chine de la seconde moitié du VIe siècle", *CRAI*, 227–264.
———. 2002a. "Zoroastrian Art in Iran under the Parthians and the Sasanians", in Godrej, P.J. and Mistree, F.P. (eds.), *A Zoroastrian Tapestry*, Middletown, 135–149.
———. 2002b. *Legends, Tales, and Fables in the Art of Sogdiana*, New York.
———. 2002c. "Pre-Islamic Painting of the Iranian People and its Sources in Sculpture and the Decorative Arts", in Sims, E. (ed.), *Peerless Images: Persian Painting and Its Sources*, New Heaven and London, 7–20.
———. 2004. "The Miho Couch and the Other Sino-Sogdian Works of Art of the Second Half of the 6th Century", *BMM* 4, 16–31.
———. 2009. *Iskusstvo Sogda [The Sogdian Art]*, Saint Petersburg.
Marshak, B.I. and Negmatov, N.N. 1996. "Sogdiana", in Litvinsky, B.A. (ed.), *History of Civilizations of Central Asia*, vol. 3, Paris, 233–281.
Marshak, B.I. and Raspopova, V.I. 1990. "Wall Paintings from a House with a Granary. Panjikent, 1st Quarter of the Eight Century A.D.", *SRAA* 1, 123–177.
———. 1991. "Cultes communautaires et cultes privés en Sogdiane", in Bernard, P. and Grenet, F. (eds.), *Histoire et cultes de l'Asie centrale préislamique*, Paris, 187–201.
———. 1994/1996. "Worshipers from the Northern Shrine of Temple II, Panjikent", *BAI* 8, 187–209.
———. 2003. "Otchet o raskopkah gorodishcha drevnego Pendzhikenta v 2002 g. [Excavations of Panjikent in 2002]", *MPAE* 5, 3–57.
Marshak, B.I., Raspopova, V.I. and Shkoda, V.G. 1999. "Otchet o raskopkah gorodishcha drevnego Pendzhikenta v 1998 g. [Excavations of Panjikent in 1998]", *MPAE* 1, 3–44.
Martinez-Sève, L. 2010. "À propos du temple aux niches indentées d'Aï Khanoum: quelques observations", in Carlier, P. and Lerouge-Cohen, Ch. (eds.), *Paysage et religion en Grèce antique*, Paris, 195–208.
Masson, M.E. and Pugachenkova, G.A. 1954. "Ottiski parfyanskikh pechatey iz Nisy [Stamp Impressions of Parthian Seals from Nisa]", *VDI* 4, 159–169.
Mayrhofer, M. 1973. *Onomastica Persepolitana. Das altiranische Namengut der Persepolis-Täfelchen*, Wien.
Mathiesen, H.E. 1993. *Sculpture in the Parthian Empire*, Aarhus.
de Menasce, P. 1938. "Autour d'un texte syriaque inédit sur la religion des Mages", *BSOS* 9/3, 587–601.
———. 1945. *Une apologétique mazdéenne du IXe siècle: Škand-Gumānīk Vičār: La solution décisive des doutes*, Fribourg.

Merrillees, P.H. 2005. *Catalogue of the Western Asiatic Seals in the British Museum, vol. 6: Pre-Achaemenid and Achaemenid Periods*, London.
Mettinger, T.N.D. 1995. *No Graven Image? Israelite Aniconism in its Ancient Near Eastern Context*, Stockholm.
———. 2006. "A Conversation with my Critics: Cultic Image or Aniconism in the First Temple?", in Amit, Y. et al. (ed.) *Essays on Ancient Israel in Its Near Eastern Context*, Winona Lake, 273–296.
Millar, F. 1998. "Dura-Europos under Parthian Rule", in Wiesehöfer, J. (ed.), *Das Partherreich und seine Zeugnisse*, Stuttgart, 473–493.
Minardi, M. 2013. "A Four Armed Goddess from Ancient Chorasmia: History, Iconography and Style of an Ancient Chorasmian Icon", *Iran 51*, 111–143.
Mitchell, S. 2007. "Iranian Names and the Presence of Persians in the Religious Sanctuaries of Asia Minor", in Matthews, E. (ed.), *Old and New Worlds in Greek Onomastics* (*PBA*), Oxford, 151–173.
Mkrtychev, T.K. 2002. *Buddiyskoe iskusstvo Sredney Azii (I–X vv)* [*The Buddhist Art of Central Asia (1st–10th c.)*], Moscow.
———. 2004. "Buddiyskoe i nebuddiyskoe iskusstvo Baktrii-Tokharistana (I–V vv. n. e.) [The Buddhist and Non-Buddhist Art of Bactria-Tokharistan (1st–5th Centuries CE.)]", in Nikonorov, V.P. (ed.), *Tsentral'naya Aziya ot Akhemenidov do Timuridov* [*Central Asia from Achaemnians to Timurids*], Saint Petersbourg, 350–353.
Mkrtychev, T.K. and Naimark, A.I. 1991. "Soghdian Ossuaries", in Abdullaev, K.A., Rtveladze, E.V. and Shishkina, G.V. (eds.), *Culture and Art of Ancient Uzbekistan: Exhibition Catalogue*, vol. 2, Moscow, 64–66.
Möbius, H. 1967. "Die Göttin mit dem Löwen", in Wiessner, G. (ed.), *Festschrift für Wilhelm Eilers: Ein Dokument der internationalen Forschung zum 27. September 1966*, Wiesbaden, 449–468.
Mode, M. 1991/1992. "Sogdian Gods in Exile—Some Iconographic Evidence from Khotan in the Light of Recently Excavated Material from Sogdiana", *SRAA 2*, 179–215.
———. 1992. "The Great God of Dokhtar-e Noshirwān (Nigār)", *EW* 42, 473–483.
———. 1996. "Doḵtar-e Nōšervān", *EIr 8*, 474–475.
Molé, M. 1967. *Le legende de Zoroastre selon les textes pehlevis*, Paris.
Moorey, P.R.S. 1979. "Aspects of Worship and Ritual on Achaemenid Seals", *Akten des VII. Internationalen Kongresses für Iranische Kunst und Archäologie München 7.-10. September 1976*, 218–226.
Morony, M.G. 1976. "The Effects of the Muslim Conquest on the Persian Population of Iraq", *Iran 14*, 41–59.
———. 2005. *Iraq After The Muslim Conquest*, Piscataway.
Mosig-Walburg, K. 2009. "Sonderprägungen Khusros II. (590–628): Innenpolitische Propaganda vor dem Hintergrund des Krieges gegen Byzanz", in Gyselen, R. (ed.), *Sources pour l'histoire et la géographie du monde iranien (224–710)* (*Res Orientales 18*), Bures-sur-Yvette, 185–209.
Movassat, J.D. 2005. *The Large Vault at Taq-i Bustan: A Study in Late Sasanian Royal Art*, Lewiston.
Mukherjee, B.N. 1969. *Nanā on Lion. A Study in Kushāna Numismatic Art*, Calcutta.
Mukherjee, B.N. 1988. *The Rise and Fall of the Kushāṇa Empire*, Calcutta.
Mukhtarov, A.M. 1982. "Shedevry v edinstvennom chisle [The Unique Masterpieces]", in Fayziev, Kh. (ed.), *Puteshestvie v Sogdianu* [*A Journey to Sogdiana*], Dushanbe, 5–49.
Murgotten, F.C. 1924. *The Origins of the Islamic State*, New York.
Mylonopoulos, J. 2010. "Divine Images versus Cult Images. An Endless Story About Theories, Methods, and Terminologies", in Mylonopoulos, J. (ed.), *Divine Images and Human Imaginations in Ancient Greece and Rome*, Leiden, 1–21.
Narten, J. 1989. "Bahman i: In the Avesta", *EIr 3*, 487–488.
Naveh, J. and Shaked, S. 2012. *Aramaic Documents from Ancient Bactria.* (*fourth century BCE.*)*; From the Khalili Collections*, London.
Naymark, A.I. 1988. "Tipy arkadnykh kompozitsyy v iskusstve Sogda VI–VIII v.v. [The Types of Arcade Compositions in the Sogdian Art of 7th–8th c.]", *Drevniy i srednevekovyy Vostok* [*Ancient and Medieval Orient*] 2, Moscow, 282–287.
Naymark, A.I. 1995. "O nachale chekanki mendoy monety v Bukhare [On the Beginning of Copper Coinage Minting in Bukhara]", *NTA 1*, 29–51.
Negmatov, N.N. 1984. "Bozhestvennyy i demonicheskiy panteony Ustrushany i ikh indoiranskie paralleli [The Divine and Demonic Pantheons of Ustrushana and their Indo-Iranian Parallels]", *Drevnie kul'tury Sredney Azii i Indii* [*Ancient Cultures of Central Asia and India*], Leningrad, 146–164.
der Nersessian, S. 1944/1945. "Une apologie des images du septième siècle", *Byzantion 17*, 58–88.
Nikitin, A.B. 1993/1994. "Parthian Bullae from Nisa", *SRAA 3*, 71–81.
Nikitin, A.B. and Roth, G. 1995. "A New Seventh-Century Countermark with a Sogdian Inscription", *Numismatic Chronicle 155*, 277–279.
Nikonorov, V.P. 1997. *The Armies of Bactria 700 BC–450 AD*, vol. 1, Stockport.

Novotny, S. 2007. "The Buddhist Monastery of Fondukistān—A Reconstruction", *JIAAA* 2, 31–37.
Oettinger, N. 2009. "Zum Verhältnis von Apąm Napāt- und *X ͮarənah-* im Avesta", in Pirart, É. and Tremblay, X. (eds.), *Zarathushtra entre l'Inde et l'Iran: études indo-iraniennes et indo-européennes offertes à Jean Kellens à l'occasion de son 65e anniversaire*, Wiesbaden, 189–196.
Olbrycht, M.J. 1997. "Parthian King's Tiara—Numismatic Evidence and Some Aspects of Arsacid Political Ideology", *Zapiski Numizmatyczne/Notae Numismaticae* 2, 27–61.
———. 1998. *Parthia et ulteriores gentes: Die politischen Beziehungen zwischen dem arsakidischen Iran und den Nomaden der eurasischen Steppen*, München.
———. 2003. "Parthia and Nomads of Central Asia. Elements of Steppe Origin in the Social and Military Developments of Arsacid Iran", in Schneider, I. (ed.), *Mitteilungen des SFB "Differenz und Integration" 5: Militär und Staatlichkeit, Orientwissenschaftliche Hefte 12.2003*, Halle, 69–109.
Ol'khovskiy, V.S. 1991. *Pogrebal'no-pominal'naya obryadnost' naseleniya Stepnoy Skifii (VII–III vv. do n.e.)* [*The Funeral and Commemorative Rites of the Population of Steppe Scythia (7–3 c. BCE)*], Moscow.
Orbeli, I.A. and Trever, K.V. 1935. *Sasanidskiy metall* [*The Sasanian Metal*], Moscow and Leningrad.
Ornan, T. 2001. "Ištar as Depicted on Finds from Israel", in Mazar, A. (ed.), *Studies in the Archaeology of the Iron Age in Israel and Jordan*, Sheffield, 235–256.
———. 2005a. *The Triumph of the Symbol: Pictorial Representations of Deities in Mesopotamia and the Biblical Image Ban*, Fribourg and Göttingen.
———. 2005b. "A Complex System of Religious Symbols: The Case of the Winged-Disc in First-Millennium Near Eastern Imagery", in Suter C.E. and Uehlinger, Ch. (eds.), *Crafts and Images in Contact: Studies on Eastern Mediterranean Minor Art of the 1st Millennium BCE*, Fribourg and Göttingen, 207–241.
———. 2007. "The Godlike Semblance of a King: The Case of Sennacherib's Rock Reliefs", in Cheng, J. and Feldman, M.H. (eds.), *Ancient Near Eastern Art in Context. Studies in Honor of Irene J. Winter by Her Students*, Leiden and Boston, 161–178.
———. 2009. "In the Likeness of Man: Reflections on the Anthropocentric Perception of the Divine in Mesopotamian Art", in Porter, B.N. (ed.), *What is God? Anthropomorphic and Non-Anthropomorphic Aspects of Deity in Ancient Mesopotamia*, Winona Lake, 93–153.
Overlaet, B. 2013. "And Man Created God? Kings, Priests and Gods on Sasanian Investiture Reliefs", *IA* 48, 313–354.
Panaino, A. 1995. *Tištrya, 2 vols.*, Roma.
———. 2000. "The Mesopotamian Heritage of Achaemenian Kingship", in Aro, S. and Whiting, R.M. (eds.), *The Heirs of Assyria. Proceedings of the Opening Symposium of the Assyrian and Babylonian Intellectual Heritage Project. Held in Tvärminne, Finland, October 8–11, 1998 (Helsinki: The Neo-Assyrian Text Corpus Project 2000)*, Helsinki, 35–49.
———. 2002a. "The 'bagān' of the Fratarakas: Gods or 'divine' Kings?", in Cereti, C., Maggi, M. and Provasi, E., (eds.), *Religious Themes and Texts of Pre-Islamic Iran and Central Asia*, Wiesbaden, 283–306.
———. 2002b. *The Lists of Names of Ahura Mazdā (Yašt I) and Vayu (Yašt XV)*, Rome.
———. 2004. "Astral Character of Kingship in the Sasanian and Byzantine Worlds", *La Persia e Bisanzio. Atti del Convegno internazionale (Roma, 14–18 ottobre 2002)*, Rome, 555–594.
———. 2005. "Tištrya", *EIr, Online Edition*, July 20, 2005, available at http://www.iranica.com/articles/tistrya-2.
———. 2005/2009. "Sheep, Wheat, and Wine: An Achaemenian Antecedent of the Sasanian Sacrifices *pad ruwān*", *BAI* 19, 111–119.
———. 2009a. "The King and the Gods in the Sasanian Royal Ideology," in Gyselen, R. (ed.), *Sources pour l'histoire et la géographie du monde iranien (224–710) (Res Orientales 18)*, Bures-sur-Yvette, 209–256.
———. 2009b. "The Bactrian Royal Title βαγ[η]-ζνογο / βαγο-ιηζνογο and the Kušān Dynastic Cult", in Sundermann, W., Hintze, A., and de Blois, F. (eds.), *Exegisti monumenta: Festschrift in Honour of Nicholas Sims-Williams*, Wiesbaden, 331–346.
———. 2012. "The Age of the Avestan Canon and the Origins of the Ritual Written Texts", in Cantera, A. (ed.), *The Transmission of the Avesta*, Wiesbaden, 70–98.
Panofsky, E. 1962. *Studies in Iconology*, New York and Evanton.
Parpola, A. 2002. "From the Dialects of Old Indo-Aryan to Proto-Indo-Aryan and Proto-Iranian", in Sims-Williams, N. (ed.), *Indo-Iranian Languages and People*, (*PBA* 116), 43–103.
Patrich, J. 1990. *The Formation of Nabatean Art*, Jerusalem.
Pavchinskaya, L.V. 1983. "Ossuariy iz Moullakurgana [The Ossuary from Mullakurgan]", *ONU* 3, 46–49.
———. 1994. "Sogdian Ossuaries", *BAI* 8, 209–227.
Pavchinskaya, L.V. and Rostovzev, O.M. 1988. "Ossuarii iz Sarytepe [The Ossuaries from Sarytepe]", *IMKU* 22, 91–101.
Peck, E.H. 1993. "Crown ii. From the Seleucids to the Islamic Conquest", *EIr* 6, 408–418.
Pellat, Ch. 1965. (ed. and tr.), *Masʿūdī, Les prairies d'or*, vol. 2, Paris.

Perevodchikova, E.V. 1994. *Yazyk zverinykh obrazov* [*The Language of Anymal Images*], Moscow.

Perikhanian, A. 1997. (ed. and tr.), *The Book of a Thousand Judgements* (*A Sasanian Law-Book*), Costa Mesa.

Pichikyan, I.R. 1991. *Kul'tura Baktrii. Akhemenidskiy i ellinisticheskiy periody* [*The Culture of Bactria. The Achaemenian and the Hellenistic Periods*], Moscow.

Polos'mak, N.V. 2004. *Vsadniki Ukoka* [*The Horsemen of Ukok*], Novosibirsk.

Pope, A.U. and Ackerman, Ph. 1964–1981. (ed.), *A Survey of Persian Art. From Prehistoric Times to the Present*, 16 vols., London and New York.

Porada, E. 1965. *Ancient Iran: The Art of the Pre-Islamic Times*, London.

Porter, B.N. 2009. "Introduction", in Porter, B.N. (ed.), *What is God? Anthropomorphic and Non-Anthropomorphic Aspects of Deity in Ancient Mesopotamia*, Winona Lake, 1–15.

Potts, D.T. 2001. "Nana in Bactria", *SRAA 7*, 23–37.

———. 2002. "An Ass for Ares", *BAI 16*, 103–117.

———. 2004. "The Numinous and the Immanent. Some Thoughts on Kurangun and the Rudkhaneh-e Fahliyan", in von Folsach, K., Thrane, H. and Thuesen, I. (eds.), *From Handaxe to Khan. Essays Presented to Peder Mortensen on the Occasion of his 70th Birthday*, Aarhus, 143–156.

———. 2007. "Foundation Houses, Fire Altars and the frataraka: Interpreting the Iconography of Some Post-Achaemenian Persian Coins", *IA 42*, 271–301.

———. 2013. (ed.), *The Oxford Handbook of Ancient Iran*, Oxford.

Provasi, E. 2003. "Sogdian *farn*", in Cereti, C.G., Maggi, M., and Provasi, E. (eds.), *Religious Themes and Texts of Pre-Islamic Iran and Central Asia: Studies in Honour of Professor Gherardo Gnoli on the Occasion of his 65th Birthday on 6th December 2002*, Wiesbaden, 305–323.

Pugachenkova, G.A. 1952. "Nekotorye izobrazitel'nye syuzhety na pamyatnikakh iskusstva drevnego Sogda [Some Themes on Monuments of Art of Ancient Sogd]", *IANTSSR 11*, 53–64.

———. 1966. *Khalchayan*, Tashkent.

———. 1971. *Skul'ptura Khalchayana* [*The Sculpture of Khalchayan*], Moscow.

———. 1977. "Gerakl v Baktrii [Heracles in Bactria]", *VDI 2*, 77–92.

———. 1979. *Iskusstvo Baktrii epokhi kushan* [*The Art of Bactria in the Kushan Period*], Moscow.

———. 1985. "Les ostothéques de Miankal", *Mesopotamia 20*, 29–65.

———. 1987. "Miankal'skie ossuarii [The Ossuaries of Miankal']" in *Iz hudozhestvennoy sokroveshchnitsy Srednego Vostoka* [*From the Artistic Treasures of the Middle East*], Tashkent, 89–124.

———. 1994. "The Form and Style of Sogdian Ossuaries", *BAI 8*, 227–245.

———. 1996. "Interpretatsiya odnogo iz personazhey na Biyanajmanskom ossuarii [Interpretation of a Personage on a Biyanajman Ossuary]", *IMKU 27*, 41–52.

———. 1999. "Shakhname, kak istochnik k poznaniyu doislamskoy material'noy i khudozhestvennoy kul'tury Irana i Turana [Shahnama, as a Sourse on pre-Islamic Material Culture and Art of Iran and Turan]", *IMKU 30*, 198–213.

Pulatov, U.P. 1975. *Chil'khudzhra* [*Chilhujra*], Dushanbe.

Pulleyblank, E.G. 1992. "Chinese-Iranian Relations i. In Pre-Islamic Times", *EIr 5*, 424–431.

Quagliotti, A.M. 2003. "An Image in the Indian Museum with Some Considerations on the Tutelary Couples in Gandharan Art", *SRAA 9*, 239–296.

Raede, J. 1995. "The Khorsabad Glazed Bricks and Their Symbolism", *Khorsabad, le palais de Sargon II, roi d'Assyrie: Actes du colloque organisé au musée du Louvre par le Service culturel les 21 et 22 janvier 1994*, Paris, 225–253.

Raevskiy, D.S. 1977. *Ocherki ideologii skifo-sakskikh plemen* [*Essays on Ideology of Scythian and Saka Tribes*], Moscow.

———. 1978. "'Skifskoe' i 'grecheskoe' v syuzhetnykh izobrazheniyakh na skifskikh drevnostyakh (k probleme antropomorfizatsii skifskogo panteona) ['Scythian' and 'Greek' in the Thematic Compositions on Scythian Antiquities (On the Problem of Anthropomorphization in the Scythian Art)]", *Antichnost' i antichnye traditsii v iskusstve i kul'ture narodov Sovetskogo Vostoka* [*Antiquity and Antique Traditions in the Art and the Culture of People of Soviet Orient*], Moscow, pp. 63–71.

———. 1983. "Skifskie kamennye izvayaniya v sisteme religiozno-mifologicheskikh predstavleniy iranoyazychnykh narodov evraziyskikh stepey [The Scythian Stone Statues in the System of Religious and Mythological Beliefs of Iranian Speaking People of Eurasian Steppes]", in Litvinskiy, B.A. (ed.), *Srednyaya Aziya, Kavkaz i zarubezhnyy Vostok v drevnosti* [*Central Asia, Caucasus and the Orient in Antiquity*], Moscow, 40–61.

Raffaelli, E.G. 2014. *The Sih-rozag in Zoroastrianism: A Textual and Historico-religious Analysis*, London and New York.

Rahbar, M. 1998. "Découverte d'un monument d'époque Sassanide à Bandian, Dargaz (Nord-Khorassan). Fouilles 1994 et 1995", *SI 27* 213–250.

———. 2004. "Le monument sassanide de Bandiān, Dargaz: un temple du feu d'après les dernières découvertes, 1996–98," *SI 33*, 7–30.

———. 2007. "A Tower of Silence of the Sasanian Period at Bandiyan: Some Observations about Dakhmas in Zoroastrian Religion", in Cribb, J. and Herrmann, G. (eds.), *After Alexander, Central Asia before Islam, (PBA 133)*, Oxford.
———. 2011. "The Discovery of a Sasanian Period Fire Temple at Bandiyān, Dargaz", in Kennet, D. and Luft, P. (eds.), *Current Research in Sasanian Archaeology, Art and History*, Oxford, 15–41.
Rapoport, Y.A. 1971. *Iz istorii religii Drevnego Khorezma (ossuarii) [From the History of the Religion of Ancient Chorasmia (Ossuaries)]*, Moscow.
———. 1994. "The Palaces of Topraq-Qal'a", *BAI 8*, 161–186.
Rapp, S.H. 2003. *Studies in Medieval Georgian Historiography: Early Texts and Eurasian Contexts*, Louvain.
———. 2009. "The Iranian Heritage of Georgia: Breathing New Life into the Pre-Bagratid Historical Tradition", *IA 44*, 645–693.
Rapp, S.H. and Crego, P.C. 2006. "*The Conversion of K'art'li*: The Shatberdi Variant, Kek.Inst. S-1141", *Le Muséon 119/1–2*, 169–226.
Raspopova, V.I. 2004. "Life and Artistic Conventions in the Reliefs of the Miho Couch", *BMM 4*, 43–58.
Rastorgueva, V.S. and Edelman, D.I. 2003. *Etimologicheskiy slovar' iranskikh yazykov [Etymological Dictionary of the Iranian Languages]*, vol. 2., Moscow.
———. 2007. *Etimologicheskiy slovar' iranskikh yazykov [Etymological Dictionary of the Iranian Languages]*, vol. 3., Moscow.
Razmjou, S. 2001. "Des traces de la déesse Spenta Armaiti à Perépolis et proposition pour une nouvelle lecture d'un logogramme élamite", *SI 30*, 7–15.
Reding-Hourcade, N. 1983. "Recherches sur l'iconographie de la déesse Anâhitâ", in Donceel, R. and Lebrun, R. (eds.), *Archéologie et religions de l'Anatolie ancienne: Mélanges en l'honneur du professeur Paul Naster*, Louvain, 199–209.
Reeder, E.D. 2001. *L'Or des rois scythes*, Paris.
Rezakhani, Kh. 2010. "The '*Unbekannter König IV*' and the Coinage of Hellenistic and Arsacid Persis", *NIB 15*.
Riboud, P. 2003. "Le cheval sans cavalier dans l'art funéraire sogdien en Chine: À la recherche des sources d'un thème composite", *Arts Asiatiques 58*, 148–161.
———. 2005. "Réflexion sur les pratiques religieuses désignées sous le nom de *xian* ?", in de La Vaissière, E. and Trombert, E. (eds.), *Les Sogdiens en Chine*, Paris, 73–93.
———. 2007/2012. "Bird-Priest in Central Asian Tombs of 6th-Century China and Their Significance in the Funerary Realm", *BAI 21*, 1–25.
Ringbom, L.I. 1957. *Zur Ikonographie der Gottin Ardvi Sura Anahita*, Abo.
Ritter, H.-W. 1965. *Diadem und Koenigsherrschaft: Untersuchungen zu Zeremonien und Rechtsgrundlagen des Herrschaftsantritts bei den Persern, bei Alexander dem grossen und im Hellenismus*, Münich.
Robinson, C.F. 2004. *Empire and Elites after the Muslim Conquest. The Transformation of Northern Mesopotamia*, Cambridge.
Rochberg, F. 2009. "'The Stars Their Likenessess': Perspectives on the Relation Between Celestial Bodies and Gods in Ancient Mesopotamia", in Porter, B.N. (ed.), *What is God? Anthropomorphic and Non-Anthropomorphic Aspects of Deity in Ancient Mesopotamia*, Winona Lake, 41–93.
Rollinger, R. 2014. "Thinking and Writing About History in Teispid and Achaemenid Persia", in Raaflaub, K.A. (ed.), *Thinking, Recording, and Writing History in the Ancient World*, Wiley-Blackwell, 187–213.
Root, M.C. 1979. *The King and Kingship in Achaemenid Art (AI 19)*, Leiden.
———. 1995. "Art and Archaeology of the Achaemenid Empire", in Sasson, J.M. (ed.), *Civilizations of the Ancient Near East*, vol. 3, New York, 2615–2639.
———. 2002. "Animals in the Art of Ancient Iran", in Collins, B.J. (ed.), *A History of the Animal World in the Ancient Near East*, Leiden, 169–211.
Rose, J. 2005. "Investiture iii. The Sasanian Period", *EIr, Online Edition*, July 25, 2005, available at http://www.iranica.com/articles/investiture.
Rosenfield, J.M. 1967. *The Dynastic Art of the Kushans*, Los Angeles.
Rostovtzeff, M. 1922. *Iranians and Greeks in South Russia*, Oxford.
Rudenko, S.I. 1970. *The Frozen Tombs of Siberia: The Pazyryk Burials of Iron Age Horsemen*, Berkeley.
Russell, J.R. 1987. *Zoroastrianism in Armenia*, Cambridge.
Rusyayeva, A.S. 2007. "Religious Interactions between Olbia and Scythia", in Braund, D. and Kryzhitskiy, S.D. (eds.), *Classical Olbia and the Scythian World from the Sixth Century BC to the Second Century AD, (PBA 142)*, Oxford, 93–103.
Sal'e, M.A. 1957. (ed. and tr.), *Biruni. Izbrannye proizvedeniya [Al-Bīrūnī. Selected Works]*, vol. 1, Tashkent.
Santoro, A. 2005. "Hands in Sleeves. A Note on Iranian-Central Asiatic Costume in Gandharan Art", *EW 55*, 279–299.

Saprykin, S.Yu. 1983. "Zolotaya plastina iz Gorgippii [A Golden Plaque from Gorgippia]", *VDI 1*, 68–79.
Schiltz, V. 1994. *Les Scythes et les nomades des steppes*, Paris.
Schindel, N. 2004. *Sylloge Nummorum Sasanidarum Bd. III/1. Shapur II.—Kawad I./ 2. Regierung*, Wien.
———. 2005. "Sasanian Coinage", *EIr, Online Edition*, August 31, 2005, available at http://www.iranicaonline.org/articles/sasanian-coinage.
———. 2008. "Jāmāsp ii. Coinage", *EIr, Online Edition*, 20 July 2002, available at http://www.iranica.com/articles/jamasp-ii-coinage.
———. 2009. "Ardashir II Kushanshah and Huvishka the Kushan: Numismatic Evidence for the Date of the Kushan King Kanishka I", *JONS 198*, 12–14.
———. 2013. "Sasanian Coinage", in Potts, D.T. (ed.), *The Oxford Handbook of Ancient Iran*, Oxford, 815–840.
Schlerath, B. and Skjærvø, P.O. 1987. "Aši", *EIr 2*, 750–751.
Schlumberger, D., Le Berre, M., and Fussman, G. 1983. *Surkh Kotal en Bactriane. Volume I. Les temples: architecture, sculpture, inscriptions (MDAFA 25)*, Paris.
Schmidt, E.F. 1970. *Persepolis III: The Royal Tombs and Other Monuments*, Chicago.
Schmidt H.-P. 2002. "Simorḡ", *EIr Online Edition*, July 20, 2002, available at http://www.iranicaonline.org/articles/simorg.
———. 2006. "Mithra i. Mitra in Old Indian and Mittra in Old Iranian", *EIr, Online Edition*, 12 August 2006, available at http://www.iranica.com/articles/mithra-i.
Schmitt, R. 1991. "Name und Religion. Anthroponomastisches zur Frage der religiösen Verhältnisse des Achaimenidenreiches", in Kellens, J. (ed.), *La religion iranienne à l'époque achéménide*, Gent, 111–128.
———. 1998. "Parthische Sprach- und Namenüberlieferung aus arsakidischer Zeit", in Wiesehöfer, J. (ed.), *Das Partherreich und sine Zeugnisse: Beiträge des internationalen Colloquiums, Eutin, (27.–30. Juni 1996)*, Stuttgart, 163–204.
Schwartz, M. 1996. "*Sasm, Sesen, St. Sisinnios, Sesengen Barpharangēs, and ... "Semanglof" ", *BAI 10*, 253–257.
———. 1998. "Sesen: A Durable East Mediterranean God in Iran", in Sims-Williams, N. (ed.), *Proceedings of the Third European Conference of Iranian Studies*, vol. 1, Wiesbaden, 9–11.
———. 2005/2009. "Appolo and Khshathrapati, the Median Nergal, at Xanthos", *BAI 19*, 145–151.
———. 2007. "Kerdīr's Clairvoyants: Extra-Iranian and Gathic Perspectives", in Macuch, M., Maggi, M. and Sundermann, W. (eds.), *Iranian Languages and Texts from Iran and Turan: Ronald E. Emmerick Memorial Volume, (Iranica 13)*, Wiesbaden, 365–377.
Scott, A.D. 1990. "The Iranian Face of Buddhism", *EW 40*, 43–79.
Shahbazi, A.S. 1974. "An Achaemenid Symbol I. A Farewell to 'Fravahr' and 'Ahuramazda' ", *AMI 7*, 135–144.
———. 1980. "An Achaemenid Symbol II. Farnah '(God Given) Fortune' Symbolized", *AMI 13*, 119–147.
———. 1983. "Studies in Sasanian Prosopography", *AMI 16*, 255–269.
———. 1985. "Iranian Notes 1–6", *Papers in Honour of Professor Mary Boyce (AI 24)*, Leiden, 497–511.
———. 1987. "Ardašīr II", *EIr 2*, 380–381.
———. 2001. "Early Sasanians' Claim to Achaemenid Heritage", *NIB 1/1*, 61–73.
———. 2002. "Shapur I", *EIr, Online Edition*, 20 July 2002, available at http://www.iranica.com/articles/shapur-i.
———. 2003/2004. "A New Picture of the Achaemenid World. Review of *From Cyrus to Alexander, A History of the Persian Empire / Pierre Briant*", *NIB 3/2*, 69–81.
Shaked, S. 1967. "Some Notes on Ahreman, the Evil Spirit, and His Creation", in Urbach, E.E., Werblowsky, R.J.Z. and Wirszubsky, C.H. (eds.), *Studies in Mysticism and Religion Presented to G.G. Scholem*, Jerusalem, 227–234.
———. 1971. "The Notions *mēnōg* and *gētīg* in the Pahlavi Texts and their Relation to Eschatology", *Acta Orientalia 33*, 60–107.
———. 1987. "First Man, First King: Notes on Semitic-Iranian Syncretism and Iranian Mythological Transformations", in Shaked, S., Shulman, D. and Stroumsa, G.G. (eds.), *Gilgul: Essays on Transformation, Revolution and Permanence in the History of Religions Dedicated to R.J.Z. Werblowsky*, Leiden, 238–256.
———. 1990. "For the Sake of the Soul: A Zoroastrian Idea in Transmission into Islam", *JSAI 12*, 15–33.
———. 1994a. *Dualism in Transformation. Varieties of Religion in Sasanian Iran*, London.
———. 1994b. "Some Islamic Reports Concerning Zoroastrianism", *JSAI 17*, 43–84.
———. 1995. "Jewish Sasanian Sigillography," in Gyselen, R. (ed.), *Au carrefour des religions: Melanges offerts à Philippe Gignoux*, Bures-sur-Yvette, 239–255.
———. 1997. "Popular Religion in Sasanian Babylonia", *JSAI 21*, 103–117.
———. 2001. "Gētīg and mēnōg", *EIr 10*, 574–576.
———. 2005. "Zoroastrian Origins: Indian and Iranian Connections", in Arnason, J.P., Eisenstadt, S.N., and Wittrock, B. (eds.), *Axial Civilizations and World History*, Leiden, 183–201.

———. 2007. "The Iranian Canon of Scriptures and Writings", in Vahman, F. and Pedersen, C.V. (eds.), *Religious Texts in Iranian Languages. Symposium held in Copenhagen May 2002*, København, 11–29.
———. 2008. "Religion in the Late Sasanian Period: Eran, Aneran, and Other Religious Designations", in Curtis, V.S. and Stewart, S.R.A. (eds.), *The Sasanian Era (The Idea of Iran 3)*, London and New York, 103–117.
Shaki, M. 1996. "Dēn", *EIr 7*, 279–281.
Shalem, A. 1994. "The Fall of al-Madā'in: Some Literary References Concerning Sasanian Spoils of War in Mediaeval Islamic Treasuries", *Iran 32*, 77–83.
Shaub, I.Yu. 2004. "Iz istorii yazycheskikh verovaniy v Severnom Prichernomor'e: kul't farna u skifov [On the History of Pagan Beliefs in Northern Black Sea Region: The Cult of farn Among Scythians]", *VPSTBI 2*, 149–158.
———. 2007. *Mif, kul't, ritual v Severnom Prichernomor'e (VII–IV vv. do n. e.) [Myth, Cult, Ritual in the North Pontic Area (7th–4th centuries B.C.)]*, Saint Petersburg.
Shayegan, R. 2003. "Approaches to the Study of Sasanian History", in Adhami, S. (ed.), *Paitimāna: Essays in Iranian, Indo-European, and Indian Studies in Honor of Hanns-Peter Schmidt*, Costa Mesa, 363–384.
———. 2013. "Sasanian Political Ideology", in Potts, D.T. (ed.), *The Oxford Handbook of Ancient Iran*, Oxford, 805–813.
Shenkar, M. 2007. "Temple Architecture in the Iranian World before the Macedonian Conquest", *Iran and the Caucasus 11/2*, 169–194.
———. 2011. "Temple Architecture in the Iranian World in the Hellenistic Period", in Kouremenos, A., Rossi, R., Chandrasekaran, S. (eds.), *From Pella to Gandhara: Hybridisation and Identity in the Art and Architecture of the Hellenistic East*, Oxford, 117–140.
———. 2008/2012. "Aniconism in the Religious Art of Pre-Islamic Iran and Central Asia", *BAI 22*, 239–257.
———. forthcoming a. "Rethinking Sasanian Iconoclasm", *JAOS*.
———. forthcoming b. "Images of Daēnā and Mithra on two seals from Indo-Iranian Borderlands", *SI*.
Shepherd, D.G. 1972. "The Diadem—A Clue to the Religious Iconography of Sasanian Art", *Summaries of Papers to be Delivered at the Sixth International Congress of Iranian Art and Archaeology, 10–16th, September 1972*, Oxford, 79.
———. 1980. "The Iconography of Anahita: Part 1", *Berytus 28*, 47–86.
———. 1983. "Sasanian Art", in Yarshater, E. (ed.), *The Cambridge History of Iran. vol. 3(2): The Seleucid, Parthian and Sasanian Periods*, Cambridge, 1055–1113.
Shishkin, V.A. 1963. *Varakhsha*, Moscow.
Shkoda, V.G. 1980. "K voprosu o kul'tovykh stsenakh v sogdiyskoy zhivopisi [The Cultic Scenes in Sogdian Paintings]", *SGE 45*, 60–64.
———. 1989. "Grecheskoe 'Zhilishche bogov' i sogdiyskiy khram [The Greek 'House of Gods' and the Sogdian Temple]", in Afanas'eva, V.K. and Mavleev, E.V. (eds.), *Drevniy Vostok i Antichnaya tsivilizatsya [The Ancient Near East and the Classical Civilization]*, Leningrad, 82–92.
———. 2009. *Pyandzhikenstkie khramy i problemy religii Sogda (V–VIII vv) [The Temples of Penjikent and the Problems of Sogdian Religion (5th to 8th Centuries)]*, St. Petersburg.
Secunda, S. 2009. "Talmudic Text and Iranian Context: On the Development of Two Talmudic Narratives", *AJSReview 33*, 45–69.
———. 2005/2009. "Studying with a Magus/Like Giving a Tongue to a Wolf", *BAI 19*, 151–159.
Seidl, U. 1976/1980. "Inanna/Ištar (Mesopotamien). B. In der Bildkunst", *RIA 5*, 87–89.
———. 1980. "Einige Urartäische Bronzezylinder (Deichselkappen?)", *AMI 13*, 63–83.
———. 1994. "Achaimenidische Entlehnungen aus der urartäischen Kultur", in Sancisi-Weerdenburg, H., Kuhrt, E. and Root, M. (eds.), *Continuity and Change, (Achaemenid History 8)*, Leiden, 107–129.
———. 1999. "Ein Monument Darius' I. aus Babylon", *Zeitschrift für Assyriologie und vorderasiatische Archäologie 89*, 101–114.
Sellwood, D. 1980. *The Coinage of Parthia*, London.
Sims-Williams, N. 1983. "Indian Elements in Parthian and Sogdian", in Röhrborn, K. and Veenker, W. (eds.), *Sprachen des Buddhismus in Zentralasien: Vorträge des Hamburger Symposions vom 2. Jul ibis 5 Juli 1981*, Wiesbaden, 132–141.
———. 1989. "Baga ii. In Old and Middle Iranian", *EIr 3*, 404–405.
———. 1991. "Mithra the Baga", in Bernard, P. and Grenet, F. (eds.), *Histoire et cultes de l'Asie centrale préislamique*, Paris, 177–187.
———. 1997a. "A Bactrian God", *BSOAS 60*, 336–339.
———. 1997b. *New Light on Ancient Afghanistan: The Decipherment of Bactrian*, London.
———. 1998. "Further Notes on the Bactrian Inscription of Rabatak, with an Appendix on the Names of Kujula Kadphises and Vima Taktu in Chinese", in Sims-Williams, N. (ed.), *Proceedings of the Third European Conference of Iranian Studies*, vol. 1, Wiesbaden, 79–93.

———. 1997/1998. "A Bactrian Deed of Manimission", *SRAA* 5, 191–213.
———. 2000. "Some Reflections on Zoroastrianism in Sogdiana and Bactria", in Christian, D. and Benjamin, C. (eds.), *Realms of the Silk Roads: Ancient and Modern* (*Silk Road Studies* 4), Turnhout, 1–13.
———. 2001/2005. "Bactrian Legal Documents from 7th- and 8th-Century Guzgan", *BAI* 15, 9–31.
———. 2002. "Ancient Afghanistan and Its Invaders: Linguistic Evidence From the Bactrian Documents and Inscriptions", in Sims-Williams, N. (ed.), *Indo-Iranian Languages and People*, (*PBA* 116), 225–243.
———. 2004/2008. "The Bactrian Inscription of Rabatak: A New Reading", *BAI* 18, 53–69.
———. 2007. *Bactrian Documents from Northern Afghanistan II: Letters and Buddhist Texts*, London.
———. 2010. *Bactrian Personal Names*, Wien.
———. 2009/2013. "Some Bactrian Inscriptions on Silver Vessels", *BAI* 23, 191–199.
Sims-Williams, N. and Cribb, J. 1996. "A New Bactrian Inscription of Kanishka the Great", *SRAA* 4, 75–142.
Sinisi, F. 2008. "Tyche in Parthia: The Image of the Goddess on Arsacid Tetradrachms", *Numismatische Zeitschrift* 116/117, 231–249.
Skjærvø, P.O. 1983. "Kirdir's Vision: Translation and Analysis", *AMI* 16, 269–306.
———. 1987. "Ard Yašt", *EIr* 2, 355–356.
———. 1995/1997. "The Manichean Polemical Hymns in M 28 I", *BAI* 9, 239–255.
———. 2002. "Ahura Mazdā and Ārmaiti, Heaven and Earth, in the Old Avesta", *JAOS* 122/2, 399–410.
———. 2008. "Jamšid i. Myth of Jamšid", *EIr* 14, 501–522.
———. 2011a. "Kartīr", *EIr, Online Edition*, May 27, 2011, available at http://www.iranicaonline.org/articles/kartir
———. 2011b. "Zoroastrian Dualism. Appendix: The Sources of Zoroastrianism", in Lange, A. et al. (eds.), *Light Against Darkness: Dualism in Ancient Mediterranean Religion and the Contemporary World*, Göttingen, 55–92.
———. 2011c. "Zarathustra: A Revolutionary Monotheist?", in Pongratz-Leisten, B. (ed.), *Reconsidering the Concept of Revolutionary Monotheism*, Winona Lake, 317–351.
———. 2011d. *The Spirit of Zoroastrianism*, New Heaven and London.
———. 2012. "The Zoroastrian Oral Tradition as Reflected in the Texts", in Cantera, A. (ed.), *The Transmission of the Avesta*, Wiesbaden, 3–49.
———. 2013a. "Anāhitā-: Unblemished or Unattached? (Avestica IV)", in Choksy, J.K. and Dubeansky. J. (eds.), *Gift to a Magus. Indo-Iranian Studies Honoring Firoze Kotwal*, New York, 113–125.
———. 2013b. "Avesta and the Zoroastrianism under the Achaemenids", in Potts, D.T. (ed.), *The Oxford Handbook of Ancient Iran*, Oxford, 547–566.
Slanski, K.E. 2007. "The Mesopotamian 'Rod and Ring' Icon of Righteous Kingship and Balance of Power Between Palace and Temple", in Crawford, H. (ed.), *Regime Change in The Ancient Near East and Egypt*, 37–61.
Smirnov, Ya.I. 1909. *Vostochnoe serebro* [*The Oriental Silver*], Saint Petersburg.
Smirnova, L.P. 1974. (ed. and tr.), *Tārīkh-i Sīstān*, Moscow.
Smirnova, O.I. 1971. "Mesta domusul'manskikh kul'tov v Sredney Azii [Places of Pre-Islamic Worship in Central Asia]", *Strani i narodi Vostoka* 10 [*Lands and People of the Orient* 10], 90–121.
———. 1981. *Svodnyy katalog sogdiyskikh monet* [*The Joint Catalogue of Sogdian Coins*], Moscow.
Smith, R.R.R. 1988. *Hellenistic Royal Portraits*, Oxford.
Sokolovsky, V.M. 2009. *Monumental'naya zhivopis' dvortsovogo kompleksa Bundzhikata* [*Monumental Painting of the Palace Complex of Bunjikat*], Saint Petersburg.
Soudavar, A. 2003. *The Aura of Kings. Legitimacy and Divine Sanction of Iranian Kingship*, Costa Mesa.
———. 2009. "The Vocabulary and Syntax of Iconography in Sasanian Iran", *IA* 44, 417–460.
———. 2010. "Farr(ah) ii. Iconography of farr(ah)/x^varənah", *EIr, Online Edition*, August 24, 2010, available at http://www.iranica.com/articles/farr-ii-iconography.
———. 2012. "Looking through The Two Eyes of the World: A Reassessment of Sasanian Rock Reliefs", *Iranian Studies*, 1–30.
Stausberg, M. 2002–2004. *Die Religion Zarathushtras. Geschichte—Gegenwart—Rituale*, 3 vols., Stuttgart.
Staviskiy, B.Y. 1961. "Ossuarii iz Biya-Najmana [The Ossuaries from Biya-Najman]" *TGE* 5, 162–176.
———. 1974. *Iskusstvo Sredney Azii. Drevniy period: VI v. do n. e—VIII v. n. e* [*The Art of Central Asia: The Ancient Period: 6th c. BCE to 7th CE*], Moscow.
———. 1977. *Kushanskaya Baktriya: problemy istorii i kul'tury* [*The Kushan Bactria: Issues of History of Culture*], Moscow.
Stein, A.M. 1907. *Ancient Khotan*, 2 vols., Oxford.
Stern, S. 2012. *Calendars in Antiquity: Empires, States and Societies*, Oxford.
Strawn, B.A. 2005. *What is Stronger than a Lion? Leonine Image and Metaphor in the Hebrew Bible and the Ancient Near East*, Fribourg.

Strootman, R. 2007. *The Hellenistic Royal Court. Court Culture, Ceremonial and Ideology in Greece, Egypt and the Near East, 336–30 BCE*, Unpublished PhD Dissertation, Utrecht University.
Subtelny, M.E. 2011. "Zoroastrian Elements in the Islamic Ascension Narrative: The Case of the Cosmic Cock", in Szuppe, M., Krasnowolska, A. and Pedersen, C.V. (eds.), *Proceedings of the 6th European Conference of Iranian Studies (Vienna 2007), Vol. 2: Mediaeval and Modern Iranian Studies*, Paris, 193–212.
Suleymanov, R.K. 2000. *Drevniy Nakhshab [Ancient Nakhshab]*, Samarkand-Tashkent.
Sundermann, W. 1986. "Bruchstücke einer manichäischen Zarathustralegende", in Schmitt, R. and Skjærvø, P.O. (eds.), *Studia Grammatica Iranica. Festschrift für Helmut Humbach*, Munich, 461–482.
———. 1988. "Kē čihr az yazdān. Zur Titulatur der Sasanidenkönige", *Archiv Orientální 56*, 338–340.
———. 1990. "Shapur's Coronation. The Evidence of the Cologne Mani Codex Reconsidered and Compared with Other Texts", *BAI 4*, 295–301.
———. 1991. "Manichaean Traditions on the Date of the Historical Buddha", in Bechert, H. (ed.), *The Dating of the Historical Buddha: (Symposien zur Buddhismusforschung, IV,1–3)*, Part 1, Göttingen, 426–441.
———. 2008. "Zoroastrian Motifs in Non-Zoroastrian Traditions", *JRAS 18/2*, 155–165.
Tanabe, K. 1984. "A Study of the Sasanian Disk-Nimbus: Farewell to its Xvarnah-Theory", *BAOM 6*, 29–51.
———. 1988. "Iranian Xvarnah and the Treasure of Shosoin at Nara in Japan", *IA 13*, 365–385.
———. 1990. "The Kushan Representations of ANEMOS/OADO and its Relevance to the Central Asian and Far Eastern Wind Gods", *SRAA 1*, 51–81.
———. 1991/1992. "OHÞO: Another Kushan Wind God", *SRAA 2*, 51–73.
———. 1993. *Silk Road Coins: The Hirayama Collection*, Kamakura.
———. 1995a. "Earliest Aspect of Kanīṣka I's Religious Ideology. A Numismatic Approach", in Invernizzi, A. (ed.), *In the Land of the Gryphons: Papers on Central Asian Archaeology in Antiquity*, Firenze, 203–217.
———. 1995b. "Nana on Lion. East and West in Sogdian Art", *Orient, 30/31*, 365–381.
———. 1995/1996. "Vishvakarman in Gandharan Art", *SRAA 4*, 175–201.
———. 2003. "The Identification of the King of Kings in the upper register of the Larger Grotte, Taq-i Bustan: Ardashir III Restated", in Compareti M., Raffetta P. and Scarcia G. (eds.), *Ēran ud Anērān. Studies presented to Boris Ilich Marshak on the Occasion of His 70th Birthday*, Venice, 583–601.
Tandon, P. 2012. "The Location and Kings of Pāradān", *SI 41*, 25–56.
Tavernier, J. 2007. *Iranica in the Achaemenid Period (ca. 550–330 B.C.): Lexicon of Old Iranian Proper Names and Loanwords, Attested in non-Iranian Texts*, Leuven.
Thomson, R.W. 1976. (ed. and tr.), *Agathangelos. History of the Armenians*, Albany.
———. 1980. (ed. and tr.), *Moses Khorenats'i. History of the Armenians*, Cambridge and London.
———. 1996. (ed. and tr.), *Rewriting Caucasian History. The Medieval Armenian Adaptation of the Georgian Chronicles*, Oxford.
———. 2004. "Armenian Ideology and the Persians," in *La Persia e Bisanzio. Atti del Convegno internazionale (Roma, 14–18 ottobre 2002)*, Rome, 373–389.
Thrope, S.F. 2012. *Contradictions and Vile Utterances: The Zoroastrian Critique of Judaism in the Škand Gumānīg Wizār*, Unpublished PhD Dissertation, University of California, Berkeley.
Tremblay, X. 2006. "Ostiran vs. Westiran: Ein oder zwei Iran vor der islamischen Eroberung?", in Eichner, H., Fragner, B.G., Sadovski, V. and Schmitt, R. (eds.), *Iranistik in Europa: Gestern, Heute, Morgen*, Vienna, 217–240.
Trever, K.V. and Lukonin, V.G. 1987. *Sasanidskoe serebro. Sobranie Gosudarstvennogo Ermitazha [Sasanian Silver. The Collection of the State Hermitage]*, Moscow.
Trokay, M. 1991. "Les origines du dieu élamite au serpent", *Mesopotamie et Elam: actes de la XXXVIème rencontre assyriologique internationale, Gand, 10–14 juillet 1989*, Ghent, 153–162.
Tsetskhladze, G.R. 2001. "Iranian Elements in Georgian Art and Archaeology", *EIr 10*, 470–480.
Tsuchiya, H. 1999/2000. "An Iconographical Study of the Buddhist Art of Shotorak, Paitāva and Kham Zargar", *SRAA 6*, 91–114.
Unvala, J.M. 1930. "The Winged Disk and the Winged Human Figure on Ancient Persian Monuments", in Sanjana D.P. et al. (ed.), *Dr. Modi Memorial Volume. Papers on Indo-Iranian and other Subjects on Honour of J. Jamshedji Modi*, Bombay, 488–513.
Ur Rahman, A. and Falk, H. 2011. *Seals, Sealings and Tokens from Gandhāra*, Wiesbaden.
Ustinova, Yu. 1999. *The Supreme Gods of the Bosporan Kingdom*, Leiden.
Ustinova, Yu. 2005. "Snake-Limbed and Tendril-Limbed Goddesses in the Art and Mythology of the Mediterranean and Black Sea", in Braund, D. (ed.), *Scythians and Greeks*, Exeter, 64–80.
Vahman, F. 1986. (ed. and tr.), *Ardā Wirāz Nāmag. The Iranian 'Divina Comedia'*, London and Malmo.
Vanden Berghe, L. 1978. "La découverte d'úne sculpture rupestre a Dārābgird", *IA 13*, 135–149.
———. 1984. *Reliefs rupestres de l'Iran ancient*, Brussels.

———. 1985. "L'état des études de l'histoire de l'art et de l'archéologie pre-islamique", in Gnoli, G. (ed.), *The First European Colloquium of Iranology*, Rome, 29–53.
———. 1987. "L'héritage parthe dans l'art sasanide", *Transition Periods in Iranian History*, Leuven, 241–253.
———. 1988. "Les scènes d'investiture sur les reliefs rupestres de l'Iran ancien: évolution et signification", in Gnoli, G. and Lanciotti, L. (eds.), *Orientalia Iosephi Tucci Memoriae Dictata*, vol. 3, Rome, 1511–1533.
Vanden Berghe, L. and Schippmann, K. 1985. *Les relief rupestres d'Elymaïde (Iran) de l'époque parthe*, Gent.
Van Buren, E.D. 1949. "The Rod and the Ring", *Archiv Orientální 17*, 434–450.
van der Toorn, K. 1997. "The Iconic Book: Analogies Between the Babylonian Cult of Images and the Veneration of the Torah", in van der Toorn, K. (ed.), *The Image and the Book: Iconic Cults, Aniconism, and the Rise of Book Religion in Israel and the Ancient Near East*, Leuven, 229–249.
Van Esbroeck, M. 1990. "La religion géorgienne pré-chrétienne", in Haase, W. (ed.), *Aufstieg und Niedergang der römischen Welt, vol. 18.4*, Berlin and New York, 2694–2725.
Van Haeperen-Pourbaix, A. 1983. "Recherche sur les origines, la nature et les attributs du dieu Mên", in Donceel, R. and Lebrun, R. (eds.), *Archéologie et religions de l'Anatolie ancienne: Mélanges en l'honneur du professeur Paul Naster*, Louvain, 221–259.
de la Vaissière, É. 2005. *Sogdian Traders: a History*, Leiden.
de la Vaissière, É., Riboud, P. and Grenet, F. 2003. "Les livres des sogdiens: Avec une note additionnelle par Frantz Grenet" *SI 32*, 127–136.
Vaynberg, B.I. 1977. *Monety drevnego Khorezma [The Coins of Ancient Chorasmia]*, Moscow.
Verardi, G. 1983. "The Kuṣāṇa Emperors as Cakravartins: Dynastic Art and Cults in India and Central Asia: History of a Theory, Clarifications and Refutations", *EW 33*, 225–295.
von Gall, H. 1984. "Globus oder Diskus auf der Krone Ḫosrow II.? Zur Datierung des grossen Iwans von Taq i Bostan", *Orientalia J. Duchesne-Guillemin Emerito Oblata (AI 29)*, Leiden, 179–191.
———. 1990. "The Figural Capitals at Taq-e Bostan and the Question of the so-called Investiture in Parthian and Sasanian Art", *SRAA 1*, 99–123.
Vyatkin, V.L. 1905. (ed. and tr.), "Kandiya Malaya [The Small Kandia]", *Spravochnaya knizhka Samarkandskoy oblasti [The Reference Book of the Samarkand District] 8*, 236–301.
Vysotskaya, T.N. 1984. "Nekotorye aspekty dukhovnoy kul'tury naseleniya Ust'-Al'minskogo gorodishcha [Some Aspects of Religious Culture of the Inhabitants of the Ust'-Al'minsk Settlement]", in Vysotskaya, T.N. (ed.), *Antichnaya drevnost' i srednie veka [Antiquity and the Middle Ages]*, Sverdlovsk, 132–140.
De Waele, É. 1989. "L'investiture et le triomphe dans la thématique de la sculpture rupestre sassanide", in de Meyer, L. and Haerinck, E. (eds.), *Archaeologia Iranica et Orientalis. Miscellanea in honorem Louis Vanden Berghe*, Gent, 811–831.
De Waele, A. 2004. "The Figurative Wall Paintings of the Sasanian Period from Iran, Iraq and Syria", *IA 39*, 349–382.
———. 2009. "Sasanian Wall Painting", *EIr, Online Edition*, 20 July, 2009, available at http://www.iranicaonline.org/articles/sasanian-wall-painting-murals-found-on-sites-within-the-territory-of-the-sasanian-empire.
Waldmann, H. 1991. *Der kommagenische Mazdaismus*, Tübingen.
Walls, N.H. 2005. (ed.), *Cult Image and Divine Representation in the Ancient Near East*, Boston.
Walter, M.N. 2009. "Buddhism and Iranian Religions Among Sogdians: Religious Interactions in Sogdian Funeral Art a Buddhist Perspective", in Pande, A. (ed.), *The Art of Central Asia and the Indian Subcontinent in Cross-Cultural Perspective*, New Delhi, 185–194.
Watters, T. 1904. *On Yuan Chwang's Travels in India, 629–645 A.D.*, London.
Weber, U. 2007. "Hormezd I., König der Könige von Ērān und Anērān", *IA 42*, 387–418.
———. 2009. "Wahrām II., König der Könige von Ērān und Anērān", *IA 44*, 559–643.
———. 2010. "Zu den Feldbildnissen des Königs Narseh", in Gyselen, R. (ed.), *Sources for the History of Sasanian and Post-Sasanian Iran, (Res Orientalis 19)*, Bures-sur-Yvette, 305–321.
Wendtland, A. 2009. "Xurmazda and Āδβaγ in Sogdian", in Allison, C., Joisten-Pruschke, A. and Wendtland, A. (eds.), *From Daēnā to Dîn. Religion, Kultur und Sprache in der iranischen Welt: Festschrift für Philip Kreyenbroek zum 60. Geburtstag*, Wiesbaden, 111–127.
Westenholz, J.G. 1997. "Nanaya: Lady of Mystery", in Finkel, I.L. and Geller, M.J. (eds.), *Sumerian Gods and Their Representations*, Groningen, 57–84.
———. 2000. "The King, the Emperor, and the Empire. Continuity and Discontinuity of Royal Representation in Text and Image", in Aro, S. and Whiting, R.M. (eds.), *The Heirs of Assyria. Proceedings of the Opening Symposium of the Assyrian and Babylonian Intellectual Heritage Project. Held in Tvärminne, Finland, October 8–11, 1998 (Helsinki: The Neo-Assyrian Text Corpus Project 2000)*, Helsinki, 99–125.
Whiston, W. 1974. *The Complete Works of Josephus*, Grand Rapids.
Wiesehöfer, J. 1994. *Die "dunklen Jahrhunderte" der Persis*, Münich.

———. 2001. "Frataraka", *EIr 10*, 195.
———. 2007. "Fars under Seleucid and Parthian Rule", in Curtis, V.S. and Stewart, S. (eds.), *The Age of Parthians, (The Idea of Iran 2)*, London, 37–50.
———. 2010a. "Frataraka Rule in Seleucid Persis: A New Appraisal", in Llewellyn-Jones, l. and Erskine, A. (eds.), *Creating a Hellenistic World*, Swansea, 107–123.
———. 2010b. "King and Kingship in the Sasanian Empire", in Lanfranchi, G.B. and Rollinger, R. (eds.), *Concepts of Kingship in Antiquity*, Padova, 135–153.
Wikander, S. 1941. *Vayu, Texte und Untersuchungen zur indo-iranischen Religionsgeschichte*, Uppsala and Leipzig.
Williams, A.V. 1990. *The Pahlavi Rivāyat Accompanying the Dādestān ī Dēnīg*, 2 vols., Copenhagen.
Winter, I.J. 1994. "Radiance as an Aesthethic Value in the Art of Mesopotamia", Saraswati, B.N., Malik, S.C. and Madhu Khanna (eds.), *Art: The Integral Vision—A Volume of Essays in Felicitation of Kapila Vatsyayan*, New Delhi, 123–132.
———. 2012. "Gold! Divine Light and Lustre in Ancient Mesopotamia", *7 ICAANE*, vol. 2, Wiesbaden, 153–173.
Wright, J.C. 1997. "Bactrian Rudra", *BSOAS 60*, 339–343.
Yakubov, Yu. 1987. "Izobrazheniya bogov na biyanajmanskikh ossuariyakh [The Depictions of Gods on the Biyanajman Ossuarues]", in *Proshloe Sredney Azii (arkheologiya, numizmatika, epigrafiya, etnografiya) [The Past of Central Asia (Archaeology, Numismatics, Epigraphy, Ethnography)]*, Dushanbe.
———. 1996. *Religiya drevnego Sogda [The Religion of Ancient Soghd]*, Dushanbe.
Yamamoto, Y. 1979. "The Zoroastrian Temple Cult of Fire in Archaeology and Literature (I)", *Orient 15*, 19–53.
———. 1981. "The Zoroastrian Temple Cult of Fire in Archaeology and Literature (II)", *Orient 17*, 67–104.
Yarshater, E. 1971. "Were the Sasanids Heirs to the Achaemenids?", *La Persia nel Medioevo*, Rome, 517–531.
———. 1983. "Iranian Common Beliefs and World-View", in Yarshater, E. (ed.), *The Cambridge History of Iran, Vol. 3(1), The Seleucid, Parthian and Sasanian Periods*, Cambridge, 343–359.
Yatsenko, S.A. 1992. "Antropomorfnye izobrazheniya Sarmatii [Anthropomorphic Images of Sarmatia]", *Alany i Kavkaz [The Alans and the Caucasus]*, Vladikavkaz, 189–214.
Zeymal, E.V. 1997. "Visha-Shiva in the Kushan Pantheon", in Allchin, F.R. (ed.), *Gandharan Art in Context: East-West Exchanges at the Crossroads of Asia Cambridge*, 245–267.
Zimansky, P. 2012. "Imagining Haldi", in Baker, H.D., Kaniuth, K. and Adelheid, O. (eds.), *Stories of Long Ago. Festschrift für Michael D. Roaf*, Münster, 713–725.
Zotenberg, H. 1867–1874. (ed. and tr.), *Moḥammad b. Jarir Ṭabari, La chronique sur la version persane d'Abou-ʿAli Mohammad Belʿami*, 4 vols., Paris.

GENERAL INDEX

INDEX OF DIVINE NAMES

FIGURES

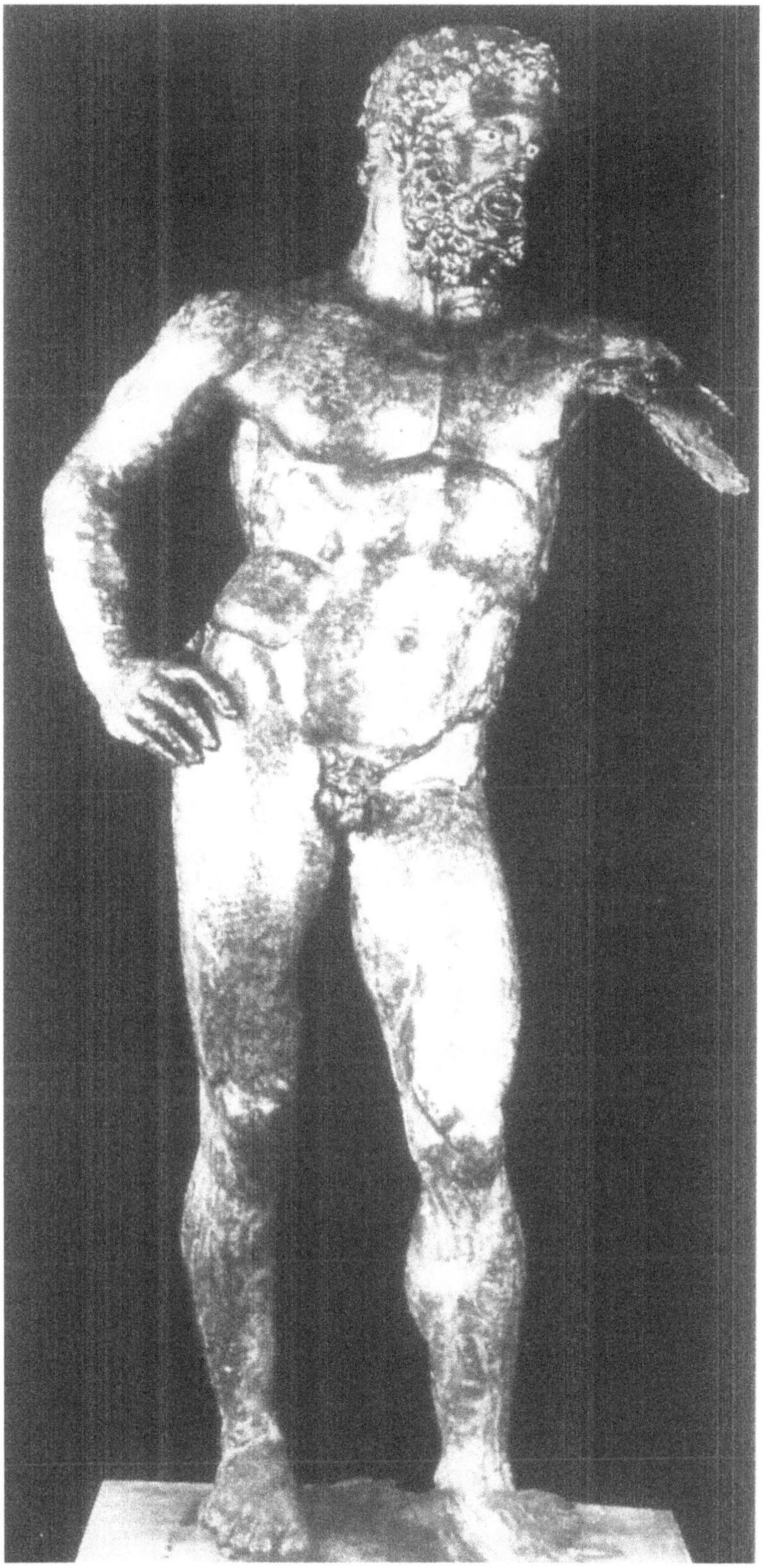

1. Statue of Heracles from Mesene (Frantz Grenet).

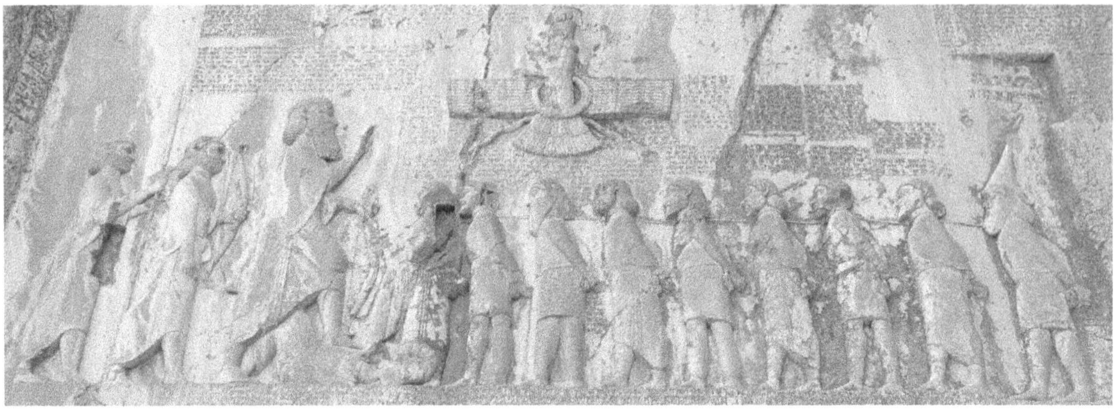

2. The Behestūn relief of Darius I (J. Breitenfeldt).

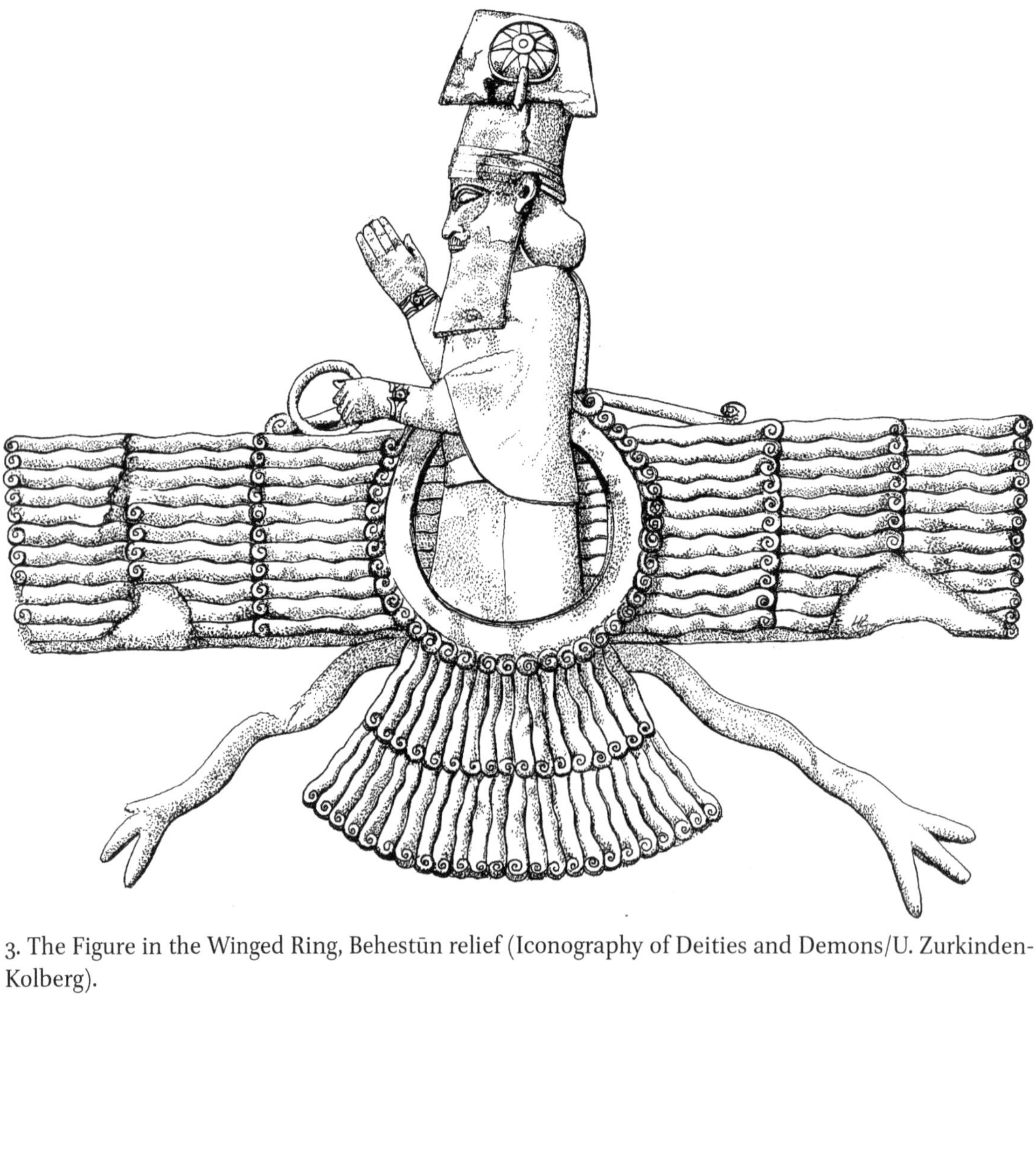

3. The Figure in the Winged Ring, Behestūn relief (Iconography of Deities and Demons/U. Zurkinden-Kolberg).

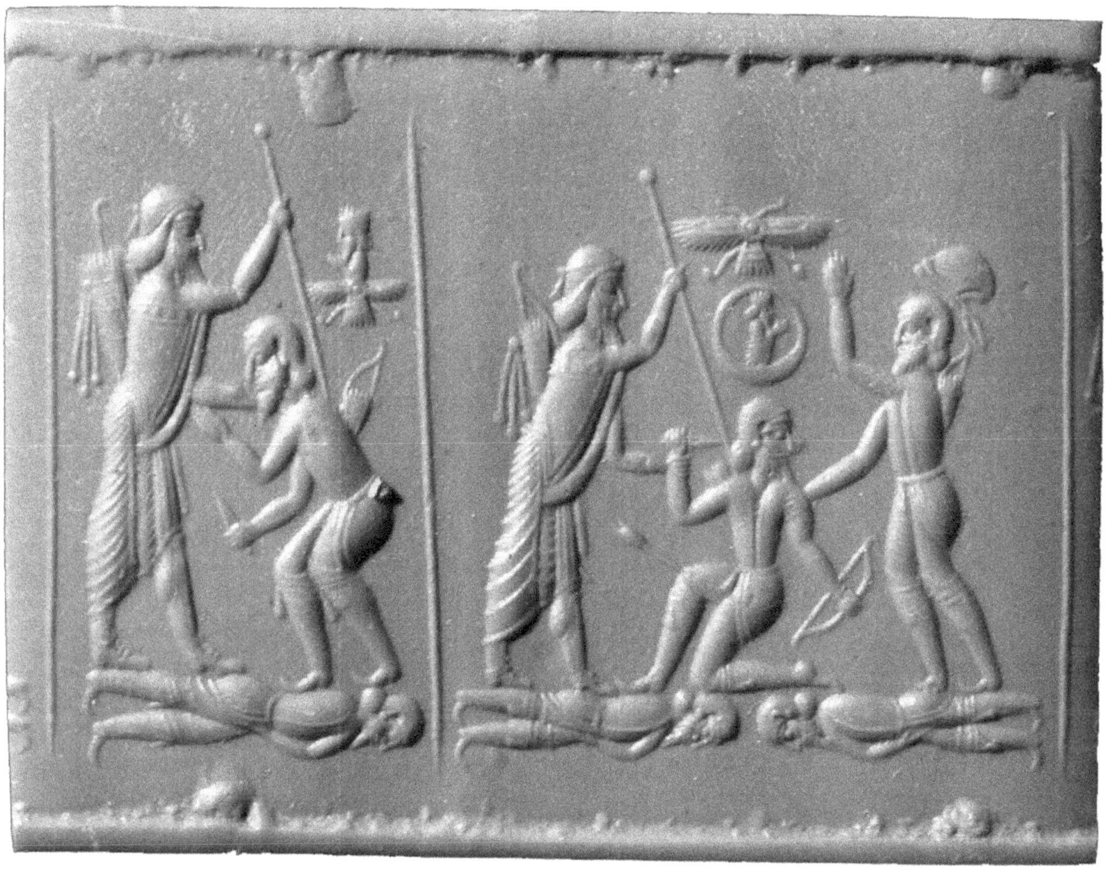

4. Achaemian cylinder seal from the Oxus Treasure (© Trustees of the British Museum).

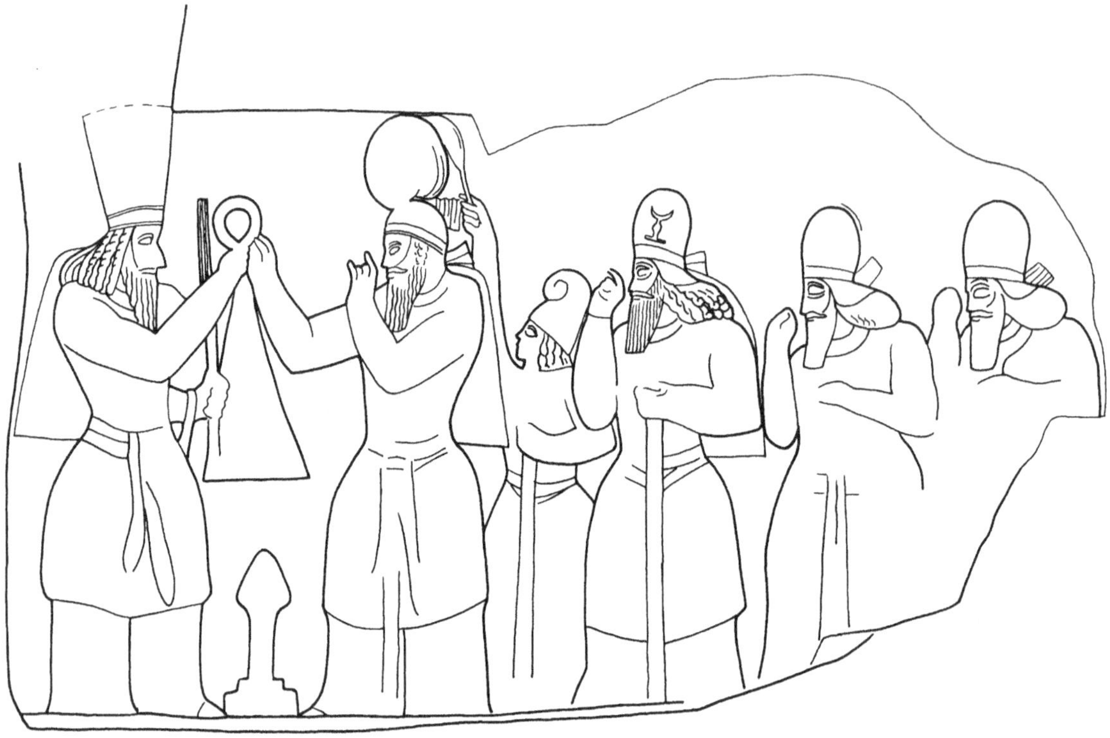

5. Investiture relief of Ardašīr I at Fīrūzābād (drawing E. Smekens © BAMI).

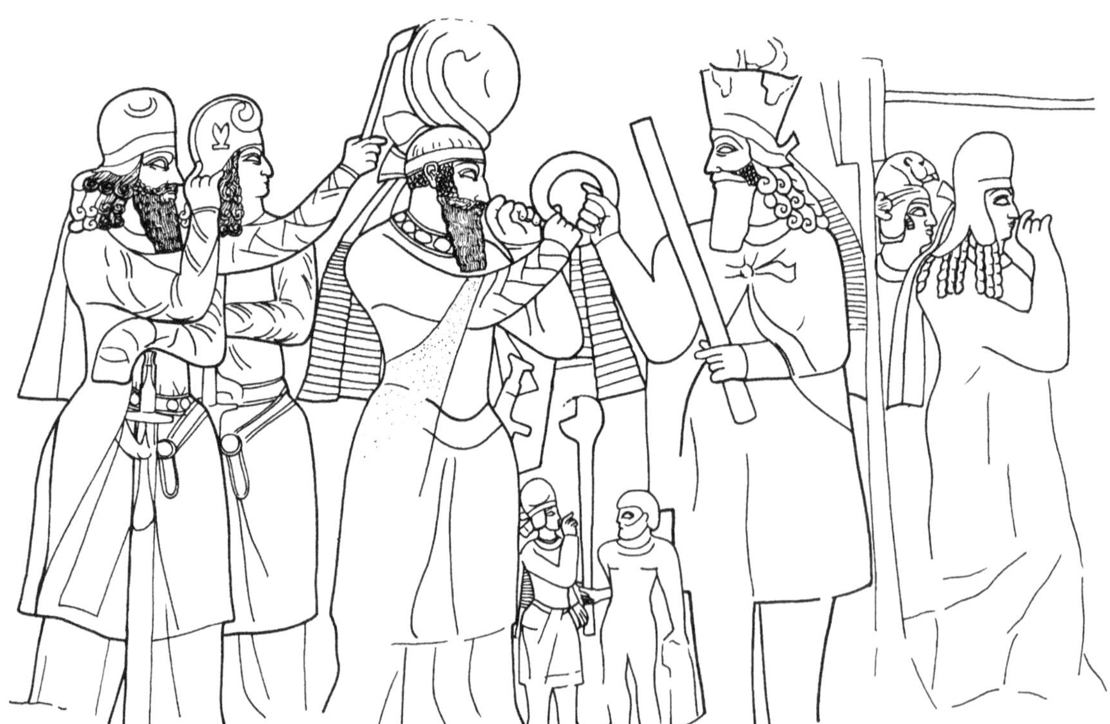

6. Investiture relief of Ardašīr I at Naqš-e Rağab (drawing E. Smekens © BAMI).

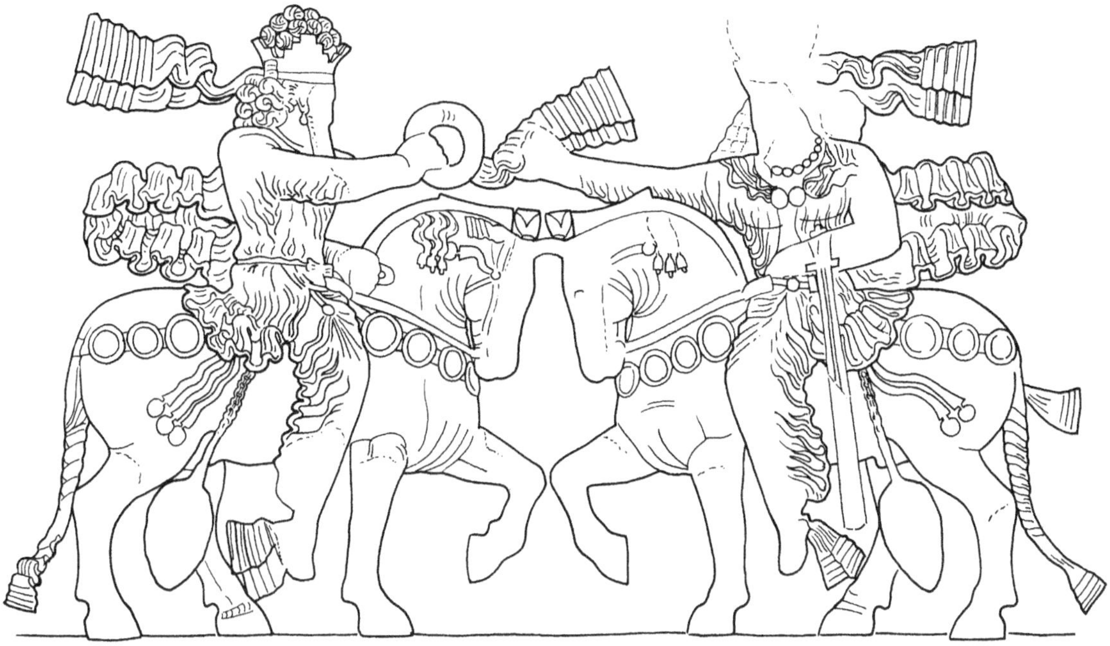

7. Investiture relief of Šāpūr I at Naqš-e Rağab (drawing E. Smekens © BAMI).

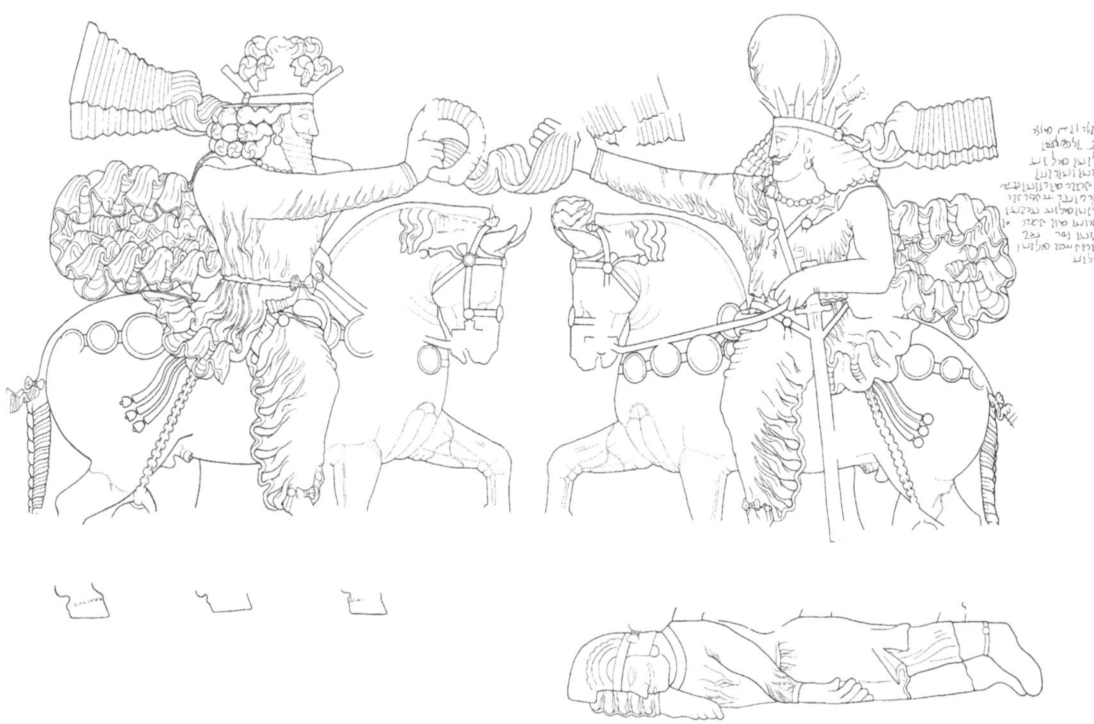

8. Investiture relief of Wahrām I at Bīšāpūr (Georginna Herrmann).

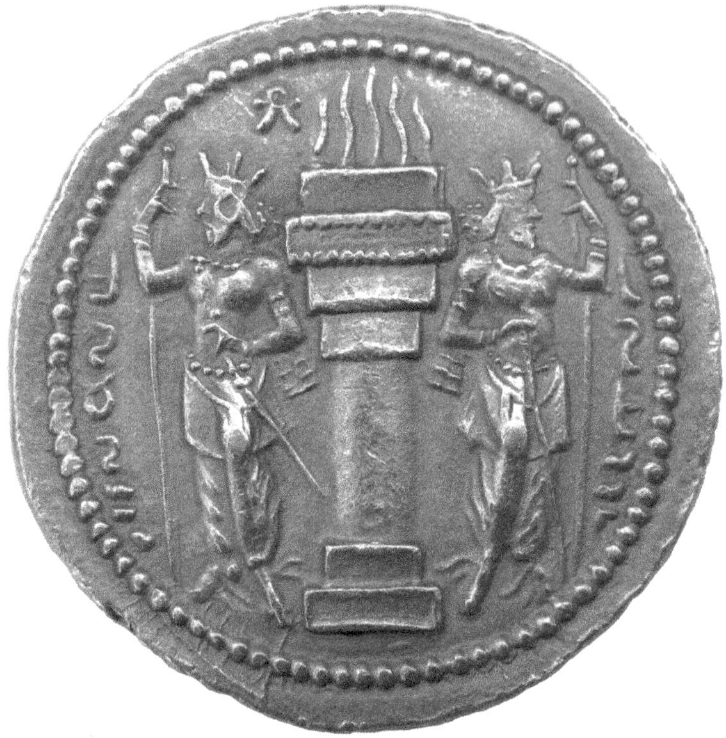

9. "Attendants" on the coin of Šāpūr I (Osmund Bopearachchi).

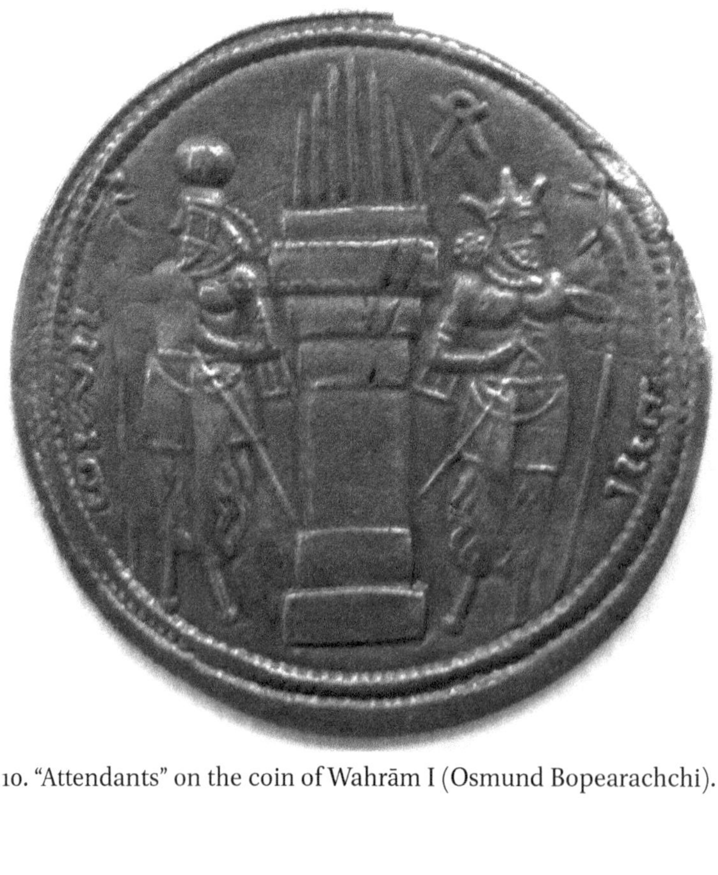

10. "Attendants" on the coin of Wahrām I (Osmund Bopearachchi).

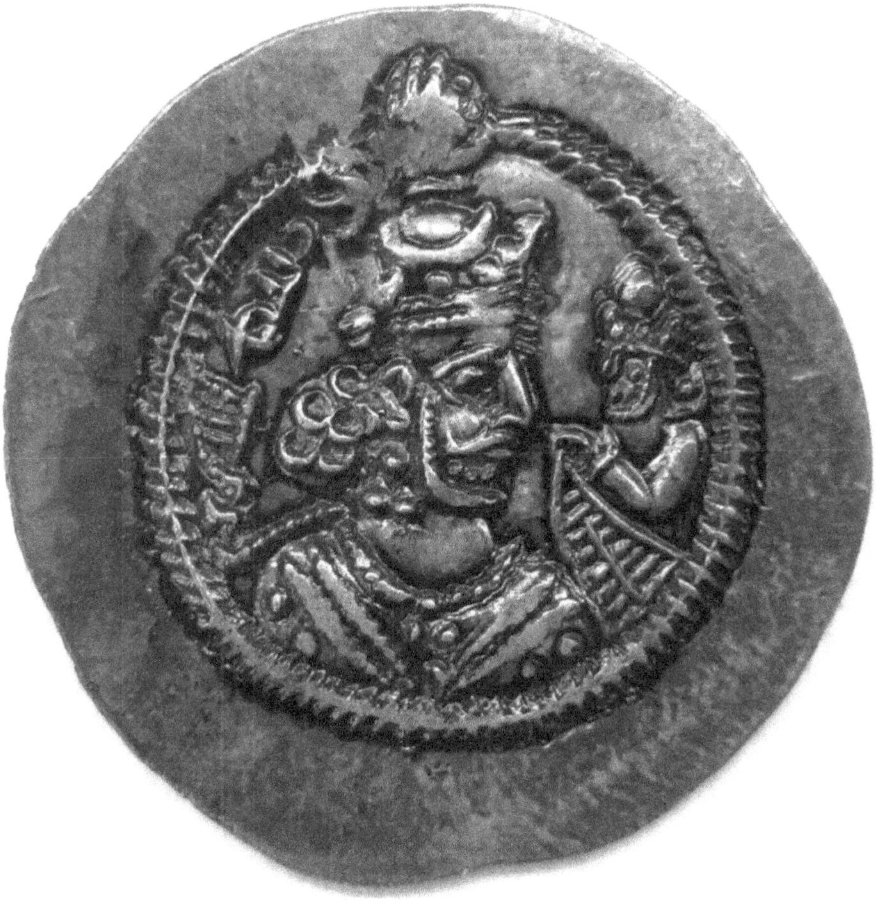

11. Bust with a diadem on the coin of Jāmāsp (Osmund Bopearachchi).

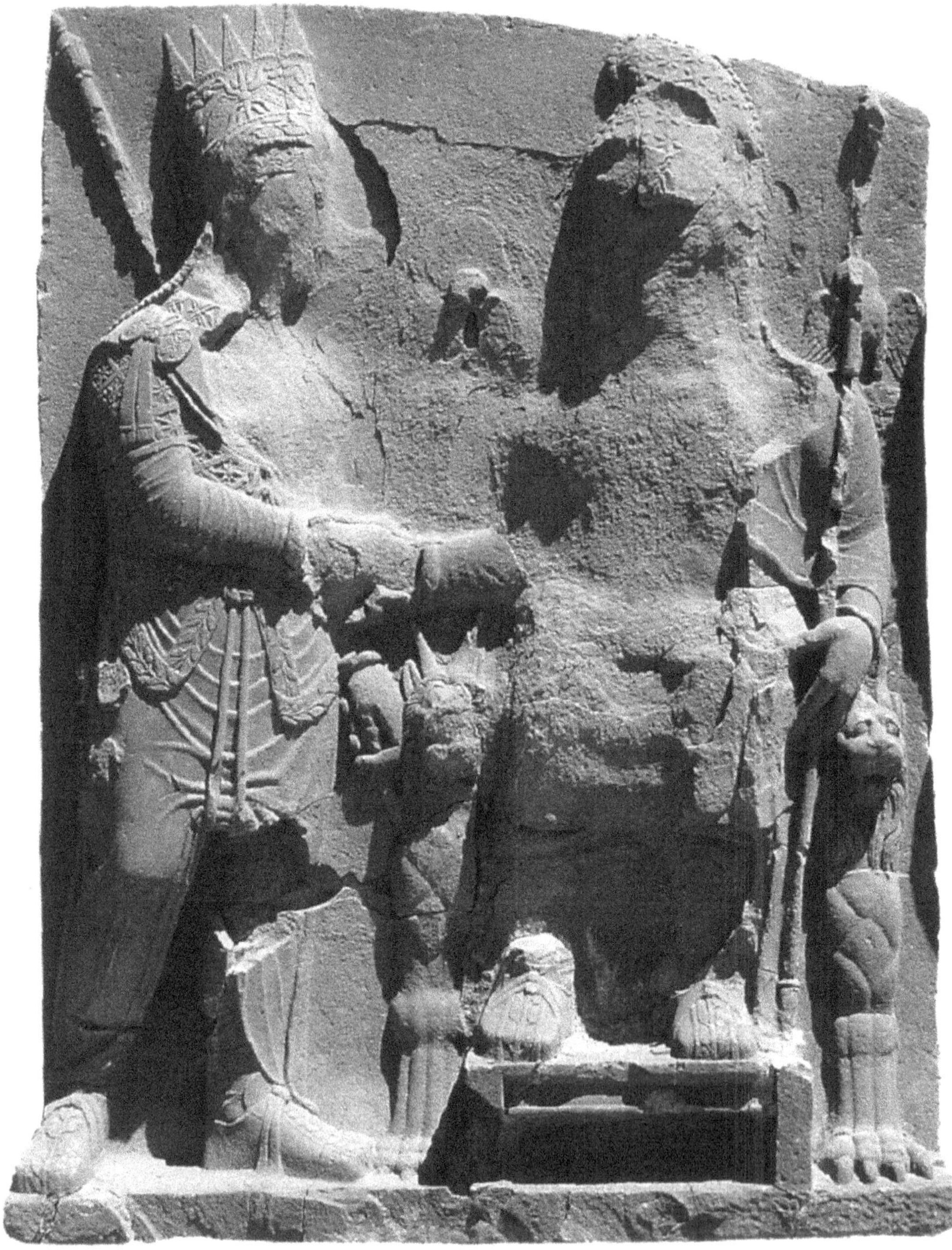

12. Antiochus I of Commagene and Zeus-Oromasdes, Nemrud Dag (Wagner 2000: fig. 39).

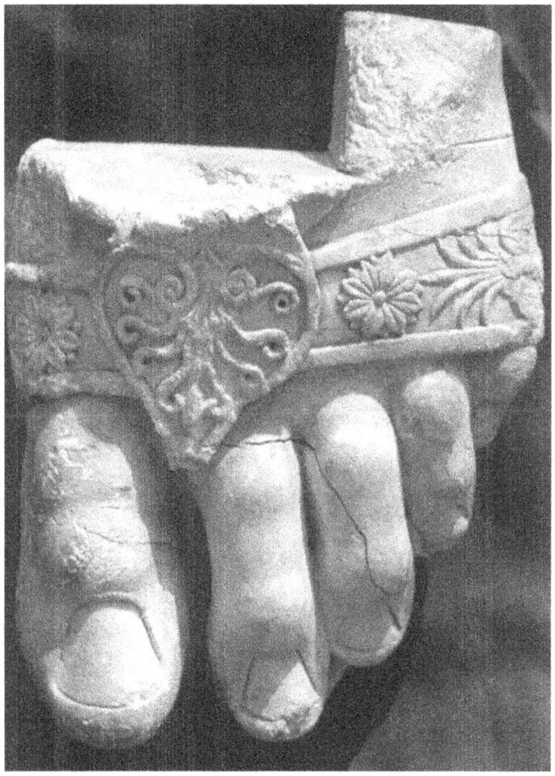

13. Fragment of a foot of a monumental statue, Ai Khanum (Frantz Grenet).

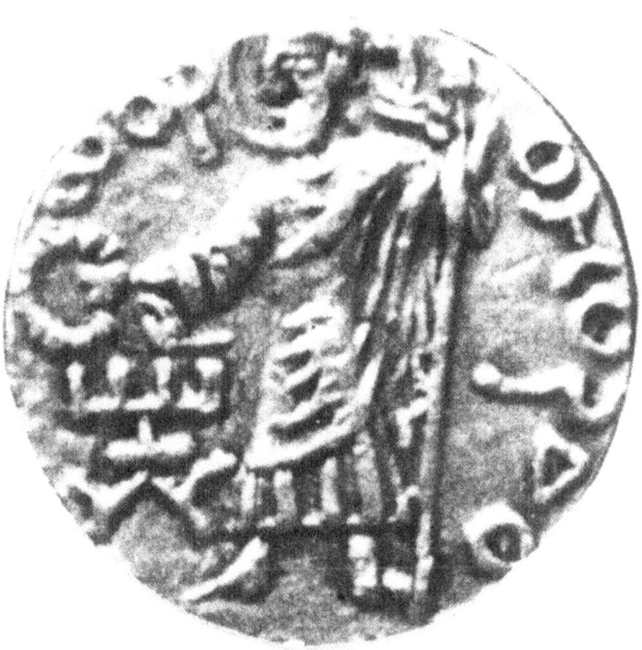

14. Ōoromozdo on a coin of Huvishka (Göbl 1984: Ōoromozdo 1).

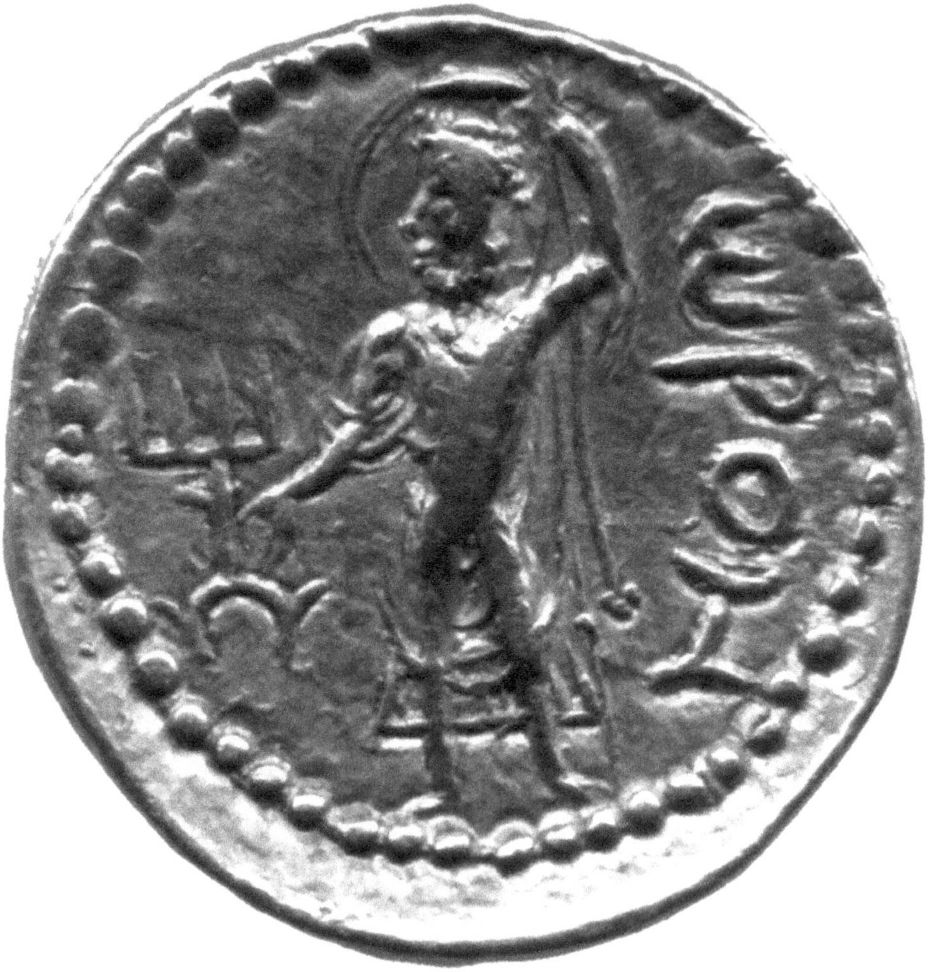

15. Ōrom on a coin of Huvishka (© Trustees of the British Museum).

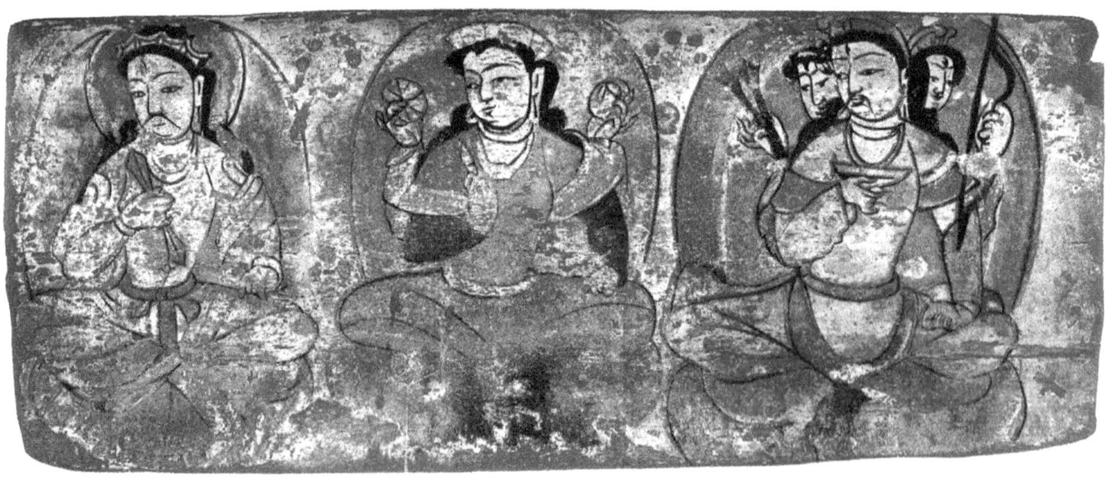

16. Wooden panel from Dandan Uiliq (Stein 1907: pl. LXIV, D.X.3).

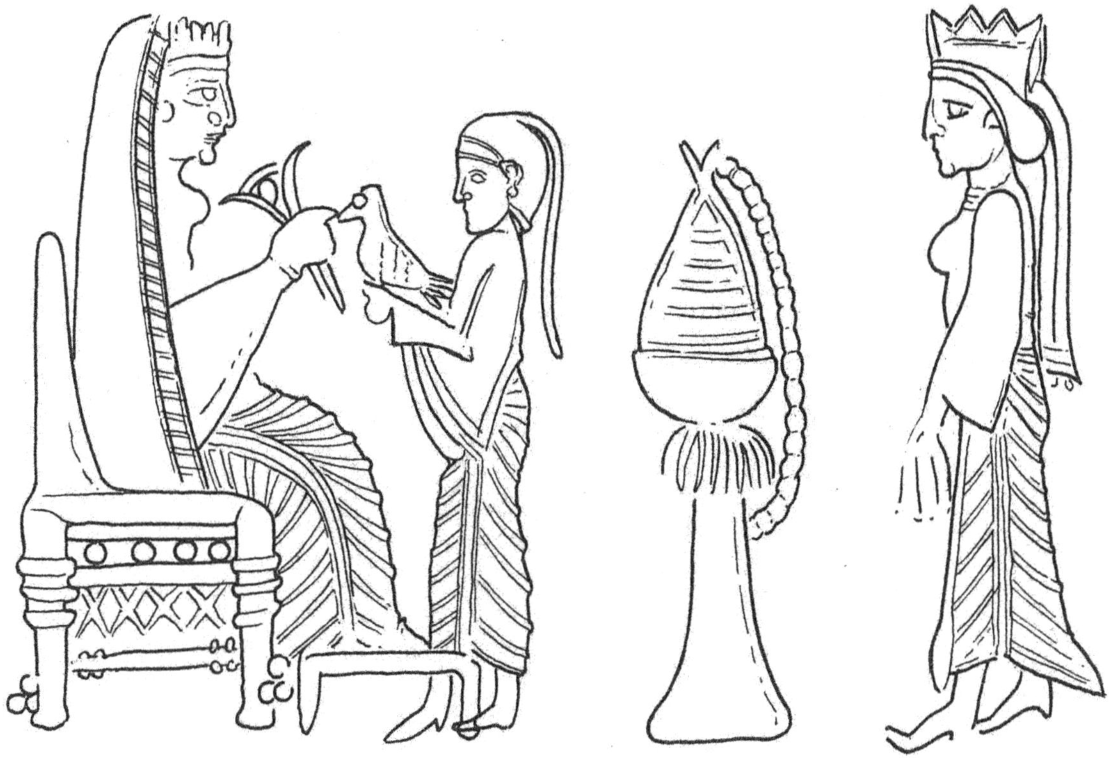

17. Enthroned woman receiving a dove (Moorey 1979: pl. 1, fig. 5).

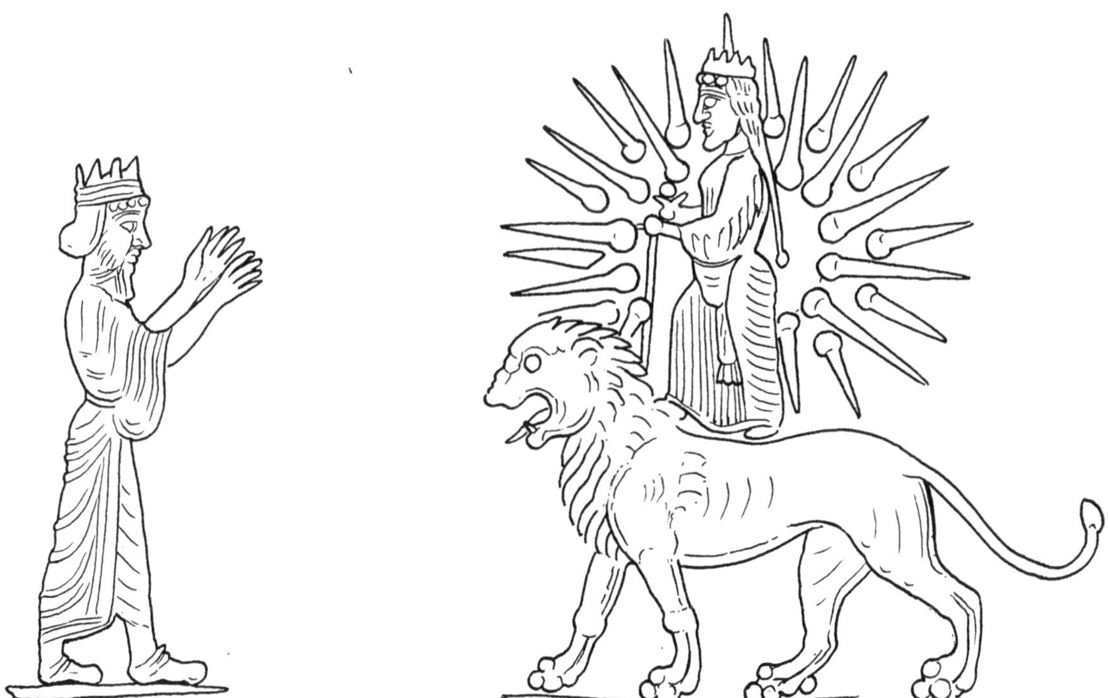

18. Rayed goddess on a lion (Moorey 1979: pl. 1, fig. 4).

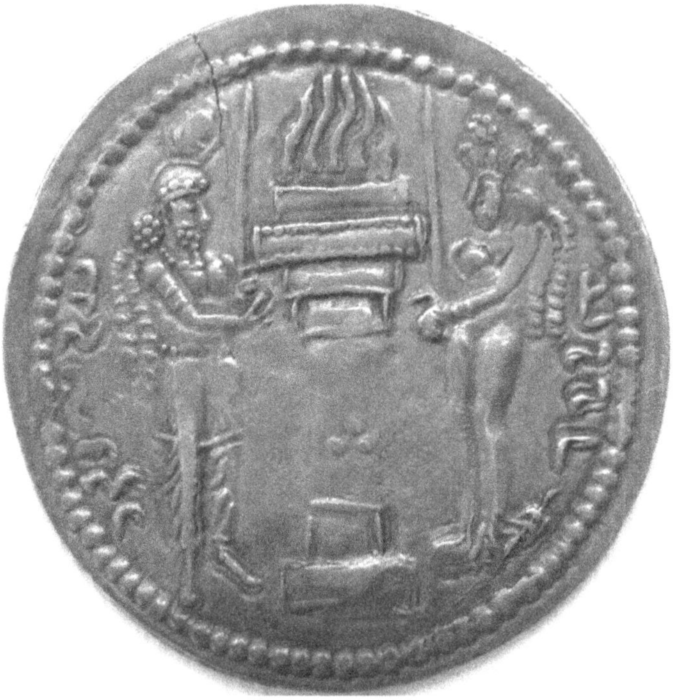

19. Female figure on the coin of Ōhrmazd I (Osmund Bopearachchi).

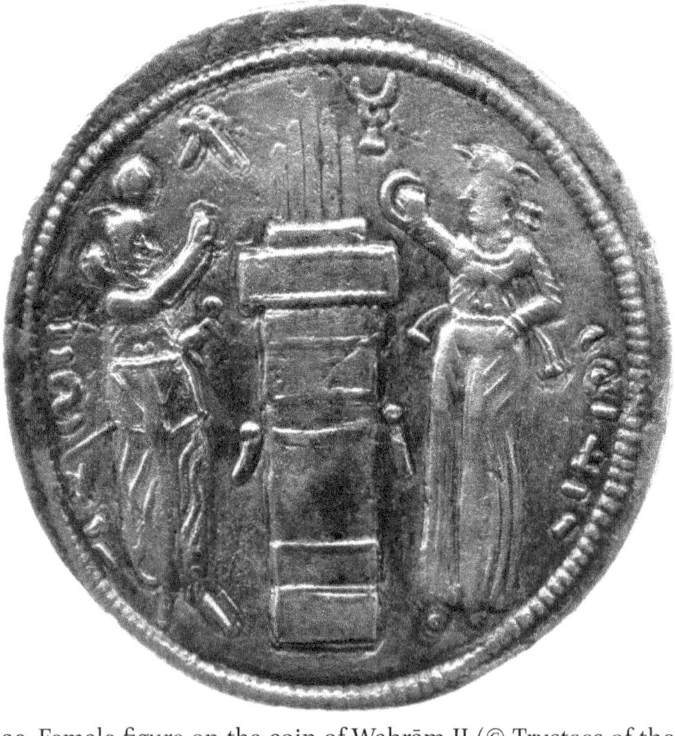

20. Female figure on the coin of Wahrām II (© Trustees of the British Museum).

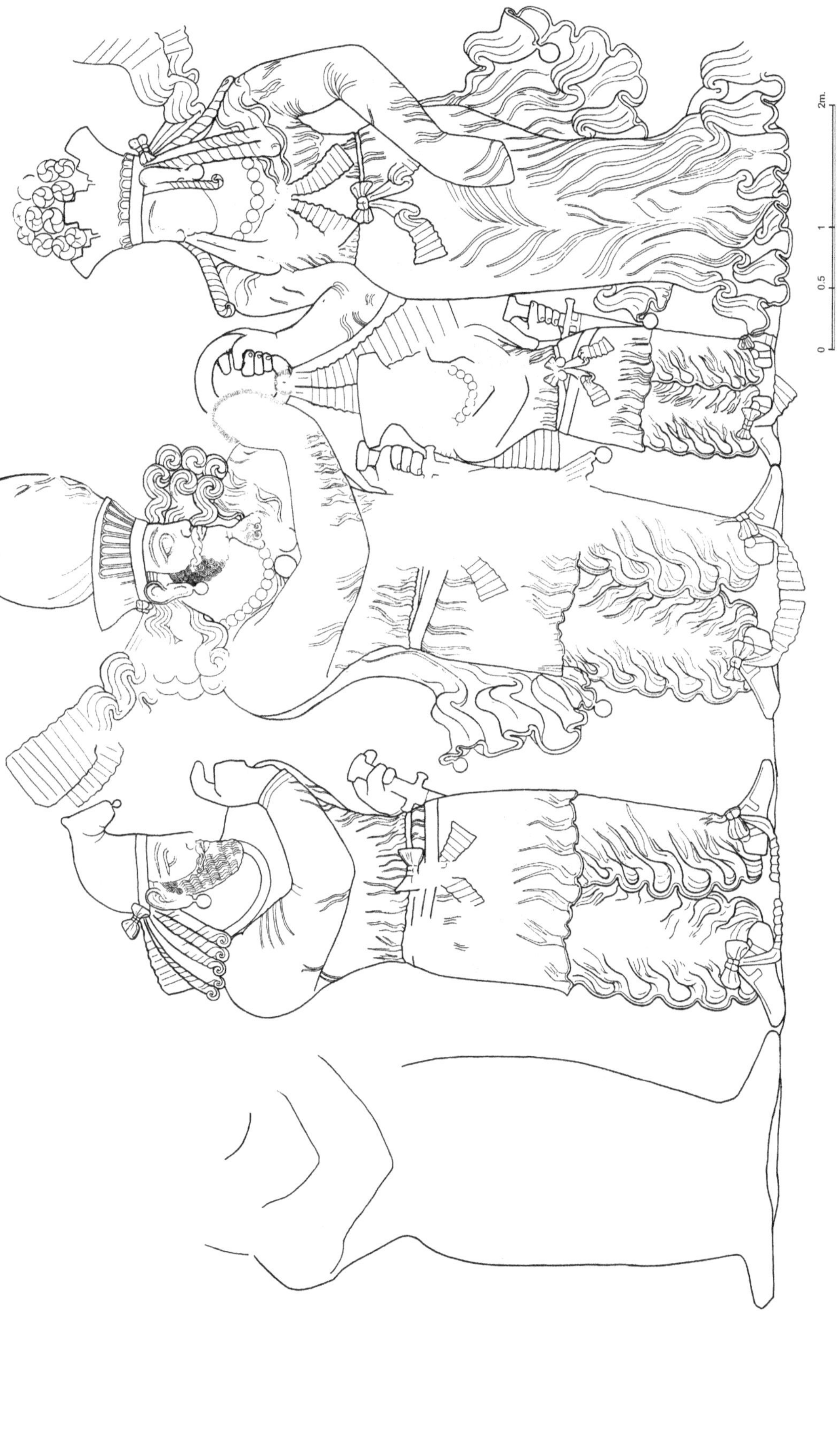

21. Investiture relief of Narseh at Naqš-e Rostam (Georginna Herrmann).

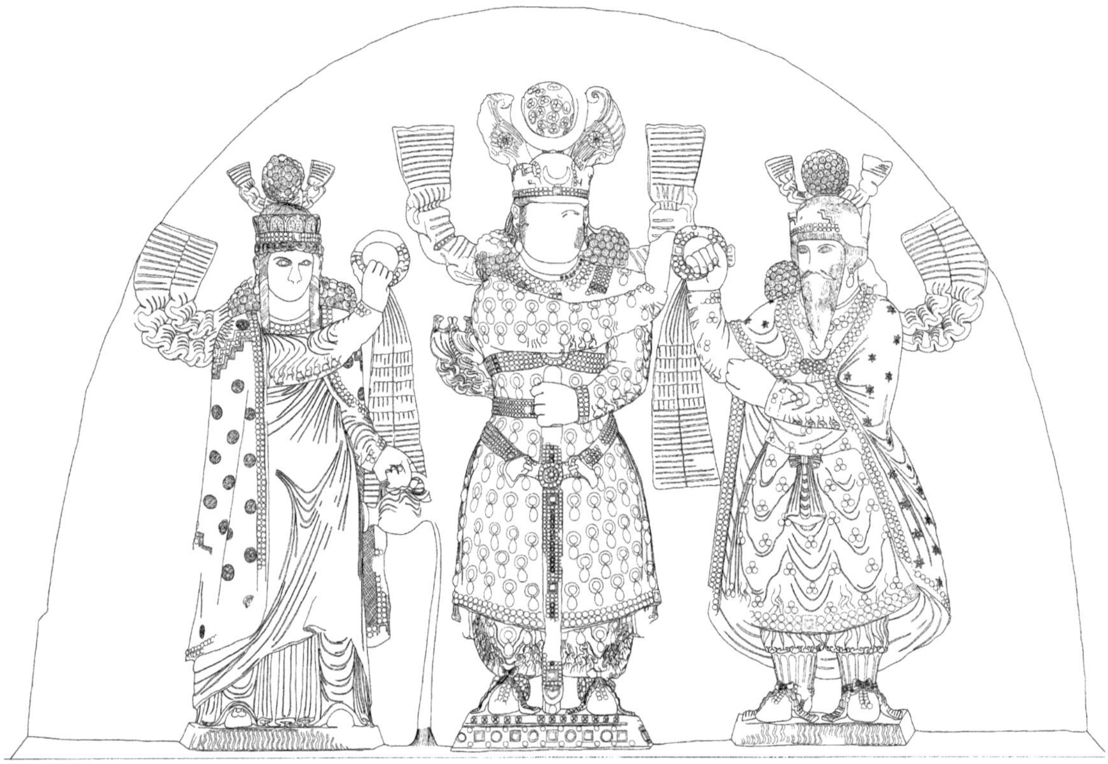

22. Investiture relief of Xusrō II at Ṭāq-i Bustān (Georginna Herrmann).

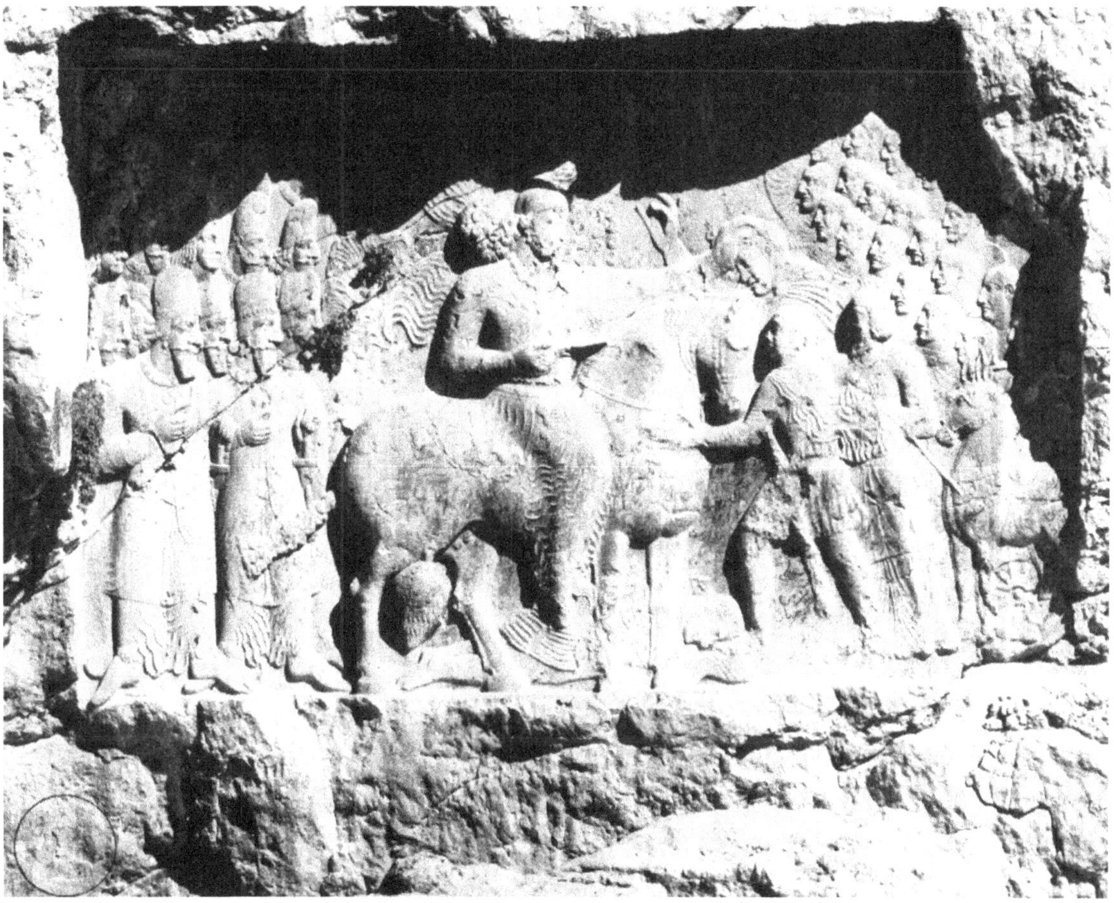

23. The Sasanian relief at Dārābgird. The female bust is encircled in the lower left corner (Vanden Berghe 1978: pl. 2).

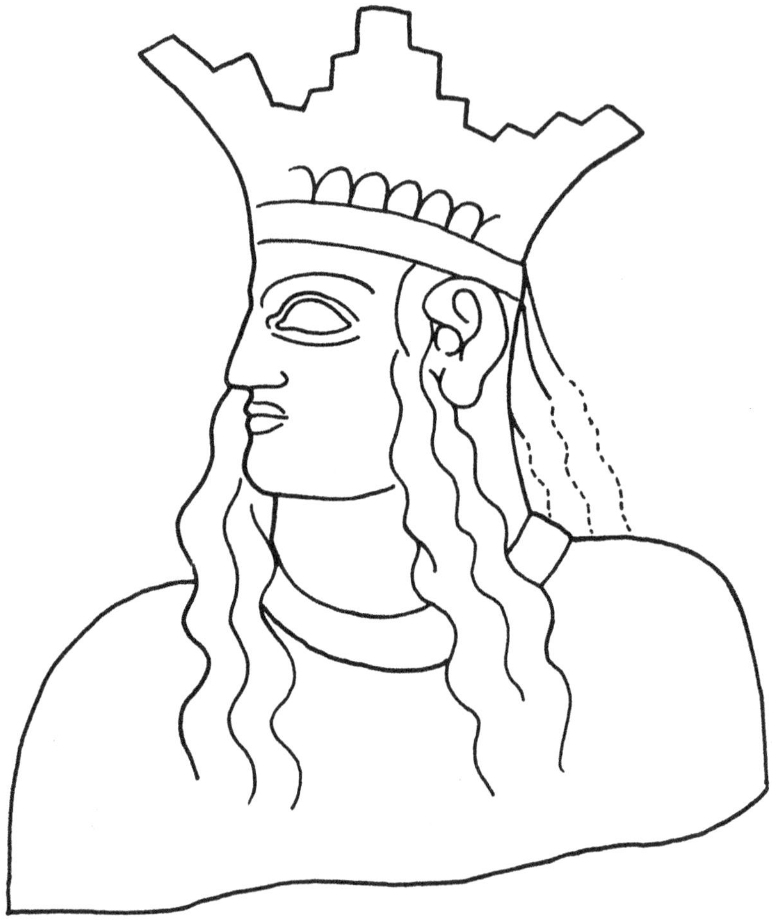

24. A female bust from Dārābgird (Vanden Berghe 1978: fig. 1).

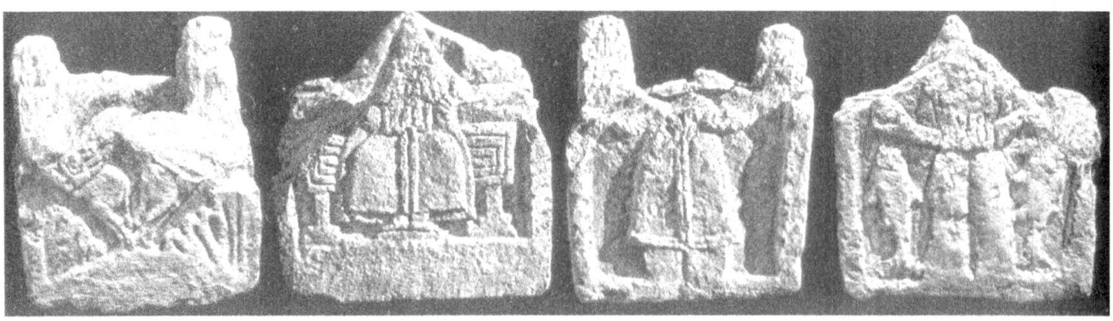

25. A stone casket from Bīšāpūr (Ghirshman 1962: fig. 210).

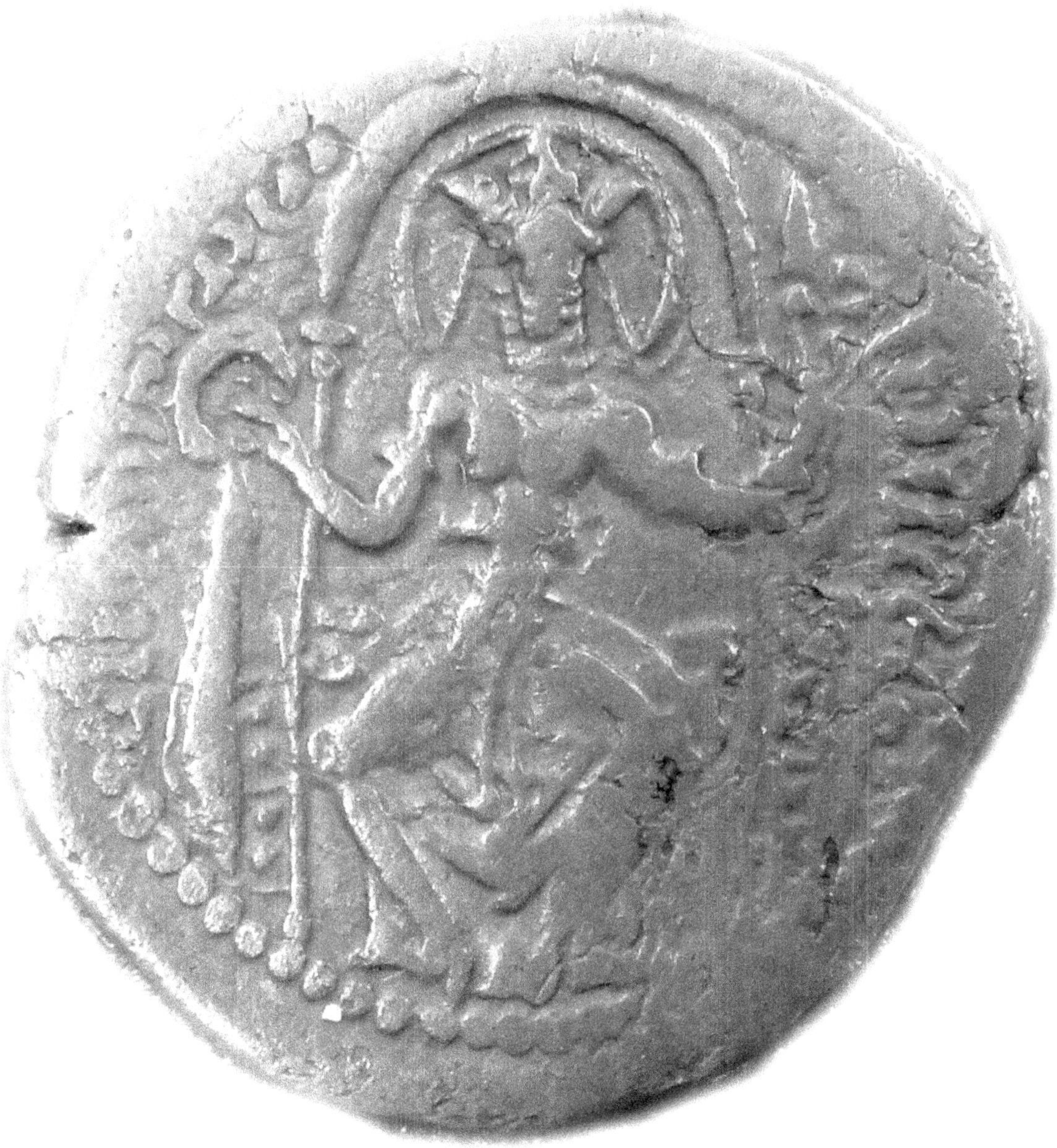

26. Enthroned goddess on a coin of Kushano-Sasanian King Ardašīr I (© Trustees of the British Museum).

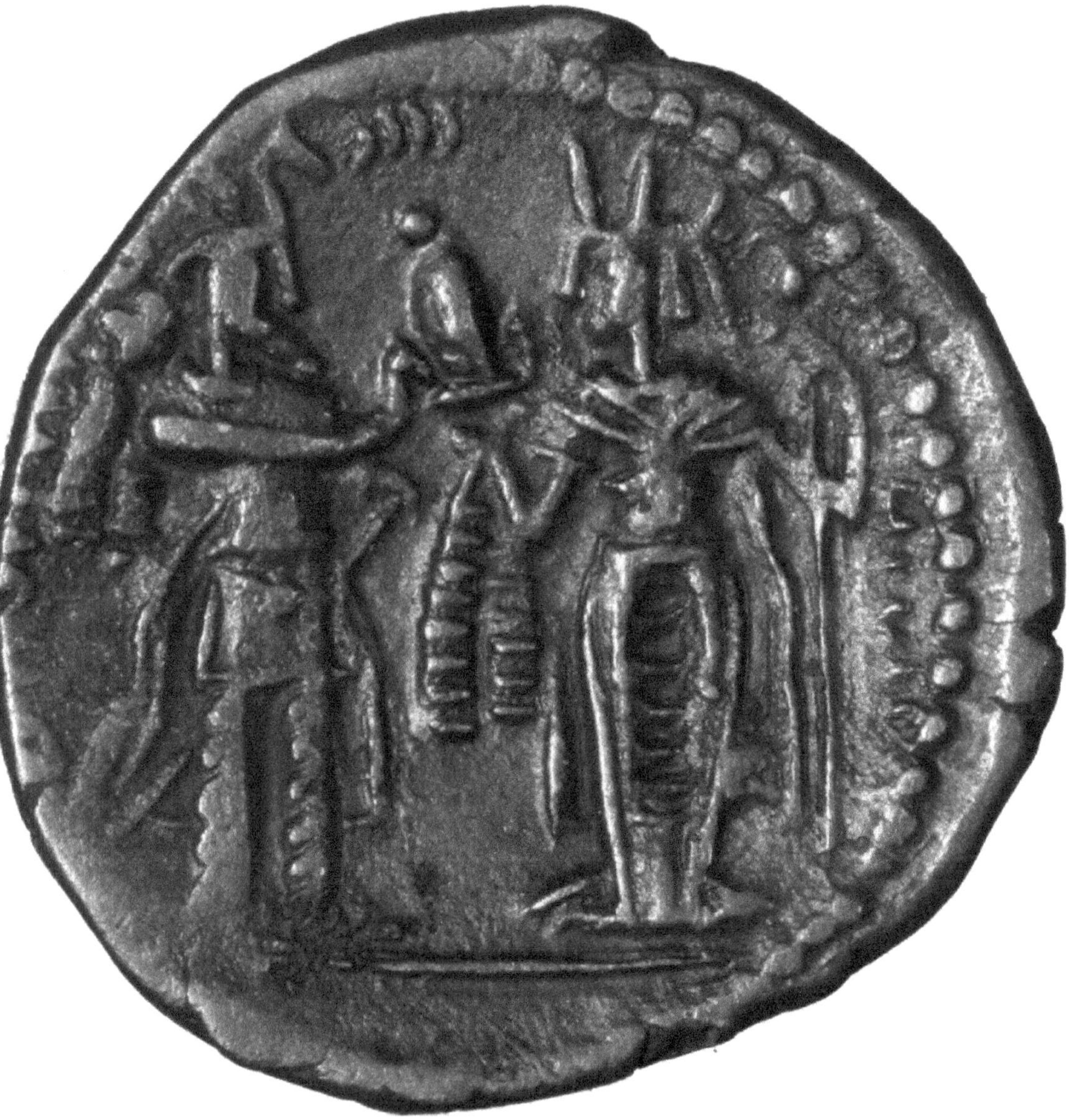

27. Kushano-Sasanian king before a goddess (Aman Ur Rahman).

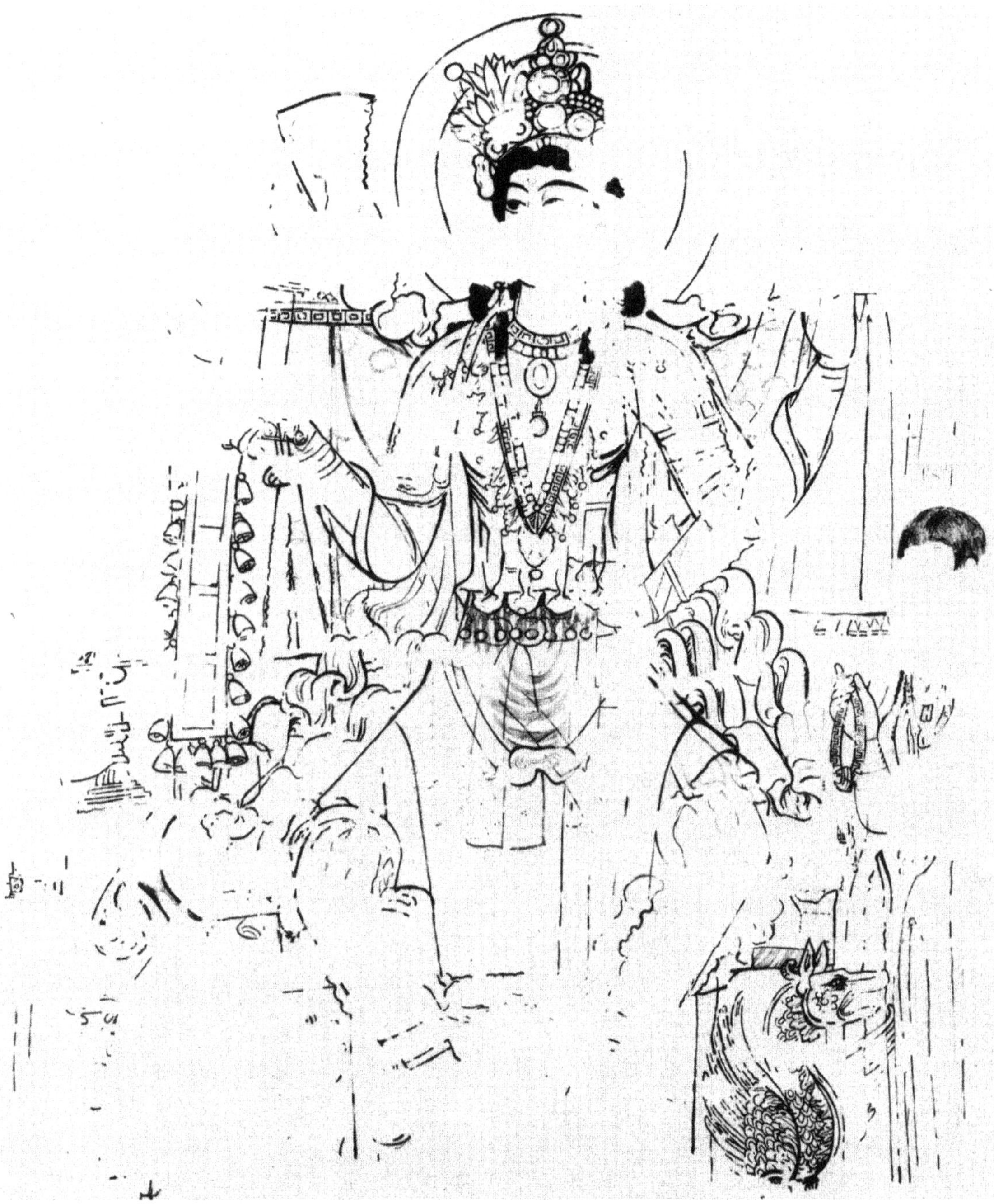

28. Enthroned goddess from Panjikent Temple II, I.5/6 (Belenitskii and Marshak 1981: fig. 34).

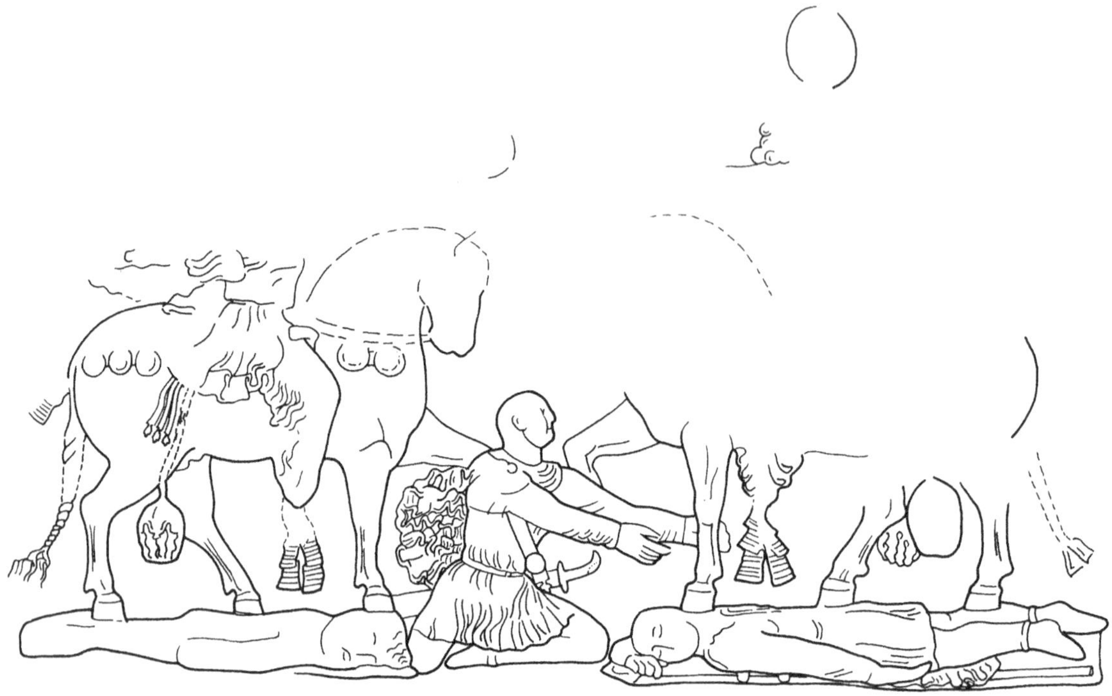

29. Investiture relief of Šāpūr I at Bīšāpūr (drawing E. Smekens © BAMI).

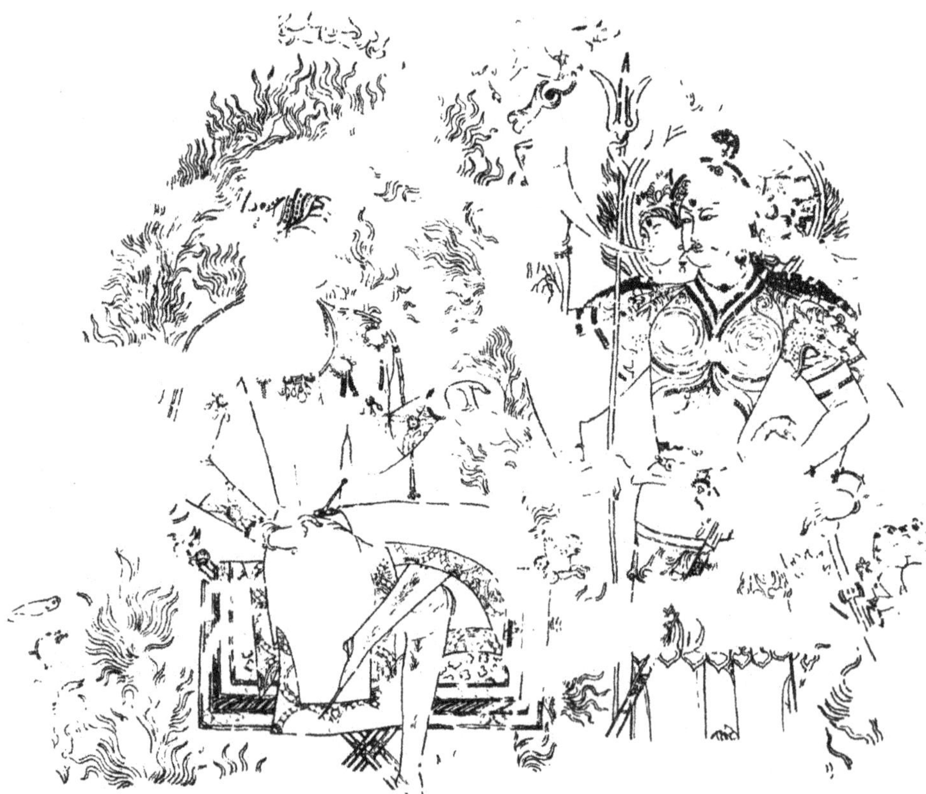

30. Two Gods, Panjikent XXII/1 (Frantz Grenet).

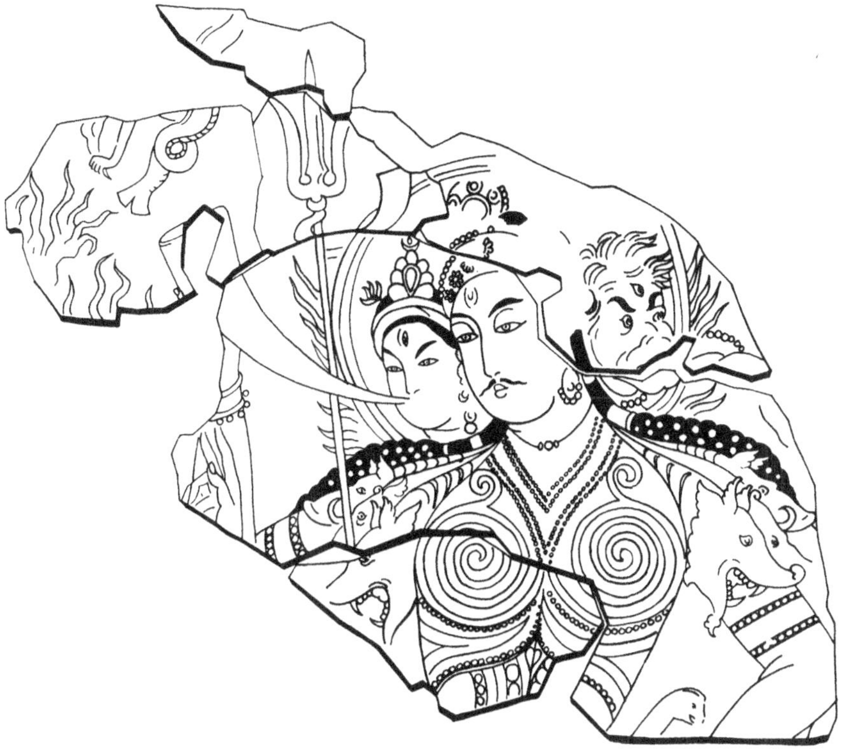

31. Wešparkar, Panjikent XXII/1 (Frantz Grenet).

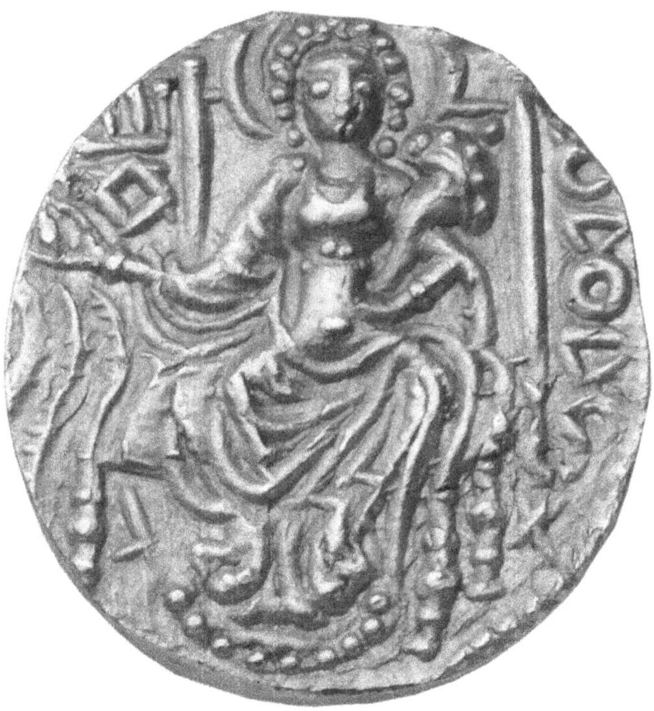

32. Enthroned Ardoxšo on a Kushan coin (Osmund Bopearachchi).

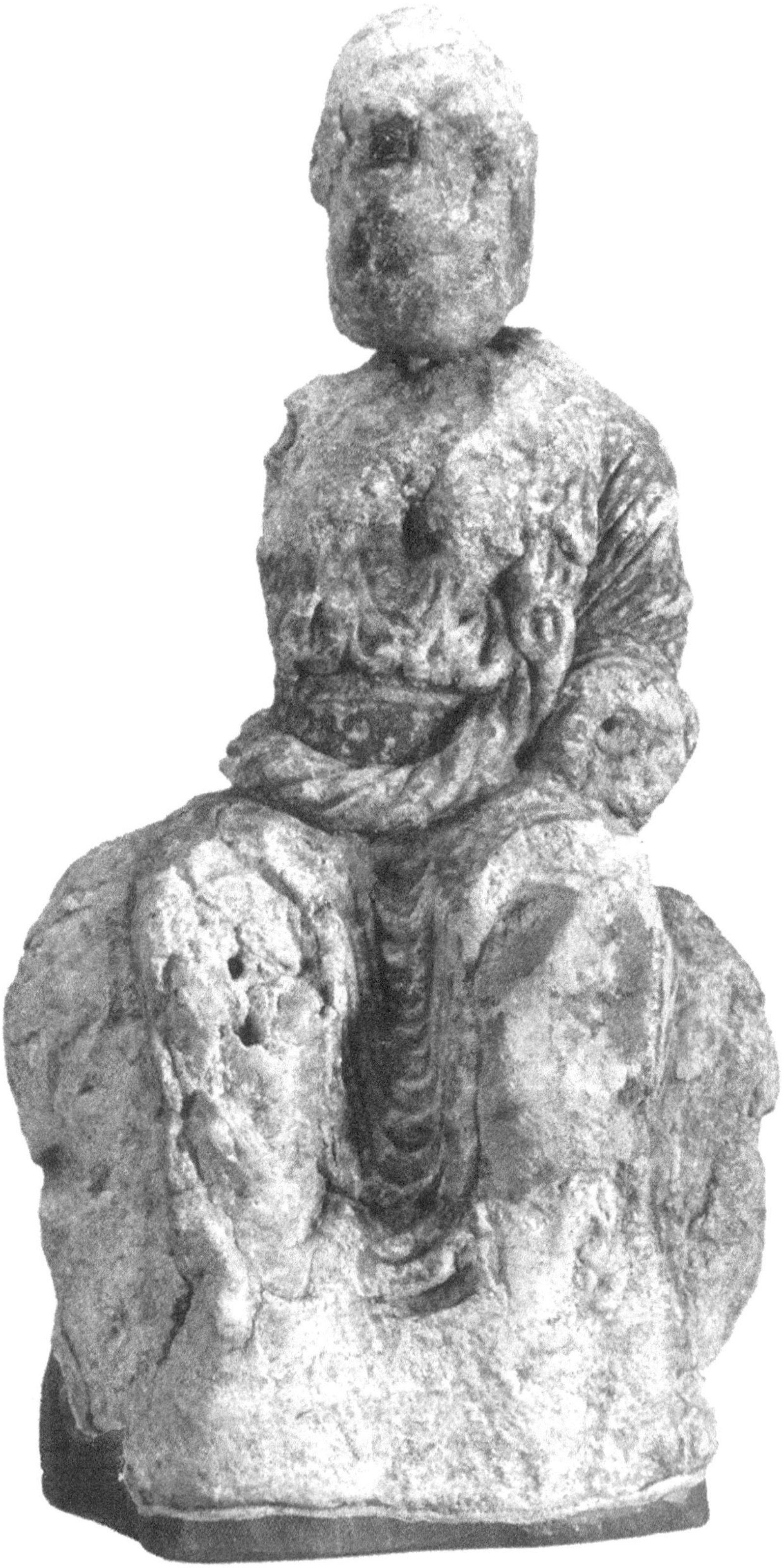

33. Female statue, Panjikent Temple II (Marshak 2009: 12).

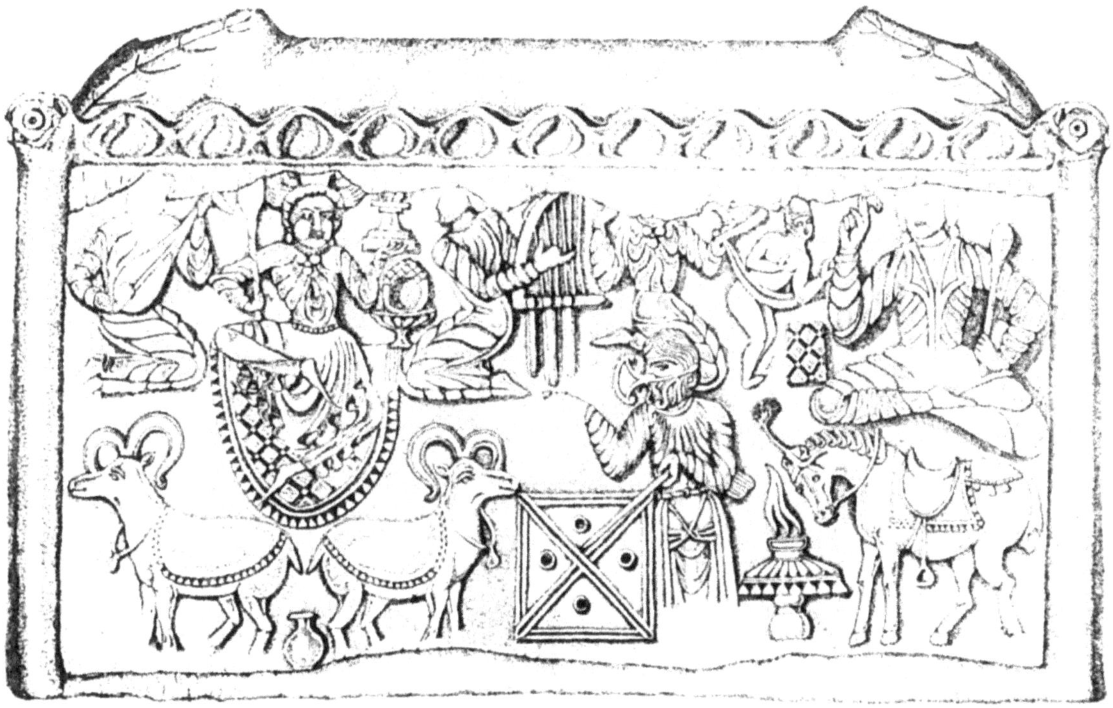

34. Ossuary from Sivaz (Frantz Grenet).

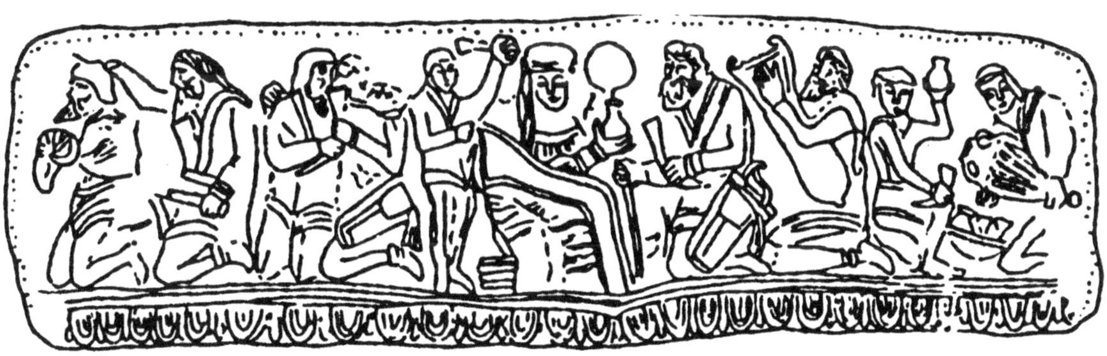

35. Sakhnovka diadem (Ustinova 1999: pl. 10.3).

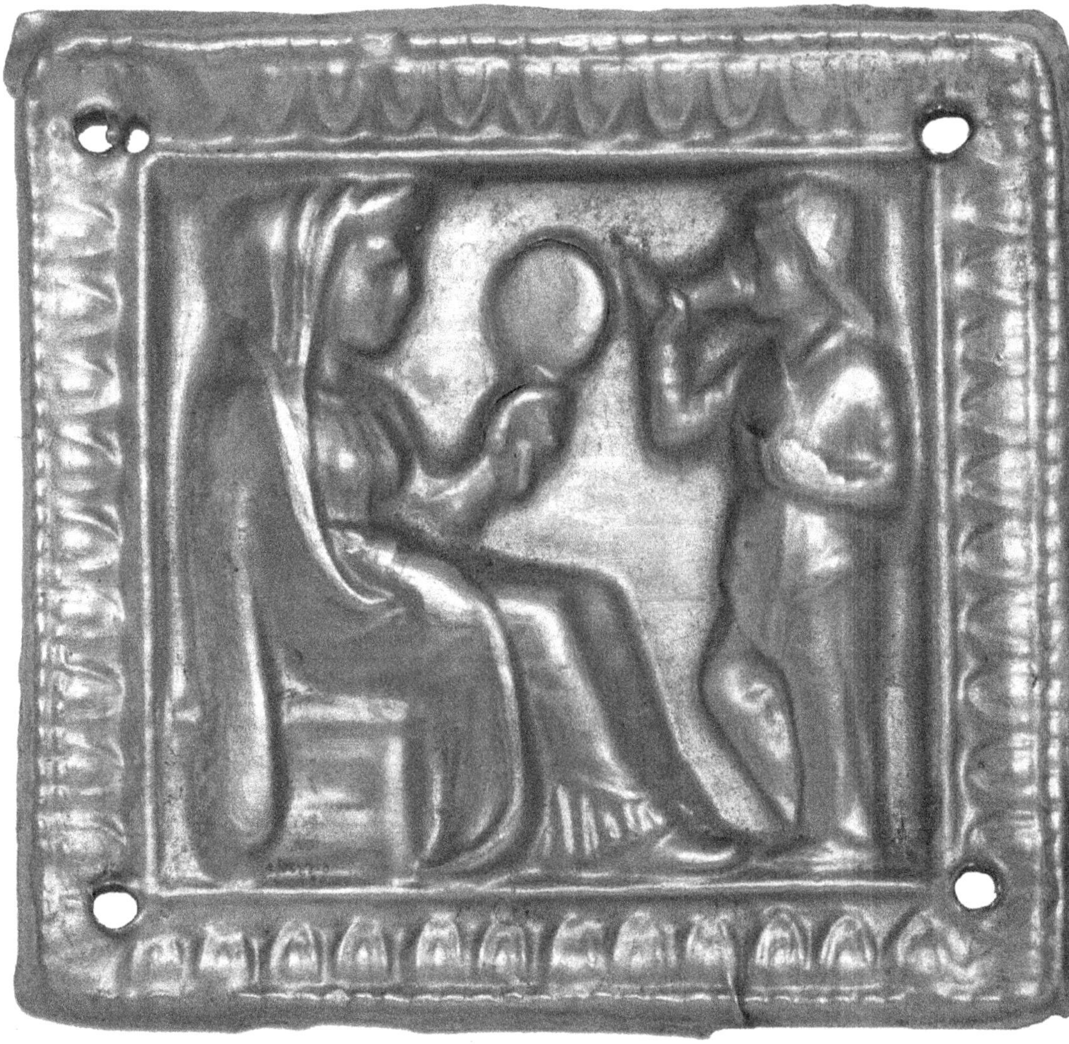

36. Golden plaque from Chertomlyk kurgan (Korol'kova 2006: fig. 48).

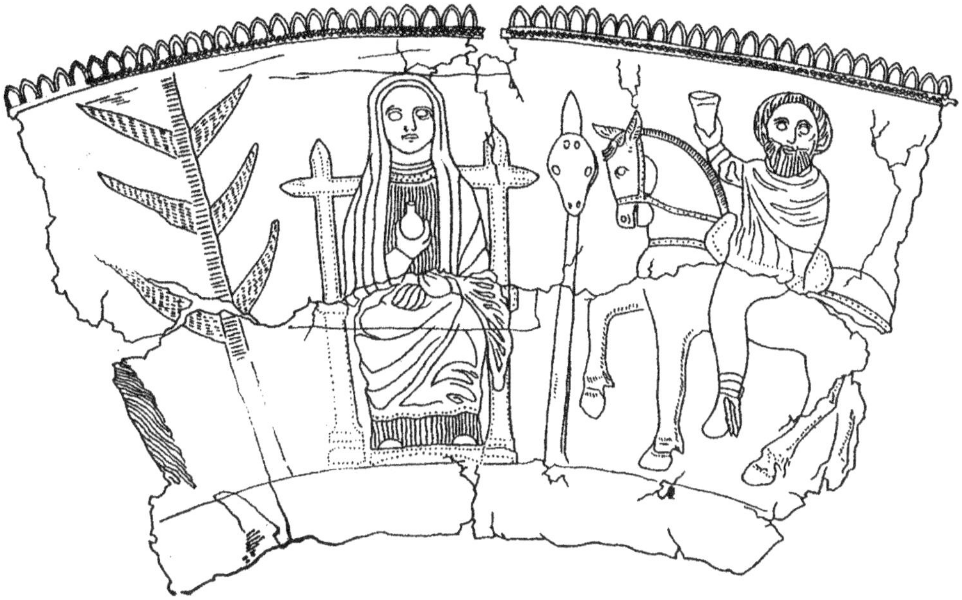

37. A goddess with a vessel, Merdzhany kurgan (Bessonova 1983: fig. 31).

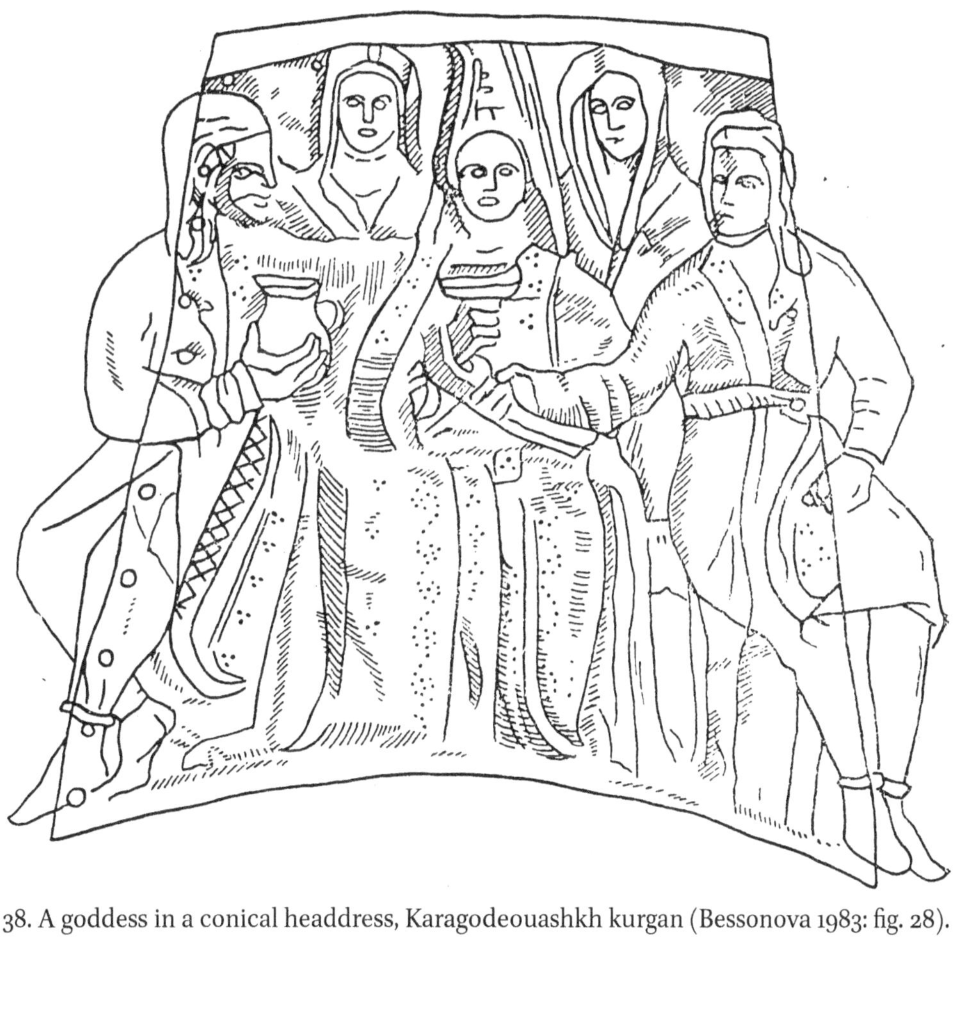

38. A goddess in a conical headdress, Karagodeouashkh kurgan (Bessonova 1983: fig. 28).

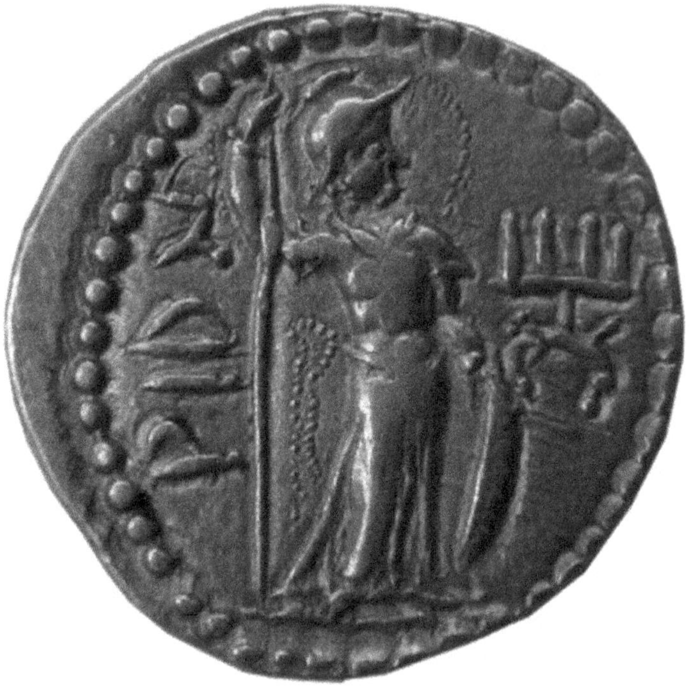

39. Rišto on a Kushan coin (© Trustees of the British Museum).

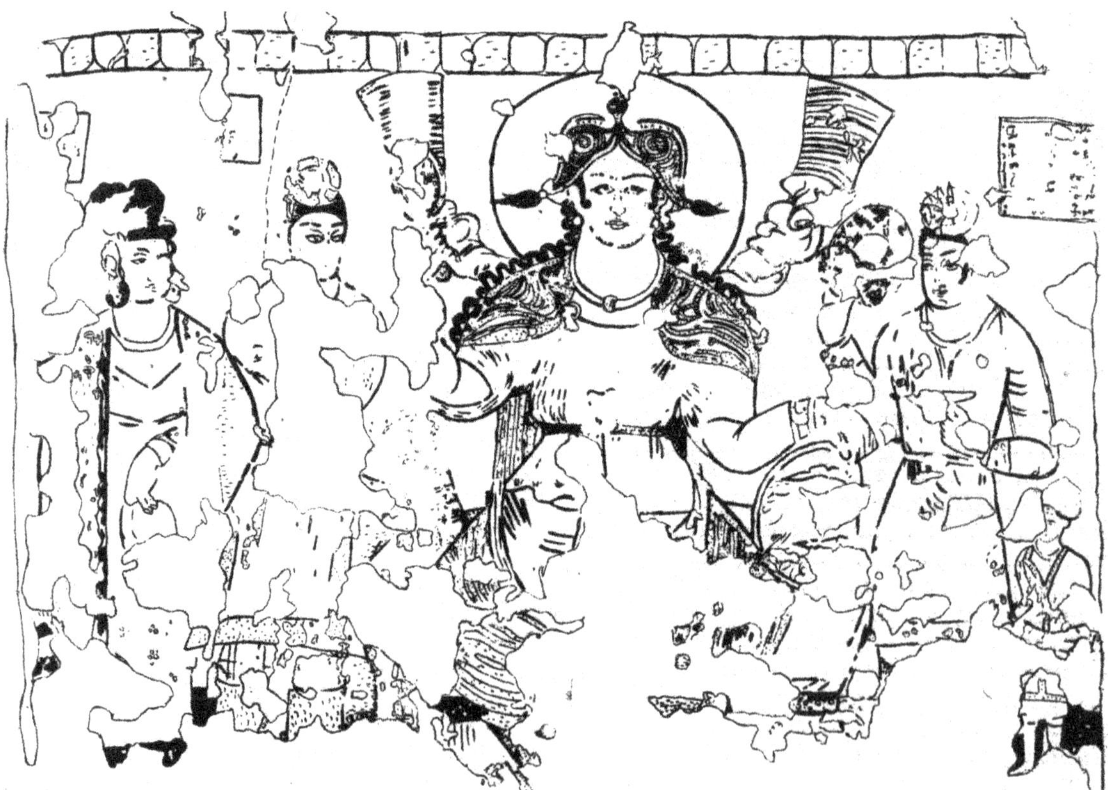

40. A goddess wearing a helmet, Dilberjin 12 (Kruglikova 1976: fig. 56).

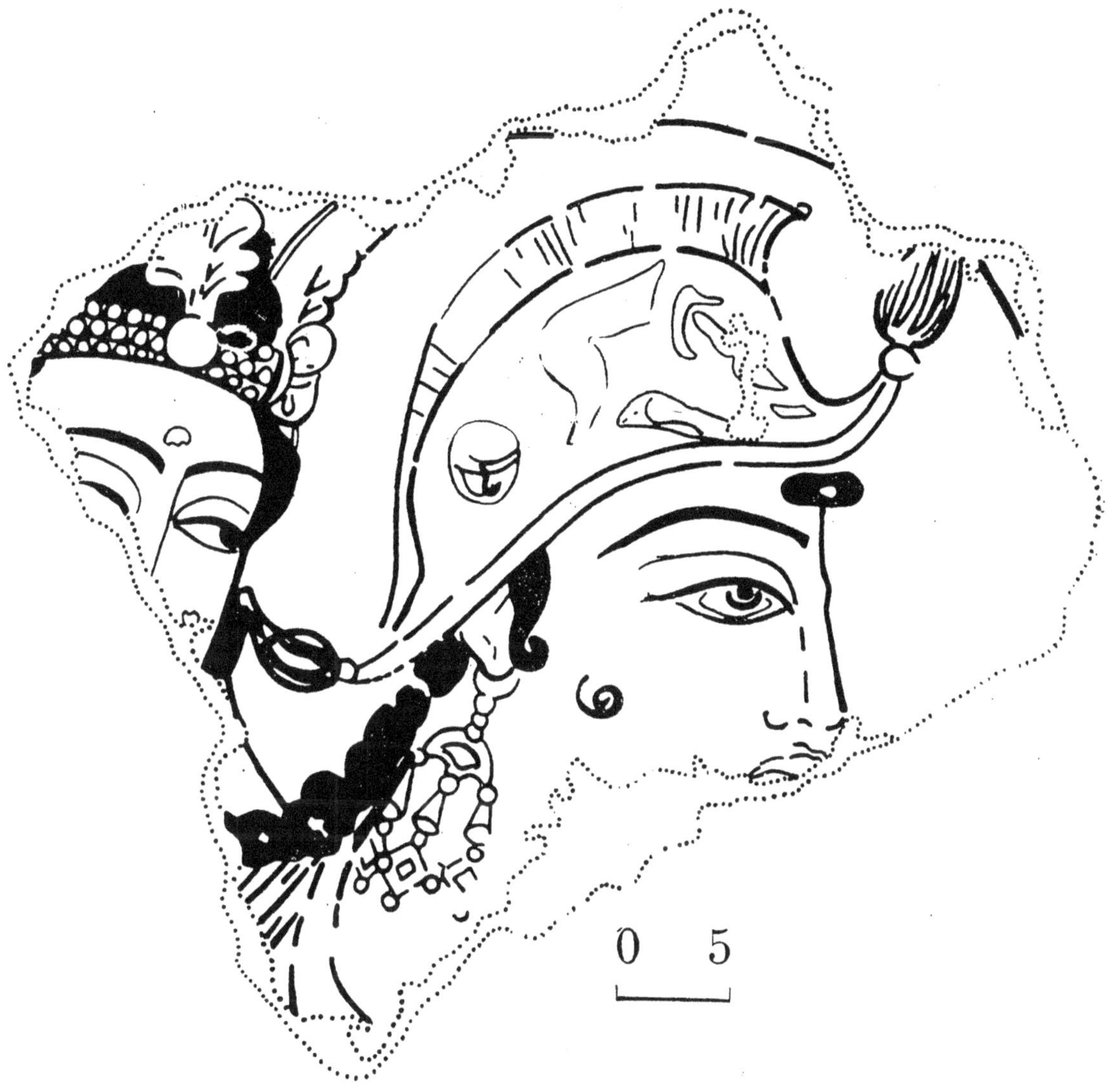

41. A goddess wearing a helmet, Dilberjin 16 (Kruglikova 1976: fig. 59).

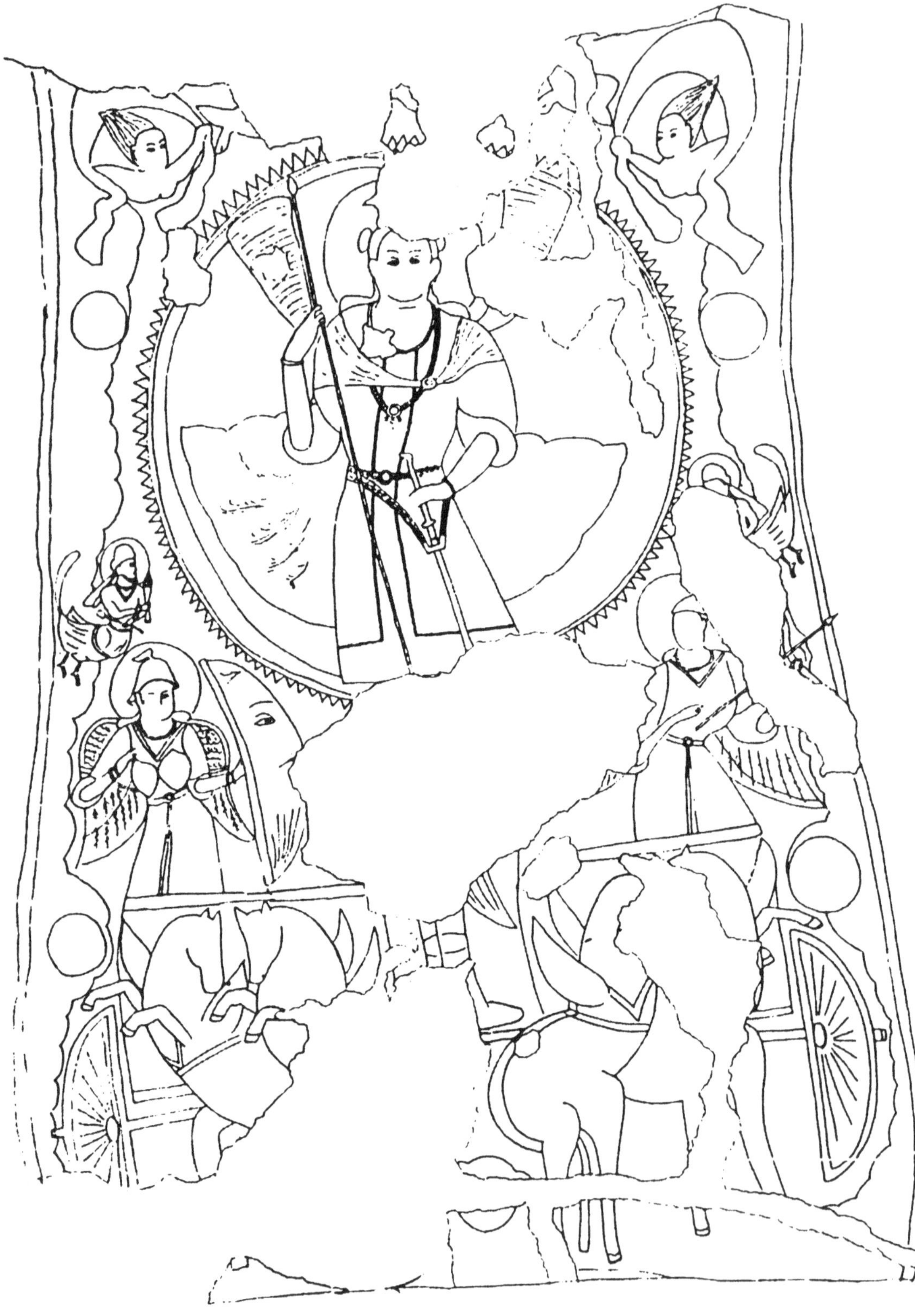

42. A solar chariot, formerly in the niche of the small Buddha, Bāmiān (Frantz Grenet).

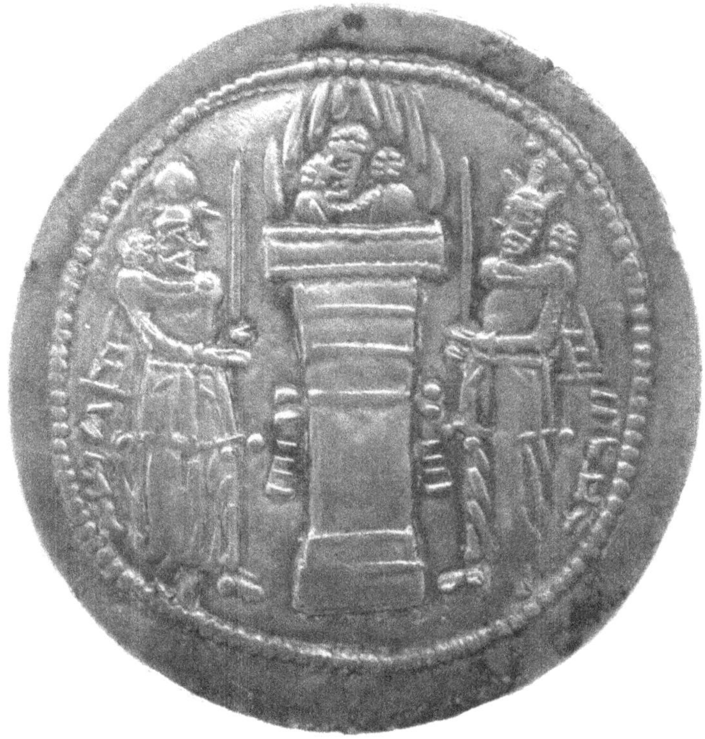

43. Bust emerging from a fire-altar on a coin of Ōhrmazd II (Osmund Bopearachchi).

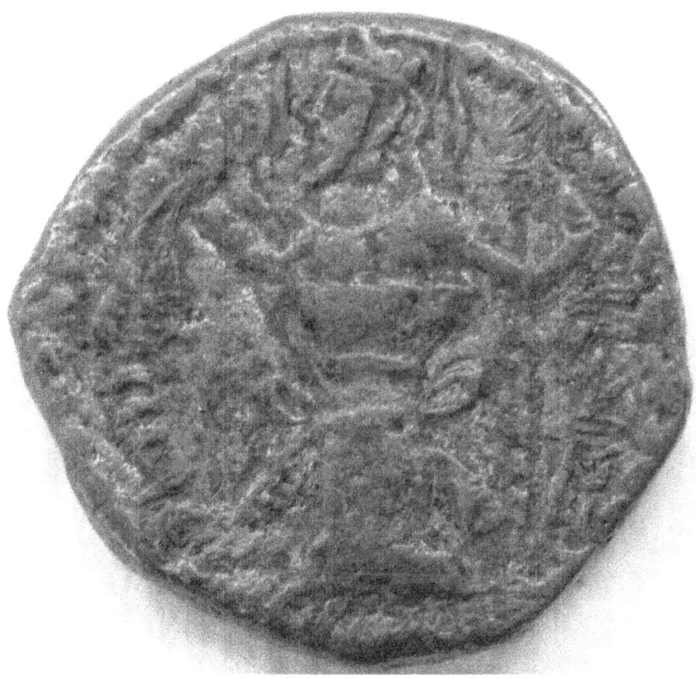

44. Flaming torso on a fire-altar, Kushano-Sasanian coin (Osmund Bopearachchi).

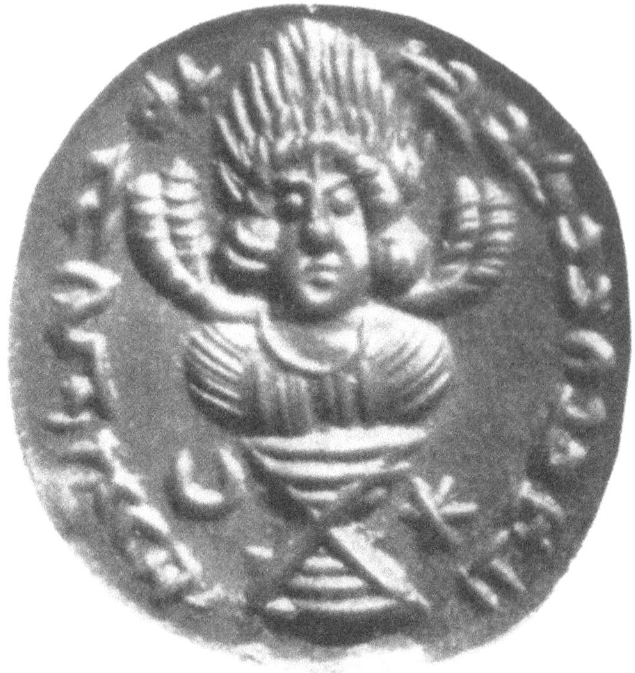

45. Bust on a fire-altar, Sasanian seal, private collection (Gyselen 1990: pl. II. 24).

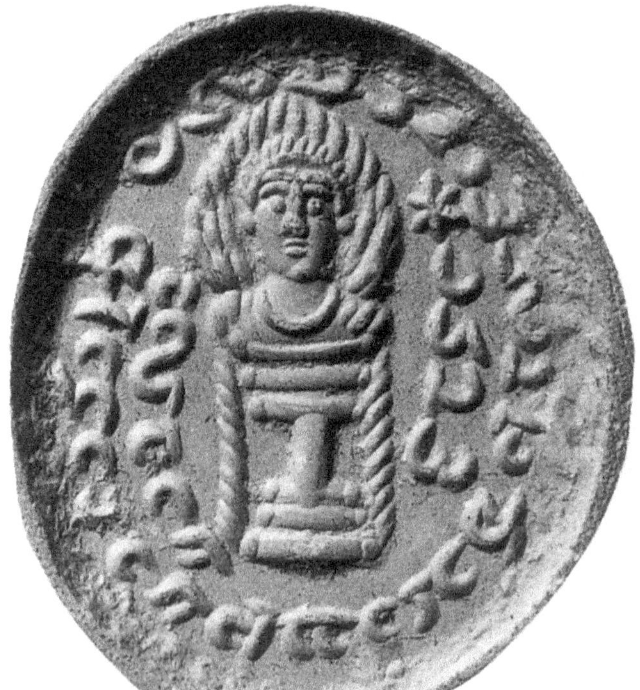

46. Bust on a fire-altar, Sasanian seal, *BnF* (Gyselen 1993: 20.I.8).

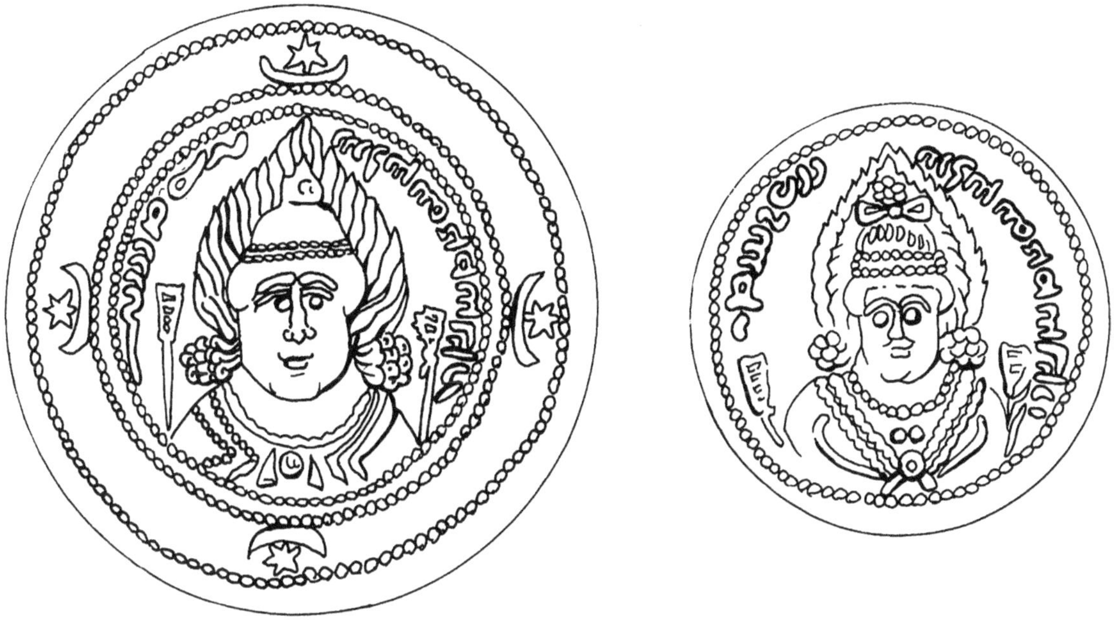

47. Two types of a flaming bust on the coins of Xusrō II (Gyselen 2000: fig. b).

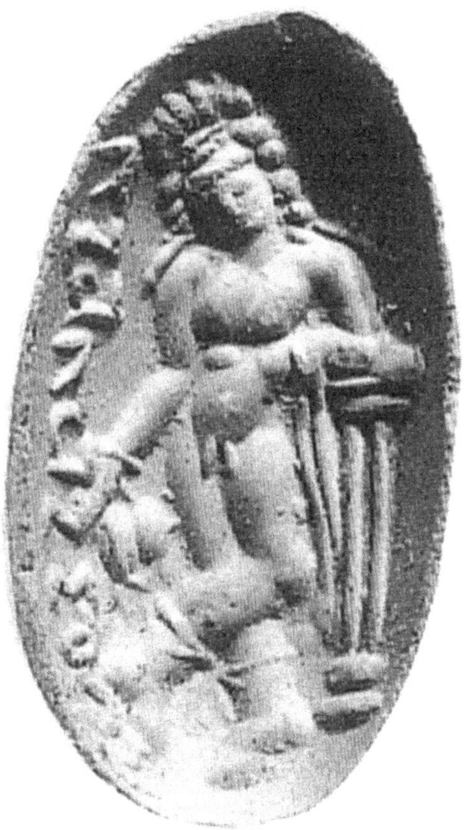

48. Naked standing figure in flames on a Sasanian seal (Gyselen 1993: 10.B).

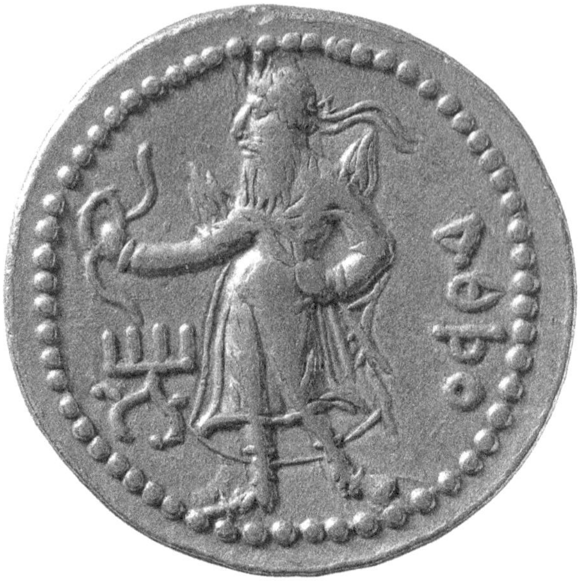

49. Athšo on a Kushan coin, type 1 (Frantz Grenet).

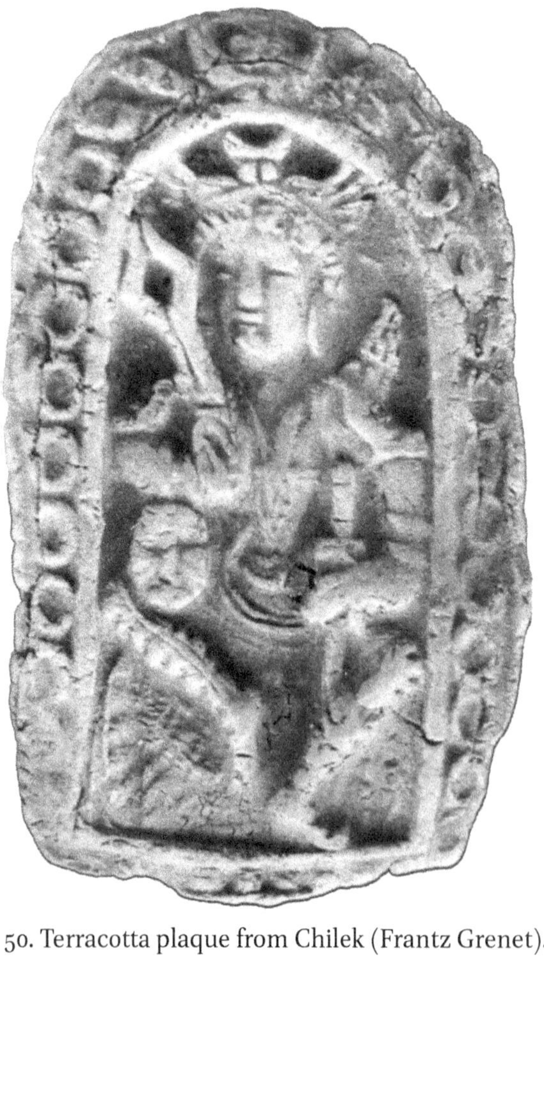

50. Terracotta plaque from Chilek (Frantz Grenet).

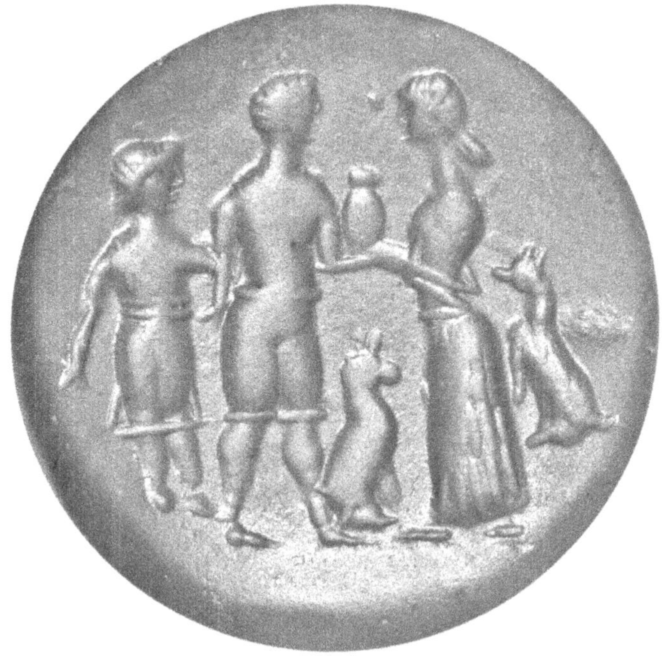

51. A seal depicting a lady with two dogs (Aman Ur Rahman).

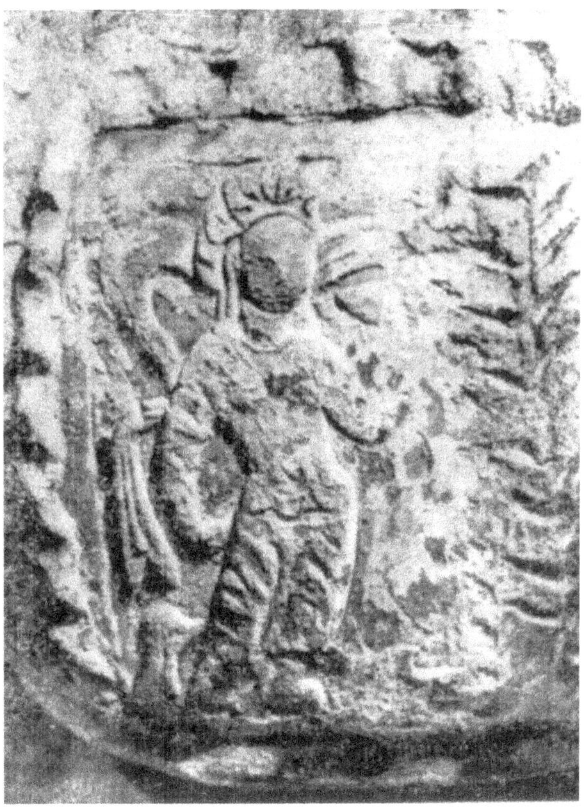

52. A female figure depicted on the ossuary from Changi (Frantz Grenet).

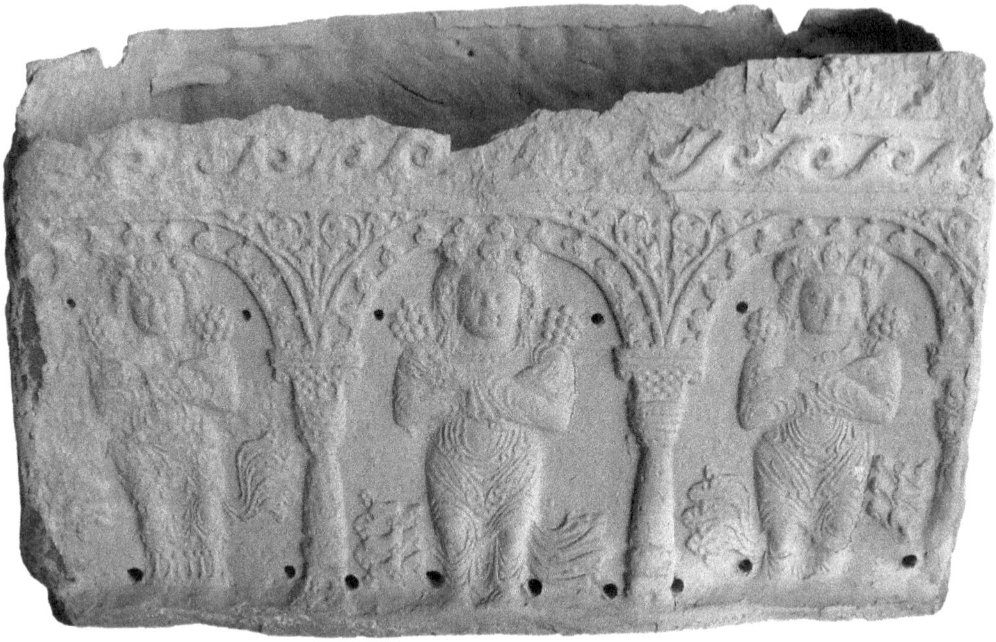

53. The ossuary from Sarytepe (Frantz Grenet).

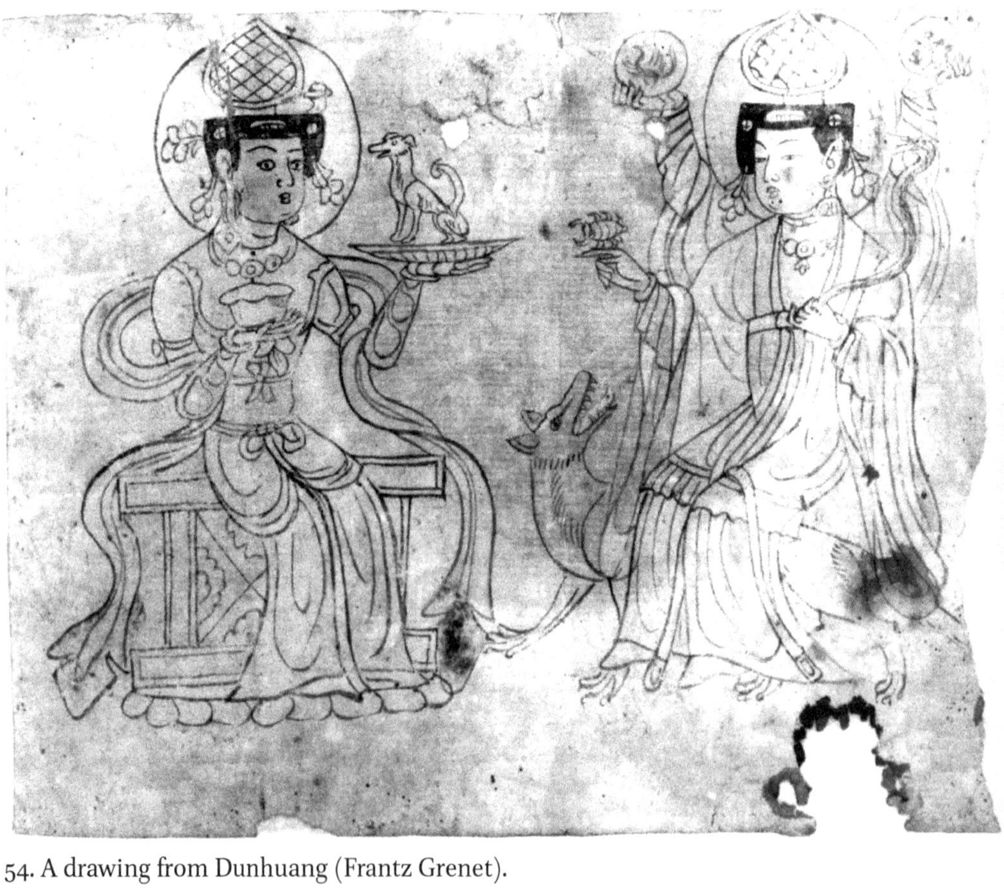

54. A drawing from Dunhuang (Frantz Grenet).

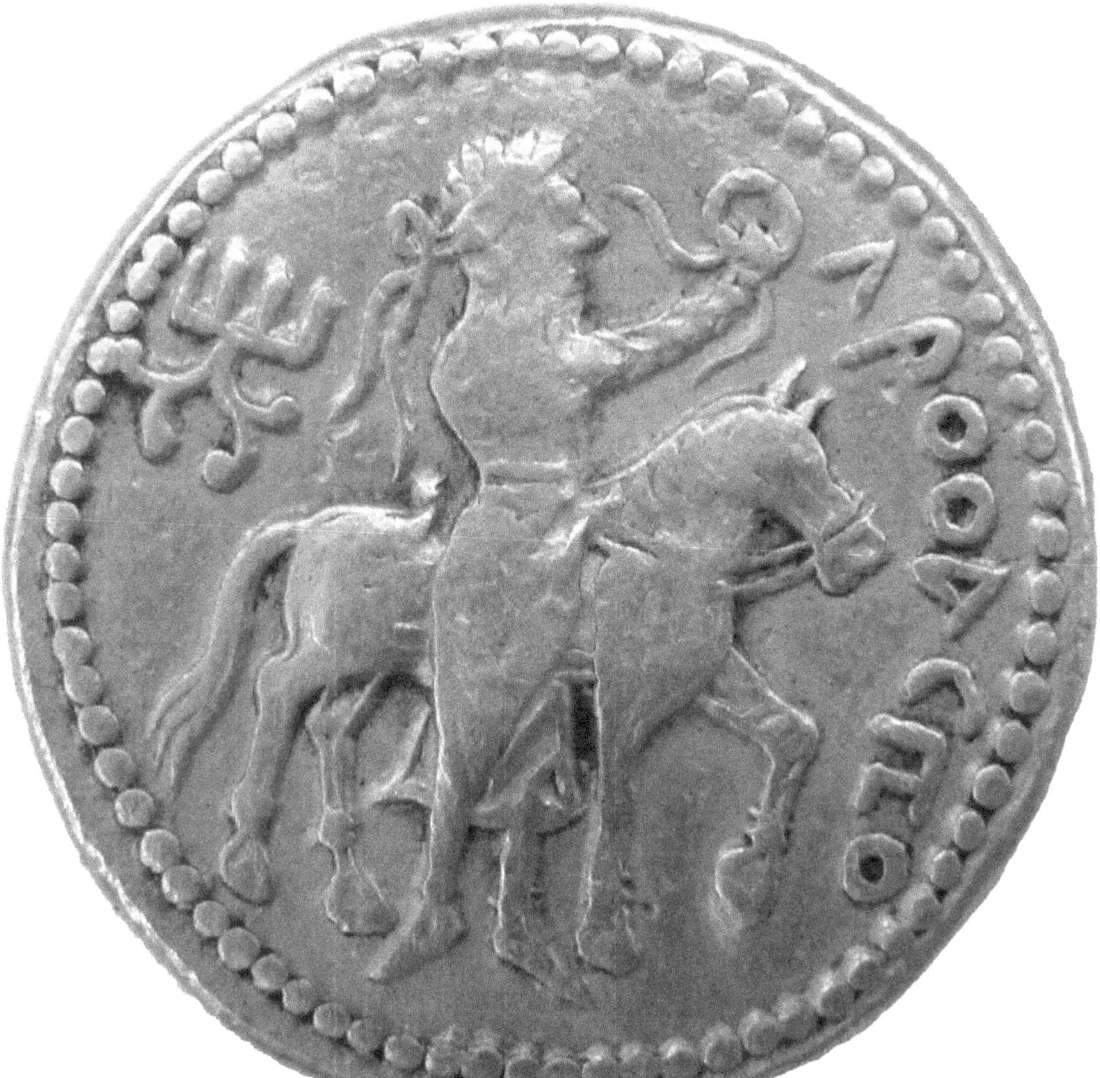

55. Lrooaspo on a Kushan coin (Osmund Bopearachchi).

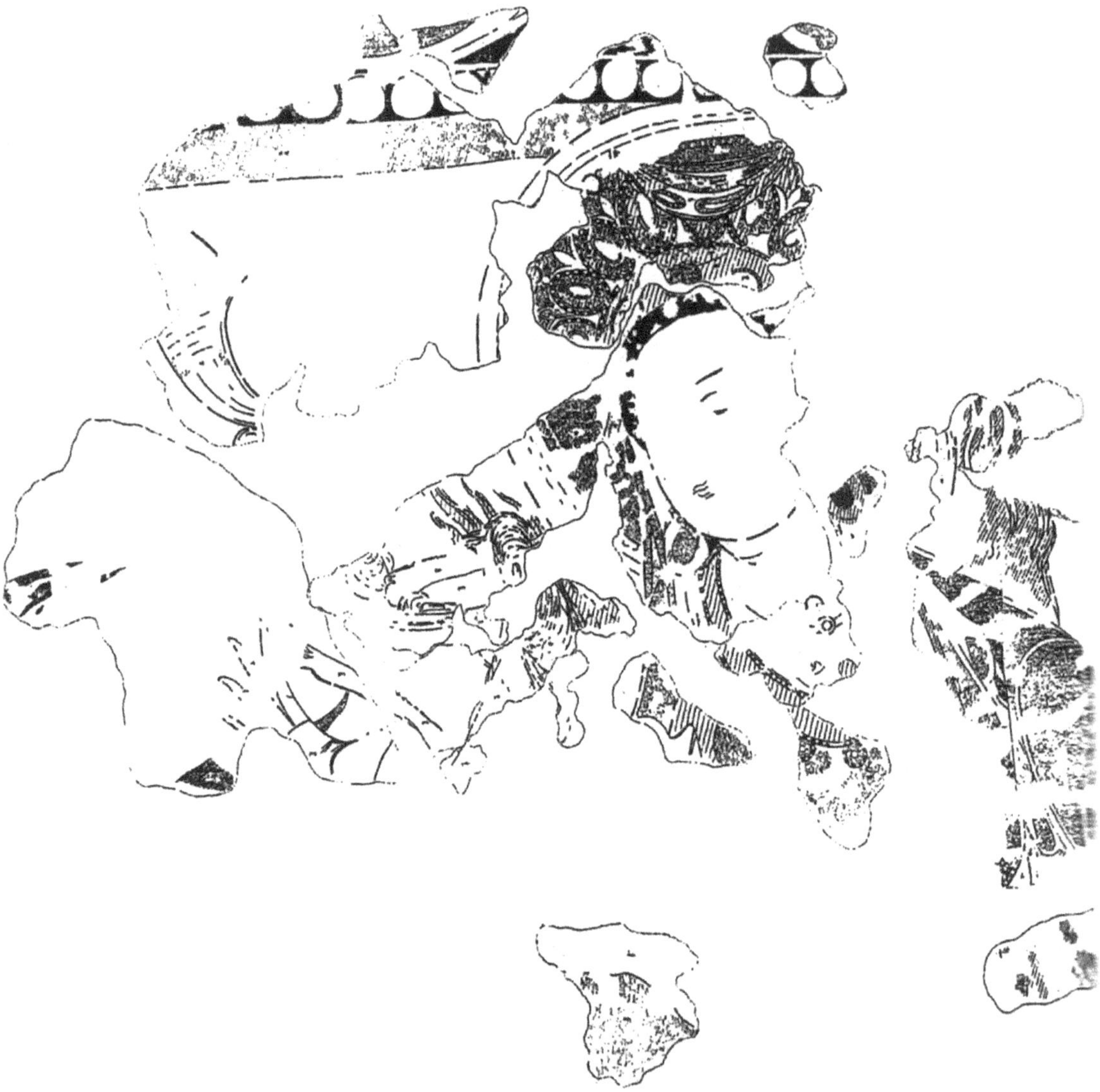

56. A goddess with a figure of a horse, Panjikent, Temple I (Frantz Grenet).

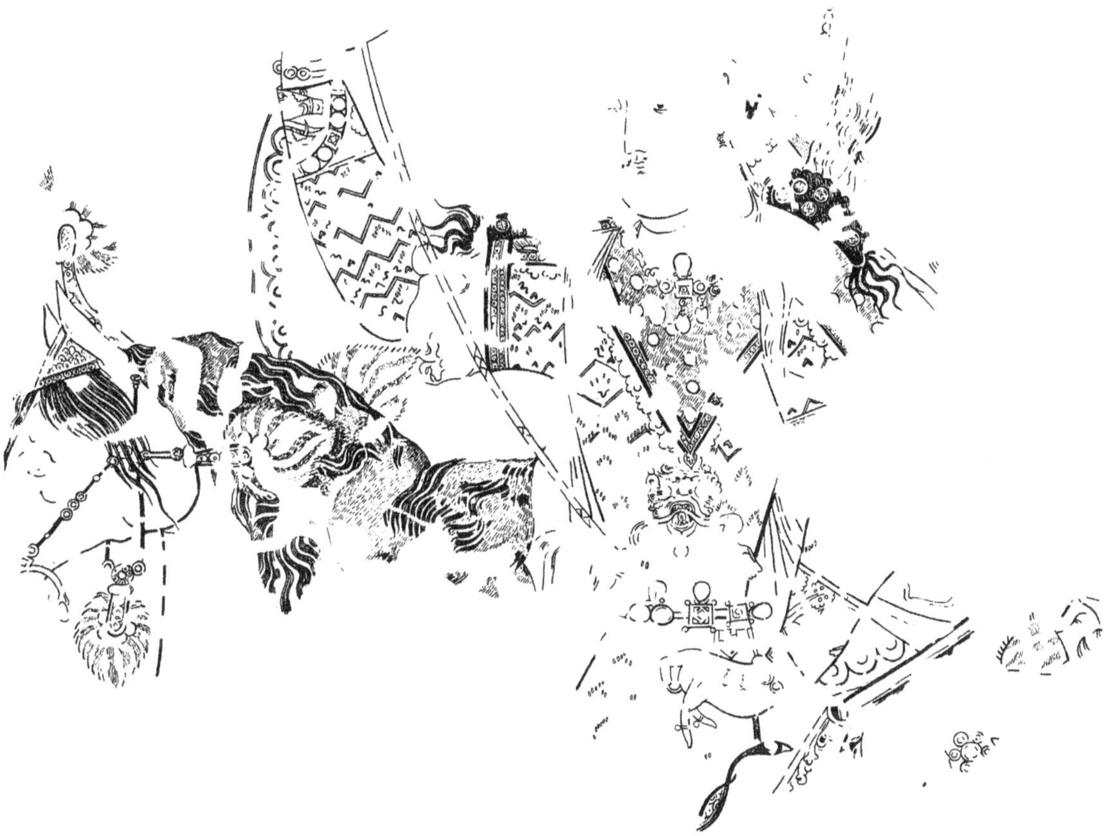

57. A god with a horse, Panjikent, Temple I (Frantz Grenet).

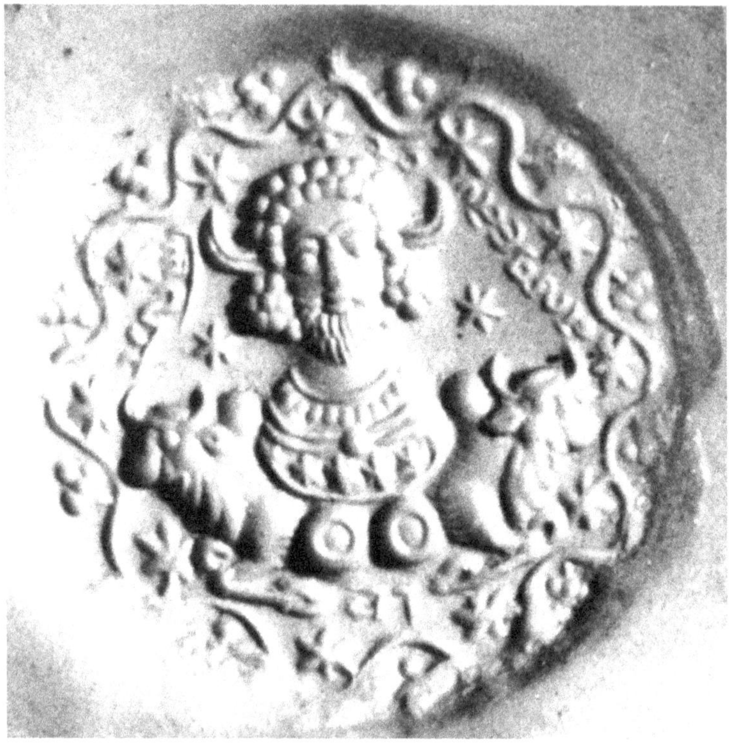

58. Chariot of the Moon god (Frantz Grenet).

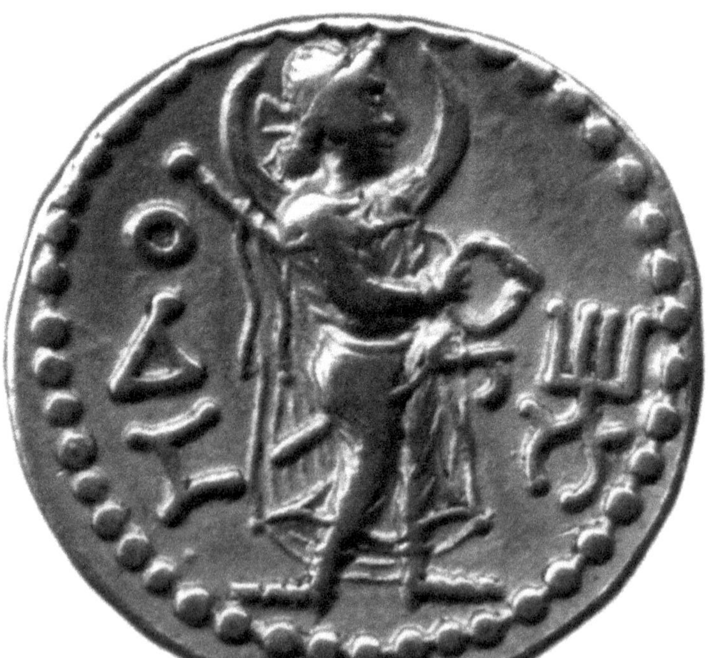

59. Mao on a Kushan coin, Göbl type 3 (© Trustees of the British Museum).

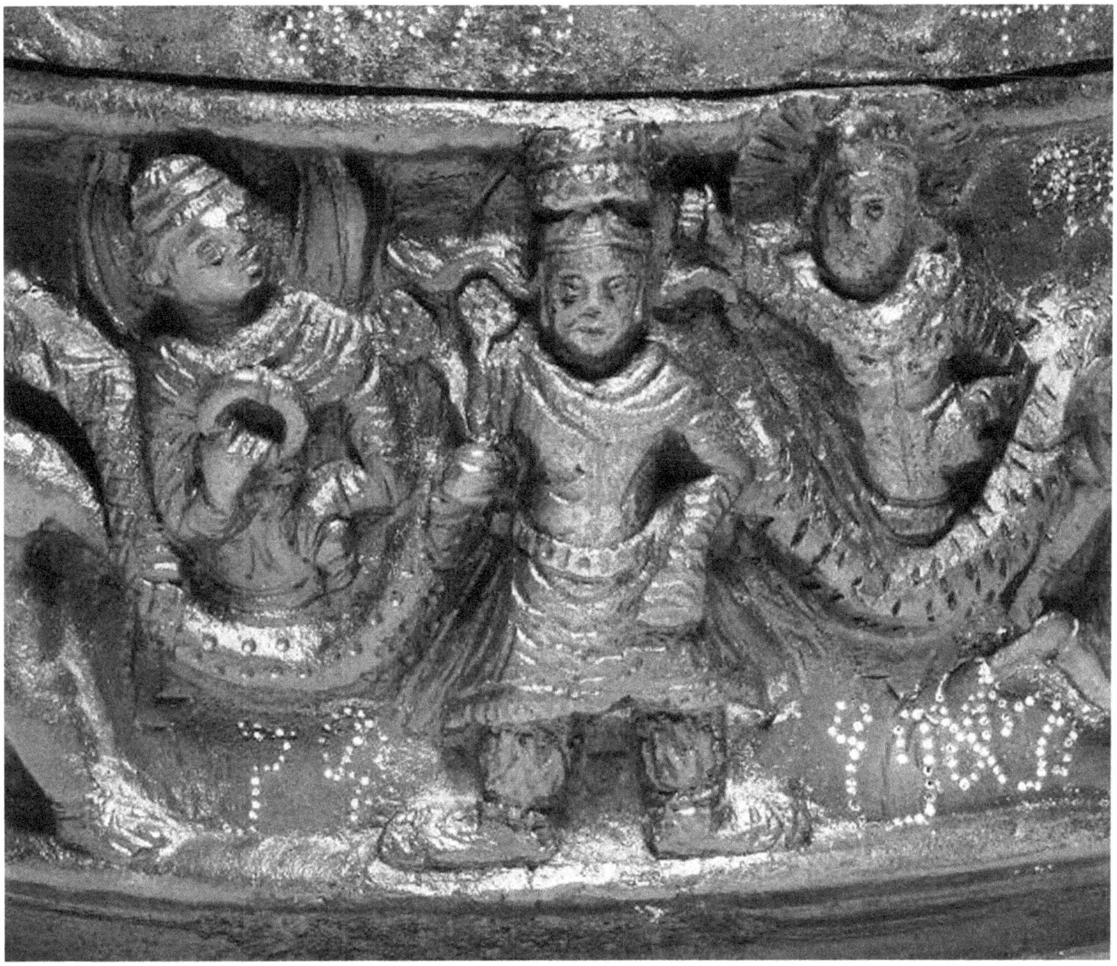

60. A fragment of the "Kanishka reliquary", replica (© Trustees of the British Museum).

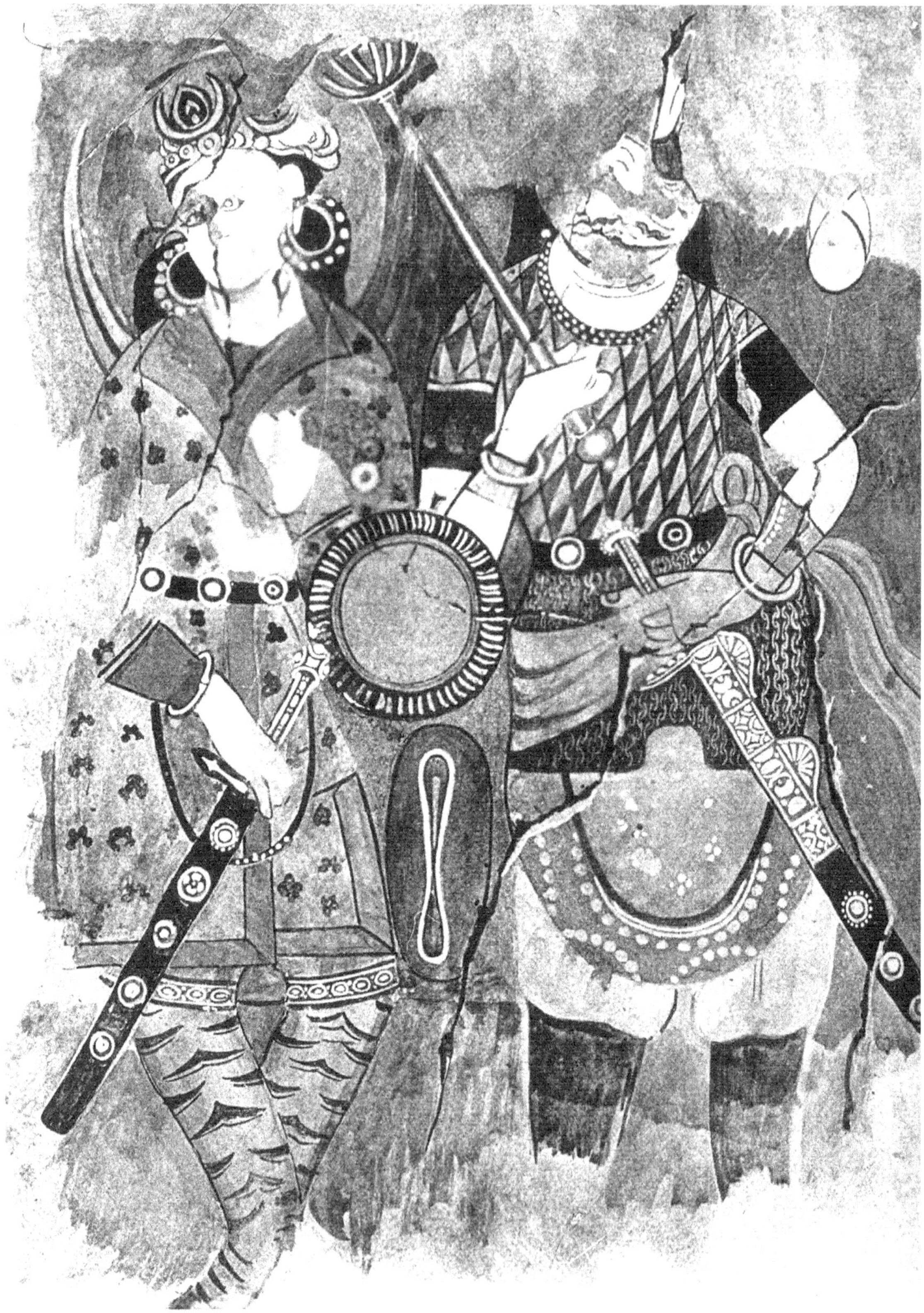

61. A pair of deities, Fondukistan (Hackin 1959: fig. 199).

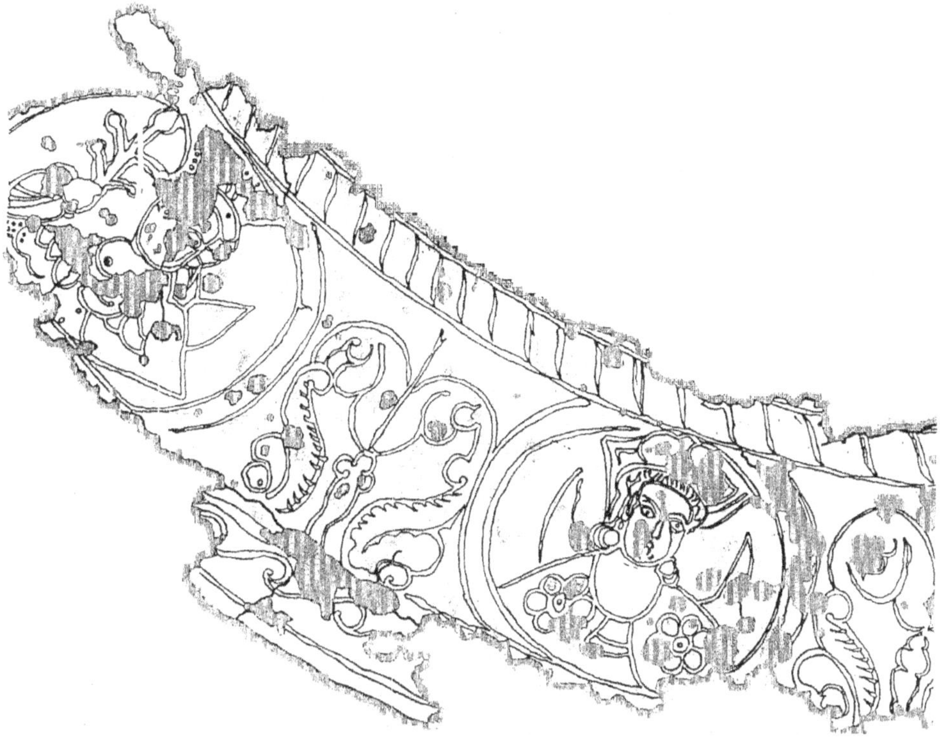

62. A bronze plaque, the first and the second medallions, Jartepa II, (Frantz Grenet).

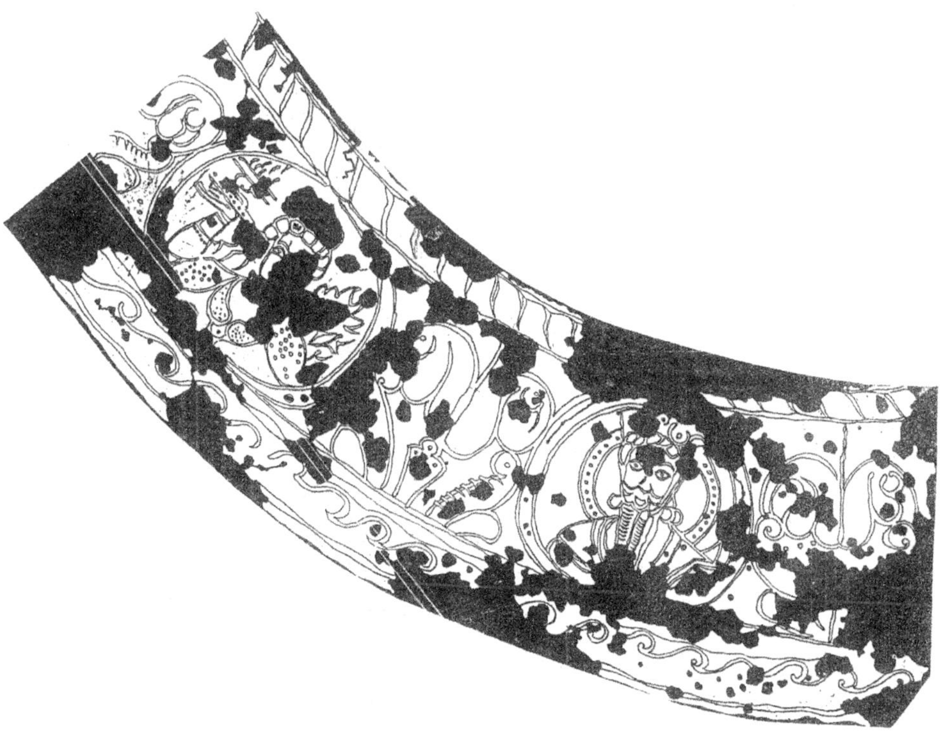

63. A bronze plaque, Jartepa II, the third and the fourth medallions (Frantz Grenet).

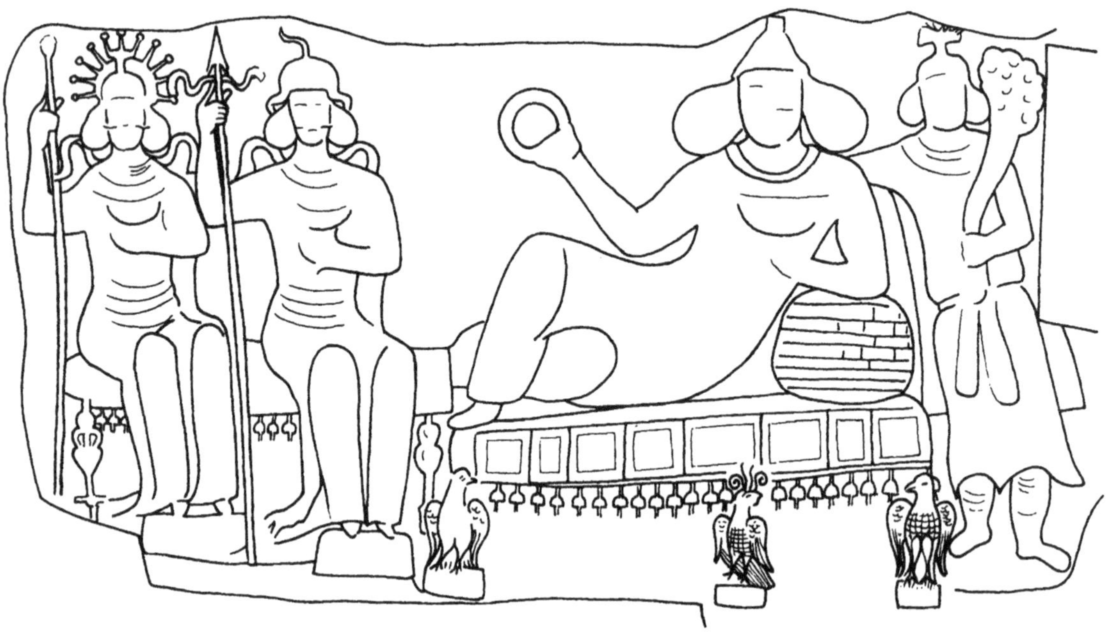

64. Tang-i Sarvak II, NE side, (drawing E. Smekens © BAMI).

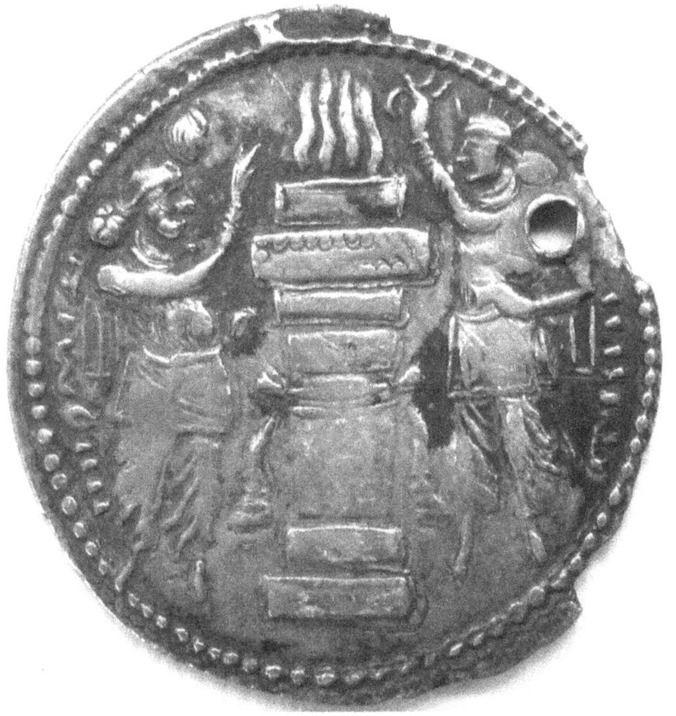

65. Mithra on a coin of Ōhrmazd I (Osmund Bopearachchi).

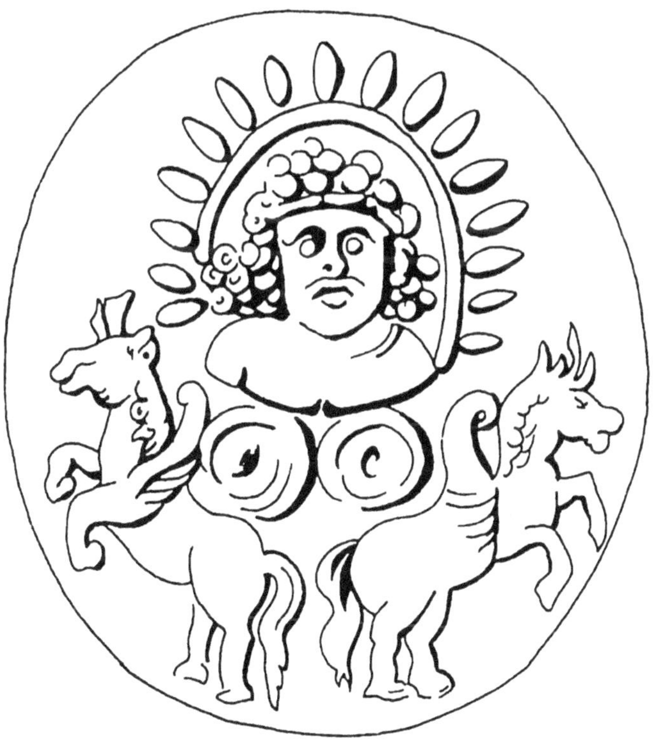

66. Mithra driving a chariot, formerly in Berlin (Gyselen 2000: fig. 14).

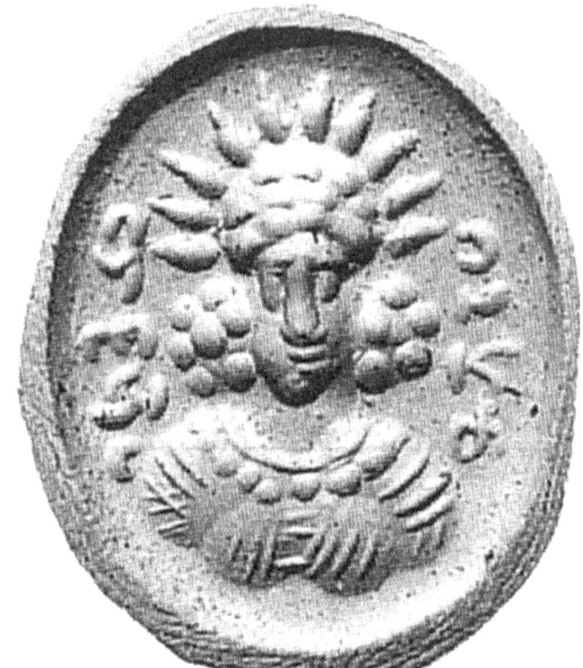

67. Radiate bust of Mithra (Gyselen 1993: 20.G.4).

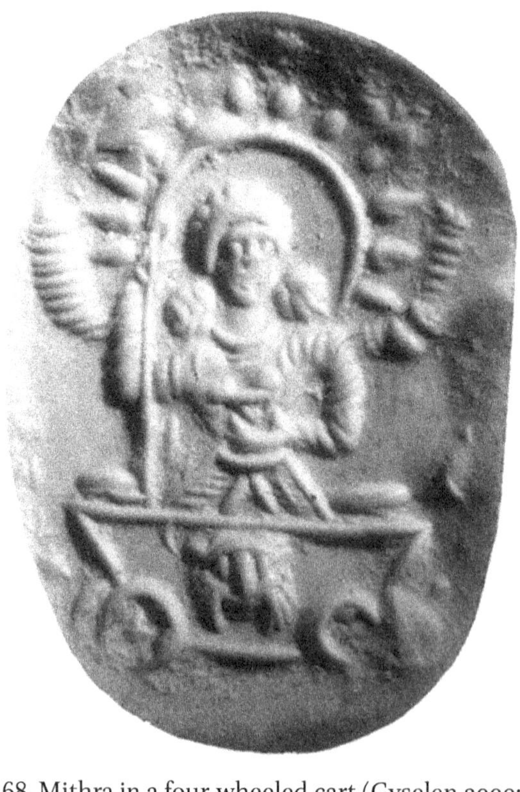

68. Mithra in a four-wheeled cart (Gyselen 2000: fig. 13).

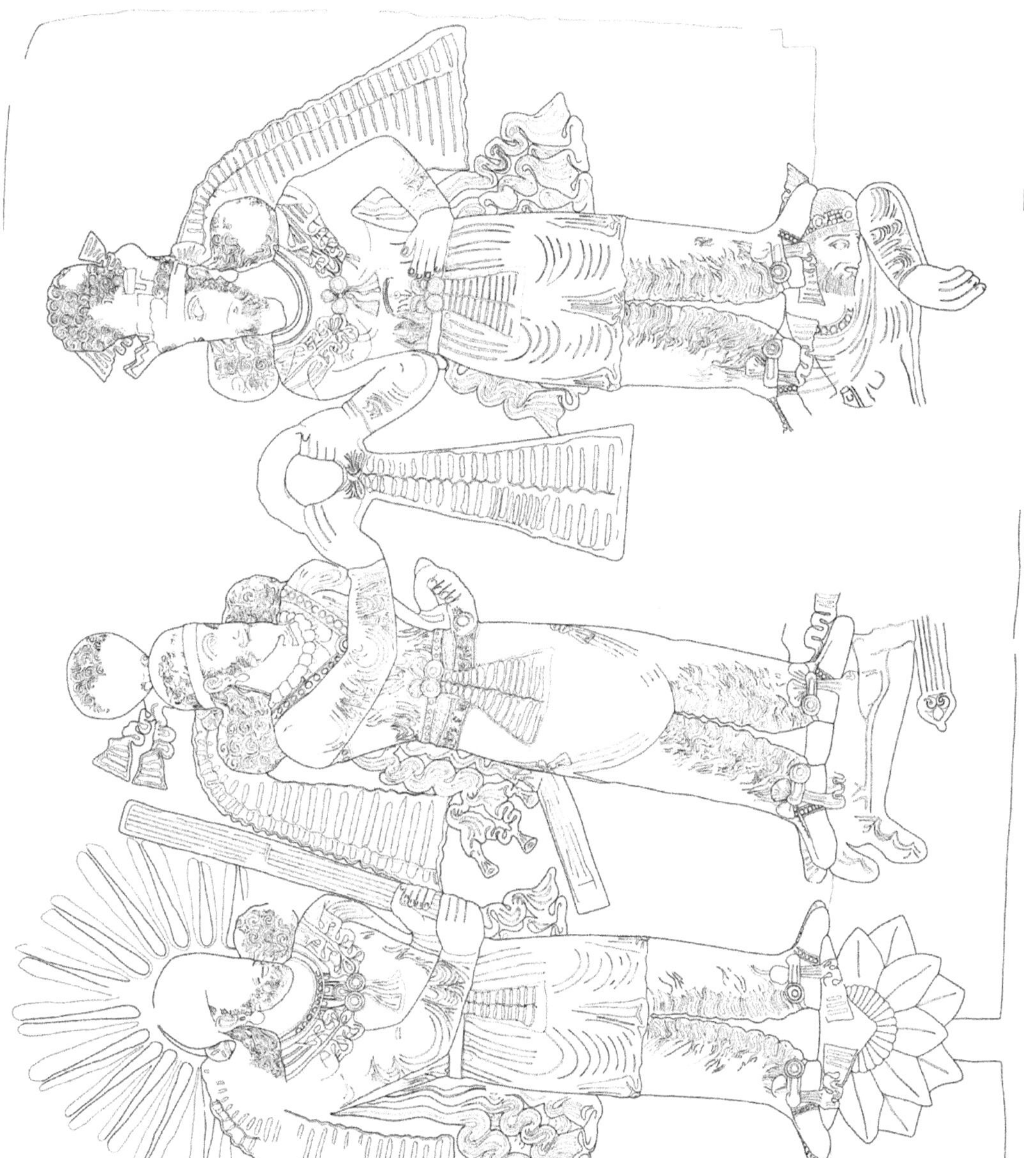

69. Investiture relief of Šāpūr II at Ṭāq-i Bustān (Georginna Herrmann).

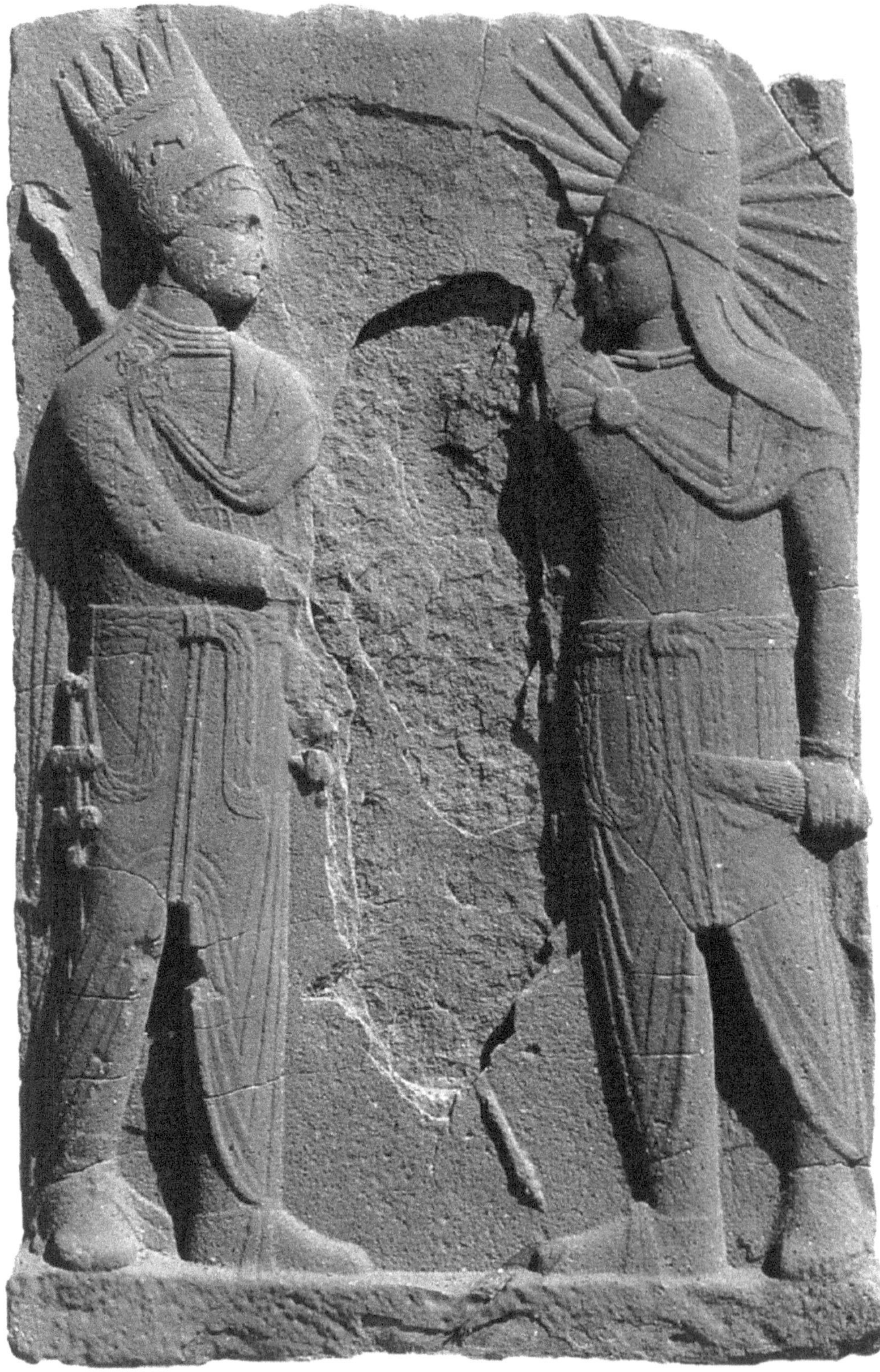

70. Antiochus I of Commagene and Apollo-Mithra-Helios-Hermes, Nemrud Dag (Wagner 2000: fig. 38).

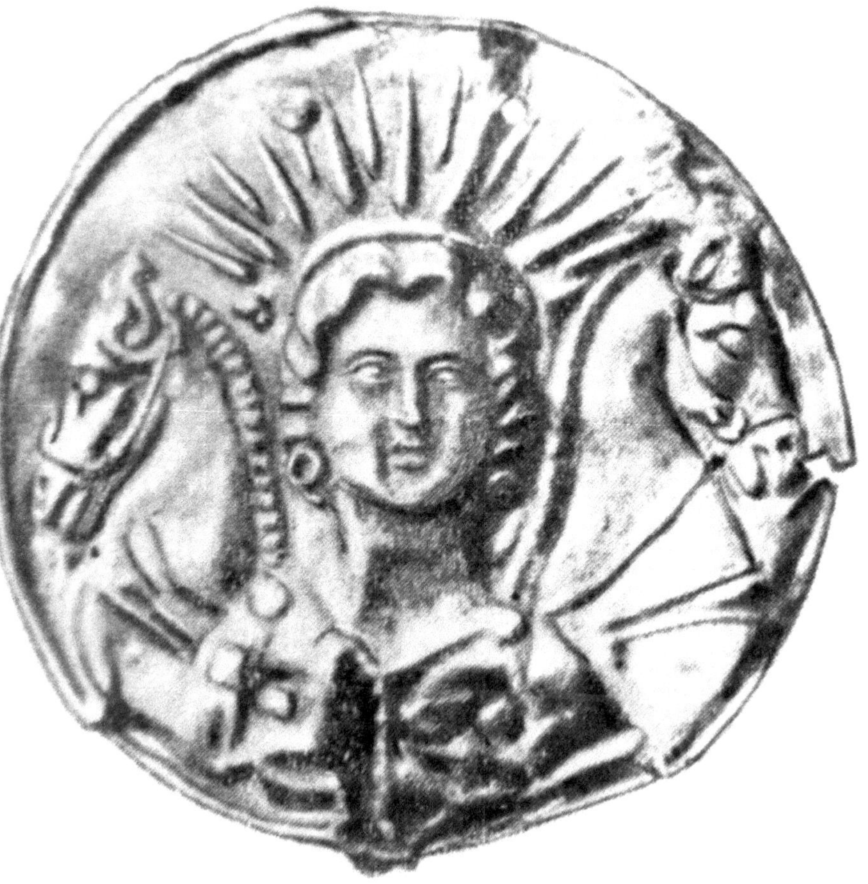

71. Detail of a horse harness from the Fedulovo hoard (Saprykin 1983: fig. 2).

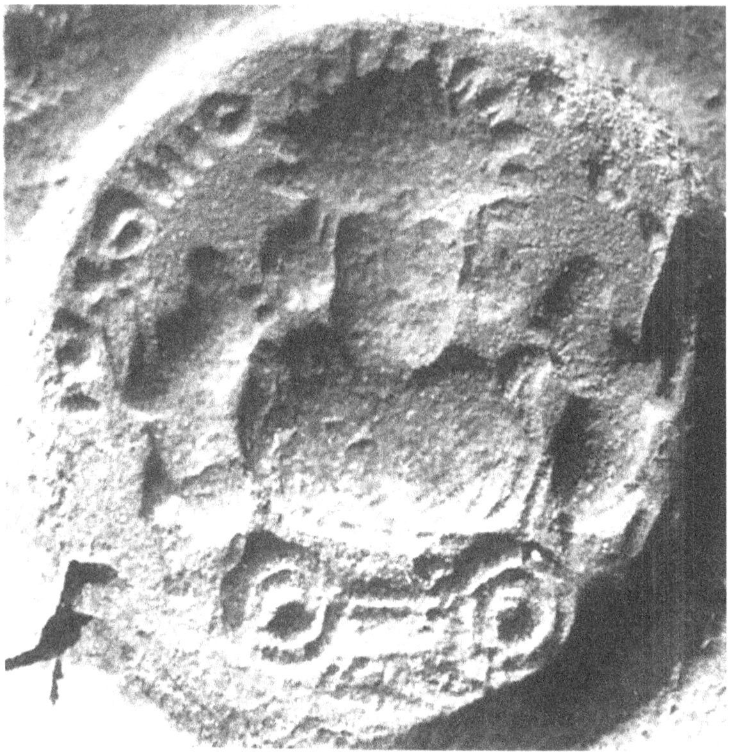

72. Radiate god driving a chariot, Ak-Depe (Gubaev, Loginov and Nikitin 1996: pl. 13).

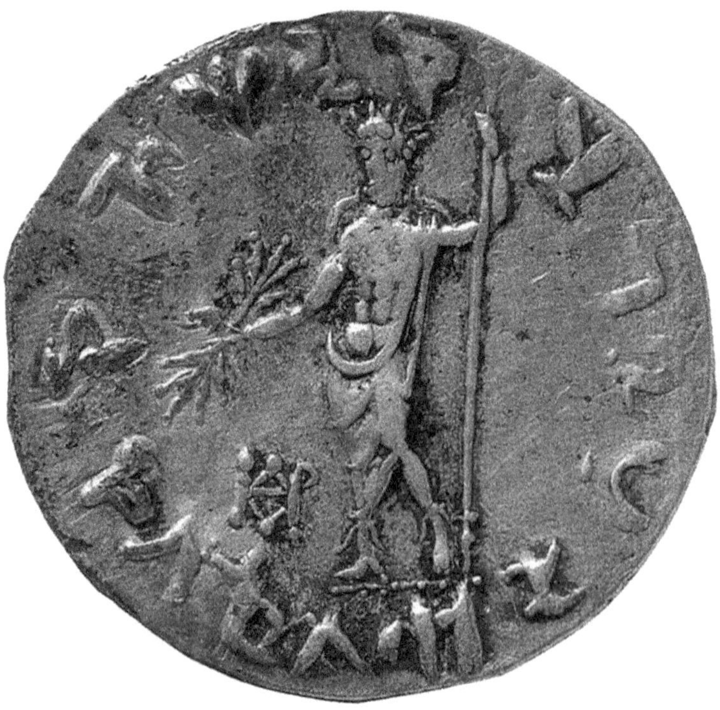

73. A Zeus-like figure on a coin of Heliocles (Frantz Grenet).

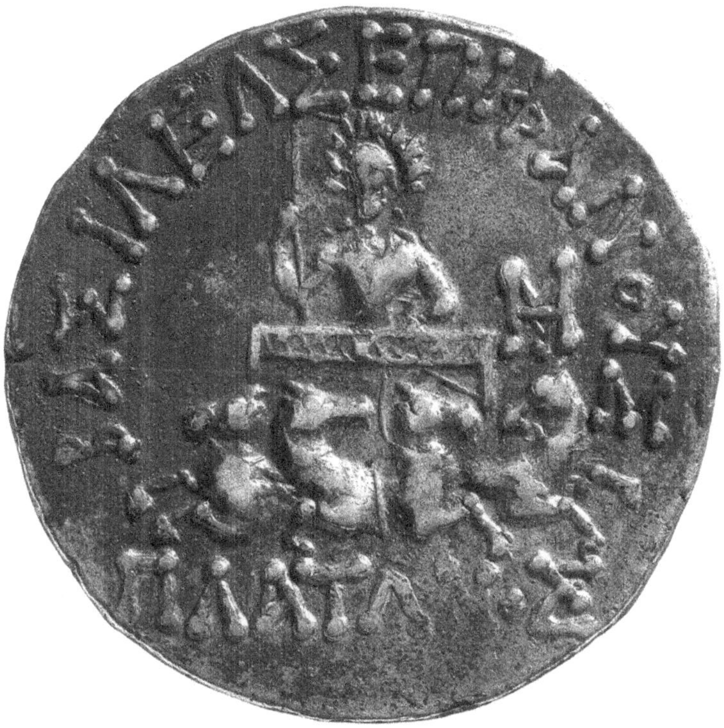

74. Helios riding a quadriga on a coin of Plato (Frantz Grenet).

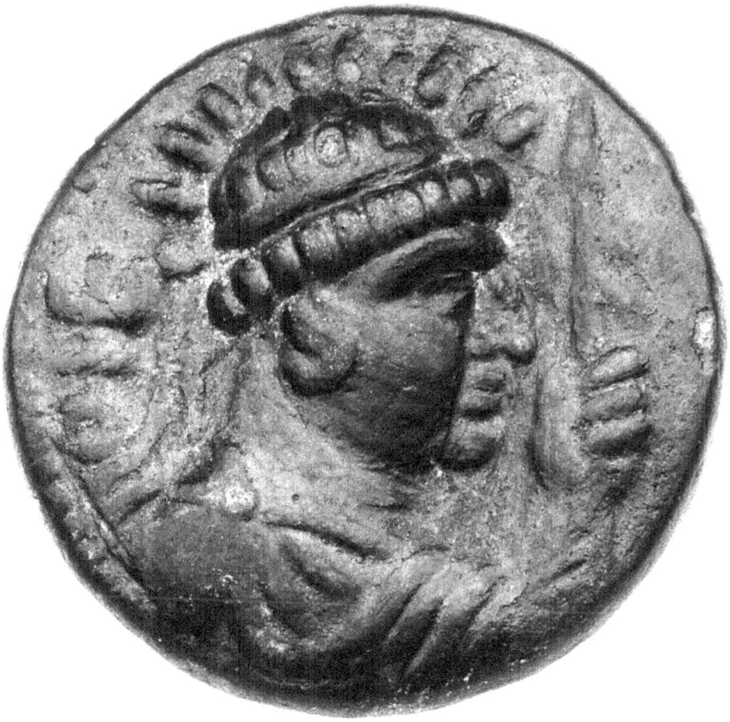

75. A radiate figure on a coin of "Soter Megas" (Osmund Bopearachchi).

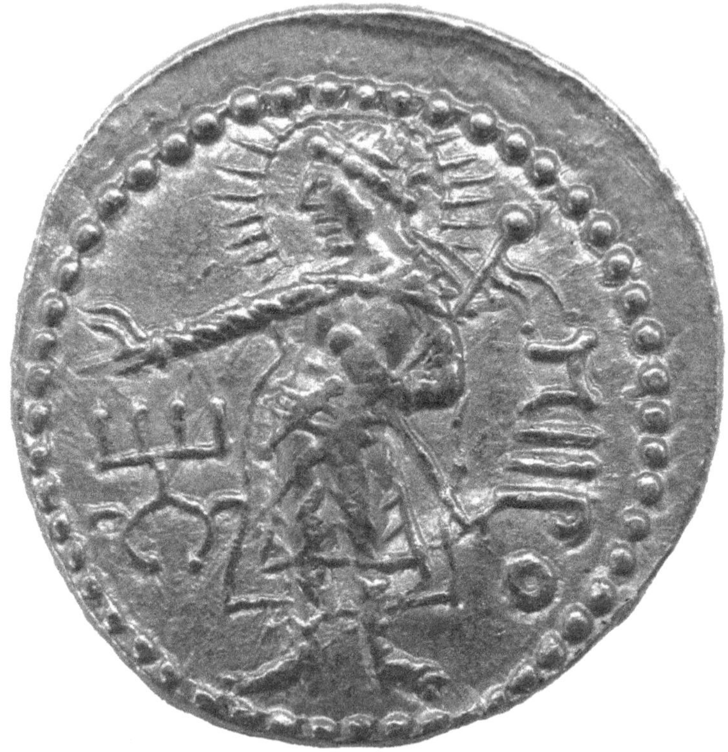

76. Miiro on a Kushan coin, type 2 (Osmund Bopearachchi).

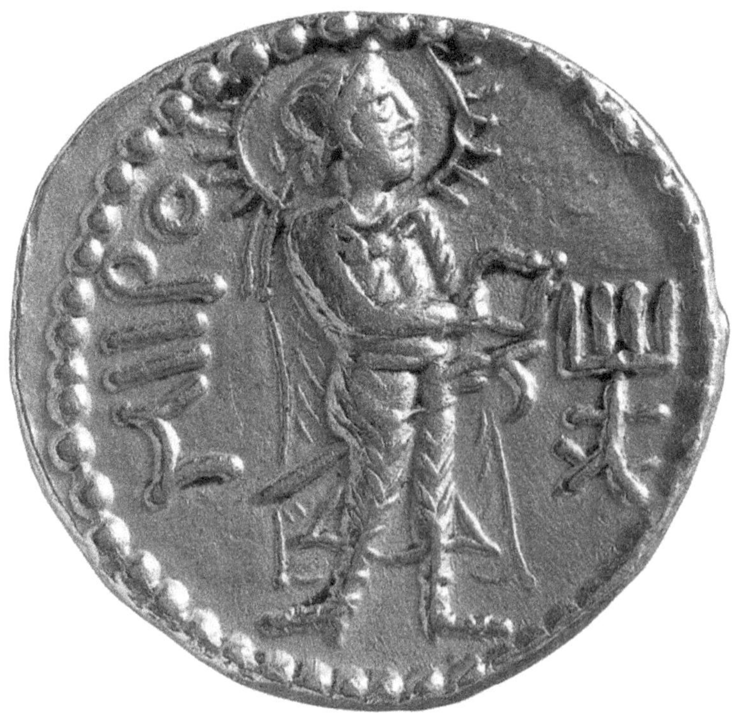

77. Miiro on a Kushan coin, type 3 (Frantz Grenet).

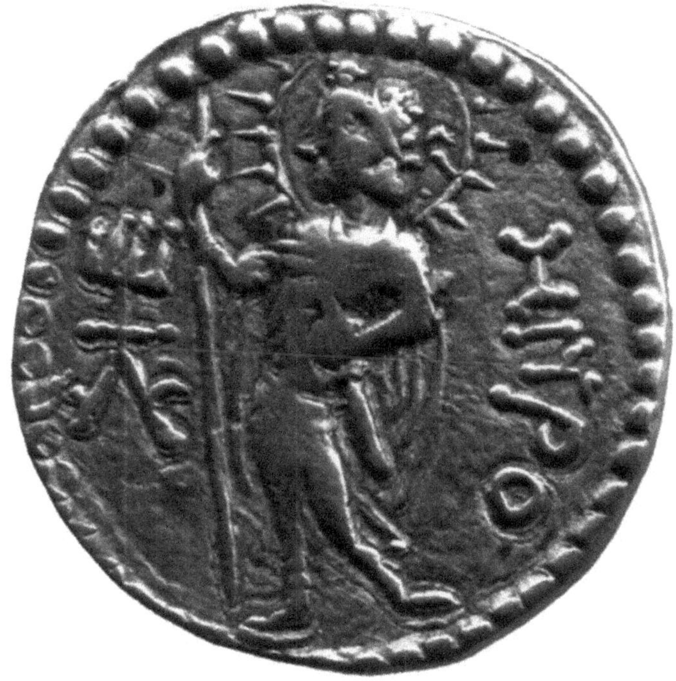

78. Miiro on a Kushan coin, type 5 (© Trustees of the British Museum).

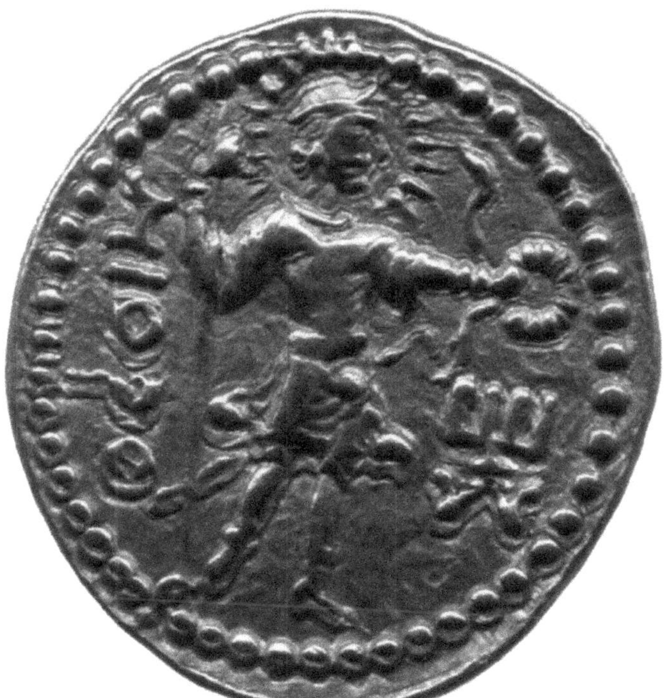

79. Miiro on a Kushan coin, type 10 (© Trustees of the British Museum).

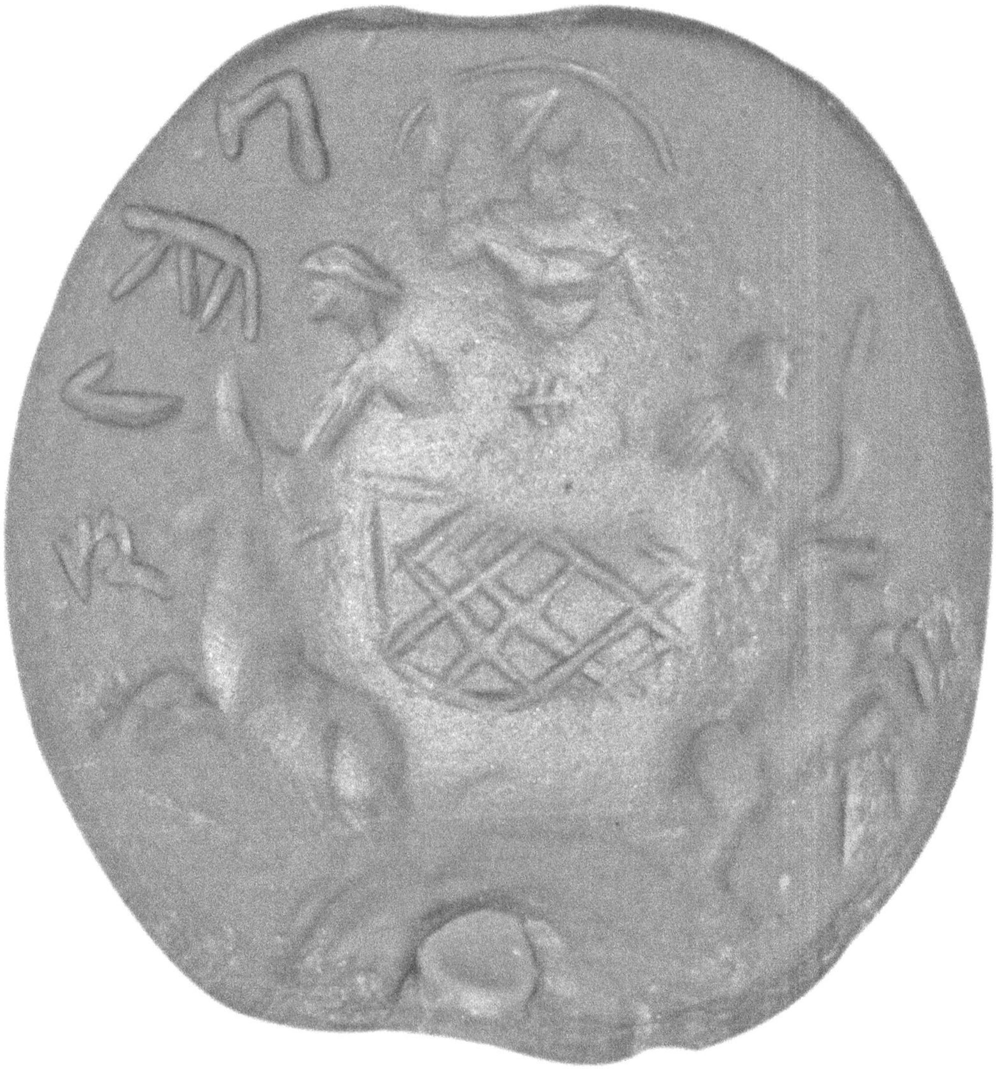

80. Mithra riding a chariot on a seal found in Gandhāra (Aman Ur Rahman).

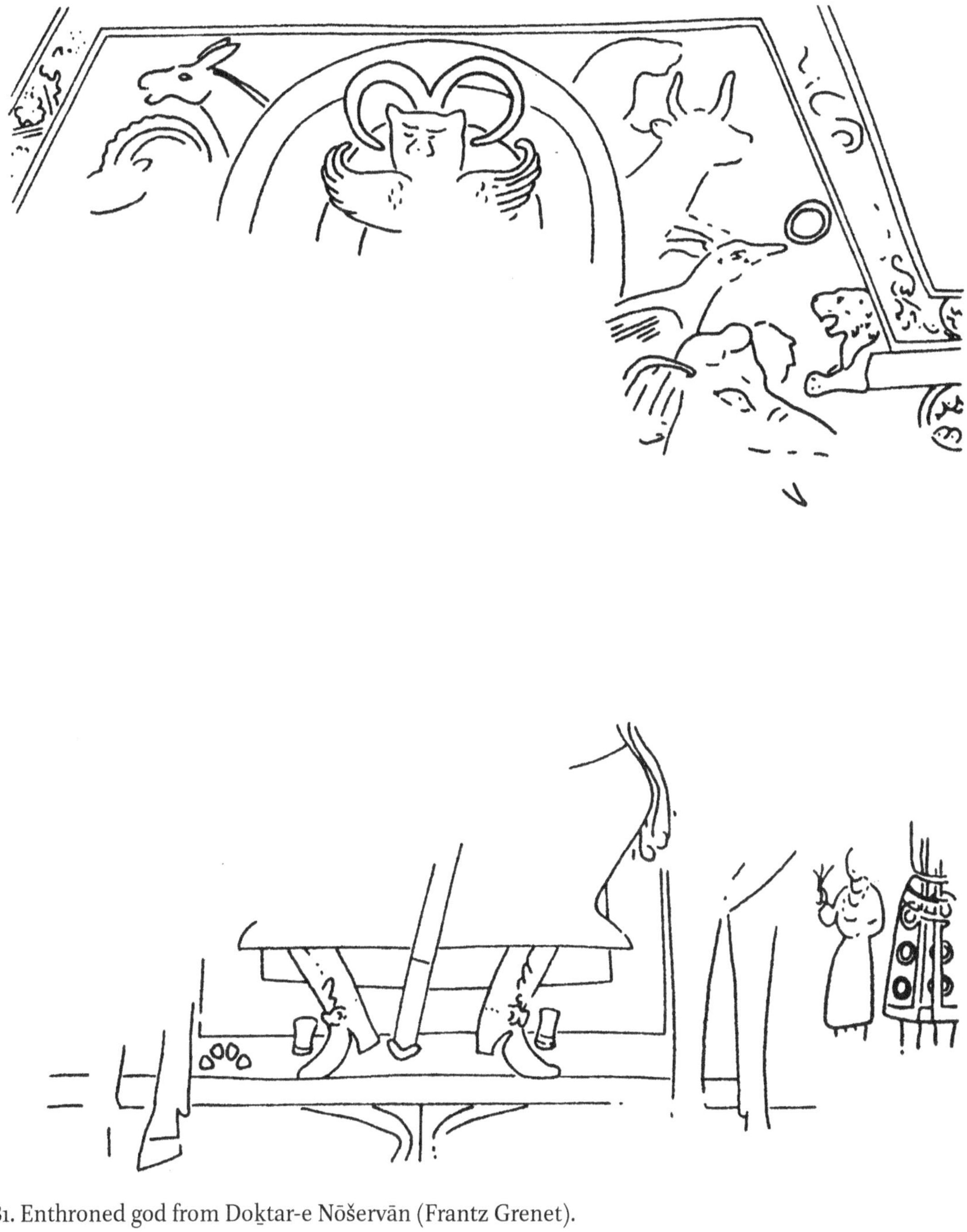

81. Enthroned god from Doḵtar-e Nōšervān (Frantz Grenet).

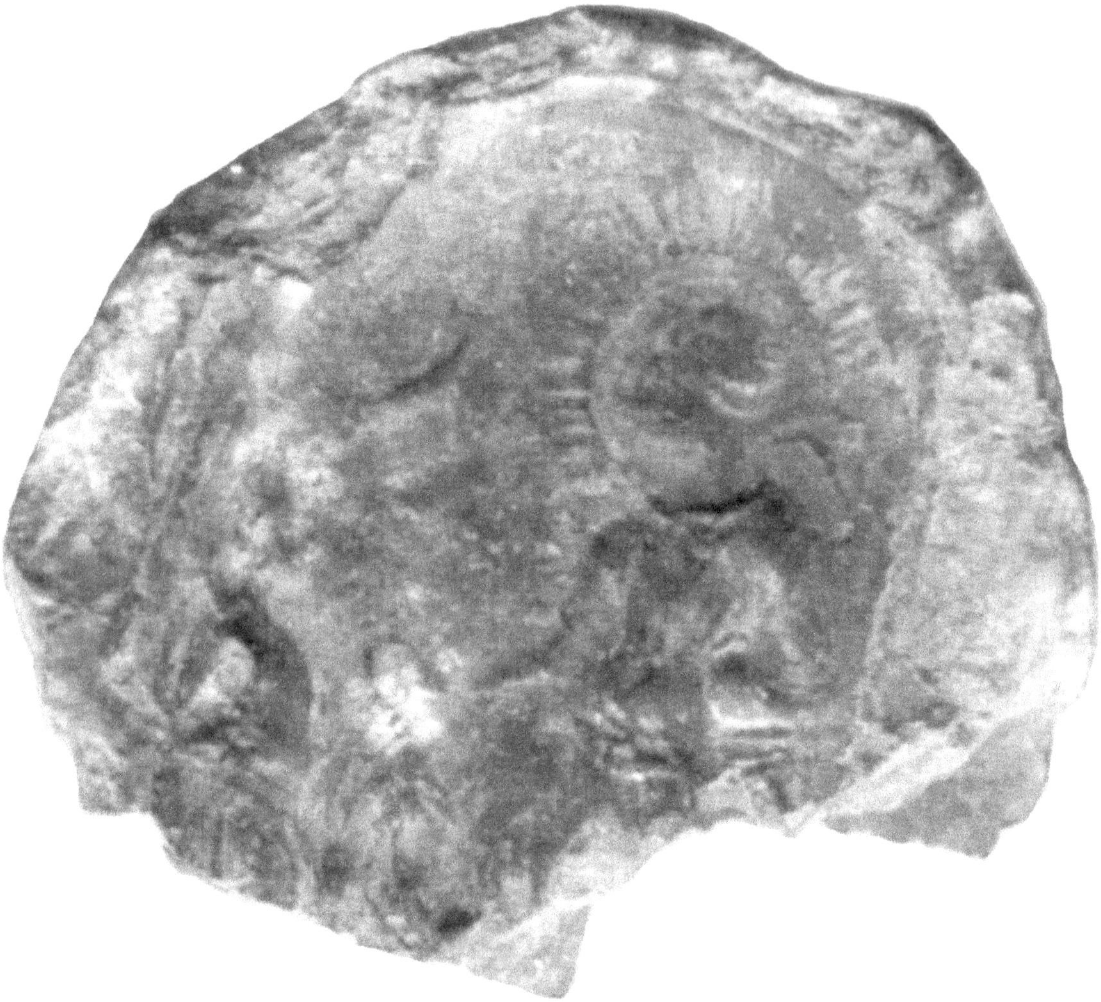

82. Radiate god before a worshipper, Kafir-Kala (Cazzoli and Cereti 2005: fig. 24).

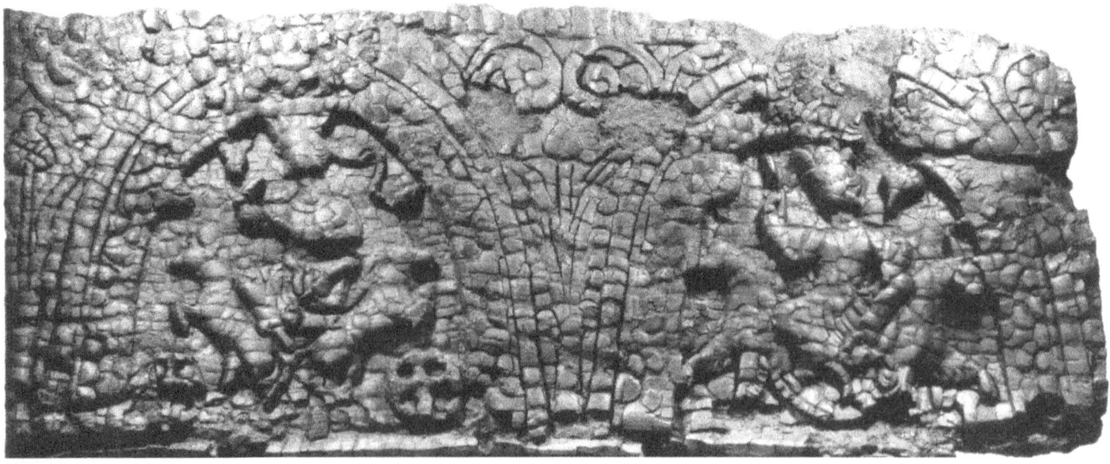

83. Detail of a wooden frieze, Panjikent, VII/11 (Frantz Grenet).

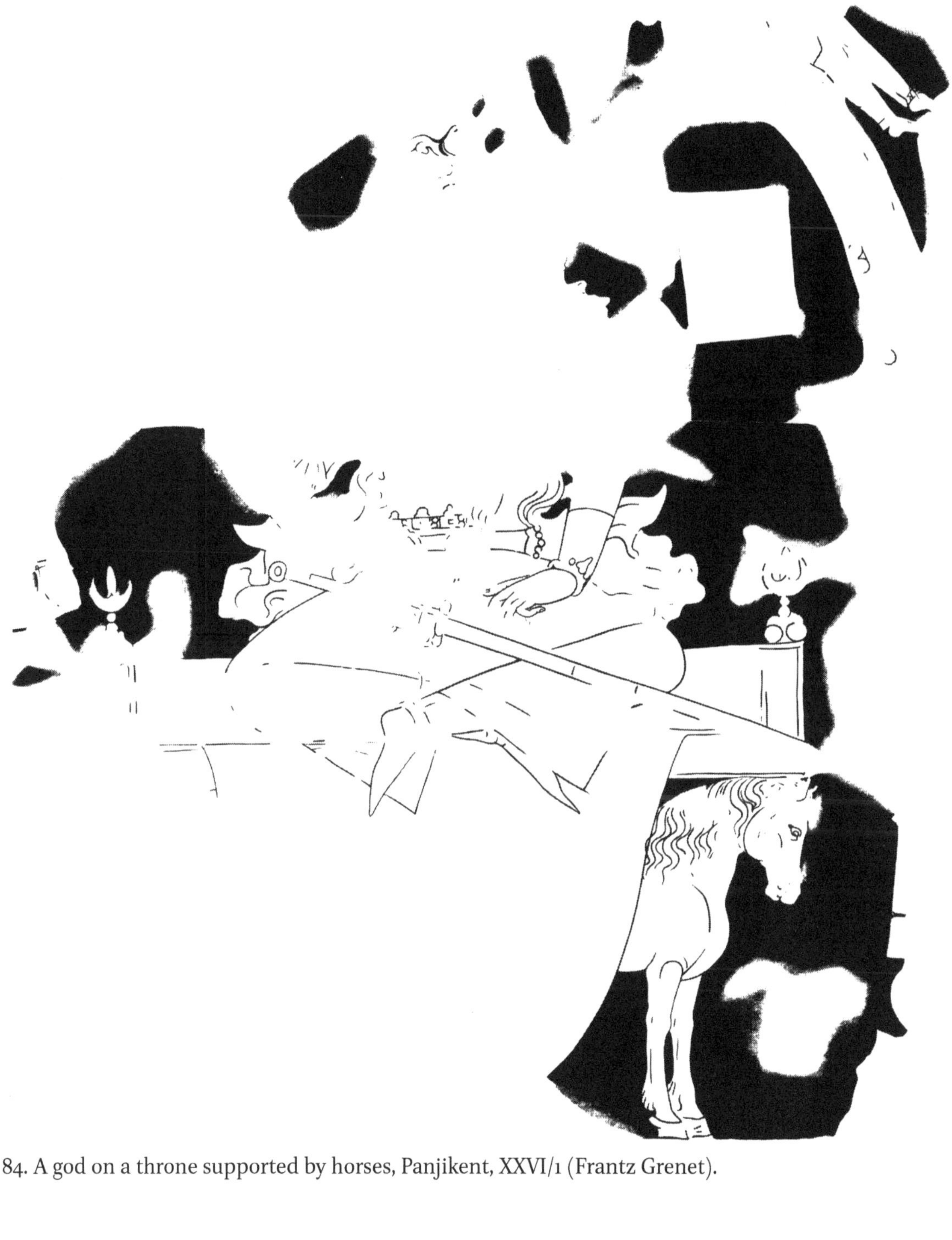

84. A god on a throne supported by horses, Panjikent, XXVI/1 (Frantz Grenet).

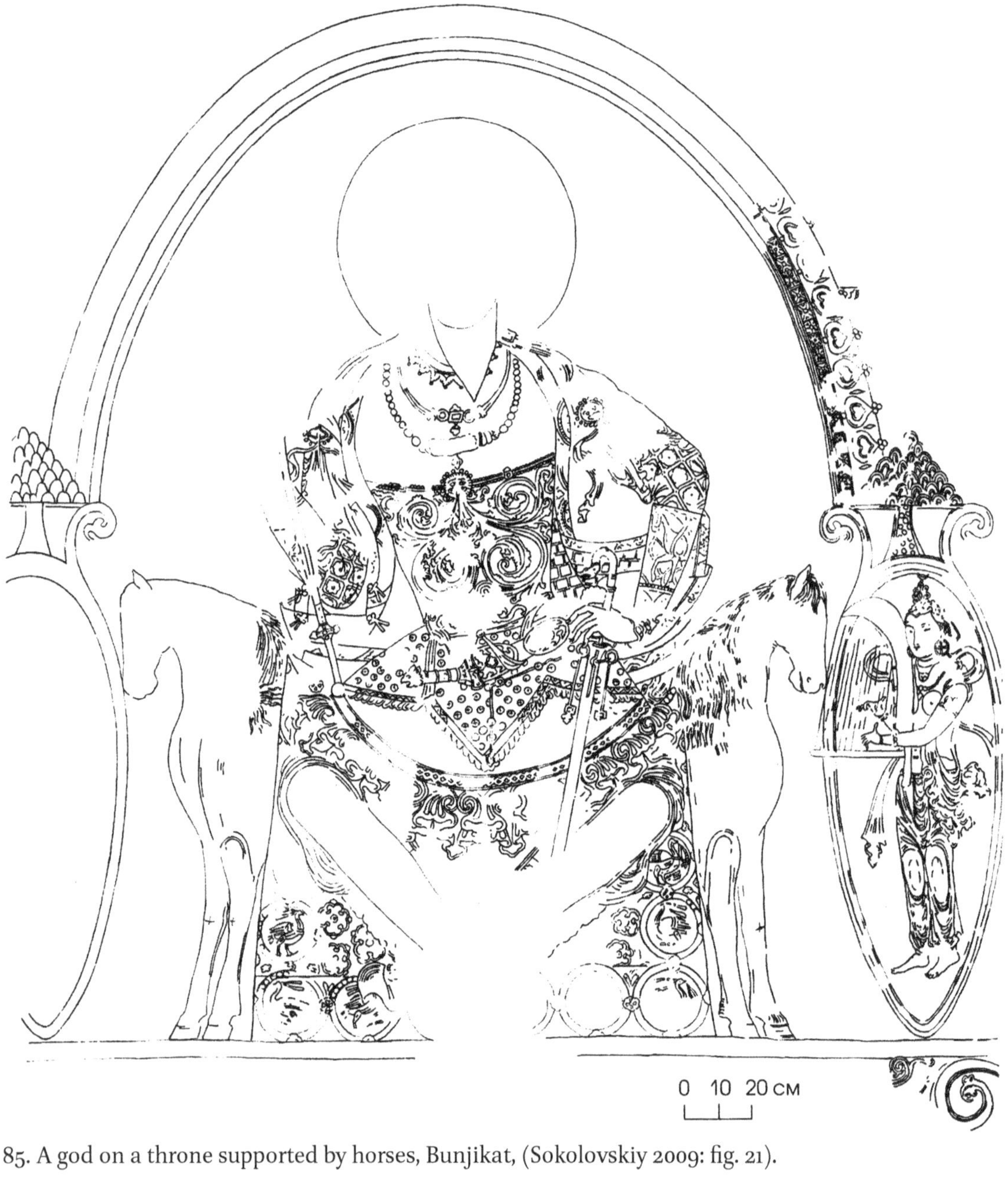

85. A god on a throne supported by horses, Bunjikat, (Sokolovskiy 2009: fig. 21).

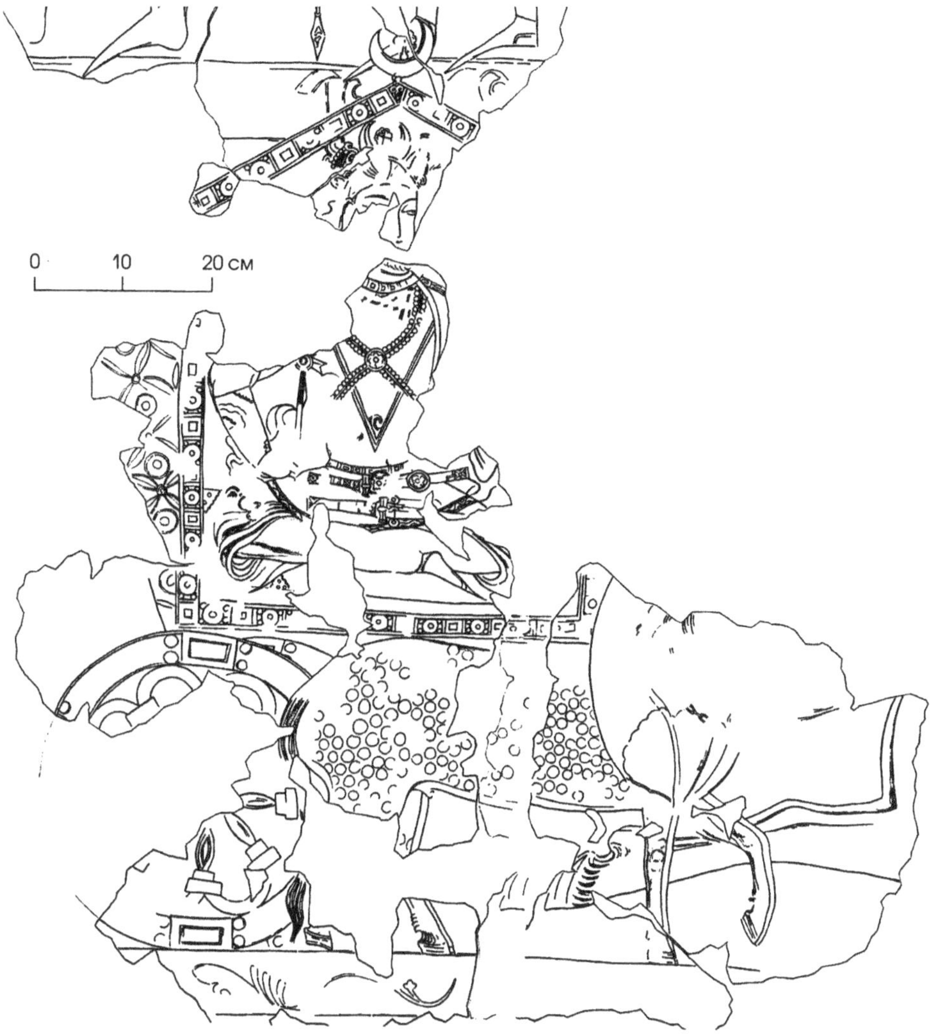

86. A male figure in a chariot, Bunjikat, northern wall, (Sokolovskiy 2009: fig. 63).

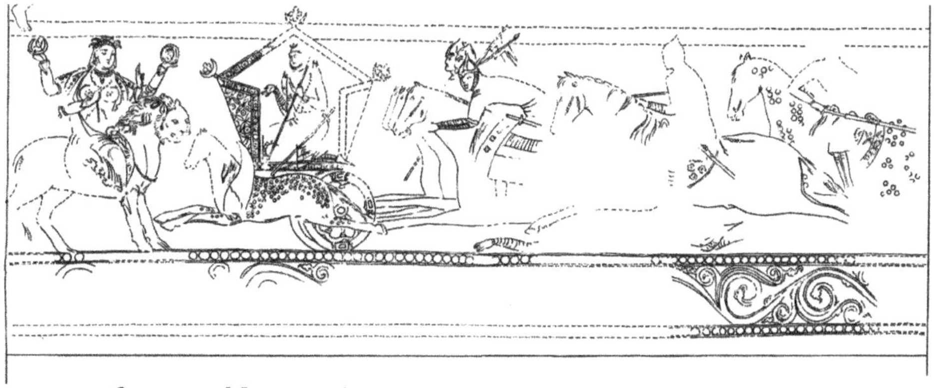

87. The lower register of the eastern wall of the "Small Hall" (left part), Bunjikat (Sokolovskiy 2009: fig. 70).

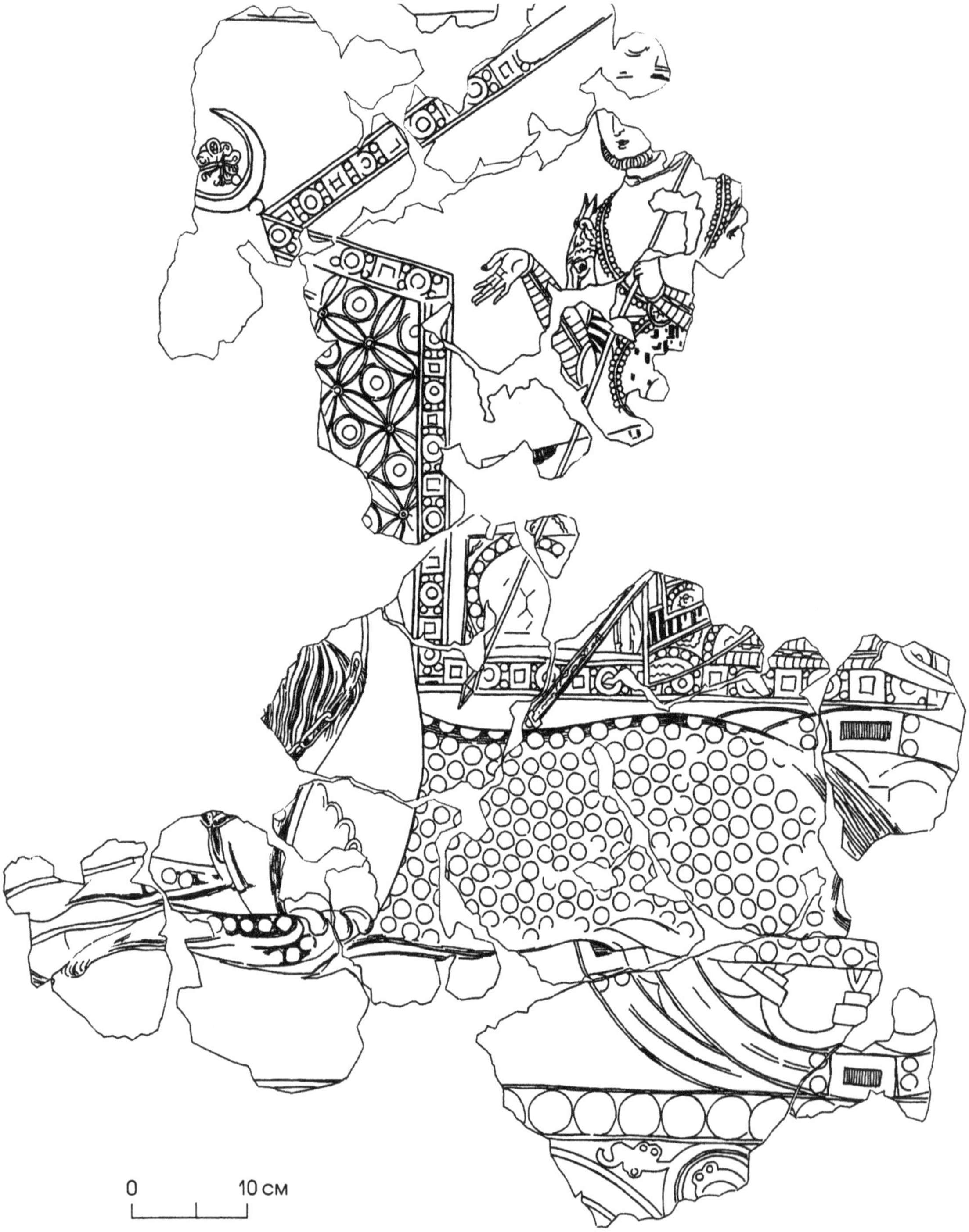

88. A male figure in a chariot, Bunjikat, eastern wall (Sokolovskiy 2009: fig. 72).

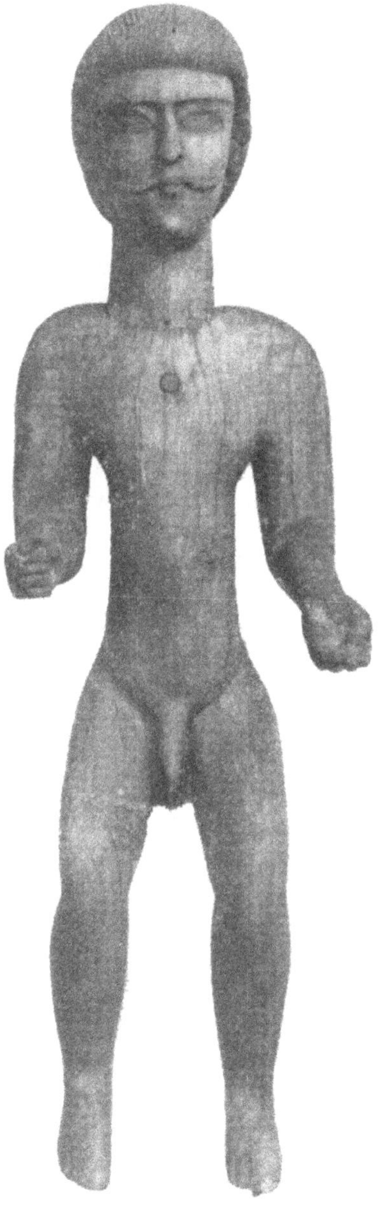

89. A wooden statue from the Surkh mountains (Zeymal' 1985: no. 595).

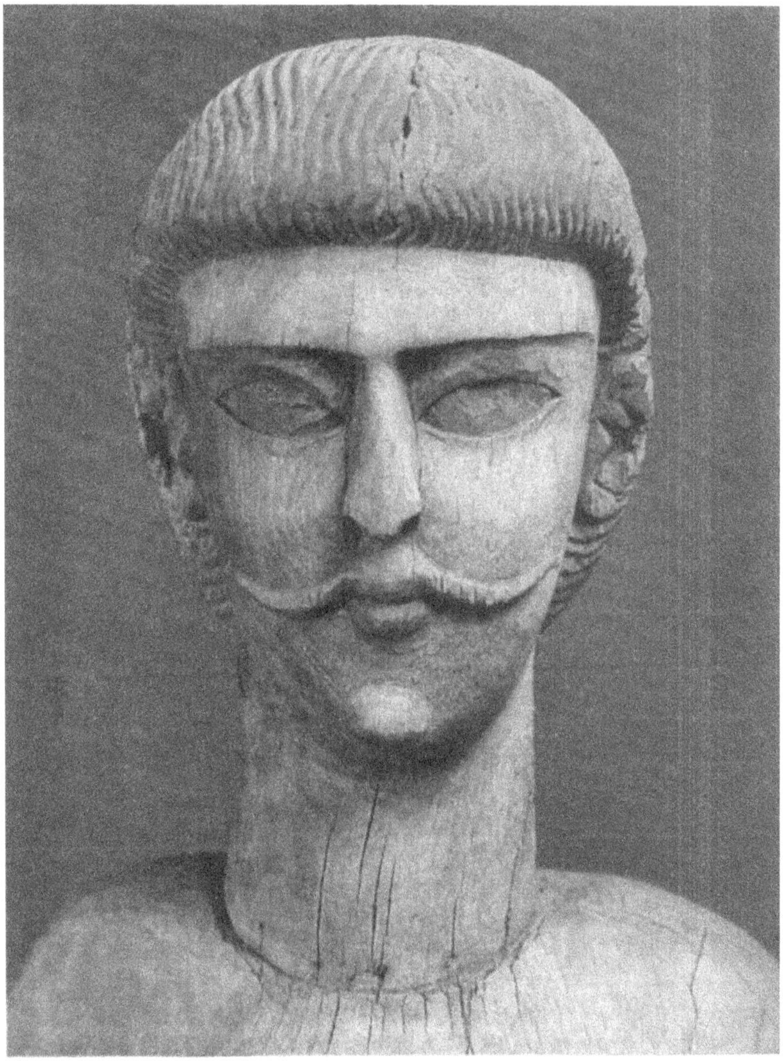

90. A wooden statue from the Surkh mountains, fragment (Zeymal' 1985: 172).

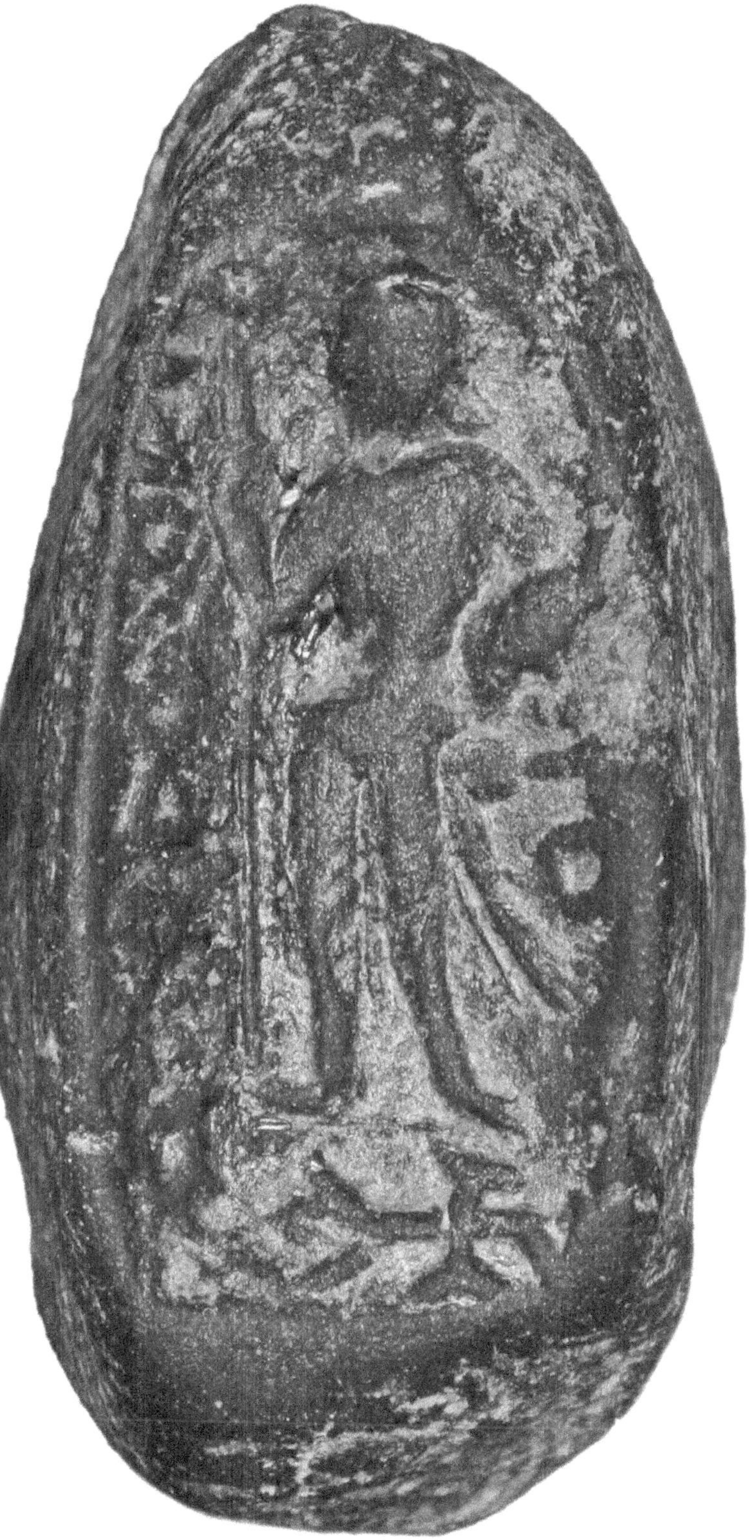

91. Standing deity on a seal found in Gandhāra (Aman Ur Rahman).

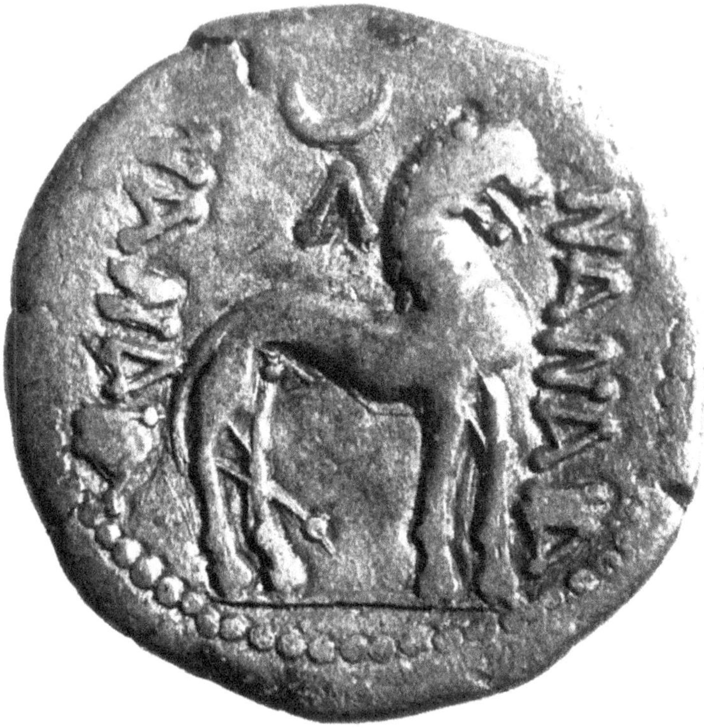

92. The lion of Nana on a coin of Sapadbizes (Tanabe 1995: fig. 2).

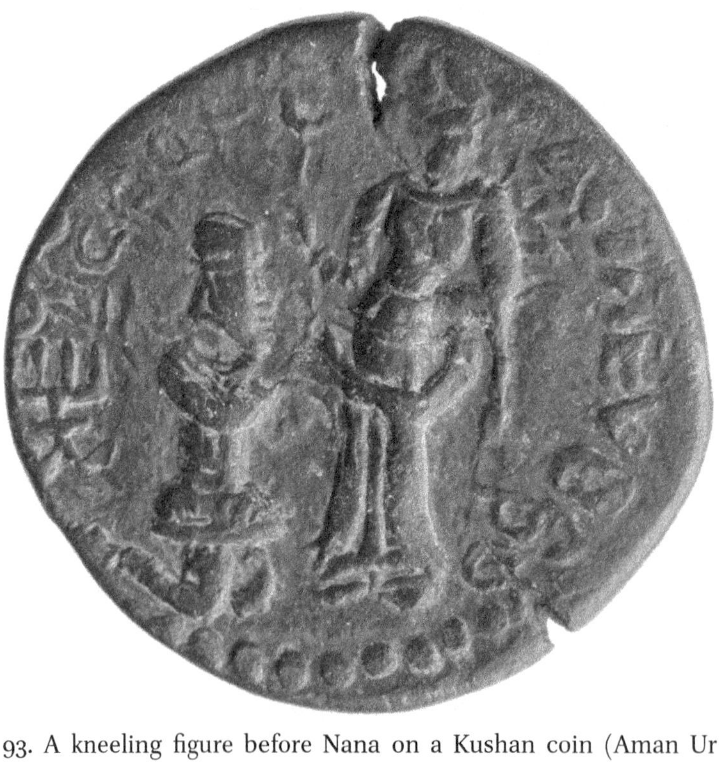

93. A kneeling figure before Nana on a Kushan coin (Aman Ur Rahman).

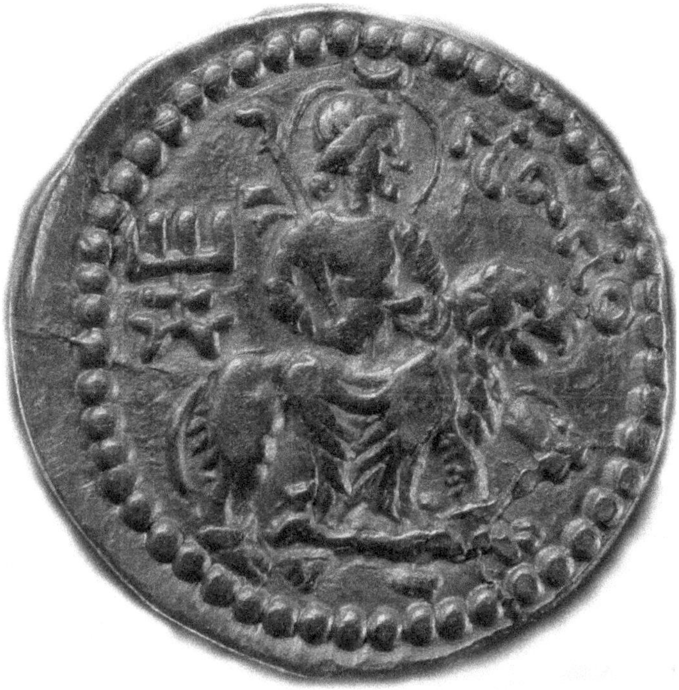

94. Nana on a lion on a Kushan coin (© Trustees of the British Museum).

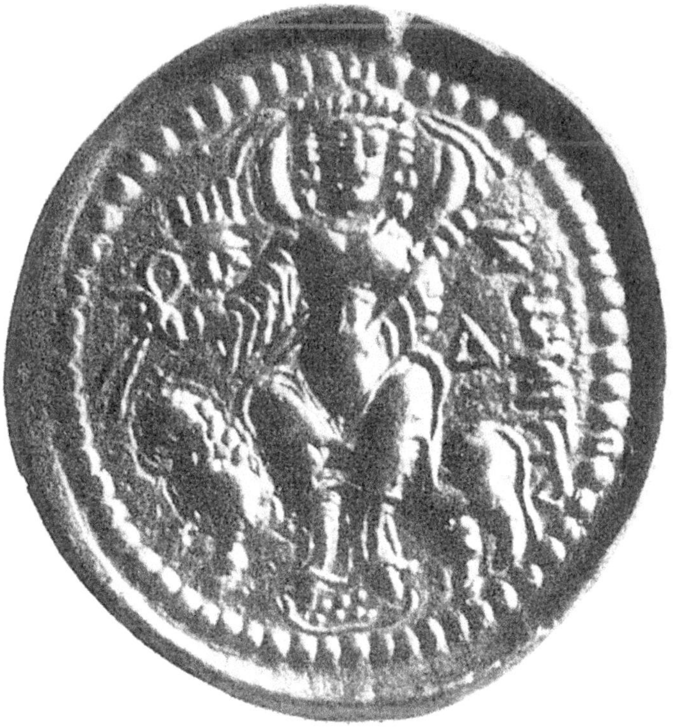

95. Nana with a crescent moon on a Kushan coin (Mukherjee 1969: pl. I, IA).

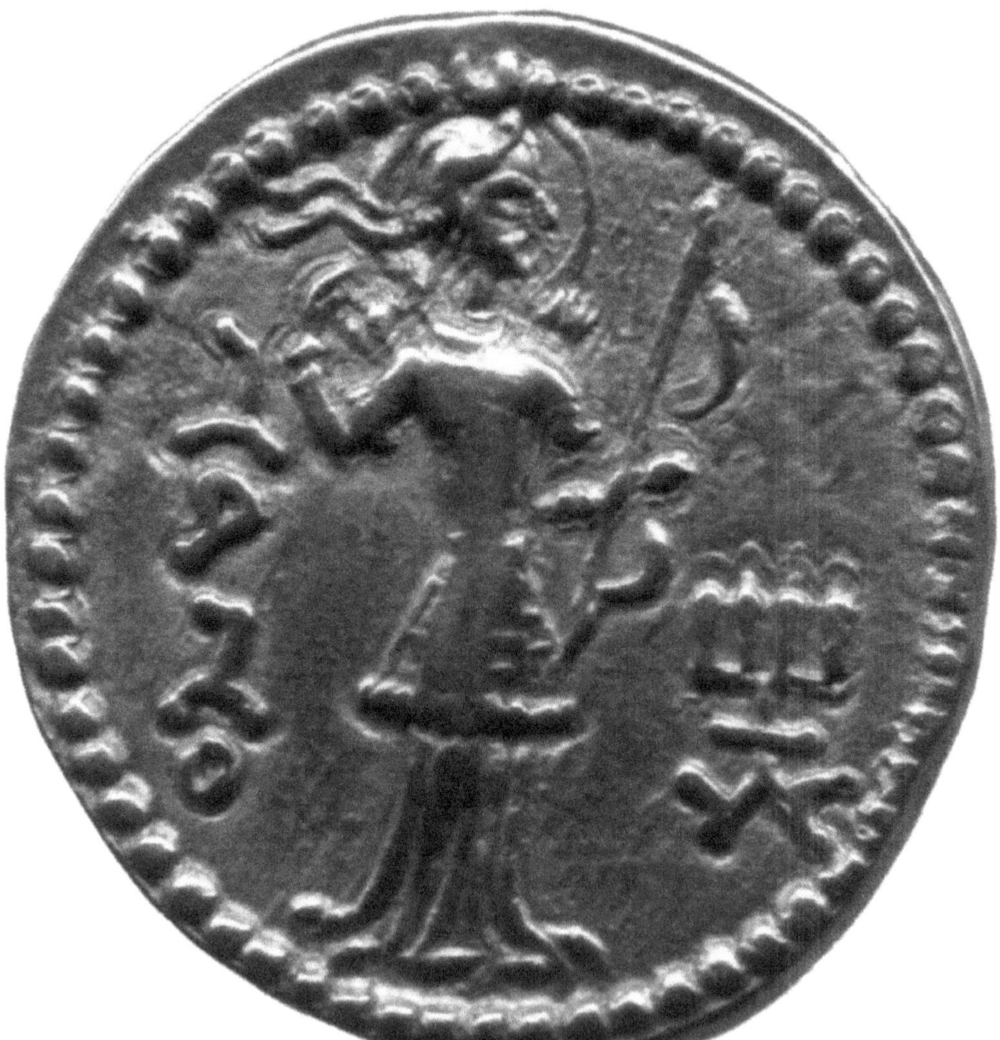

96. Nana with a bow on a Kushan coin (© Trustees of the British Museum).

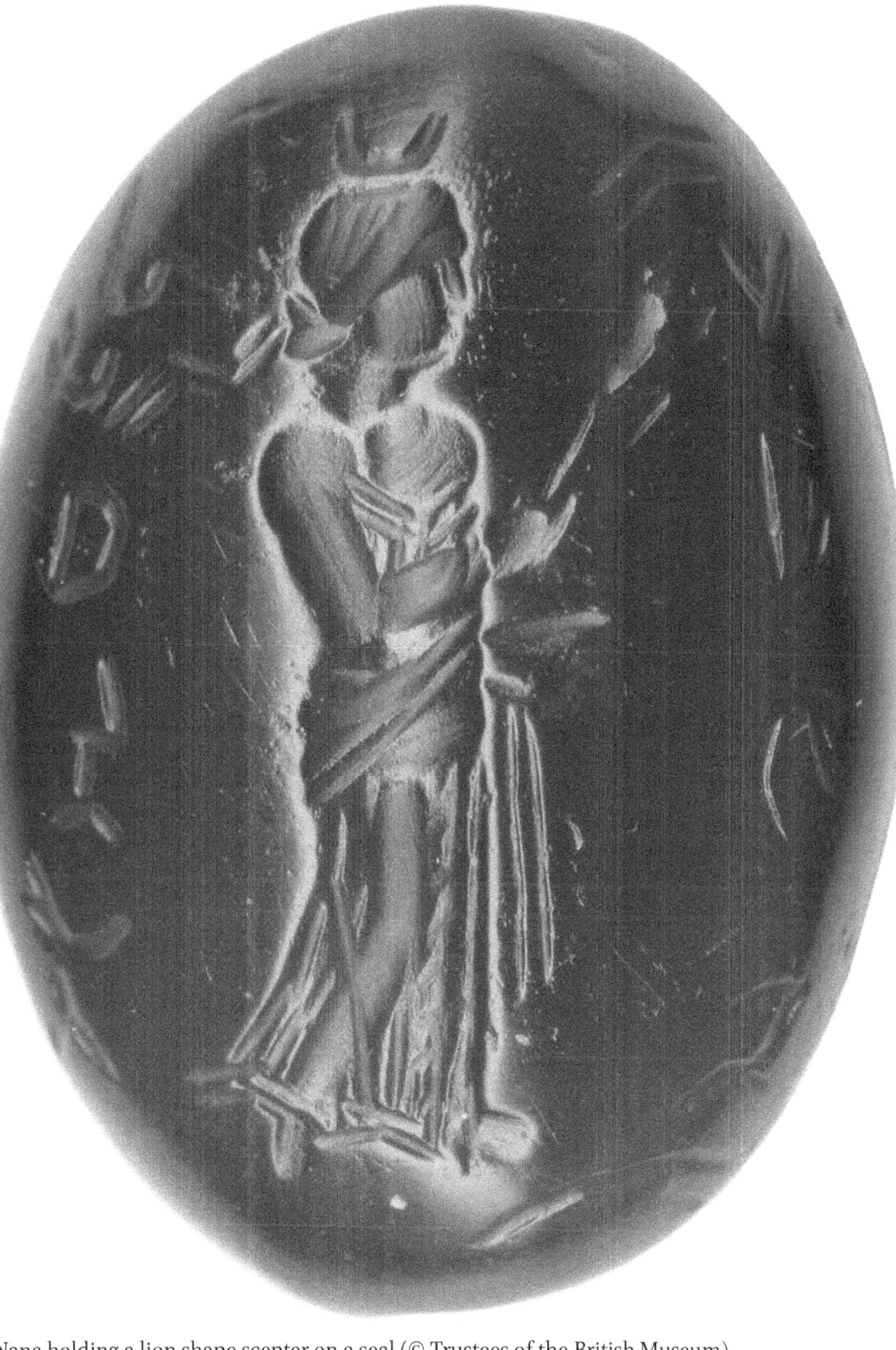

97. Nana holding a lion shape scepter on a seal (© Trustees of the British Museum).

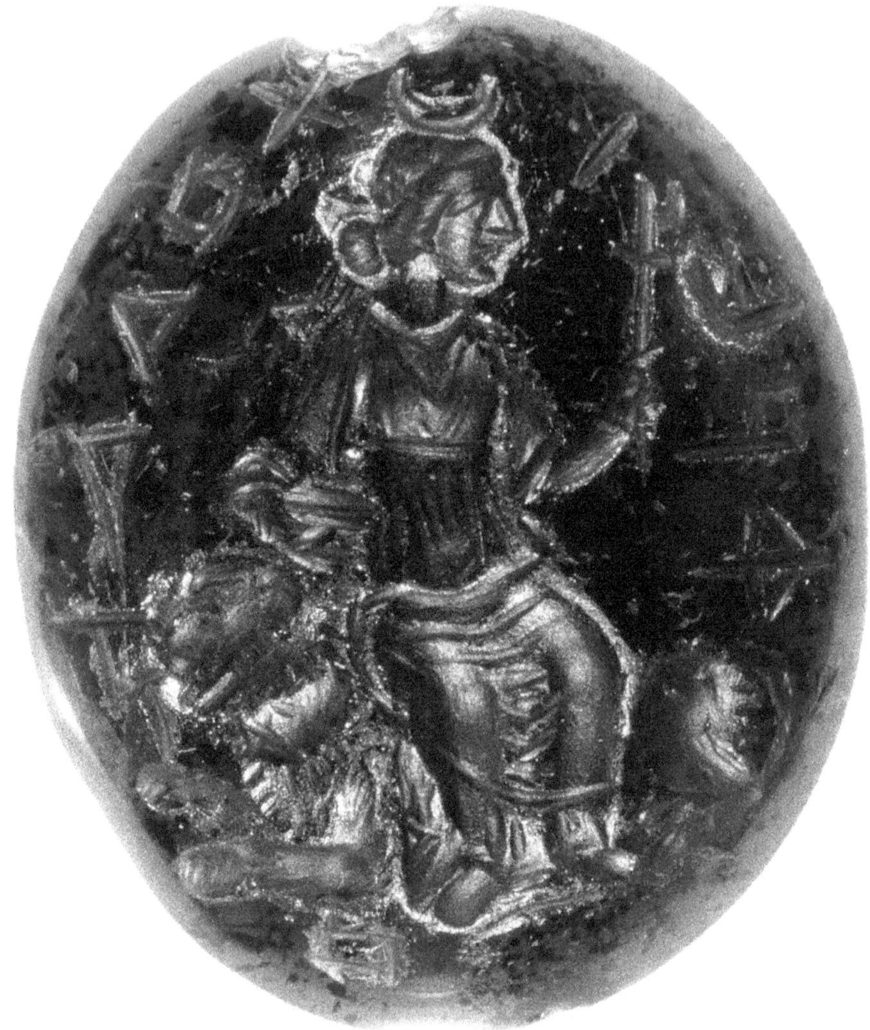

98. Nana seated on a lion (© Trustees of the British Museum).

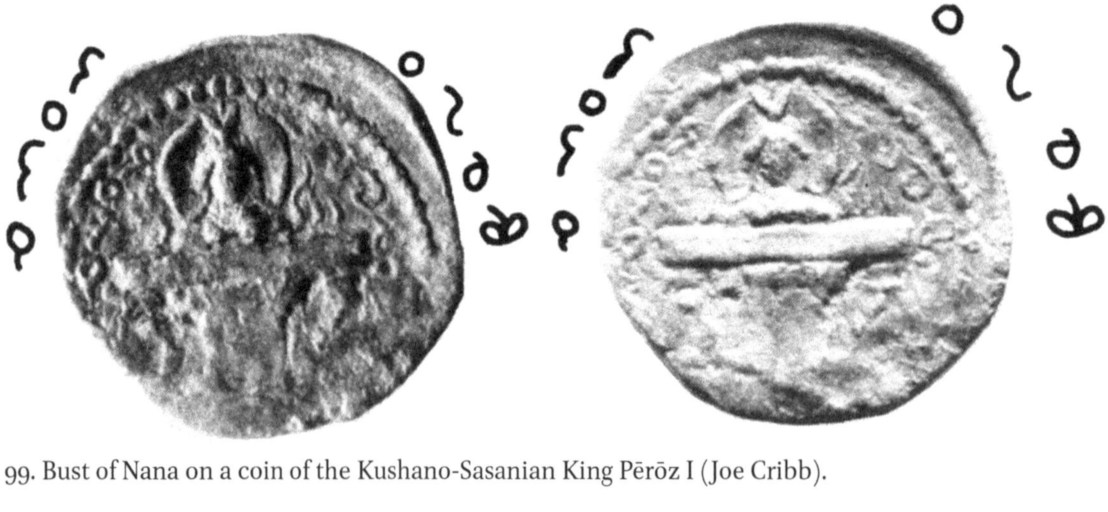

99. Bust of Nana on a coin of the Kushano-Sasanian King Pērōz I (Joe Cribb).

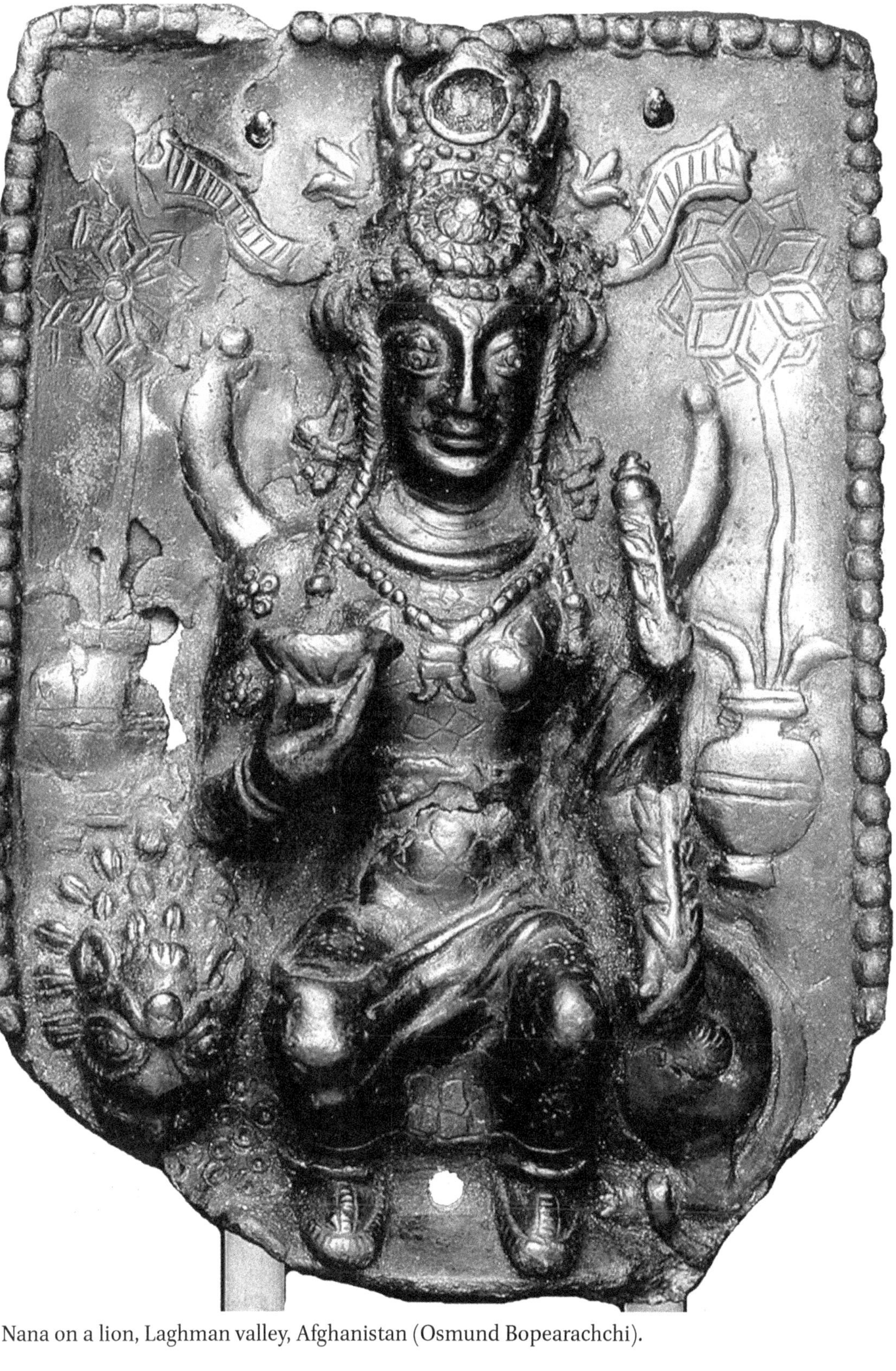

100. Nana on a lion, Laghman valley, Afghanistan (Osmund Bopearachchi).

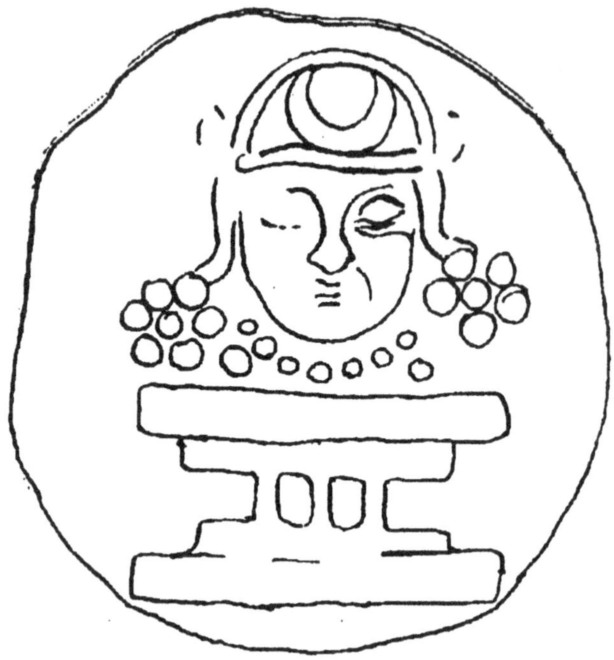

101. Bust on an altar on a Bukharan coin (Naymark 1995: 43, 3).

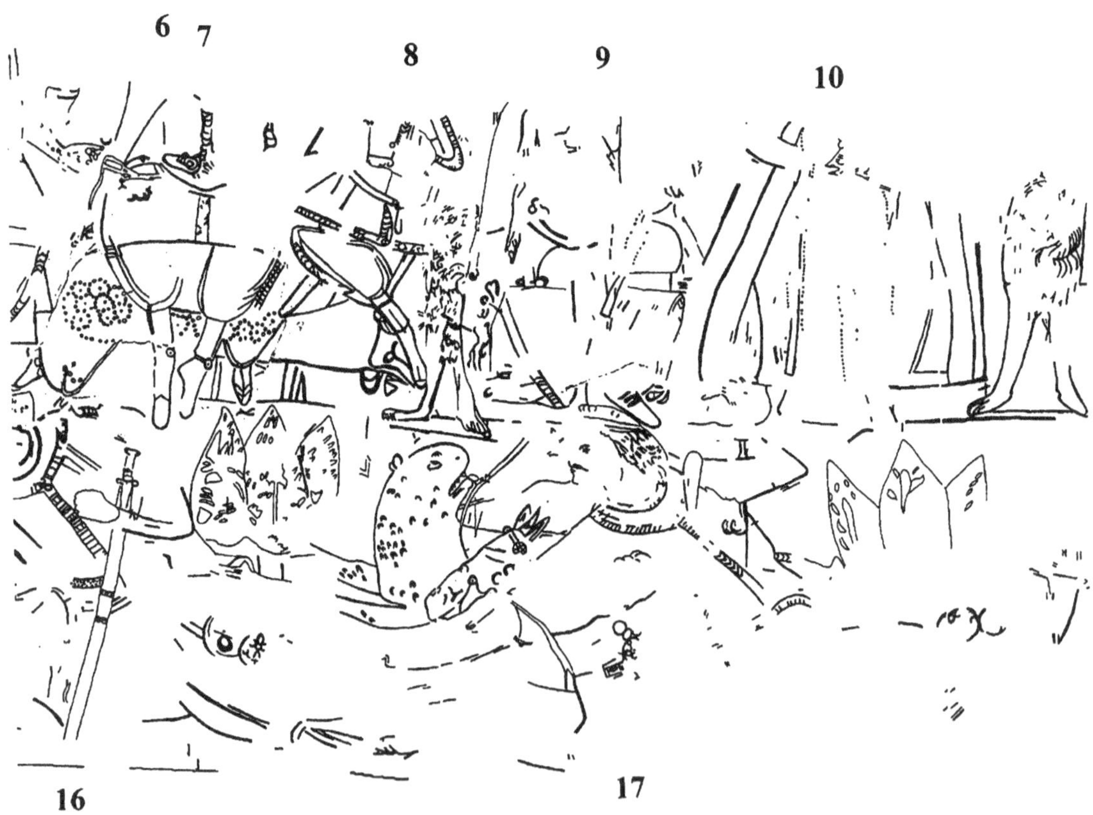

102. A divine couple on wall paintings from Jartepa II Temple (Frantz Grenet).

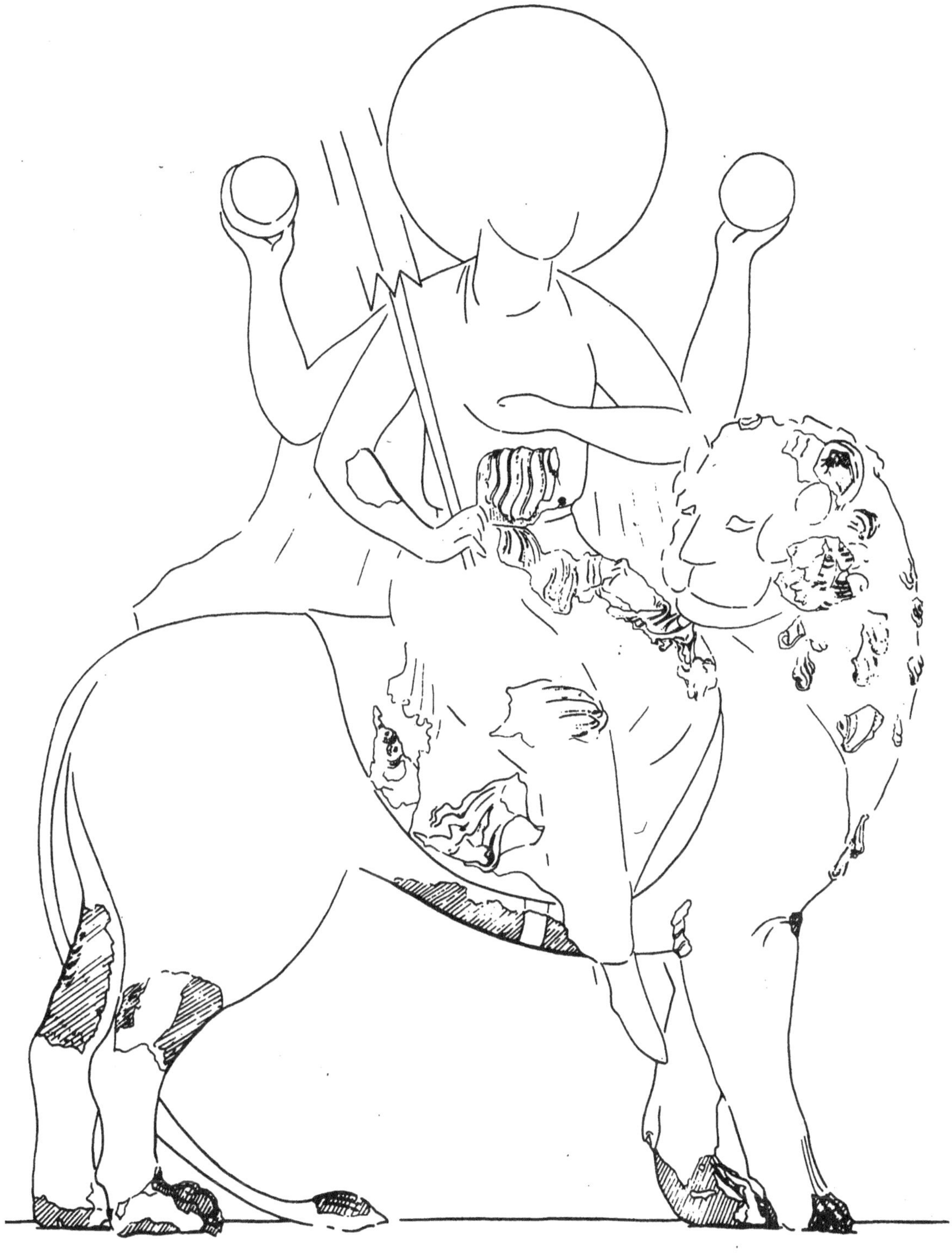

103. Nana on a lion, Panjikent, Temple II, X/13 (Shkoda 2009: fig. 121/1).

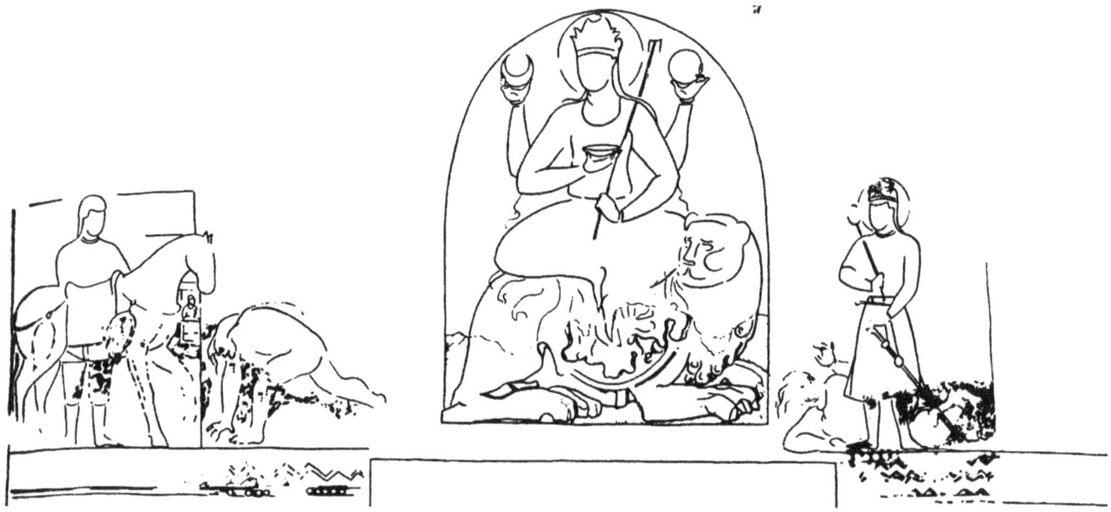

104. Nana on a lion, Panjikent, Temple II, X/14 (Shkoda 2009: fig. 121/3).

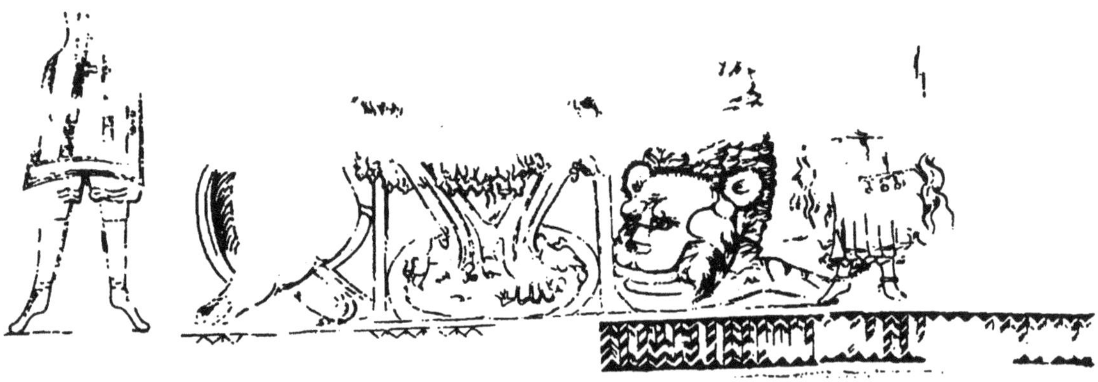

105. Nana on a lion, Panjikent, Temple II, X/14 (Shkoda 2009: fig. 121/2).

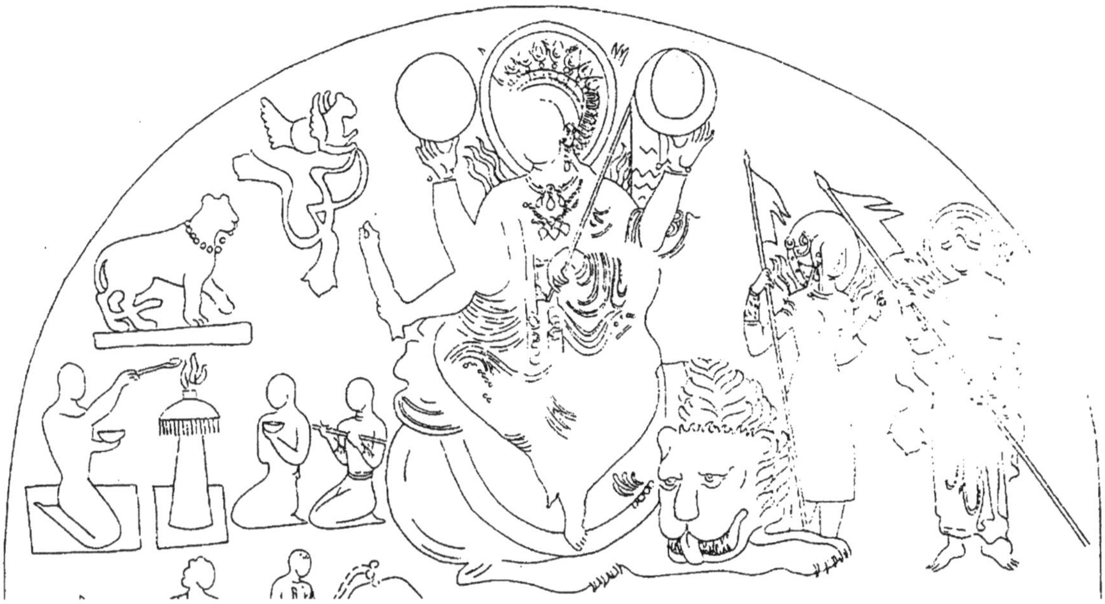

106. Nana on a lion on blue background, Panjikent, Tempe II, X (Frantz Grenet).

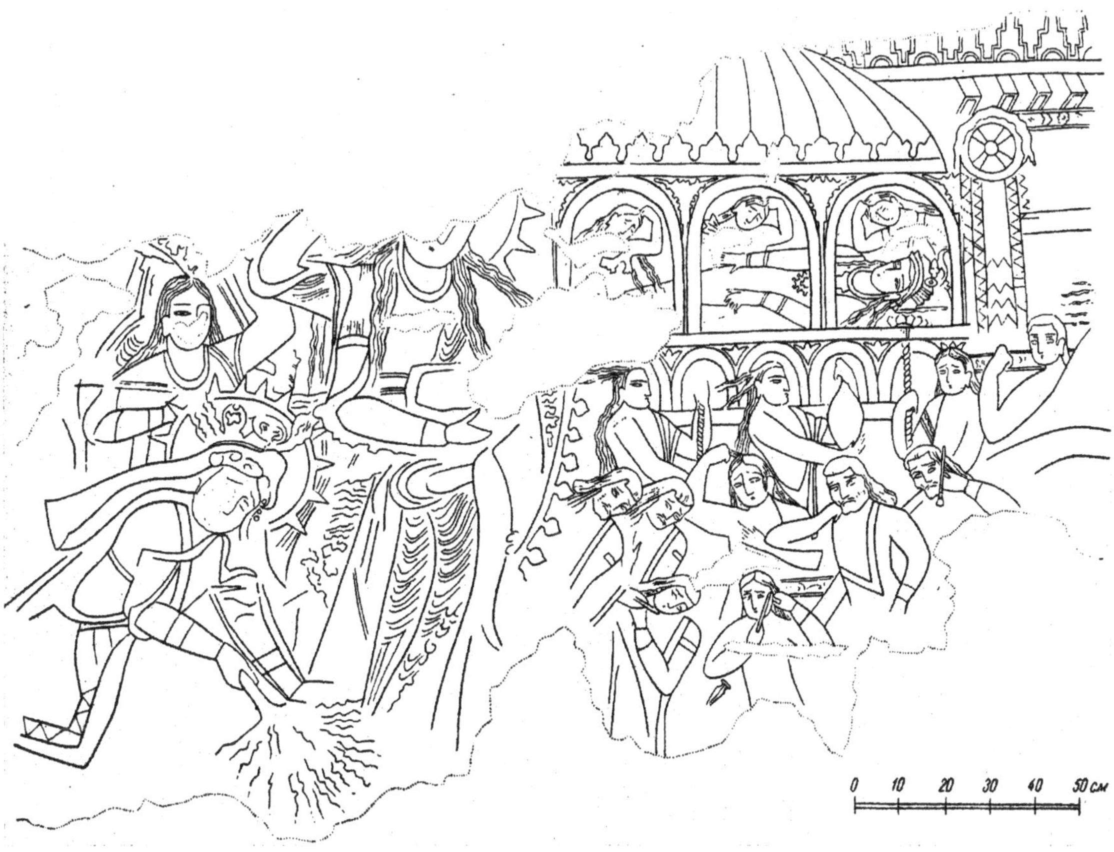

107. The "Lamentation scene", Panjikent, Temple II/5 (Frantz Grenet).

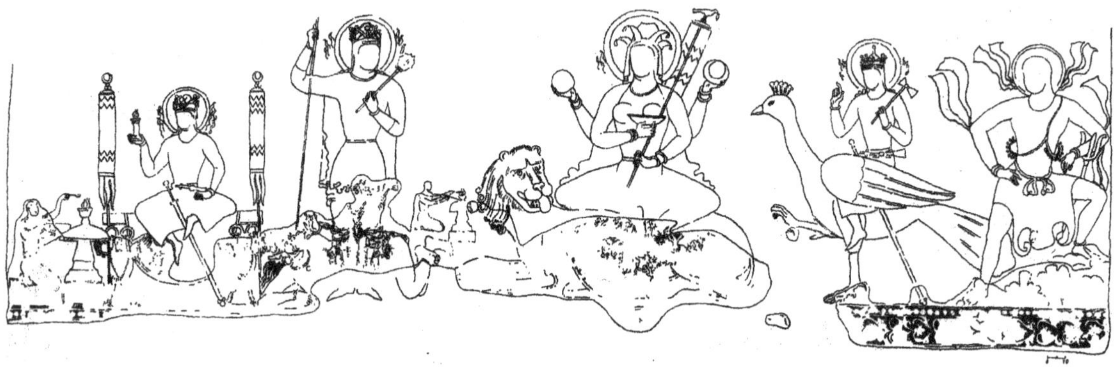

108. A group of gods, Panjikent, XXVI/2 (Frantz Grenet).

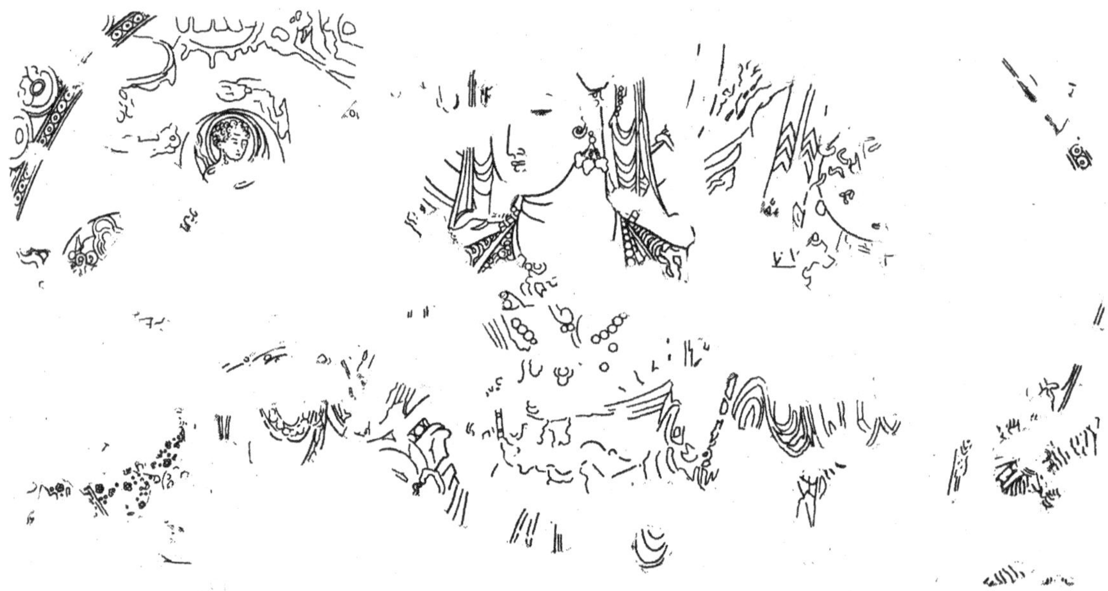

109. Nana with astral symbols, Panjikent, VI/26 (Frantz Grenet).

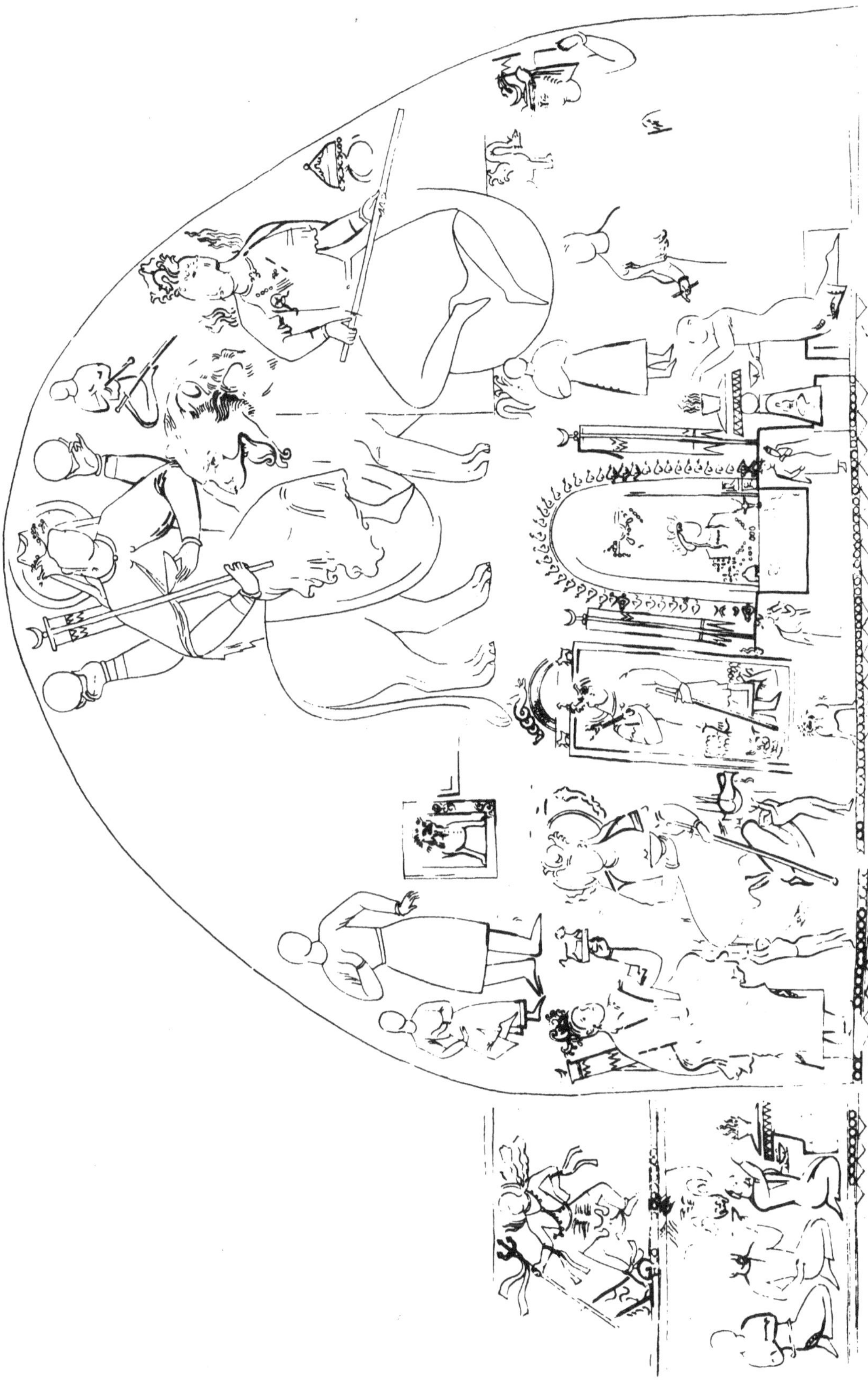

110. Nana on a lion, "Hell" and "Heaven", Panjikent XXV/12 (Frantz Grenet).

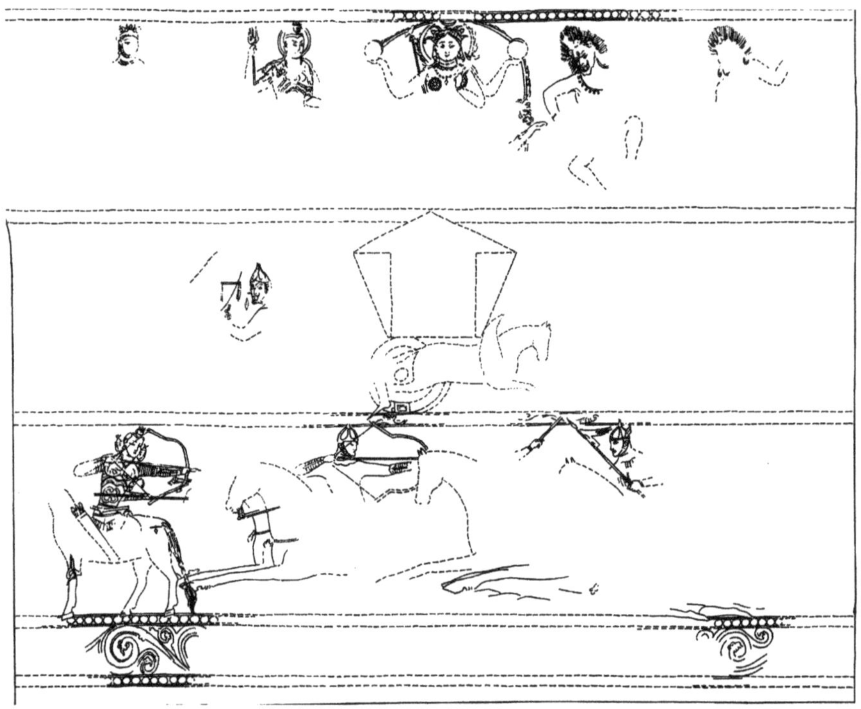

111. The eastern wall of the "Small hall" (right side), Bunjikat (Sokolovskiy 2009: fig. 70).

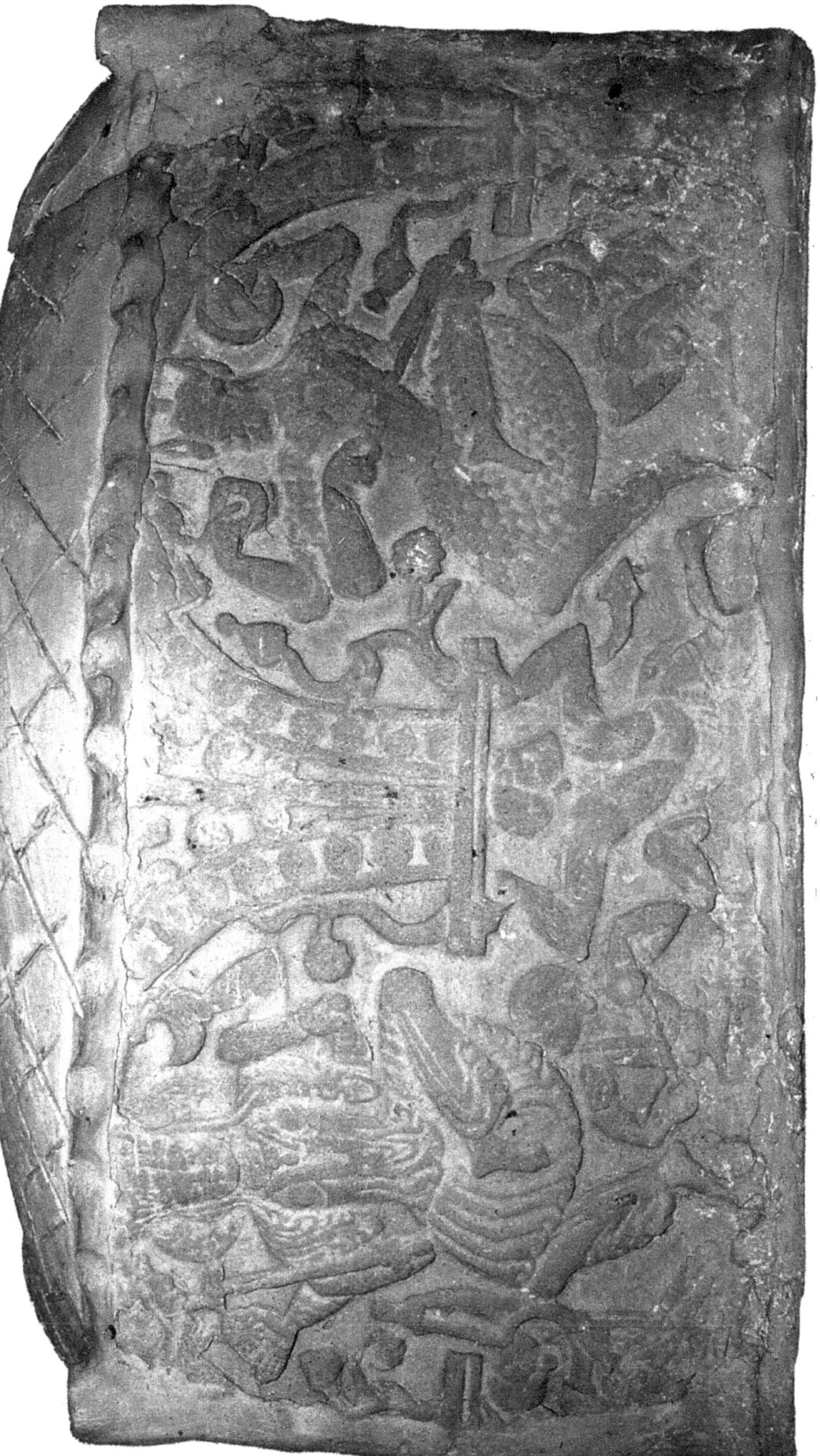

112. The ossuary from Khirmantepa (Frantz Grenet).

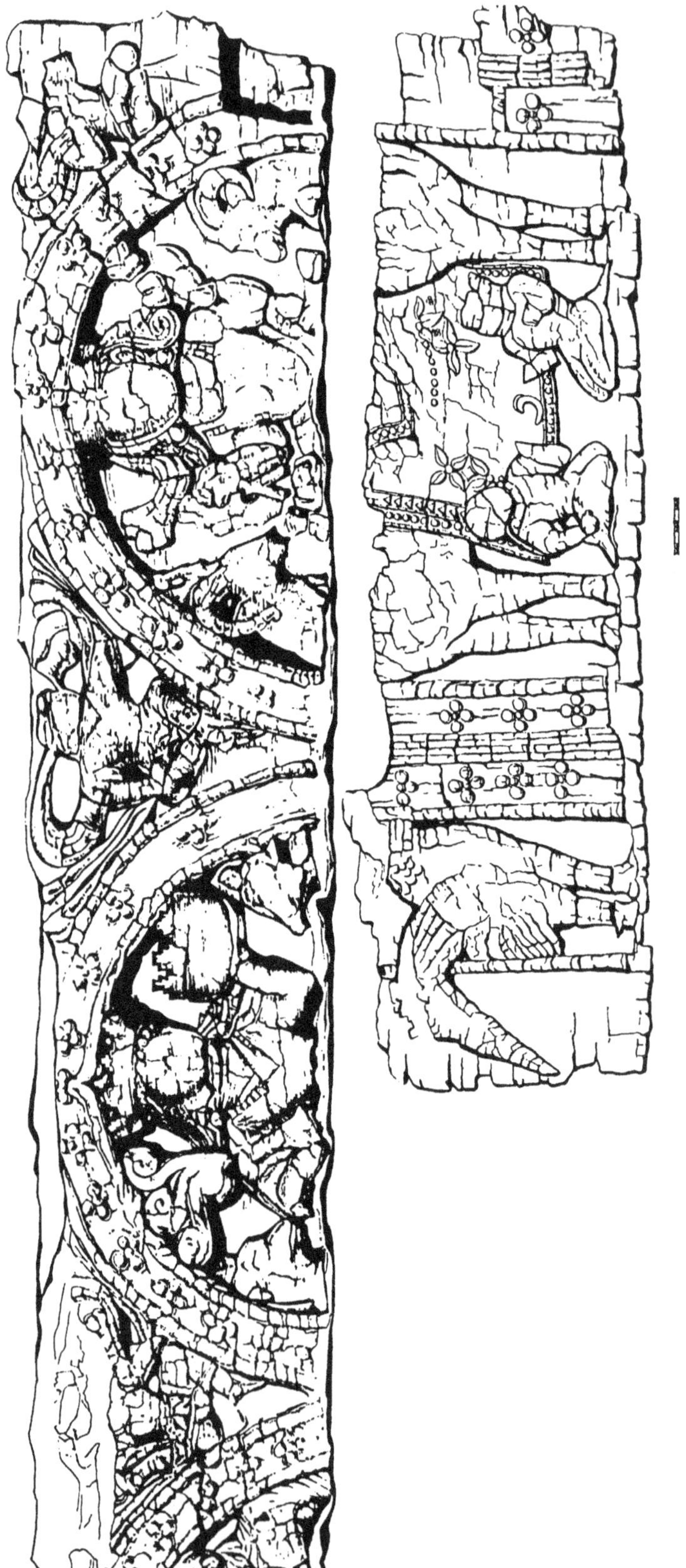

113. A wooden frieze from Kujruk-tobe, first fragment (Frantz Grenet).

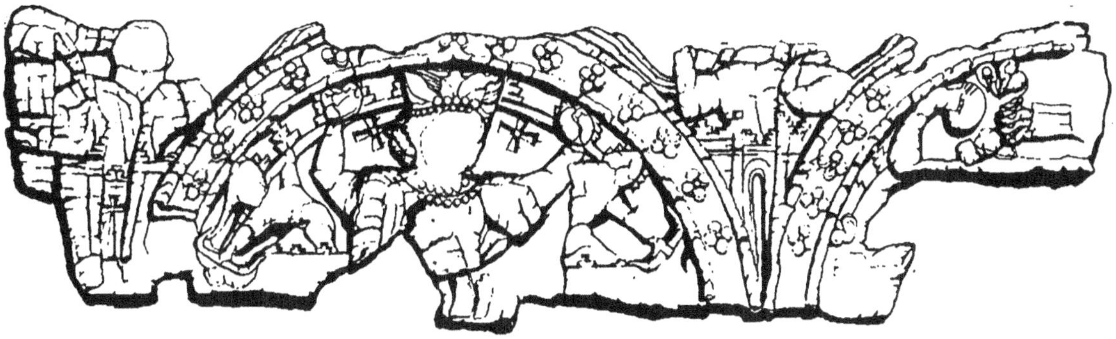

114. A wooden frieze from Kujruk-tobe, second fragment (Frantz Grenet).

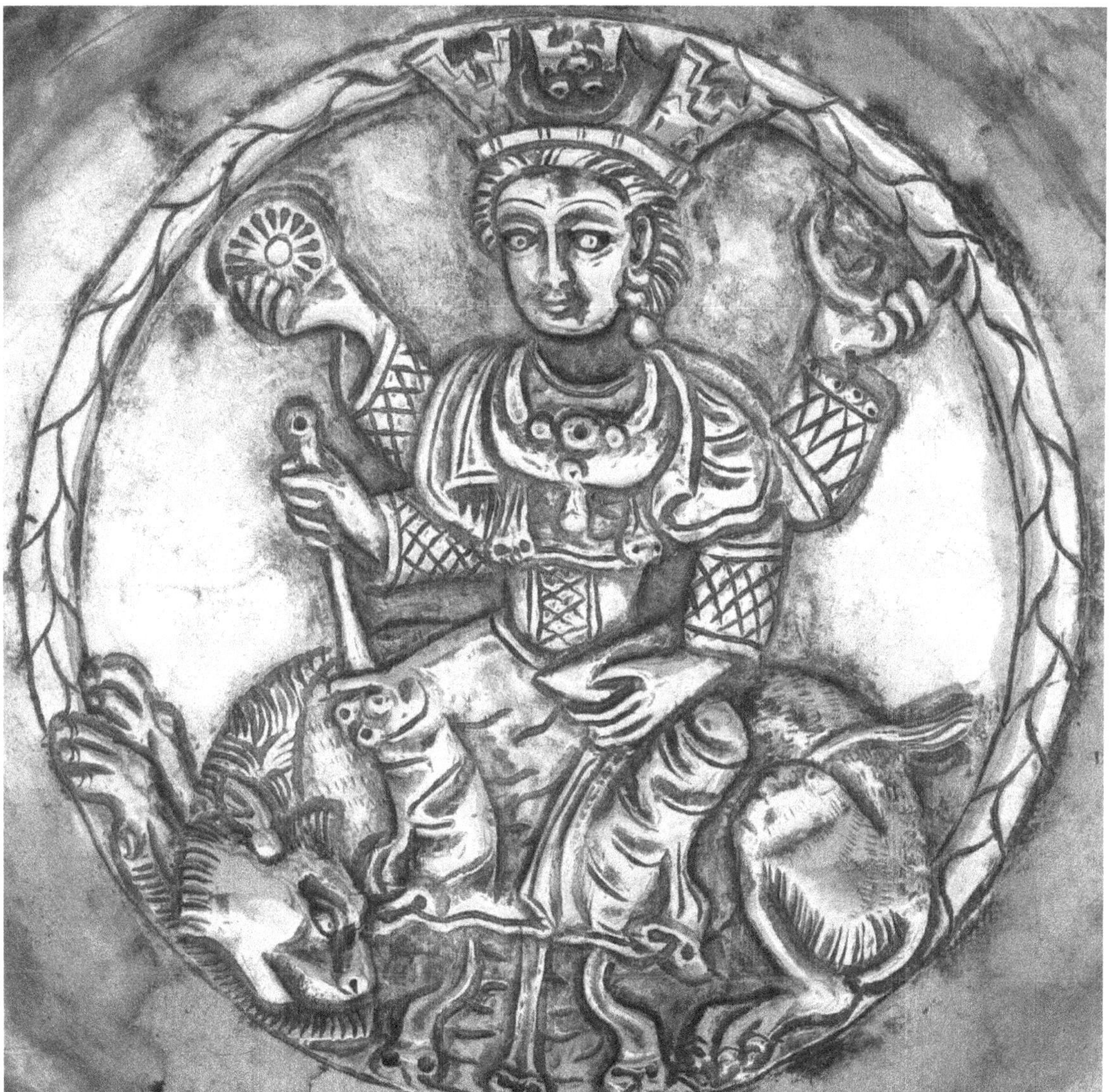

115. Nana on a Chorasmian bowl from the British Museum (© Trustees of the British Museum).

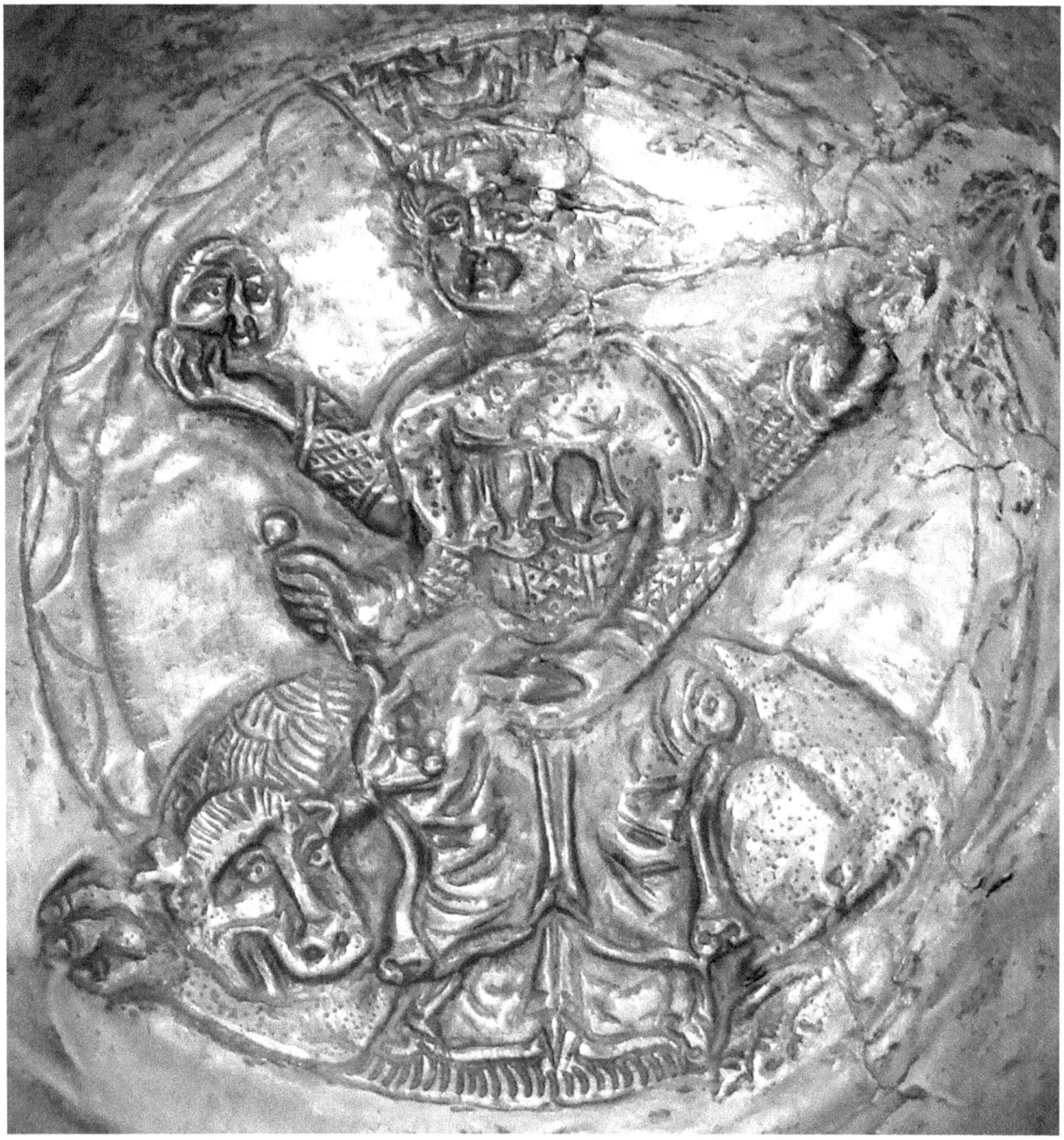

116. Nana on a prone lion, Chorasmian bowl from Bartym (Constantine Zuckerman).

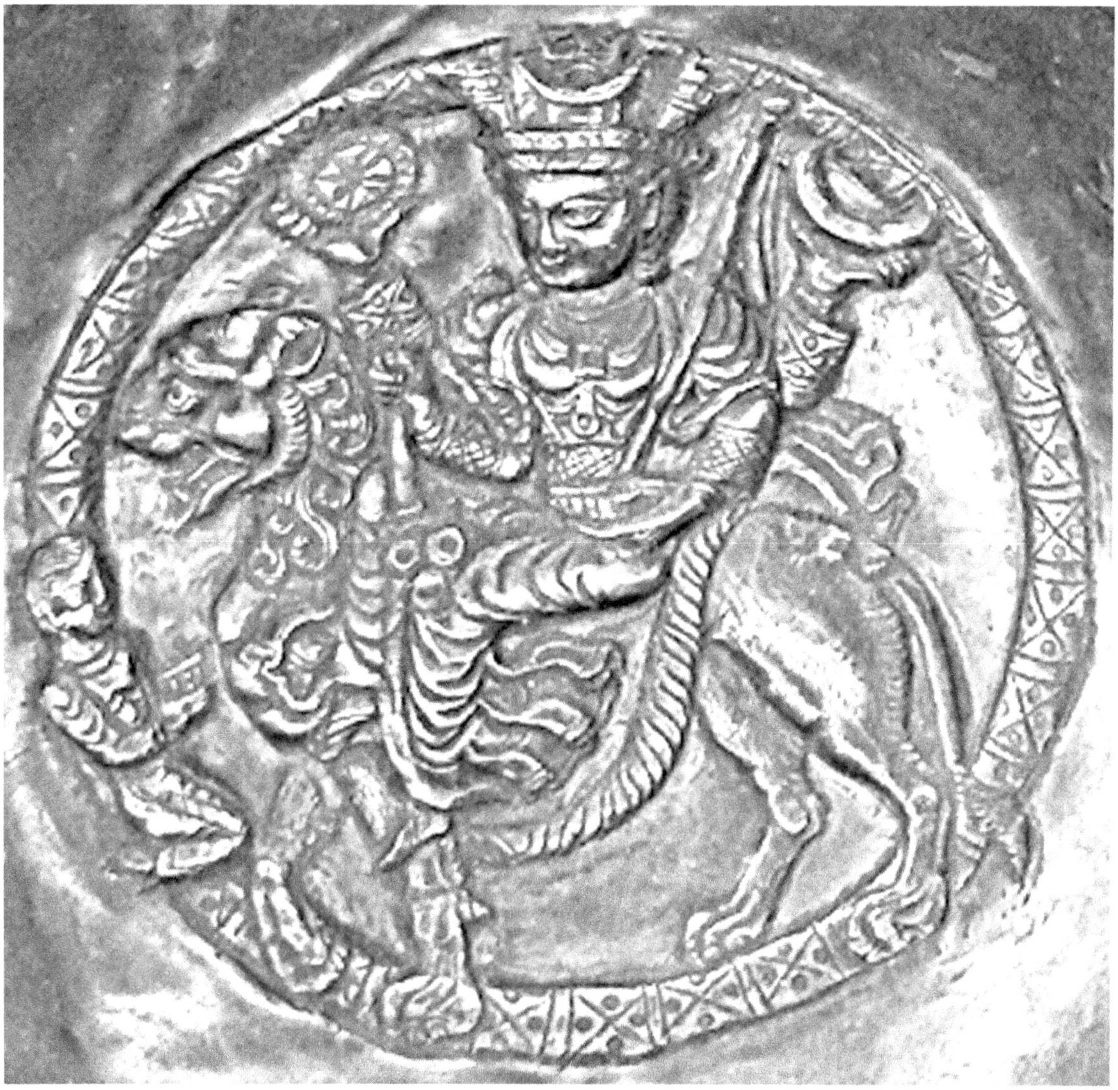

117. Nana on a marching lion, Chorasmian bowl from Bartym (Constantine Zuckerman).

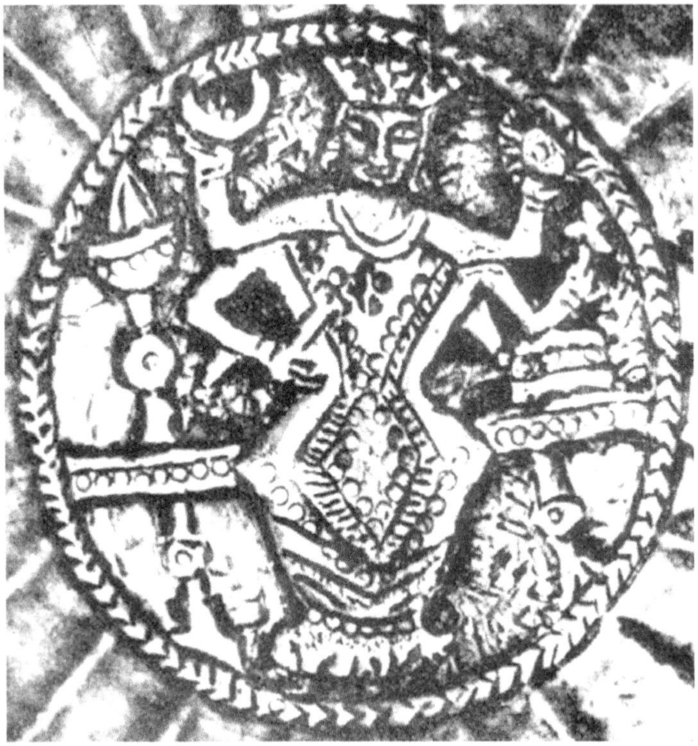

118. Standing Nana on a Chorasmian bowl (Azarpay 1969: pl. 3c).

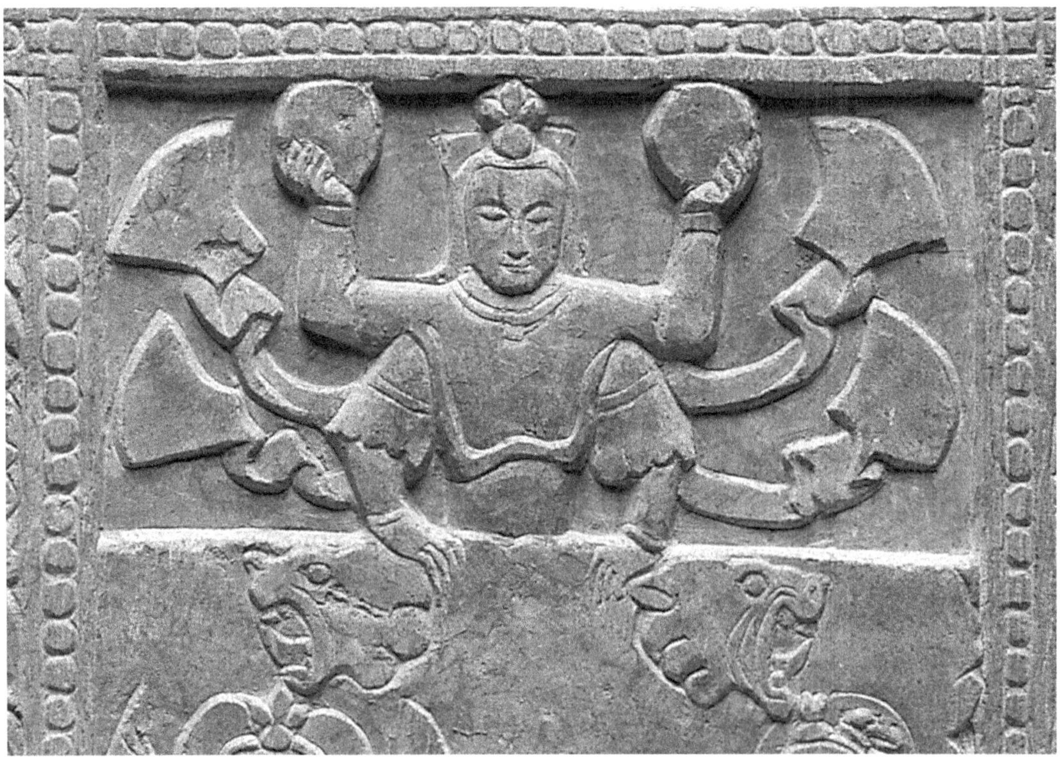

119. Nana on the "Miho couch" (© MIHO Museum).

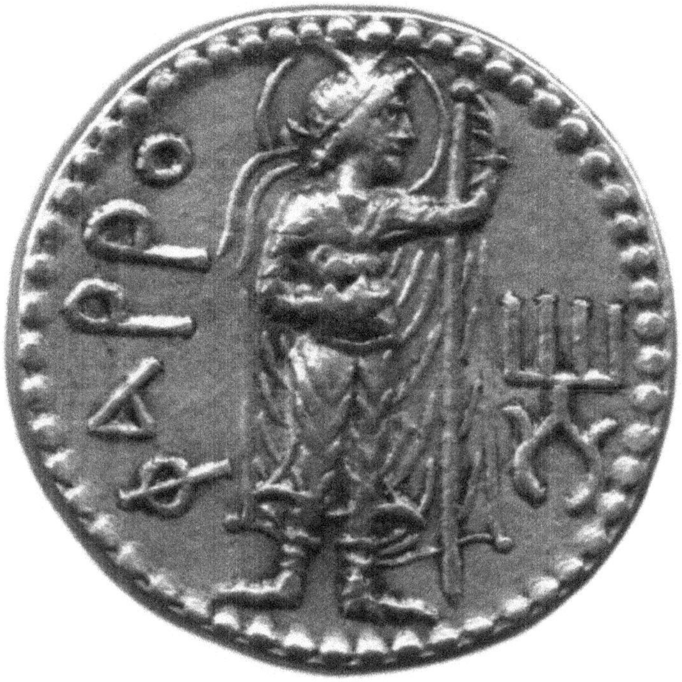

120. Pharro on a Kushan coin, type 1 (© Trustees of the British Museum).

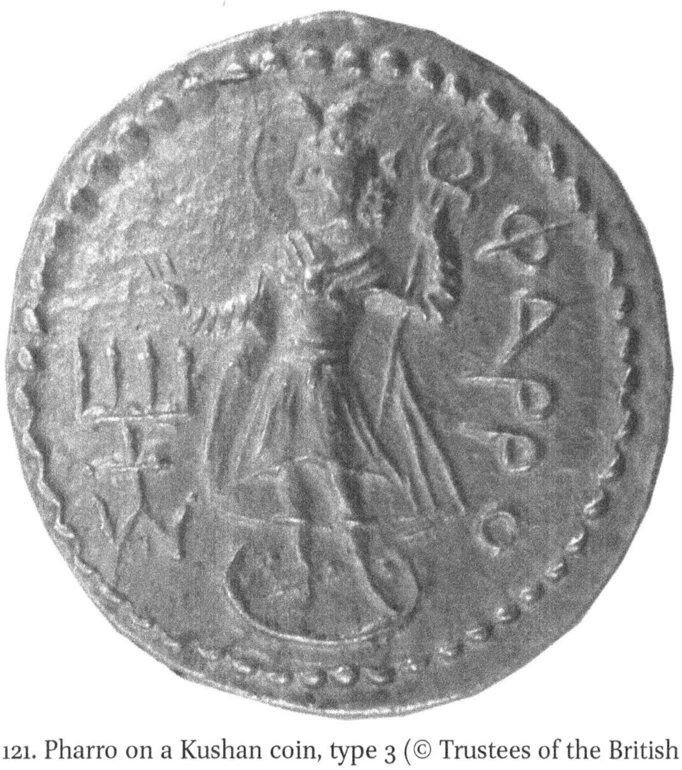

121. Pharro on a Kushan coin, type 3 (© Trustees of the British Museum).

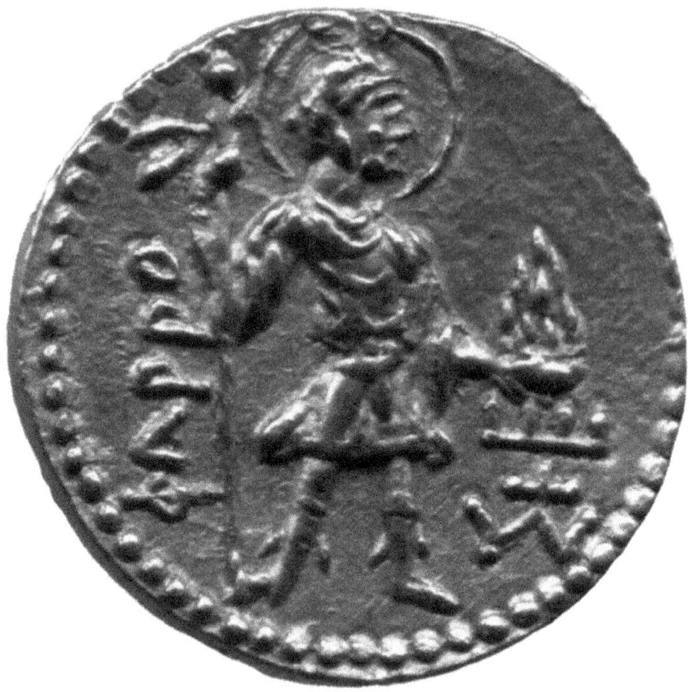

122. Pharro on a Kushan coin, type 4 (© Trustees of the British Museum).

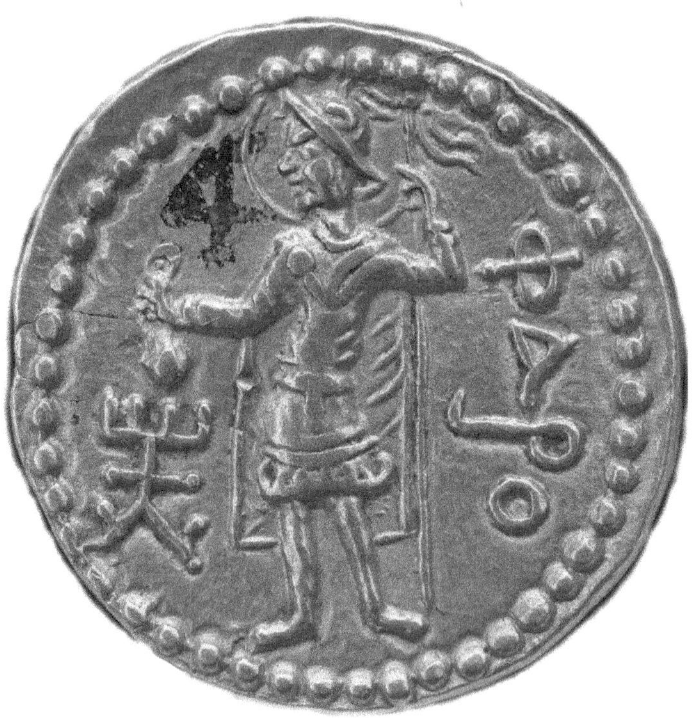

123. Pharro on a Kushan coin, type 9 (© Trustees of the British Museum).

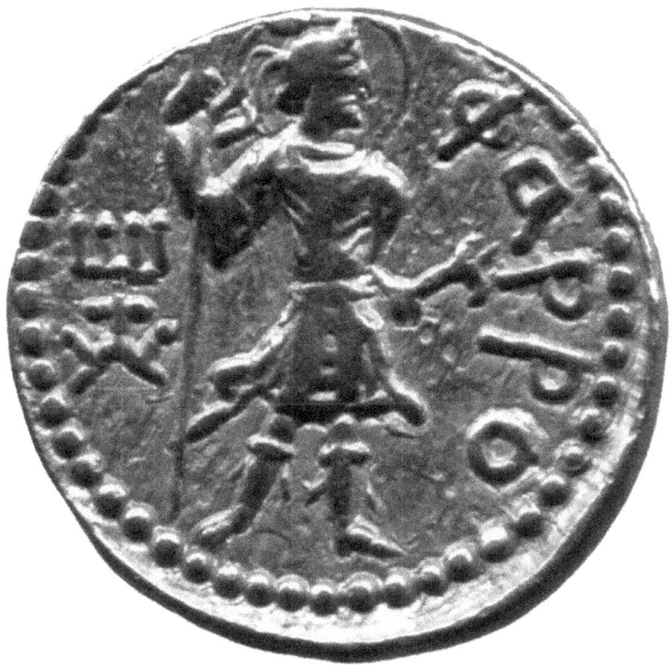

124. Pharro on a Kushan coin, type 10 (© Trustees of the British Museum).

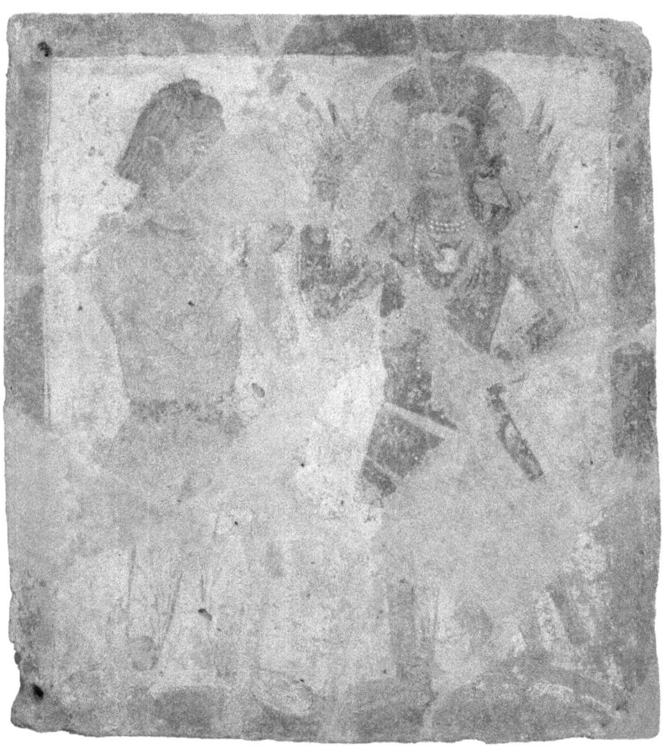

125. Terracotta panel from Afghanistan depicting a god with flaming shoulders (© The Metropolitan Museum of Art).

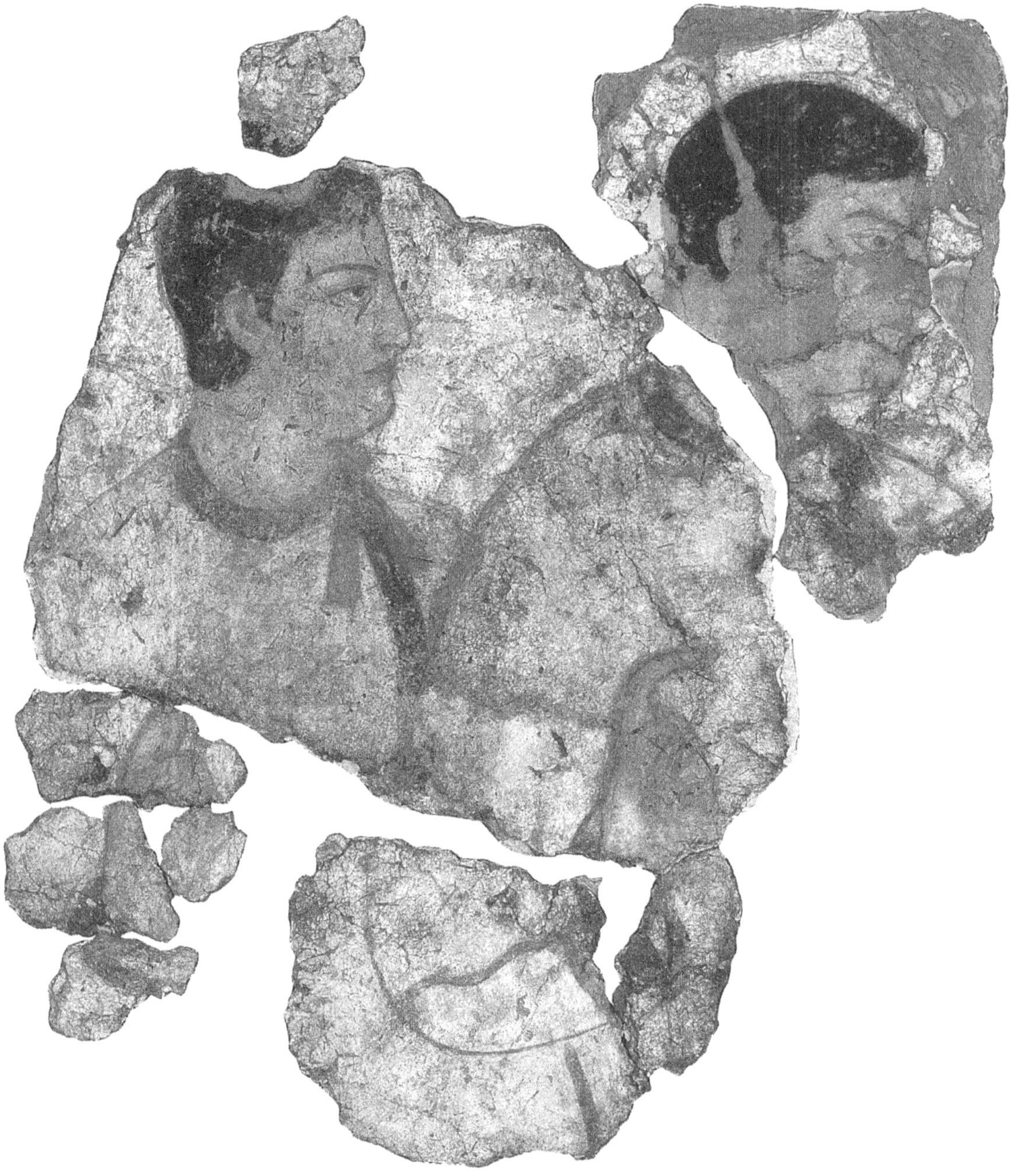

126. "Pharro" from Fayaztepa (Abdullaev, Rtveladze and Shishkina 1991: no. 119).

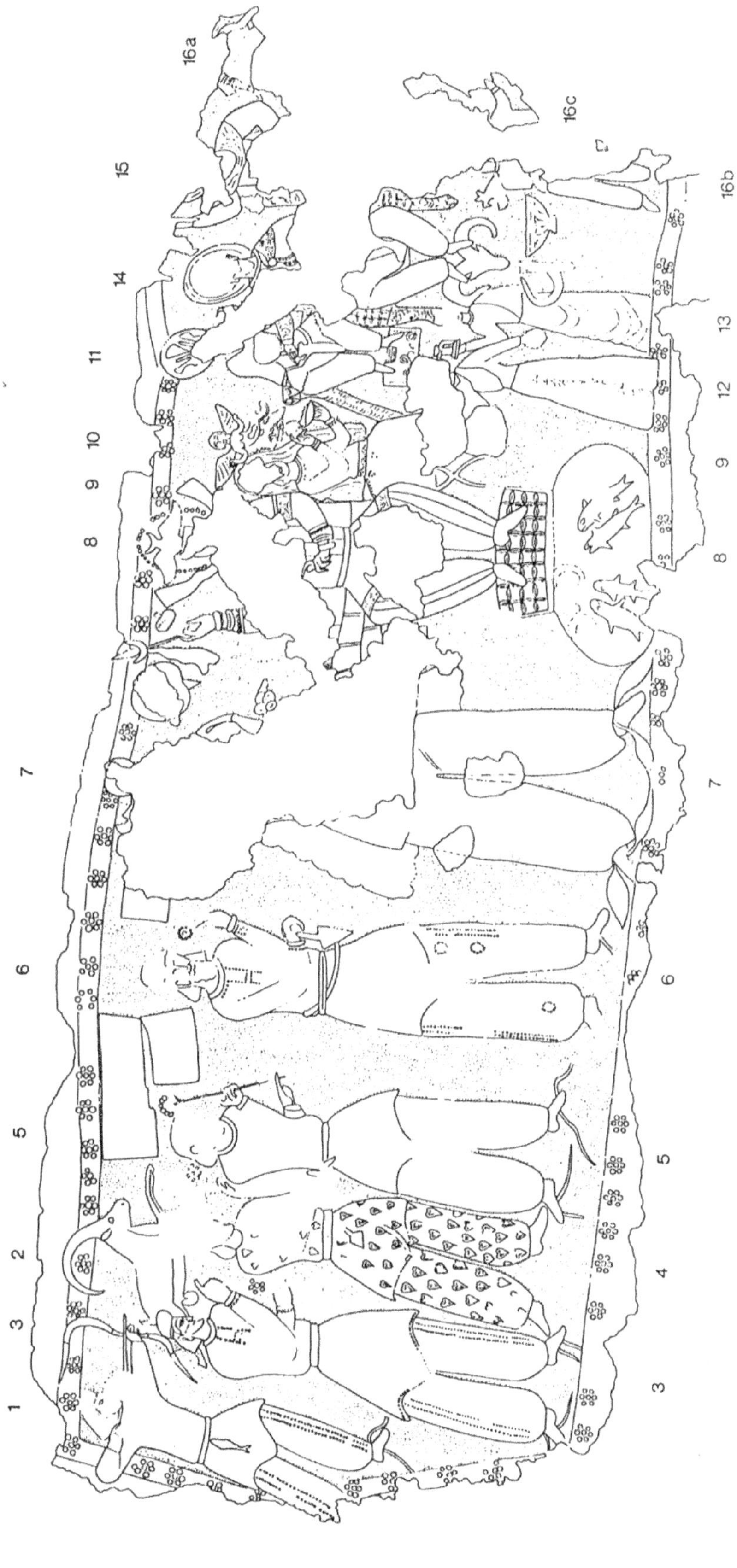

127. The Kushano-Sasanian painting from Ghulbiyan (Frantz Grenet).

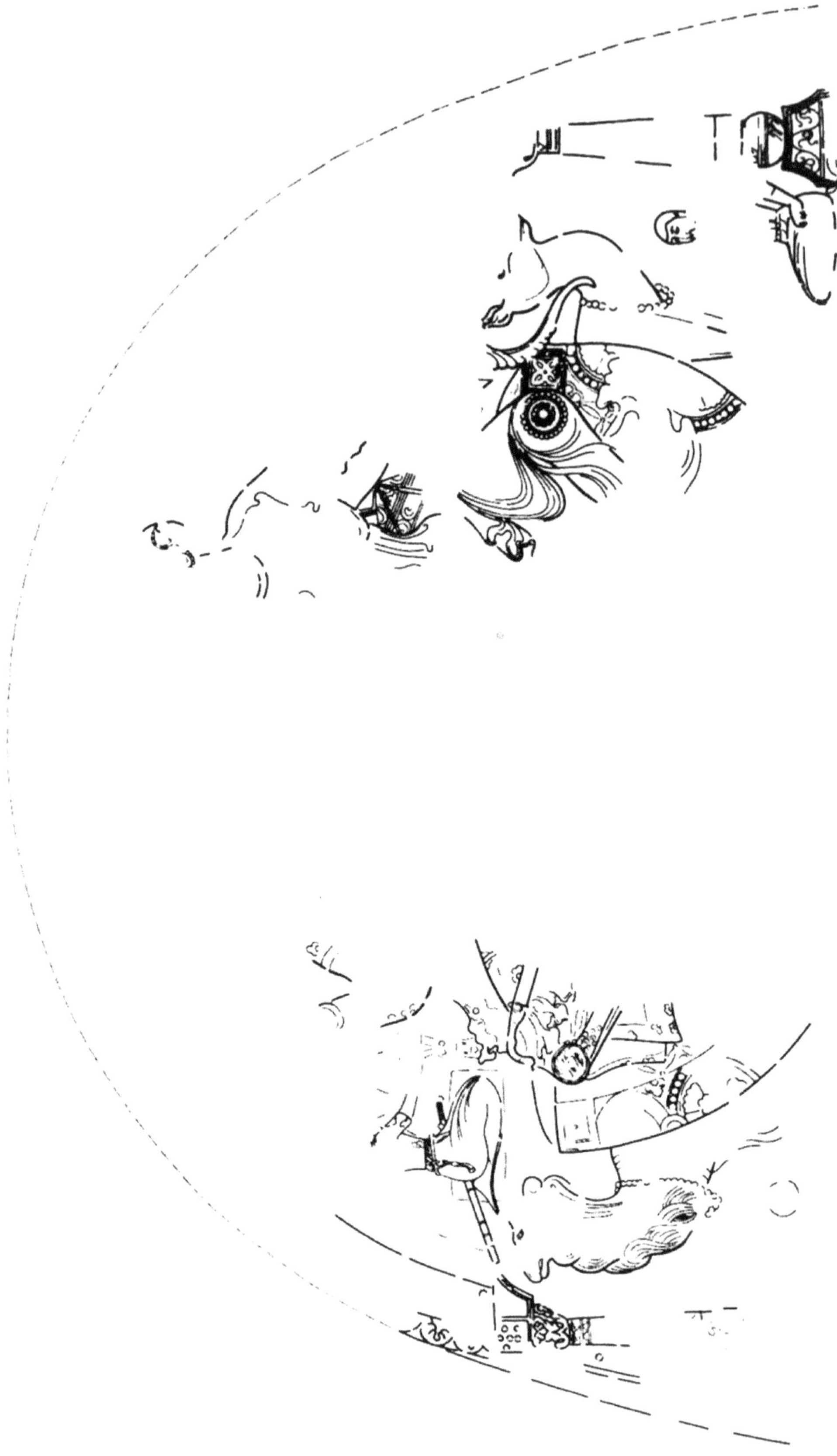

128. Enthroned divine couple, Panjikent XXIV/2 (Frantz Grenet).

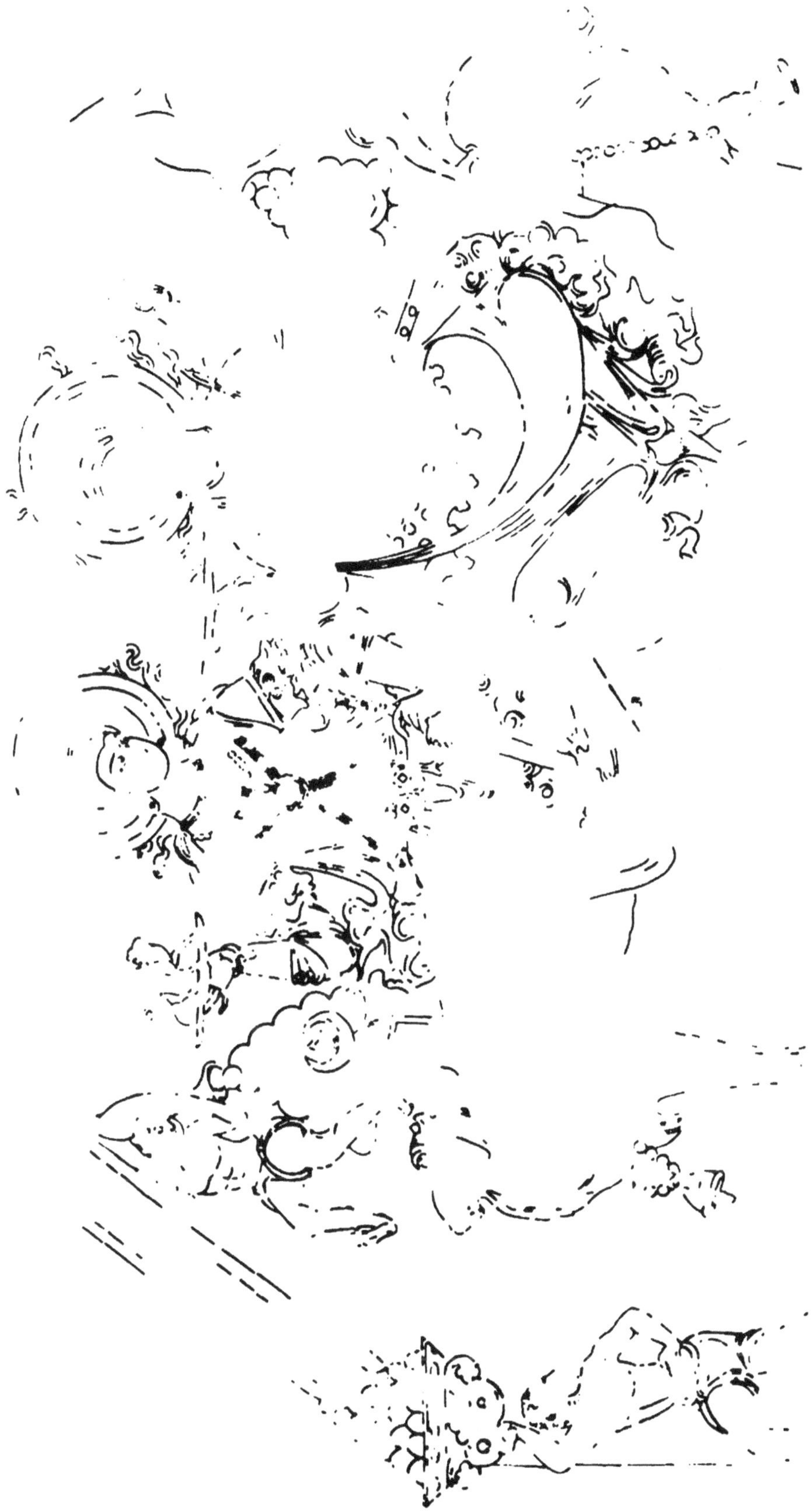

129. Enthroned divine couple, Panjikent XXIV/13 (Frantz Grenet).

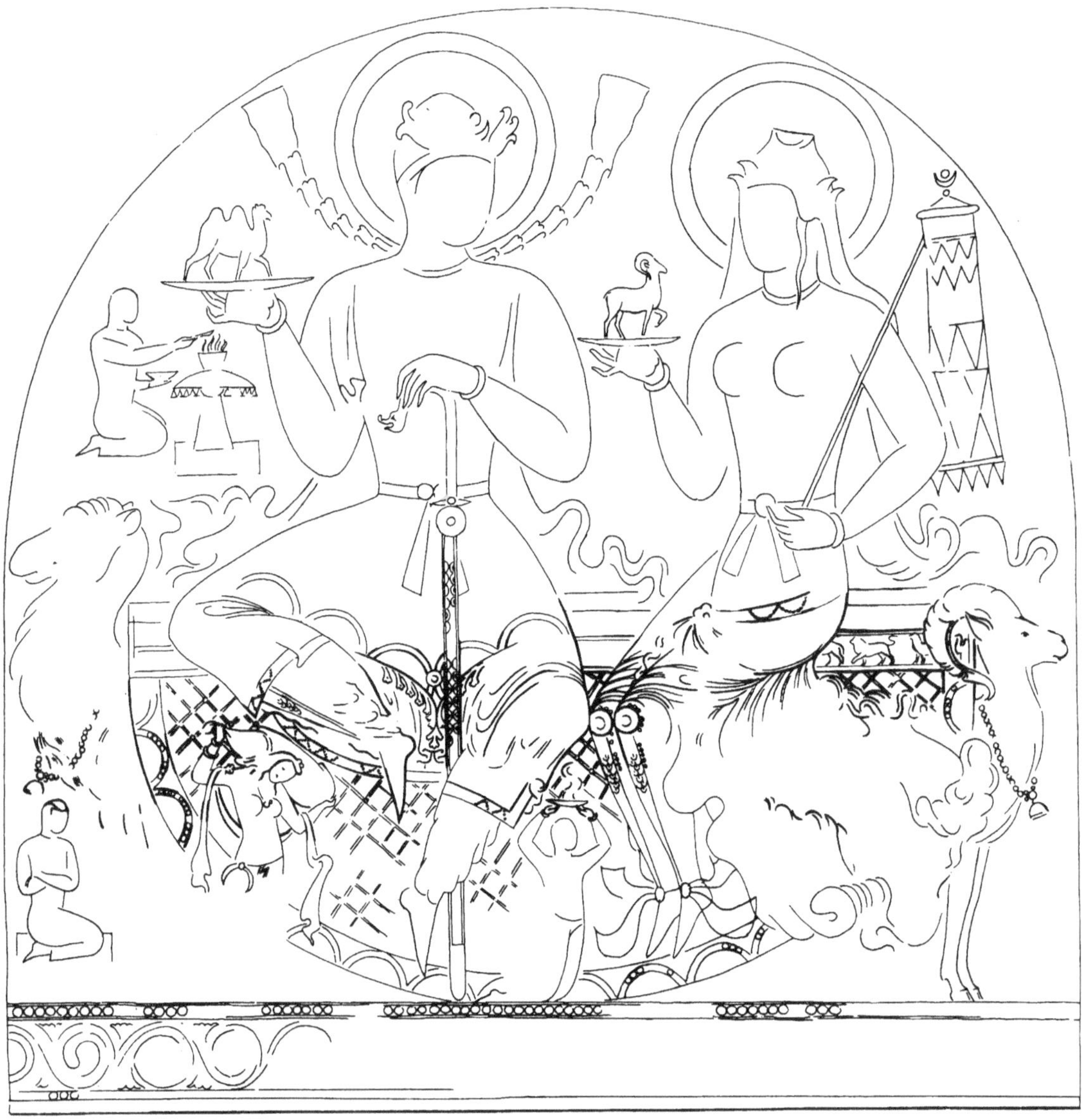

130. Enthroned divine couple, Panjikent XXV/28, southern wall (Frantz Grenet).

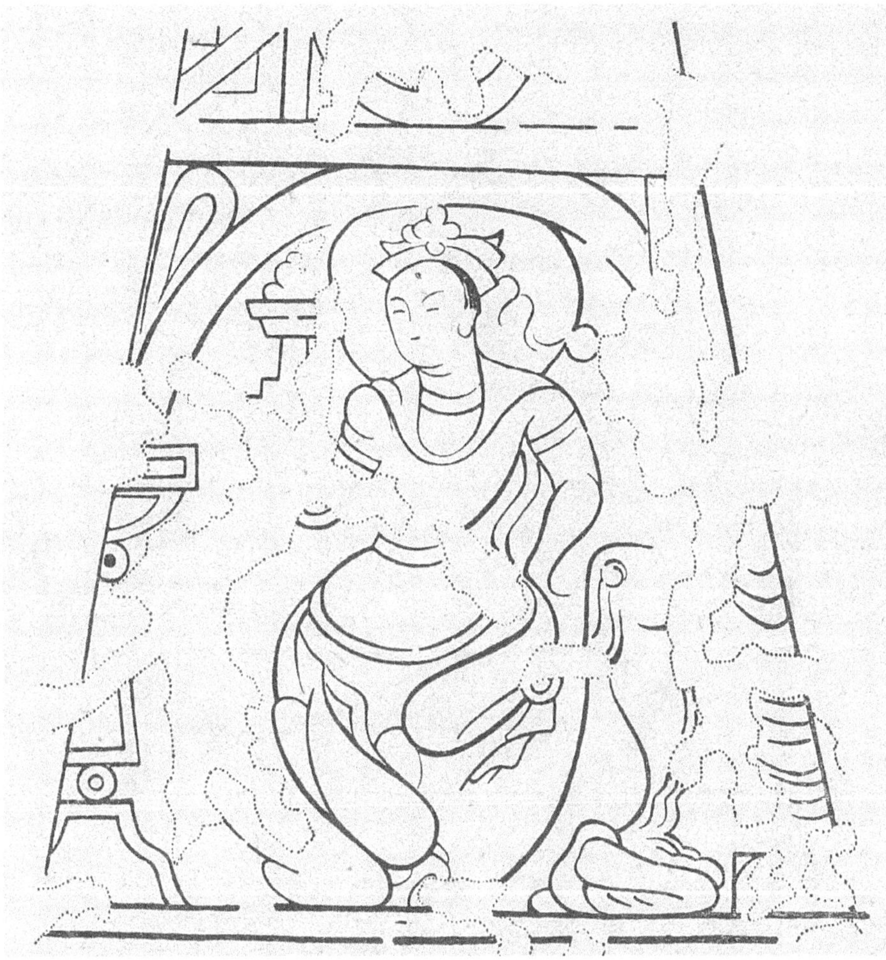

131. A male figure on a camel, Varakhsha (Frantz Grenet).

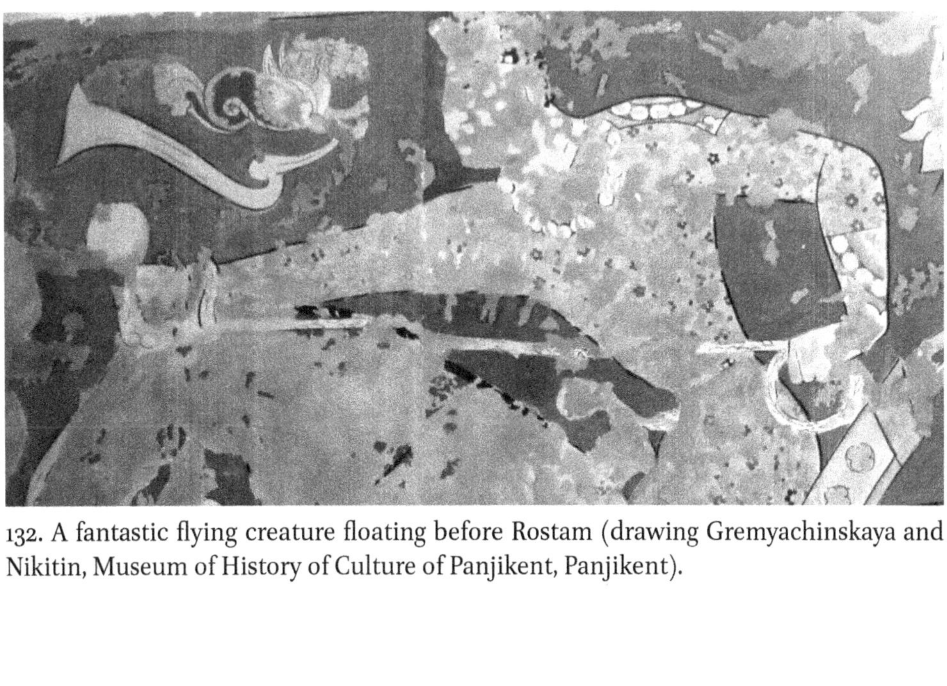

132. A fantastic flying creature floating before Rostam (drawing Gremyachinskaya and Nikitin, Museum of History of Culture of Panjikent, Panjikent).

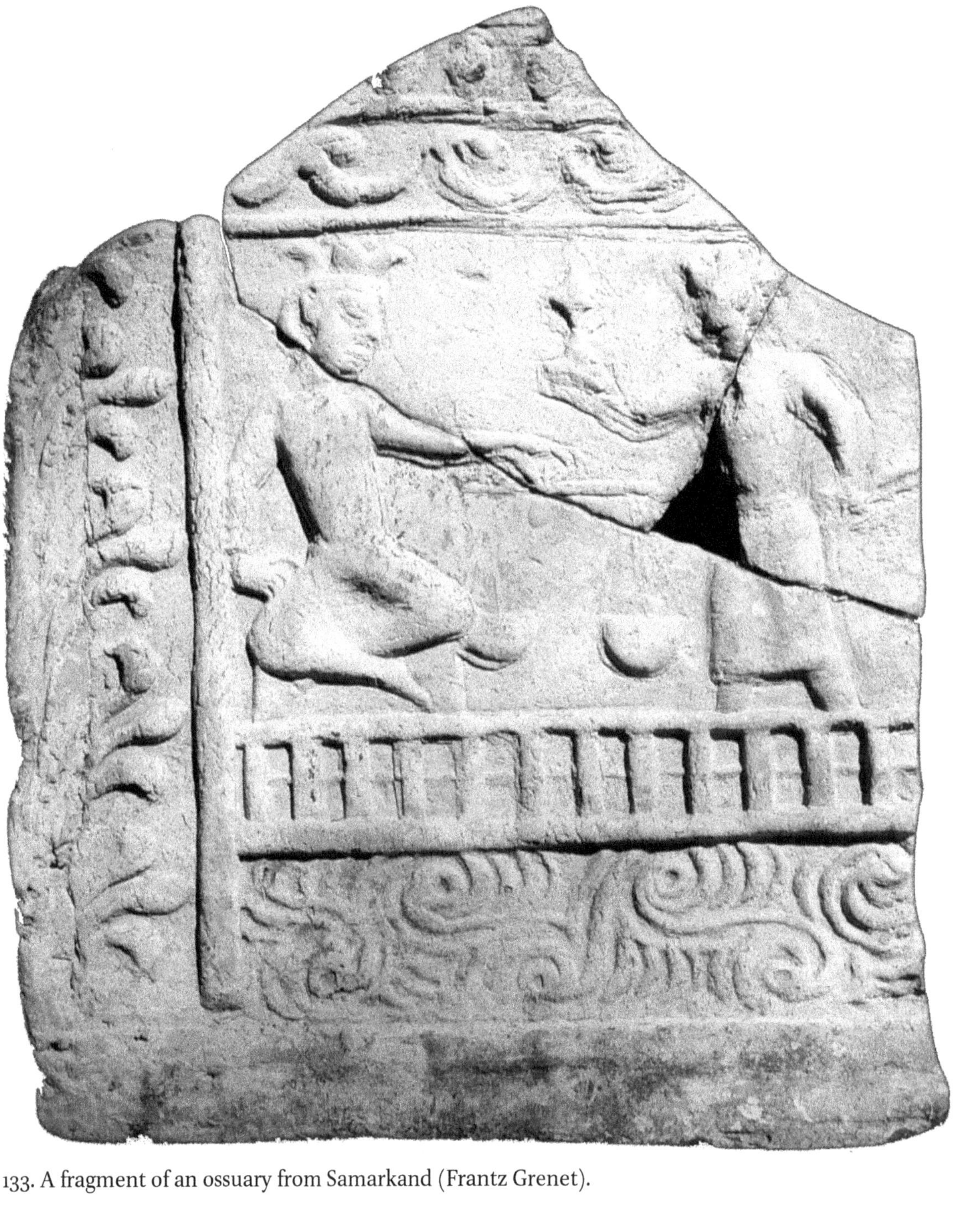

133. A fragment of an ossuary from Samarkand (Frantz Grenet).

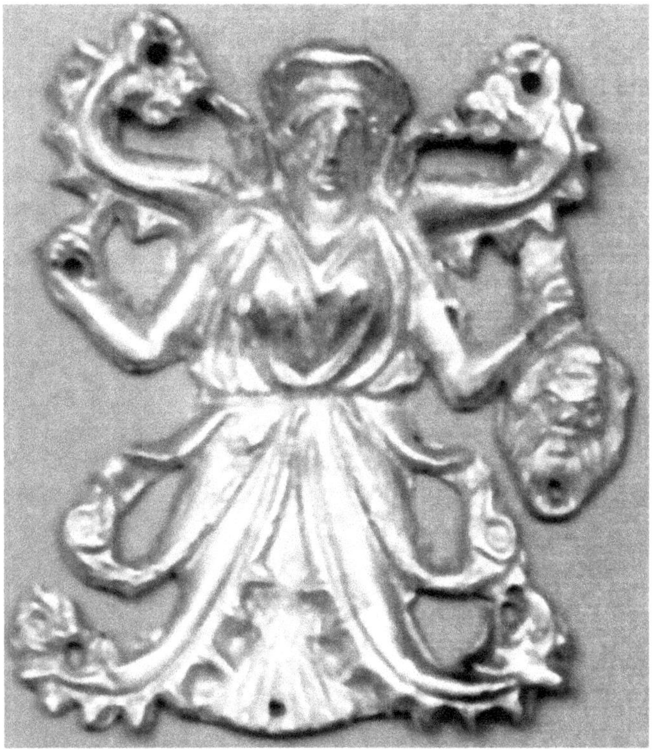

134. Anguipede goddess, Kul'-Oba Kurgan, (Korol'kova 2006: fig. 40).

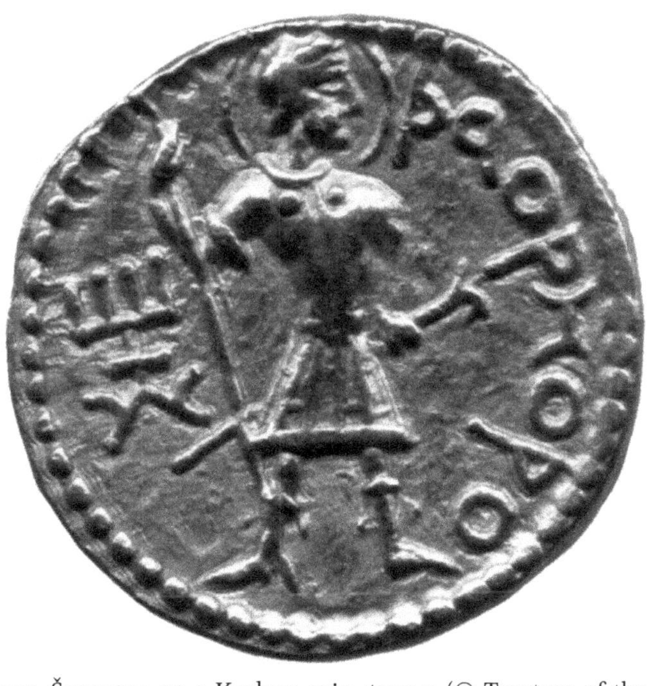

135. Šaoreoro on a Kushan coin, type 2 (© Trustees of the British Museum).

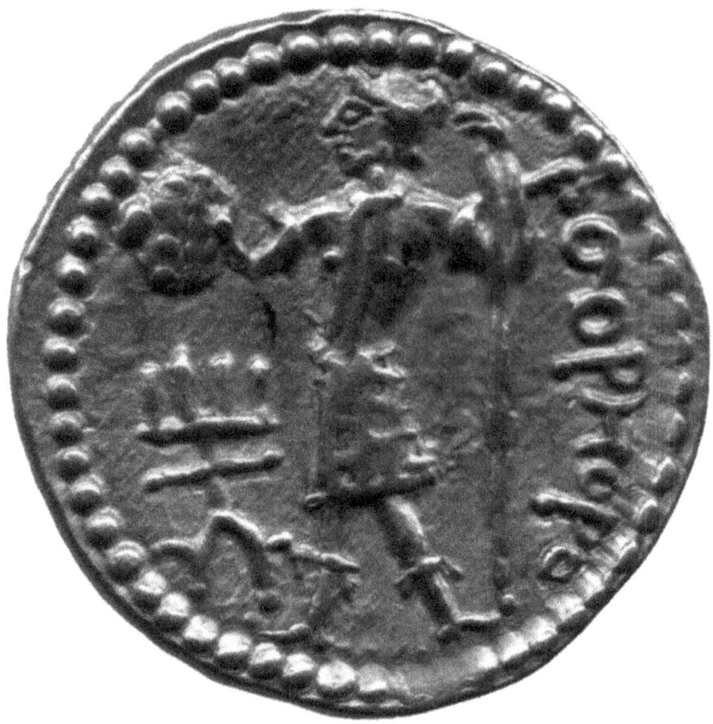

136. Šaoreoro on a Kushan coin, type 3 (© Trustees of the British Museum).

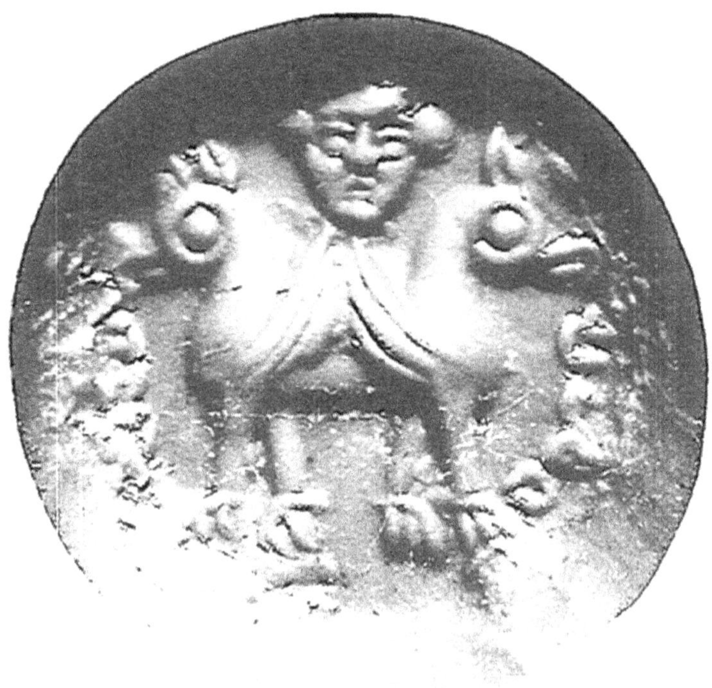

137. Chariot drawn by birds on a Sasanian seal (Frye 1971: no. 68).

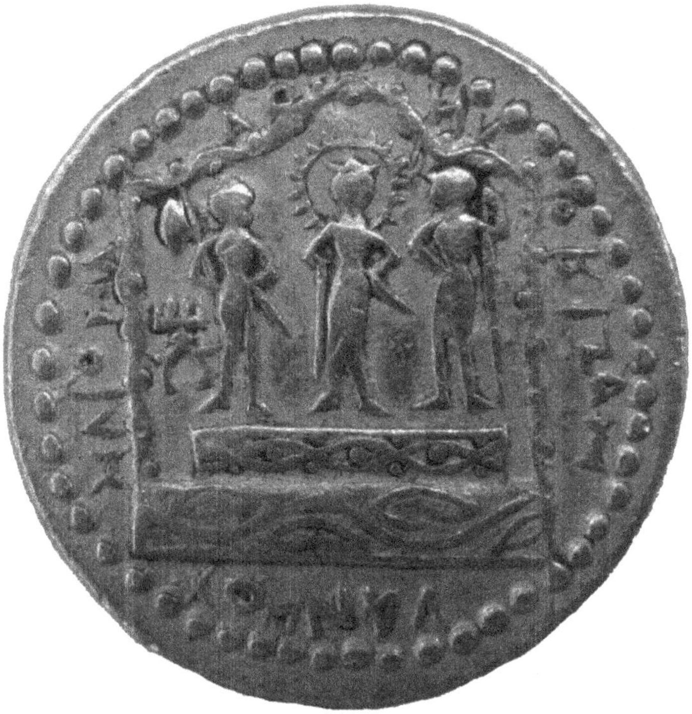

138. Maaseno, Skando-Kumaro and Bizago on a Kushan coin (Osmund Bopearachchi).

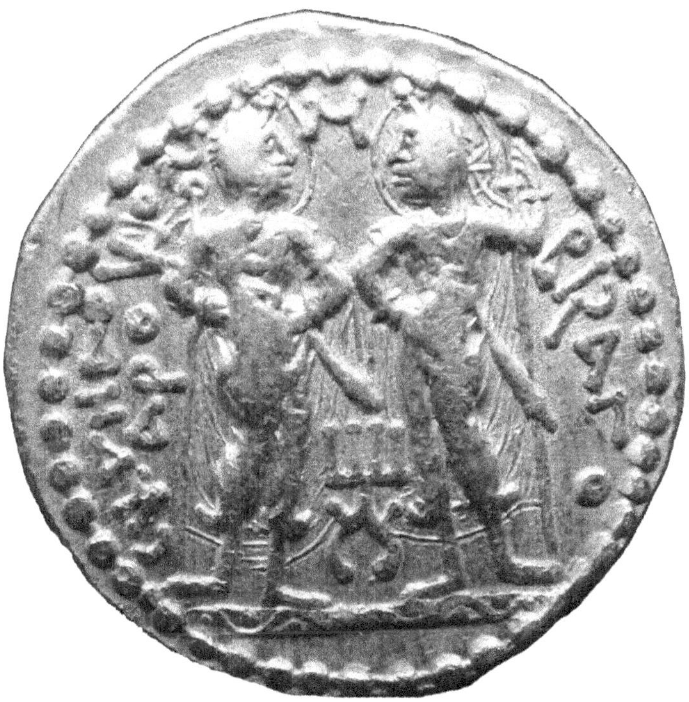

139. Skando and Bizago on a Kushan coin (© Trustees of the British Museum).

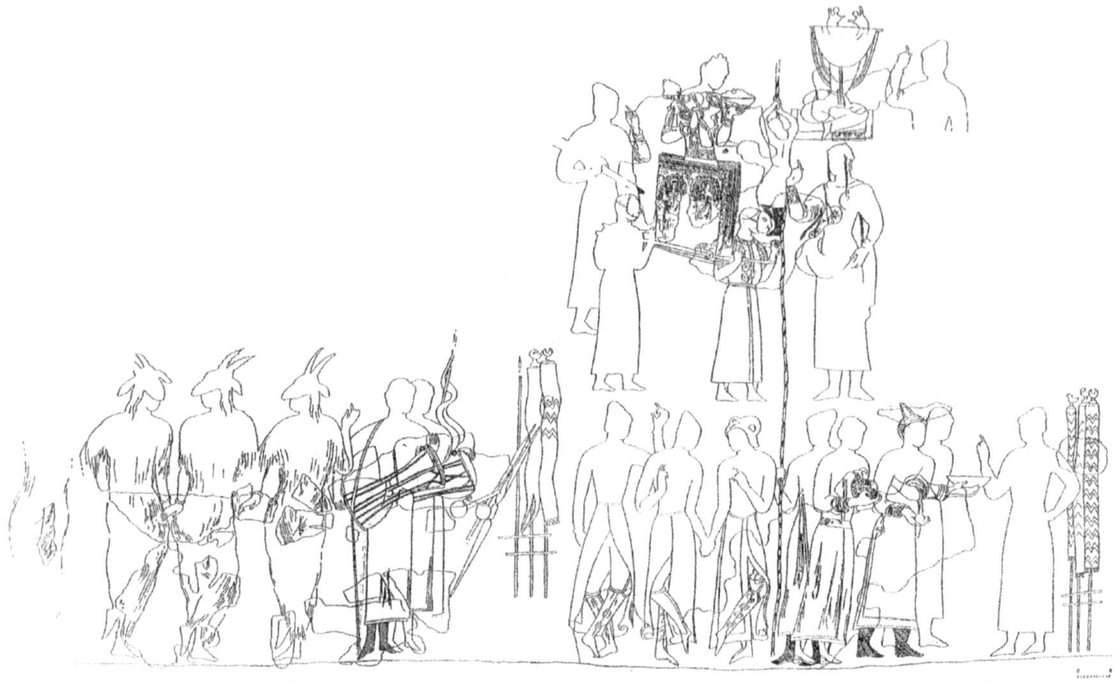

140. A golden statue carried in a procession, Panjikent XXVI/3 (Frantz Grenet).

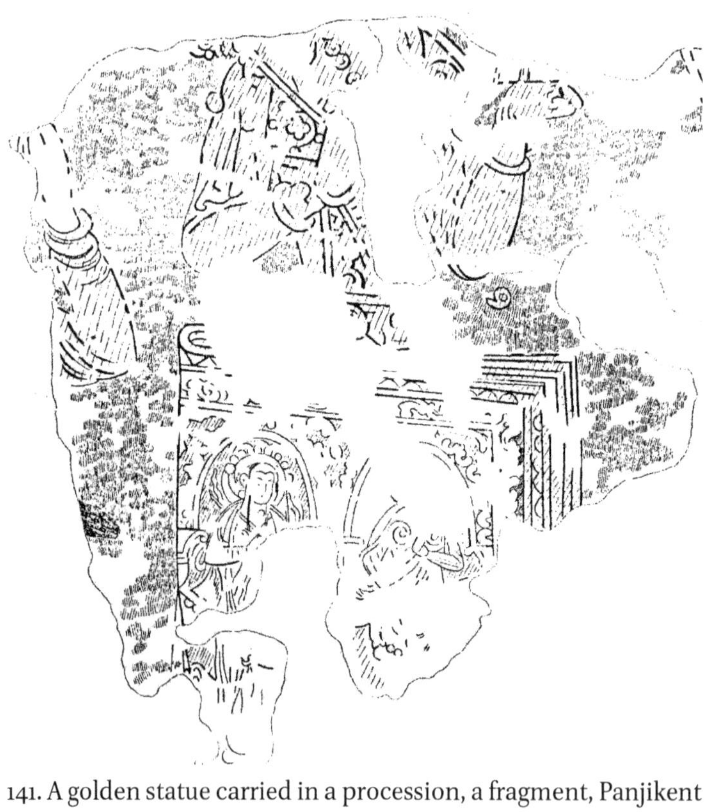

141. A golden statue carried in a procession, a fragment, Panjikent XXVI/3, (Frantz Grenet).

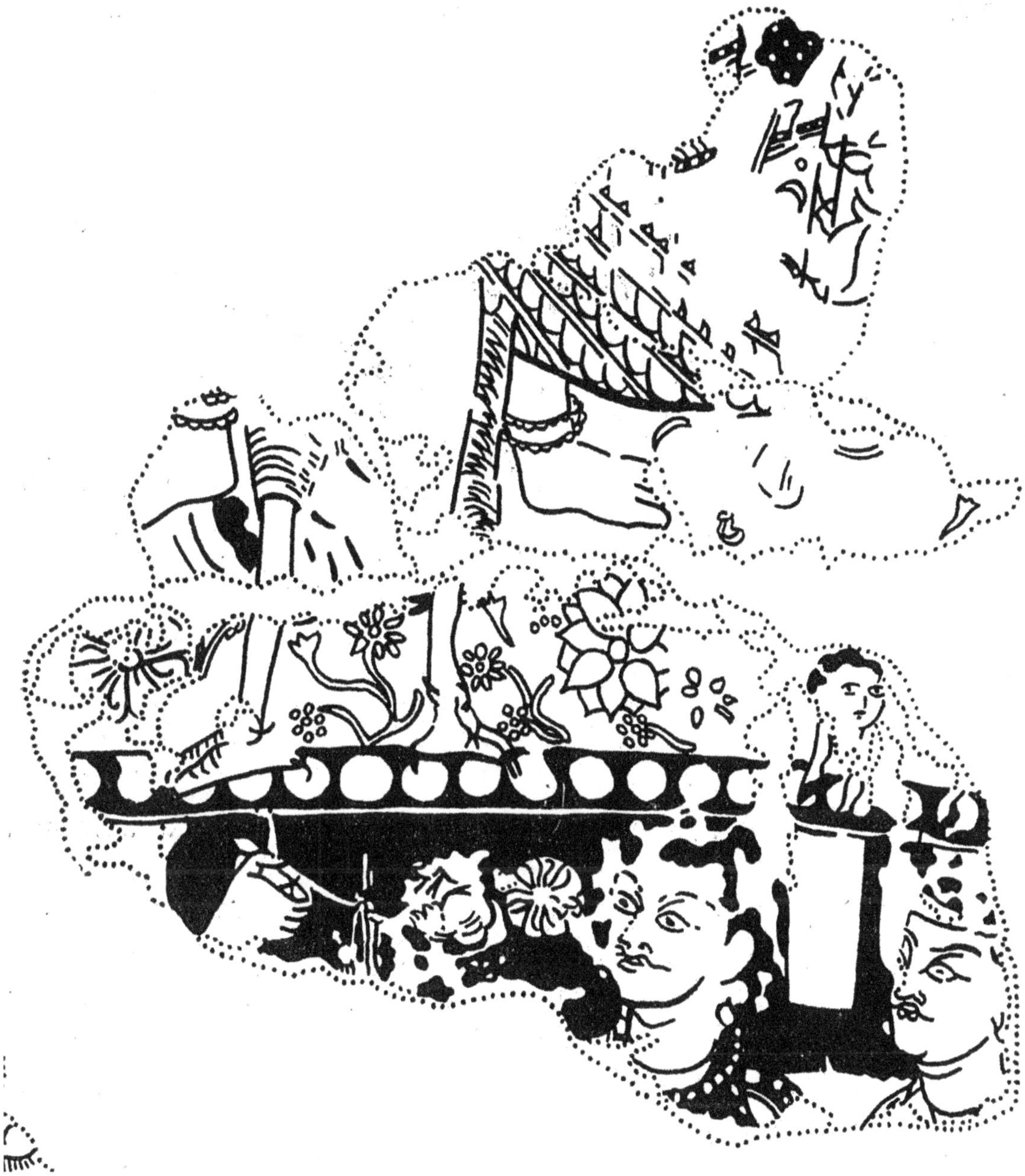

142. Skanda mounted on a peacock, room 16 of the northeastern complex, Dilberjin (Kruglikova 1979: fig. 24).

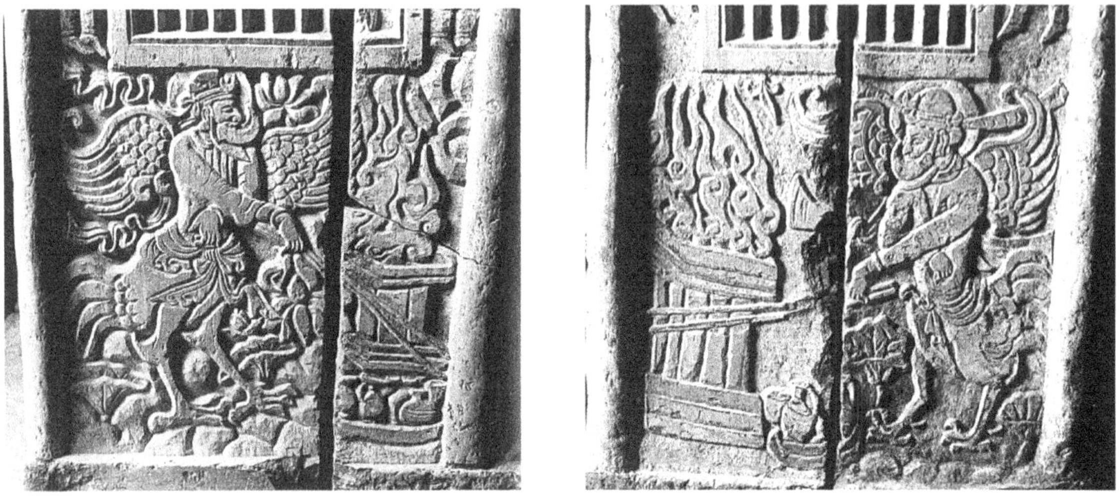

143. Bird-priests on "Lord Shi's sarcophagus" (Frantz Grenet).

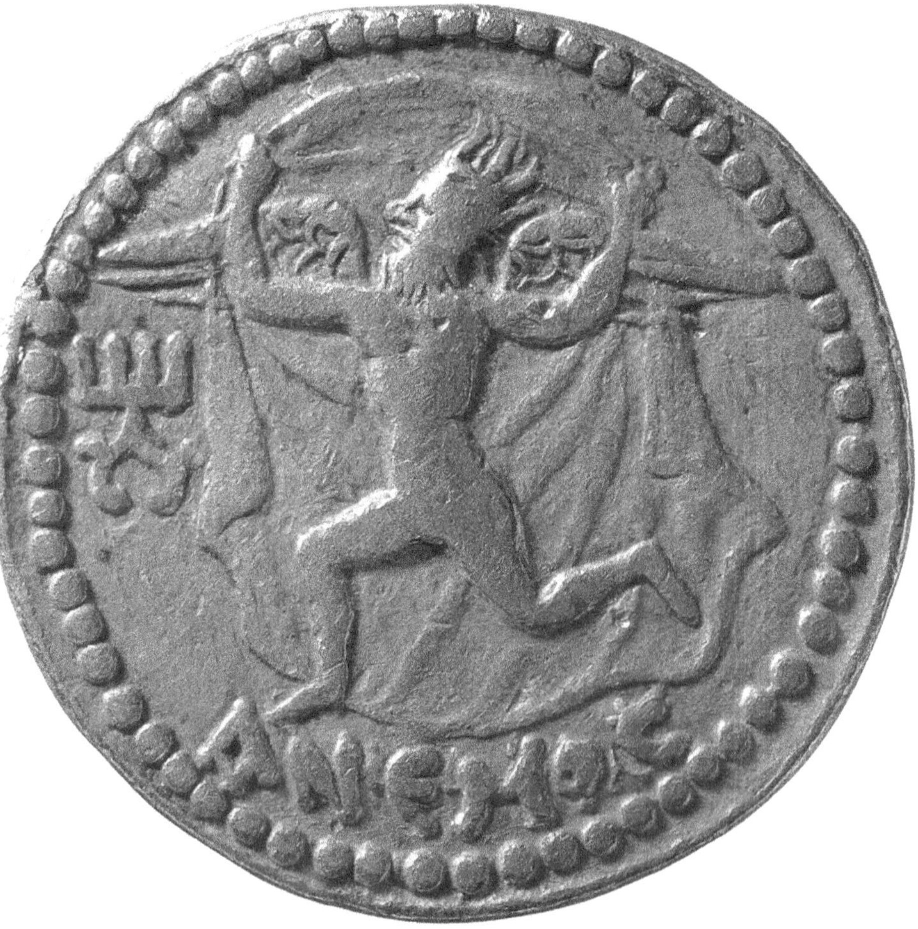

144. Anemos on a Kushan coin (Frantz Grenet).

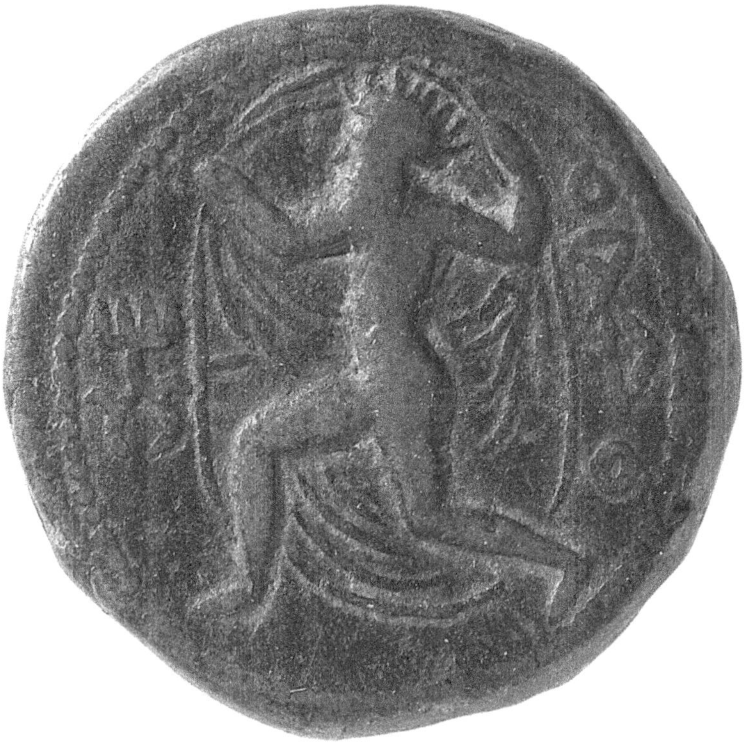

145. Oado on a Kushan coin (© Trustees of the British Museum).

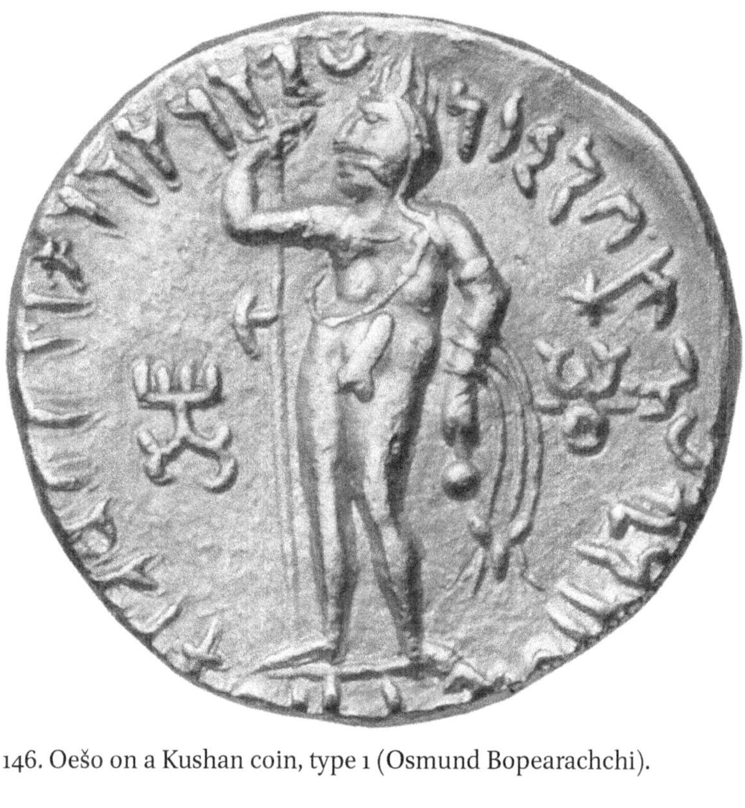

146. Oešo on a Kushan coin, type 1 (Osmund Bopearachchi).

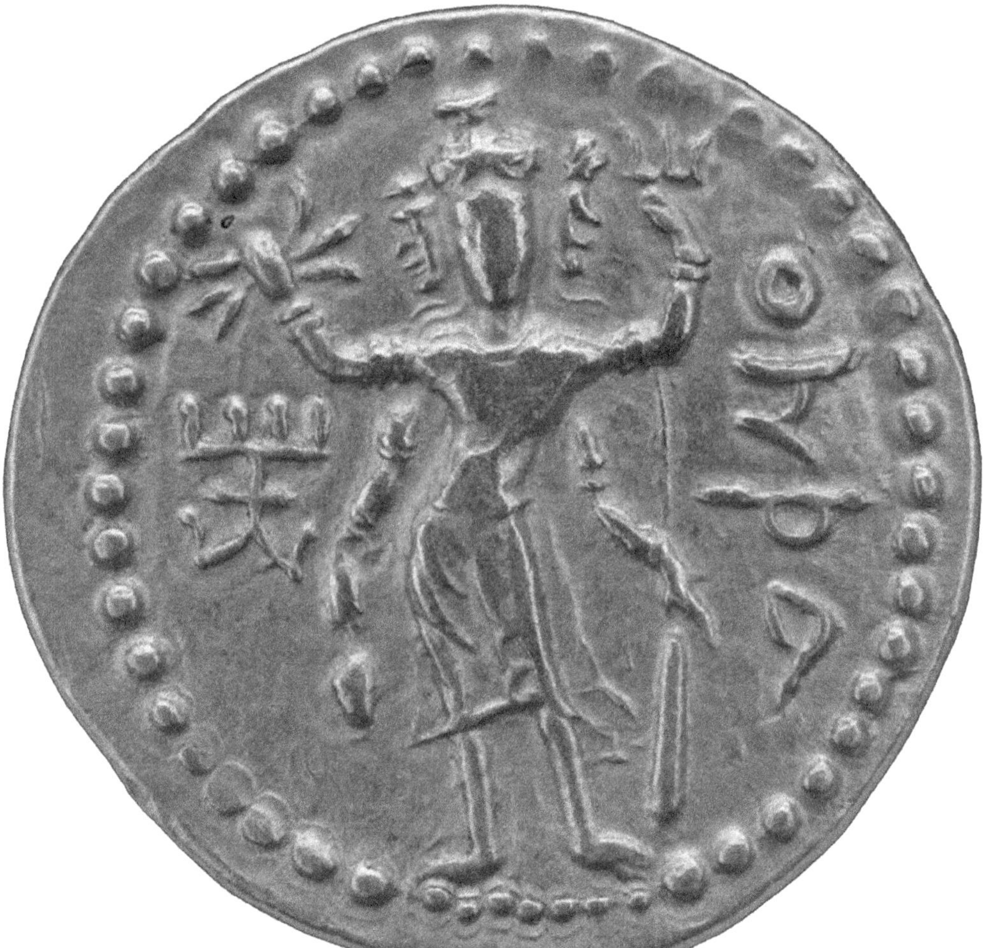

147. Oešo on a Kushan coin, type 6 (© Trustees of the British Museum).

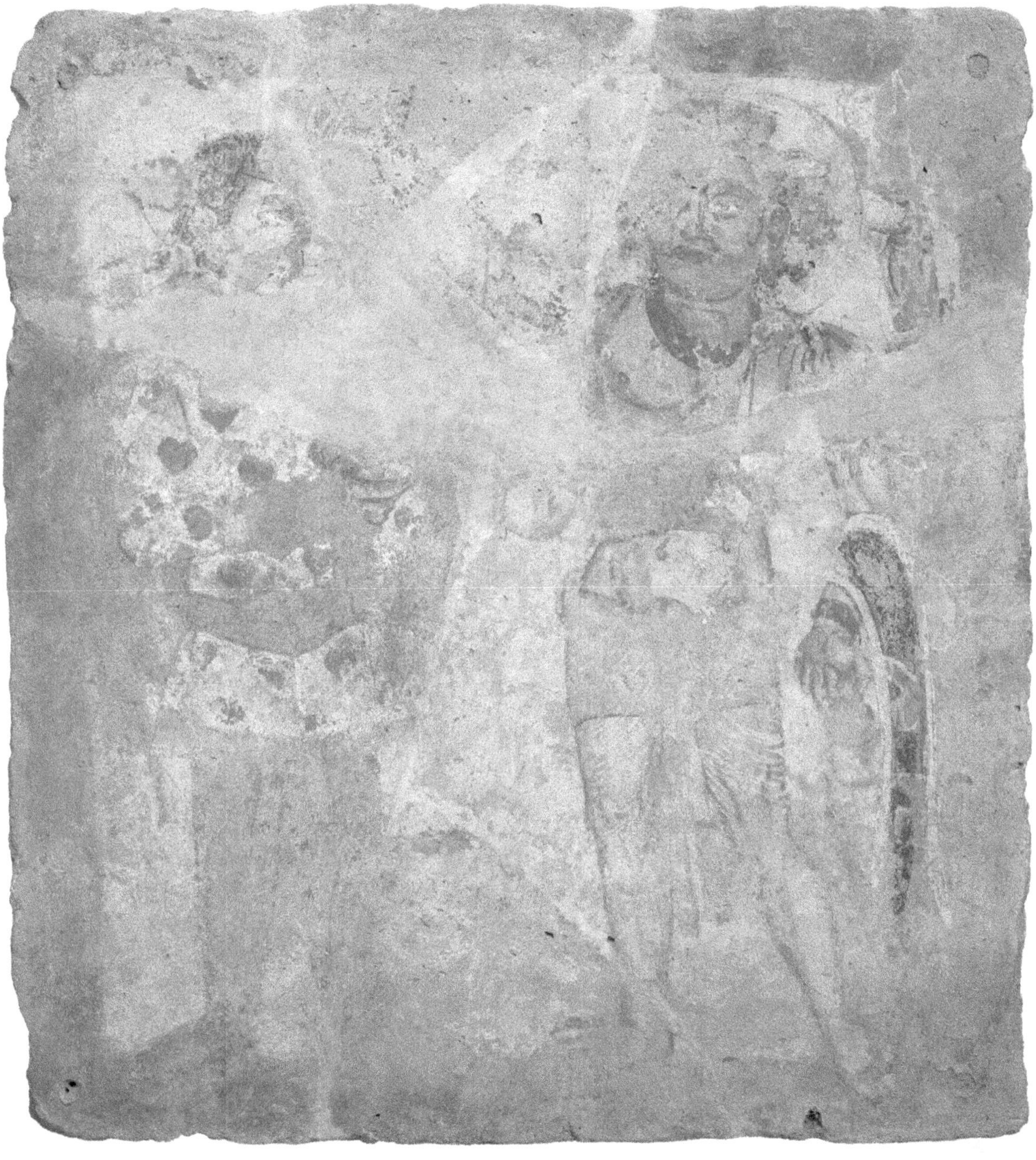

148. Oešo and a worshipper on a terracotta panel (© The Metropolitan Museum of Art).

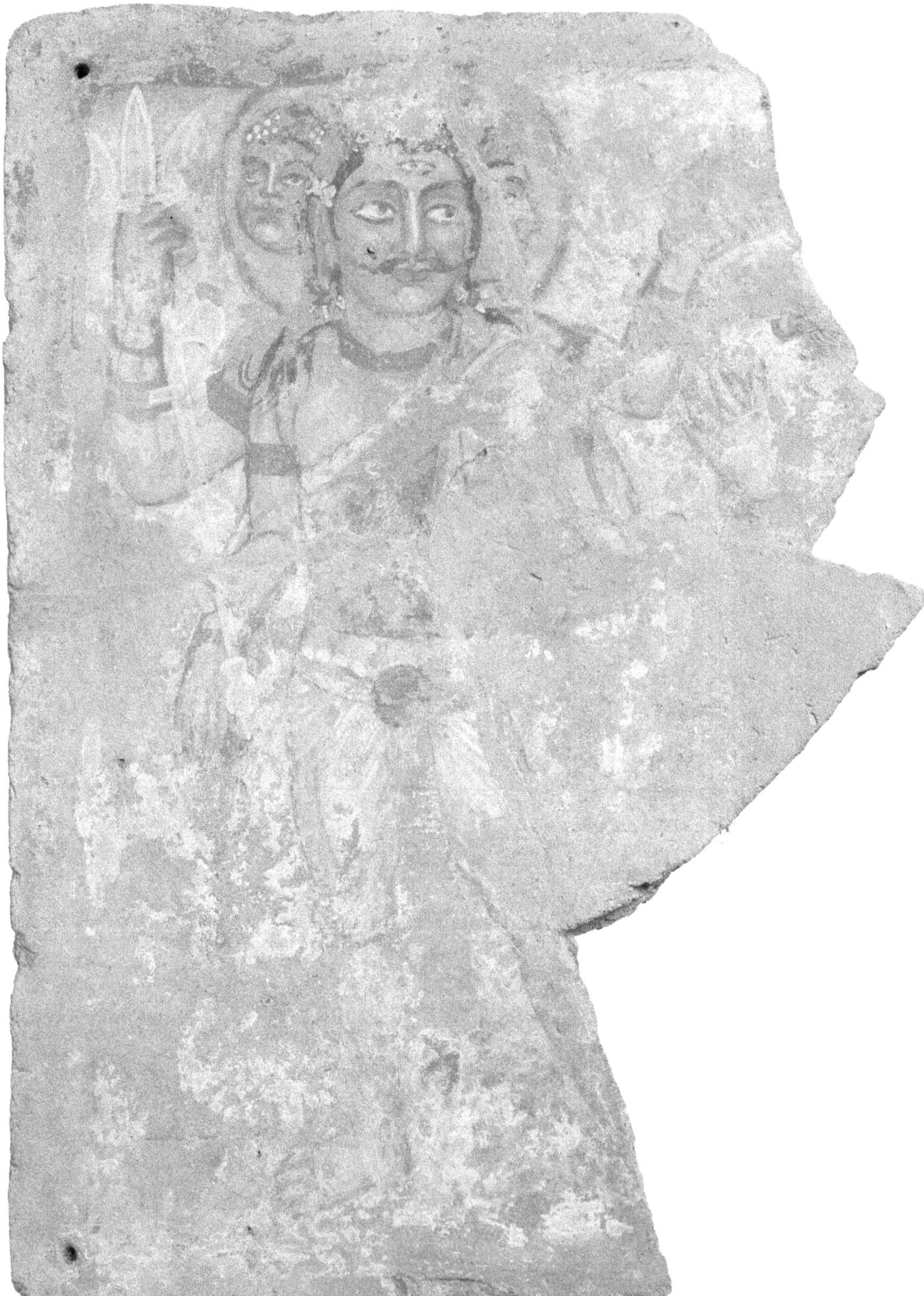

149. Oešo and a worshipper on a second terracotta panel (© The Metropolitan Museum of Art).

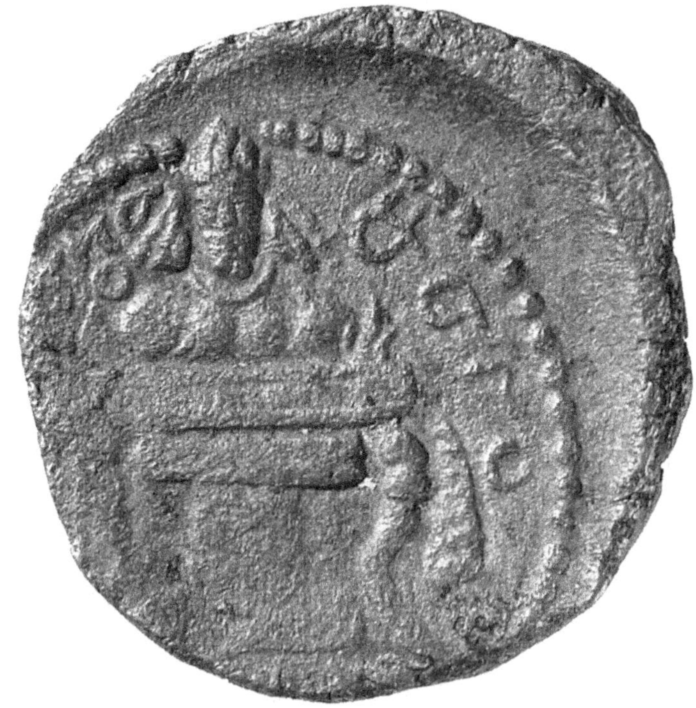

150. Bust of *Bago borzando* on a coin of the Kushano-Sasanian king Pērōz I (Joe Cribb).

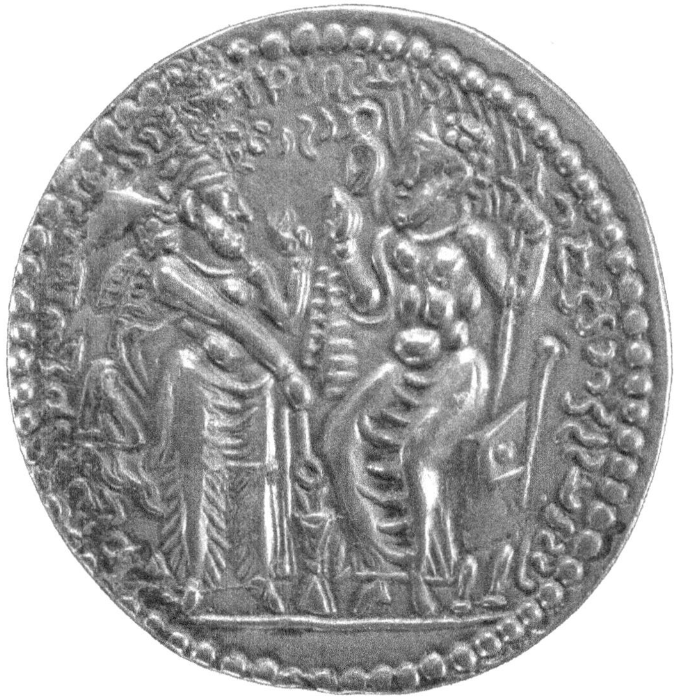

151. *Burzāwand yazad* on a coin of the Kushano-Sasanian king Ōhrmazd I (© Trustees of the British Museum).

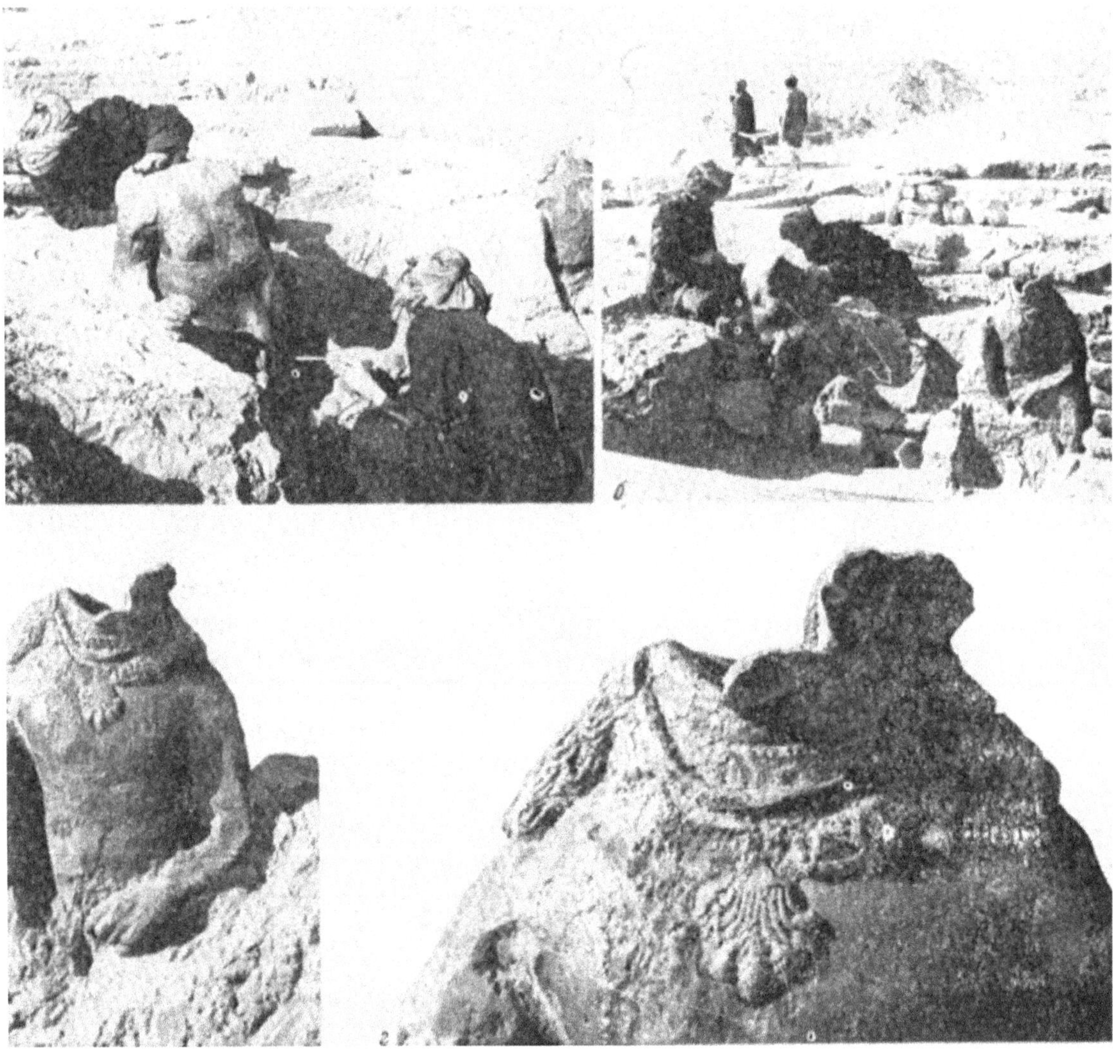

152. Statues found in sanctuary X, Dilberjin (Kruglikova 1982: fig. 7).

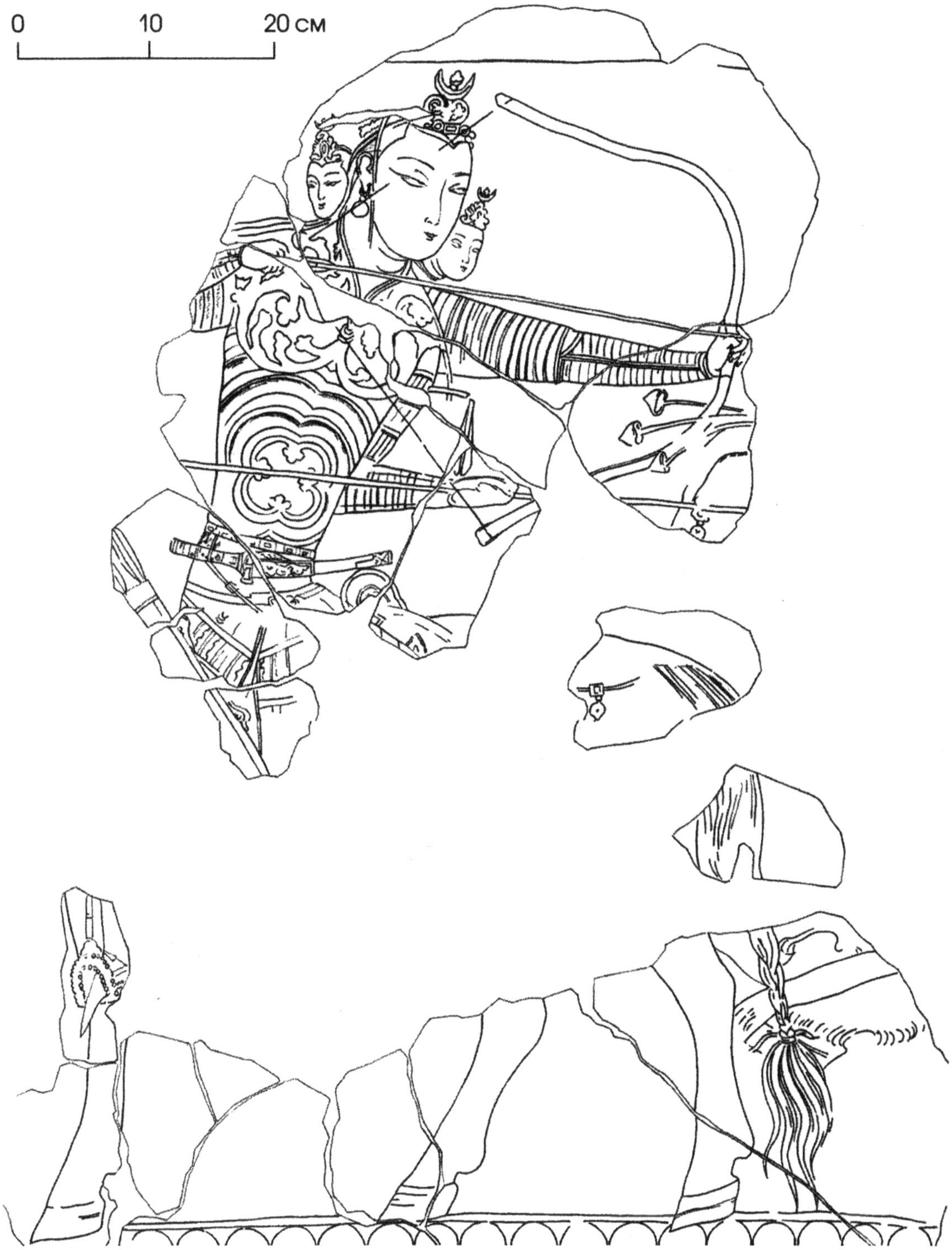

153. Wēšparkar fighting the demons, eastern wall of the "Small hall", Bunjikat (Sokolovskiy 2009: fig. 83).

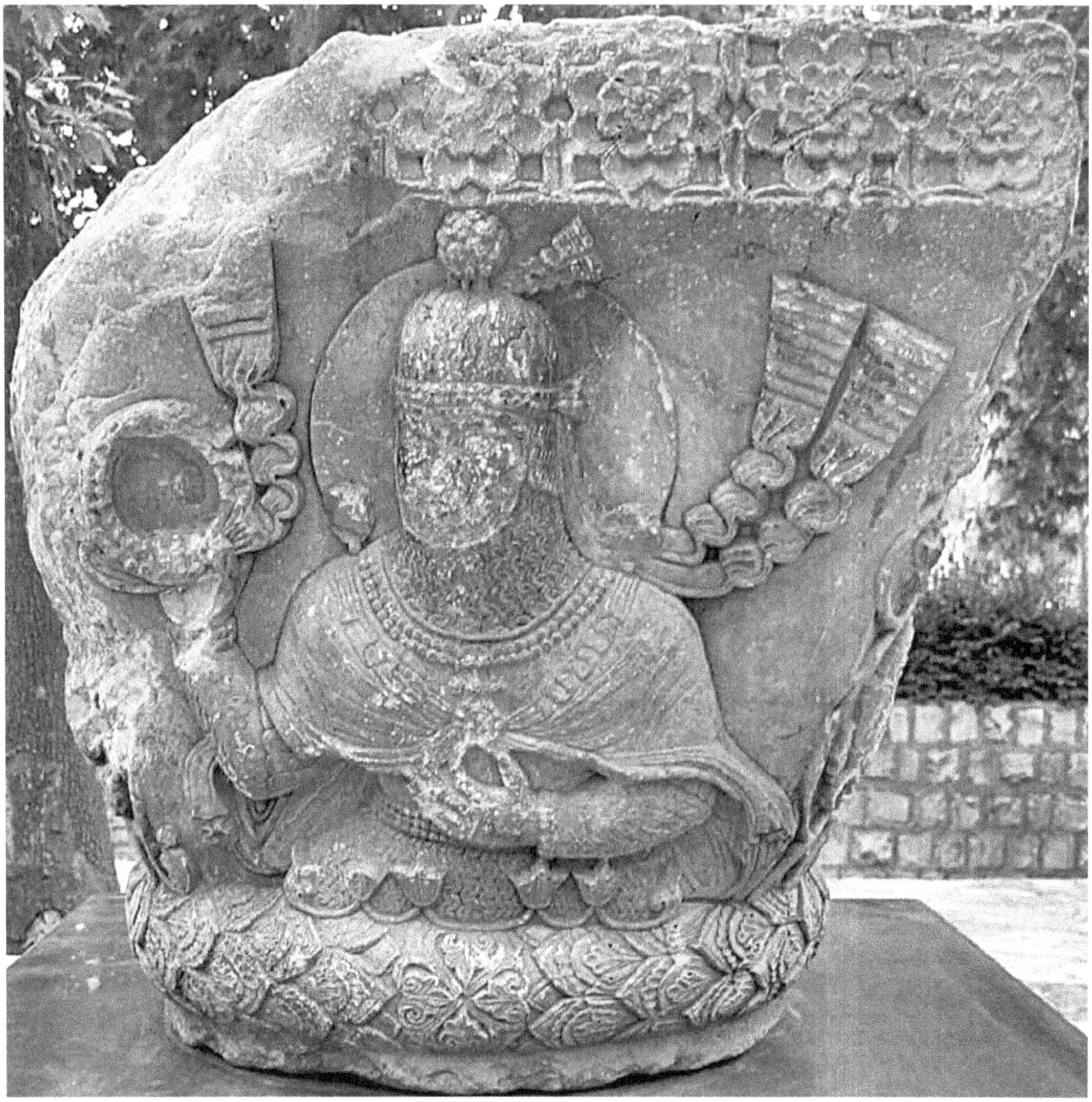

154. A Sasanian capital with figural decorations no. 1 (Matteo Compareti).

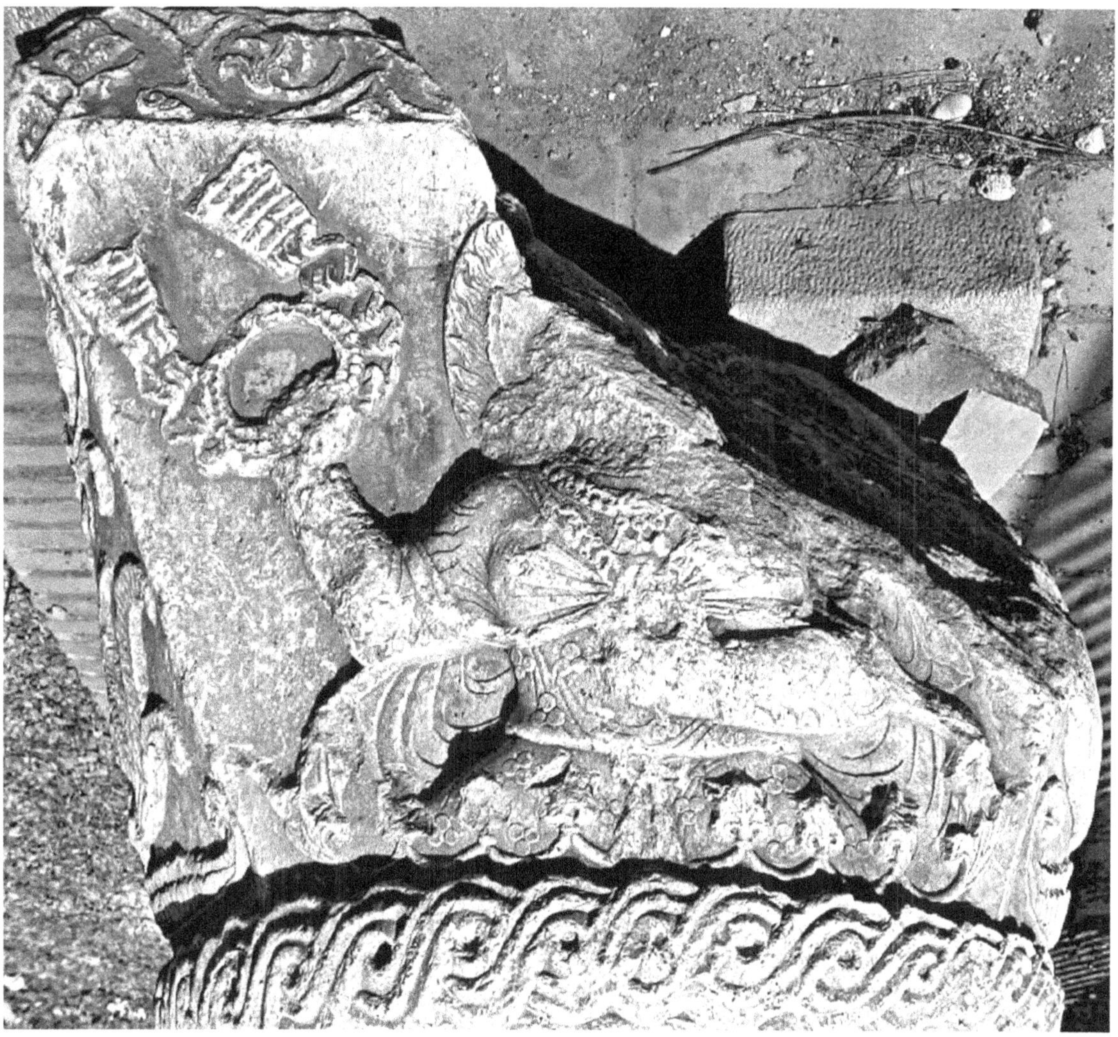

155. A Sasanian capital with figural decorations no. 2 (Matteo Compareti).

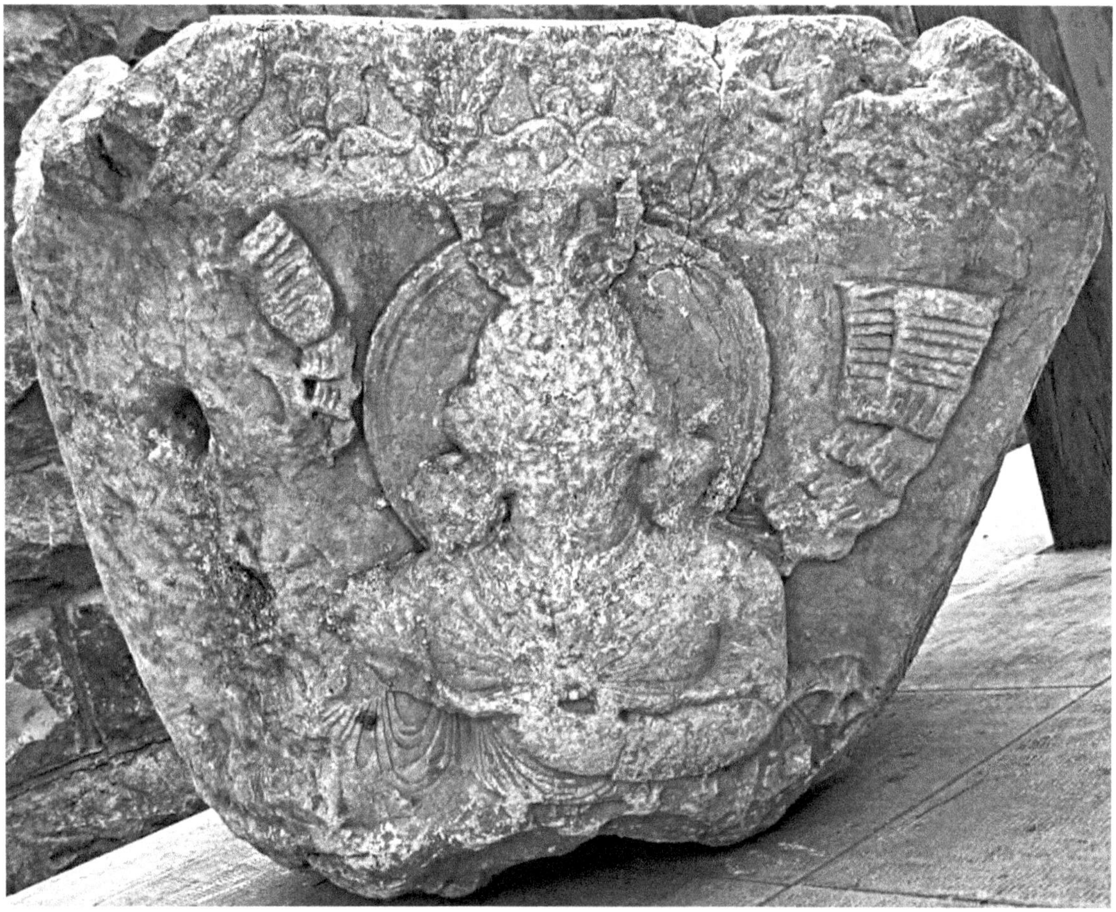

156. A Sasanian capital with figural decorations no. 3 (Matteo Compareti).

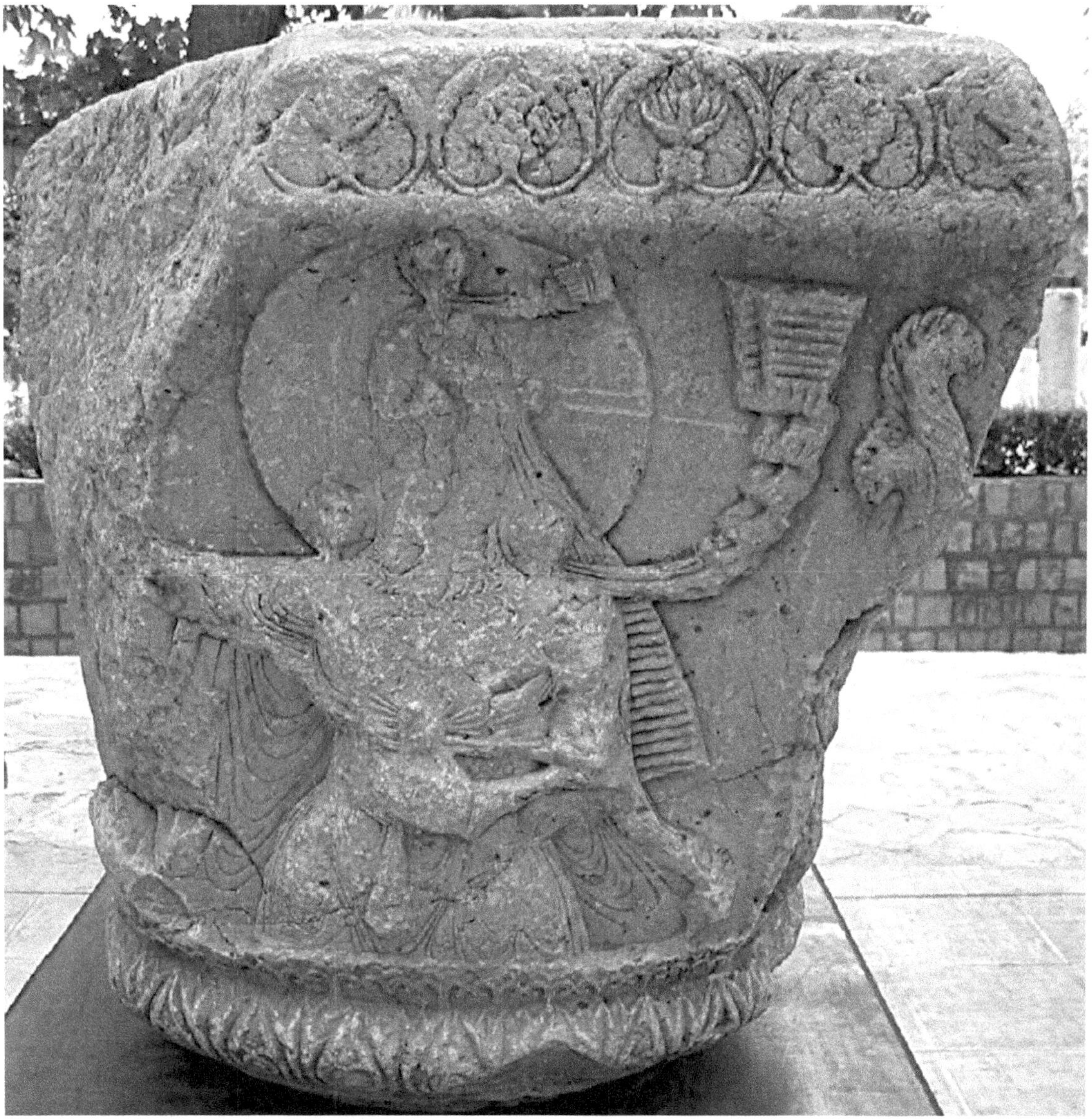

157. A Sasanian capital with figural decorations no. 4 (Matteo Compareti).

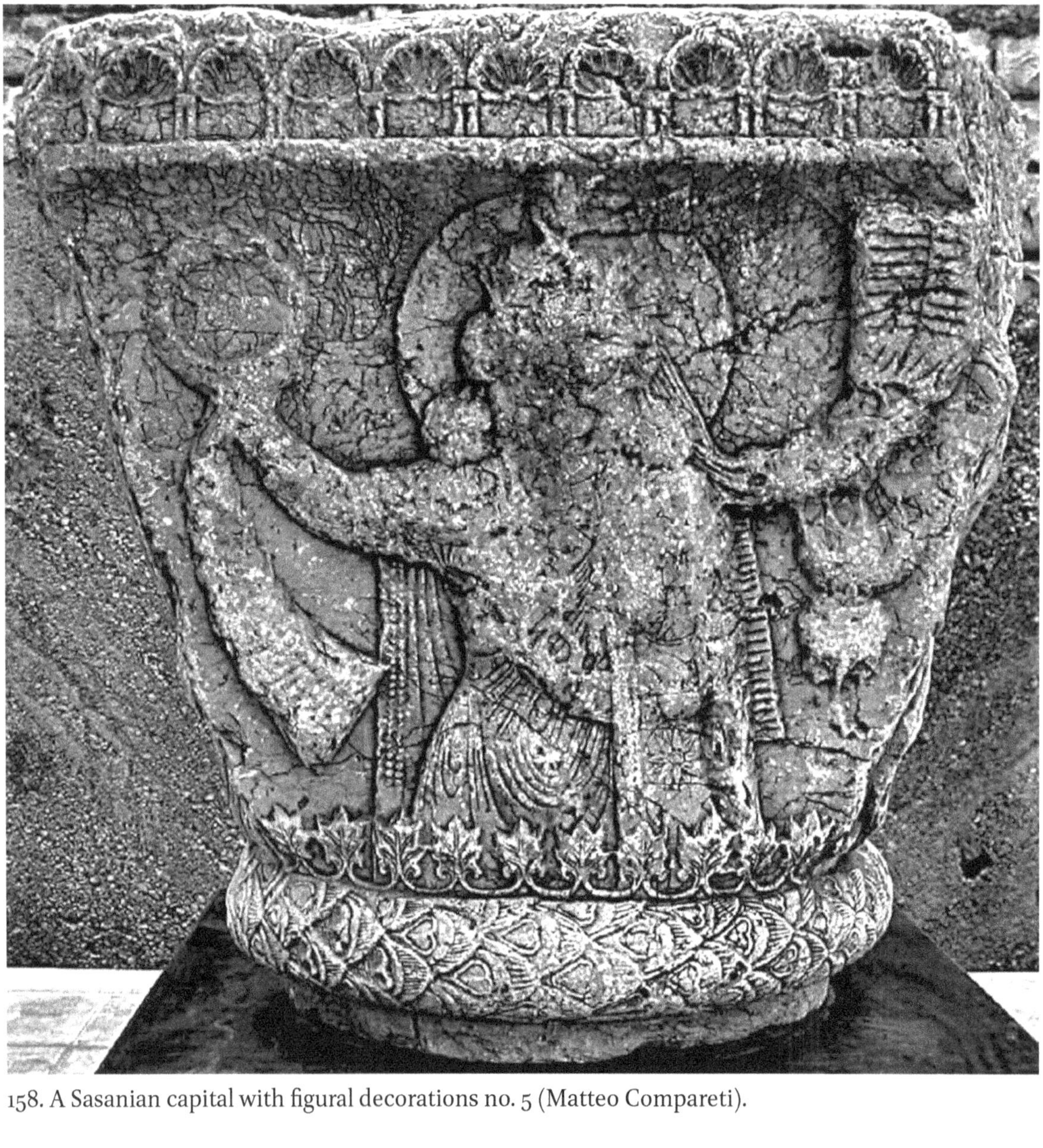

158. A Sasanian capital with figural decorations no. 5 (Matteo Compareti).

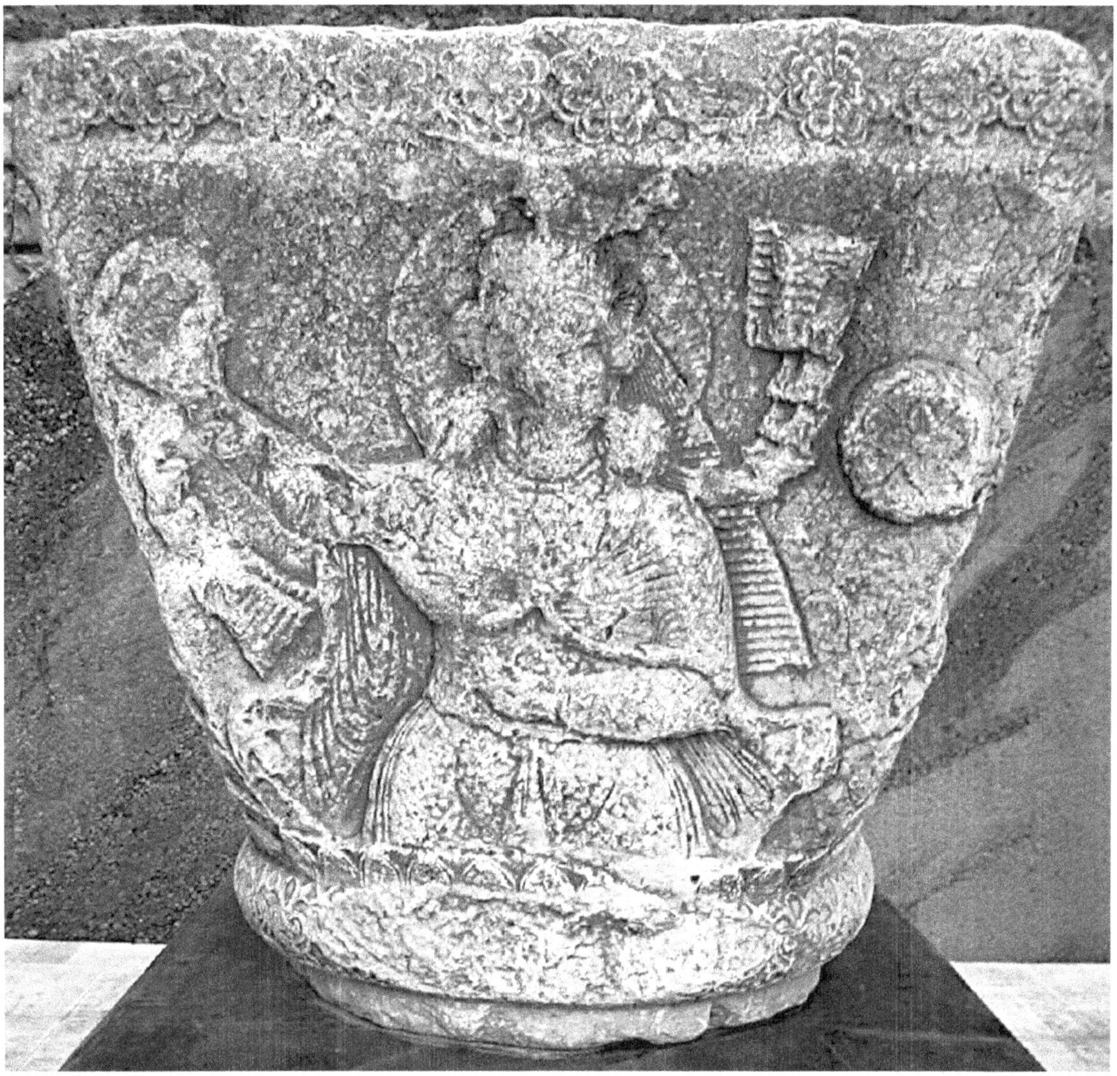

159. A Sasanian capital with figural decorations no. 6 (Matteo Compareti).

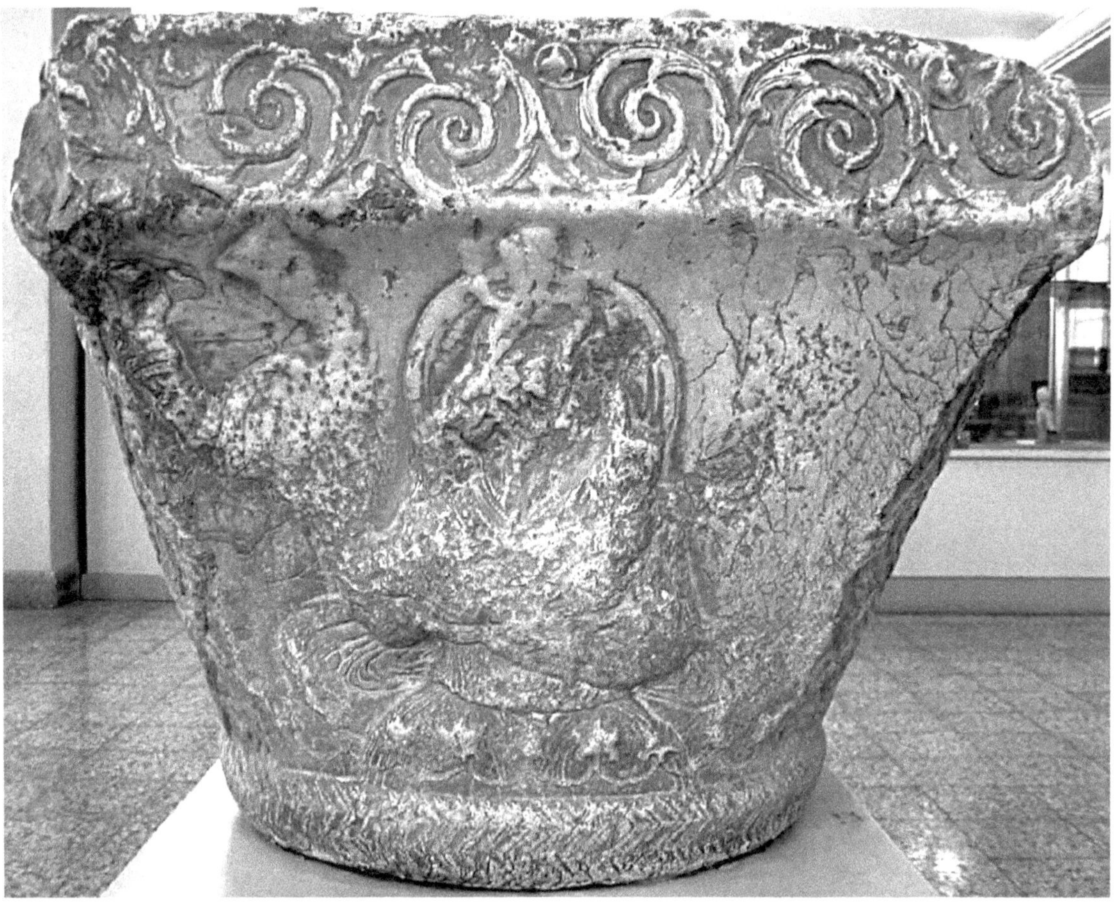

160. A Sasanian capital with figural decorations no. 7 (Matteo Compareti).

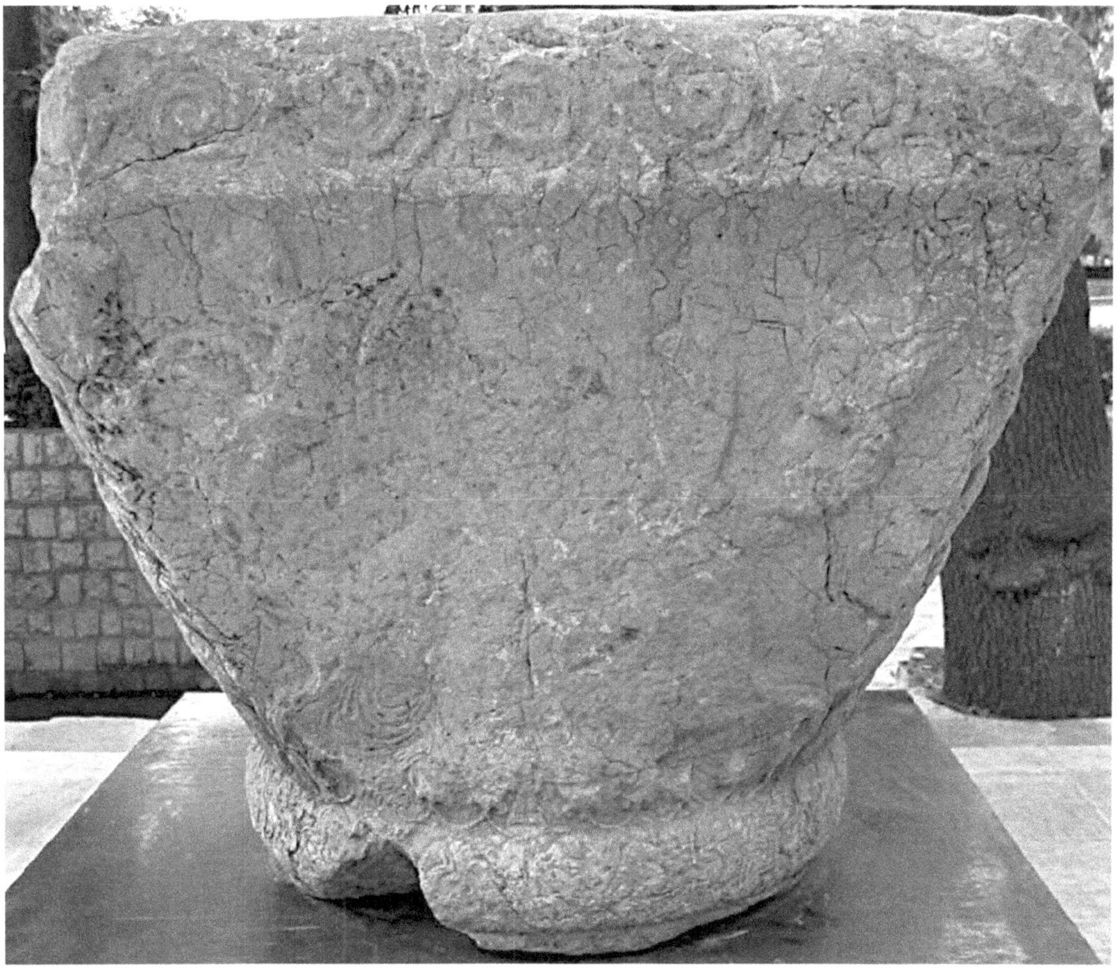

161. A Sasanian capital with figural decorations no. 8 (Matteo Compareti).

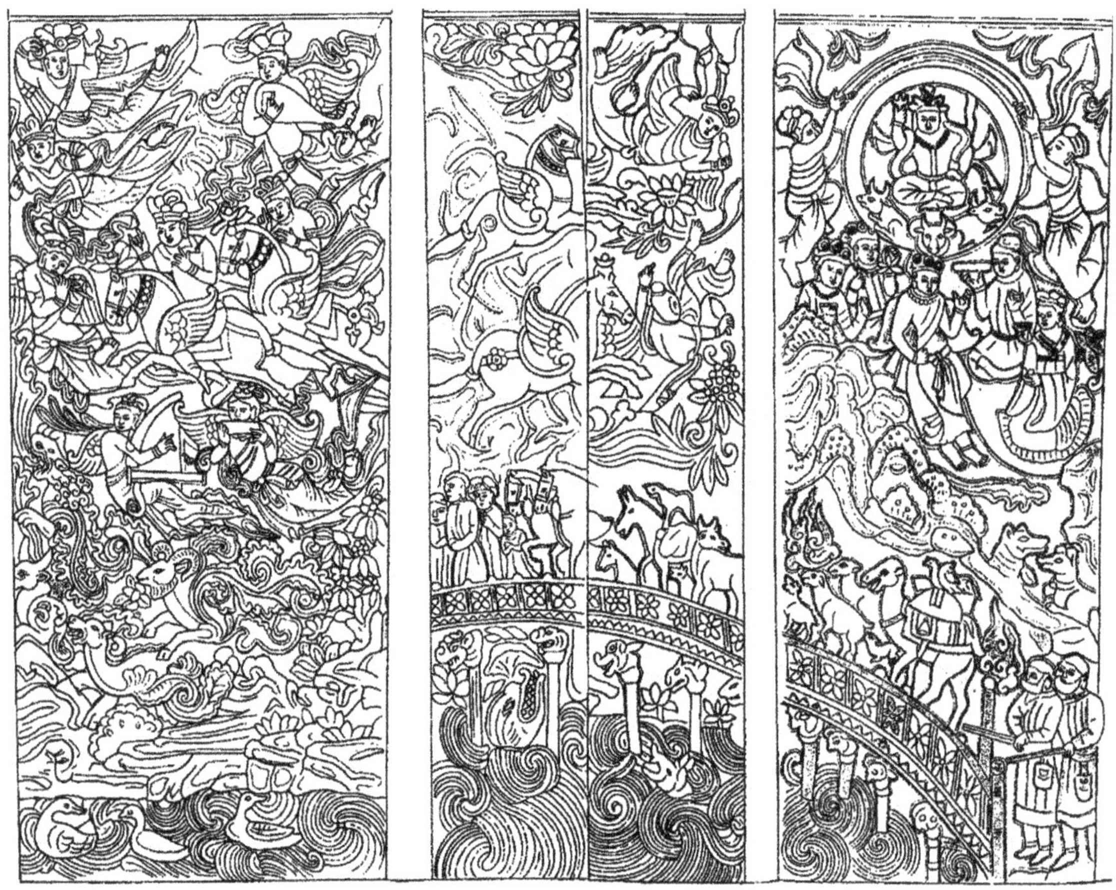

162. The sarcophagus of Wirkak, eastern side (Frantz Grenet).

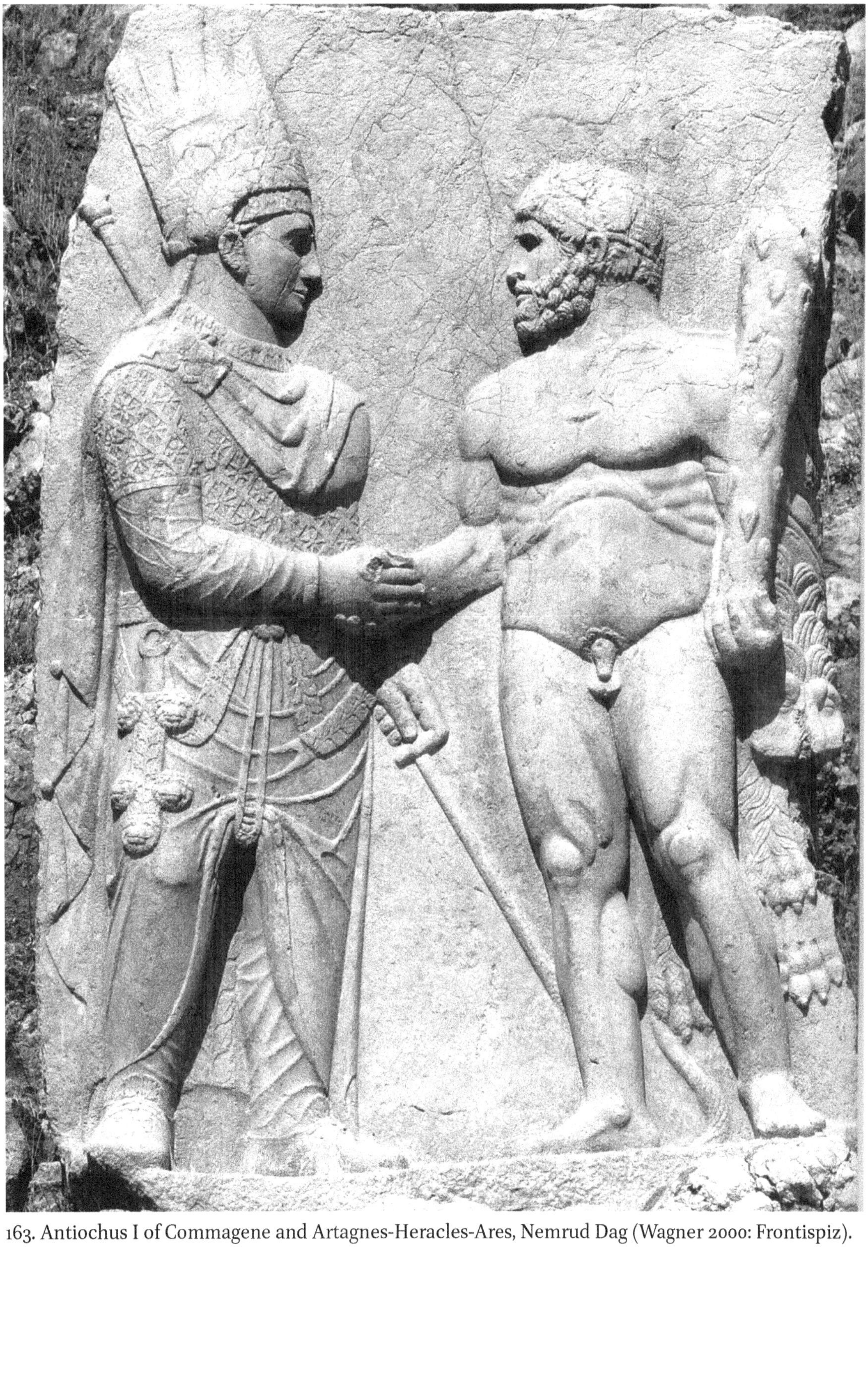

163. Antiochus I of Commagene and Artagnes-Heracles-Ares, Nemrud Dag (Wagner 2000: Frontispiz).

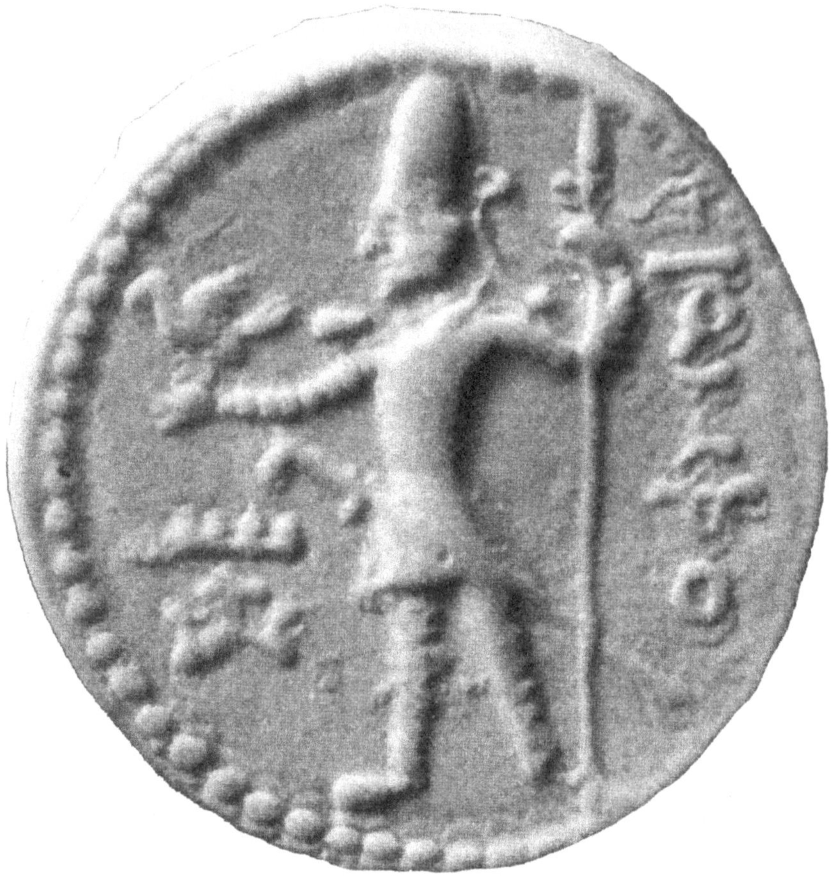

164. Iamšo on the Kushan coin (Frantz Grenet).

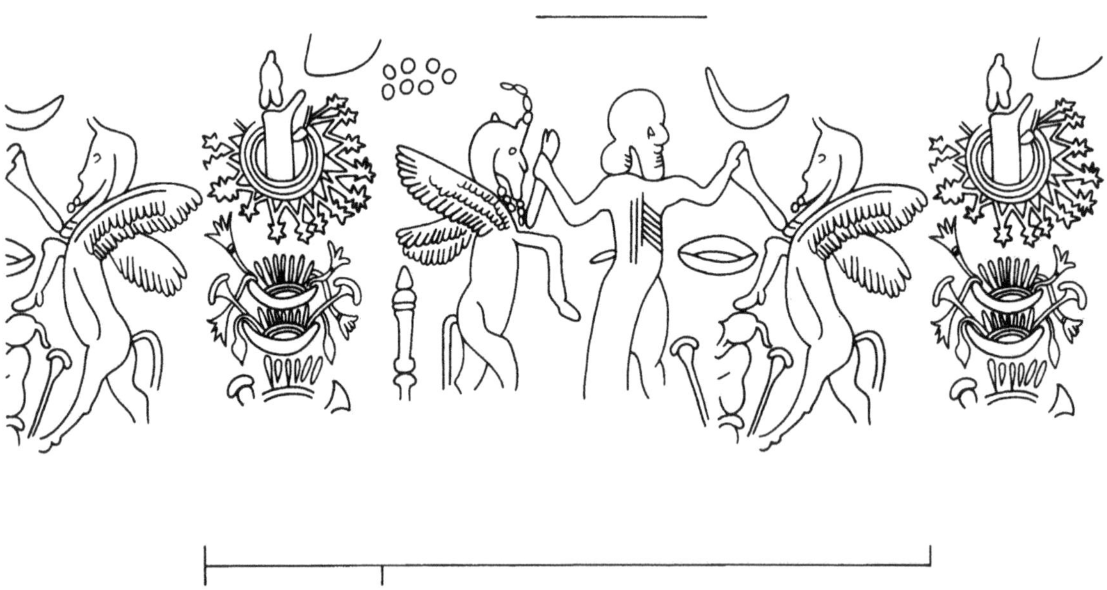

165. Composite line drawing of PFS 38 (by permission of M.B. Garrison and M.C. Root and the Persepolis Seal Project).

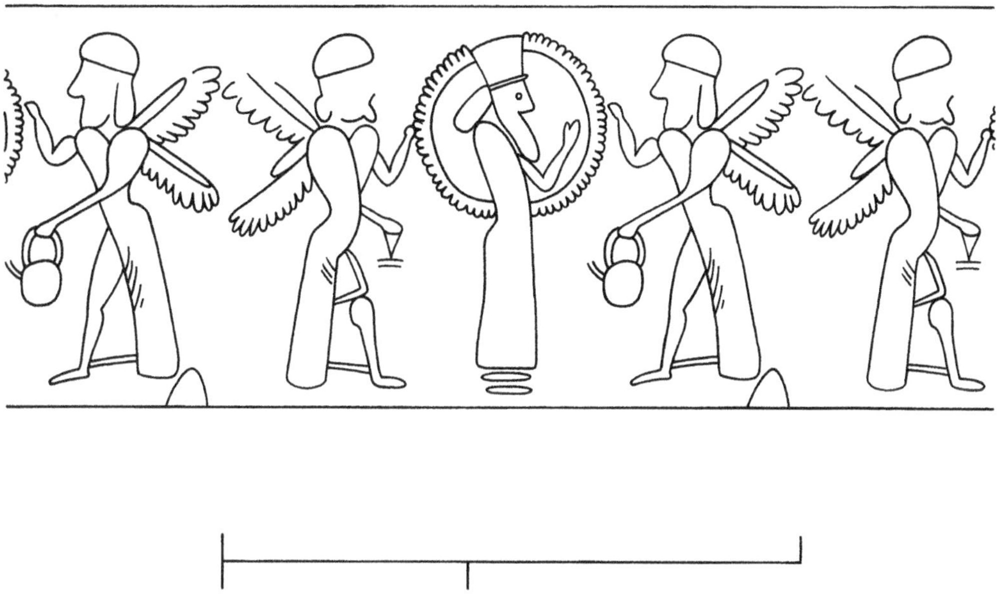

166. Composite line drawing of PFS 68 (by permission of M.B. Garrison and M.C. Root and the Persepolis Seal Project).

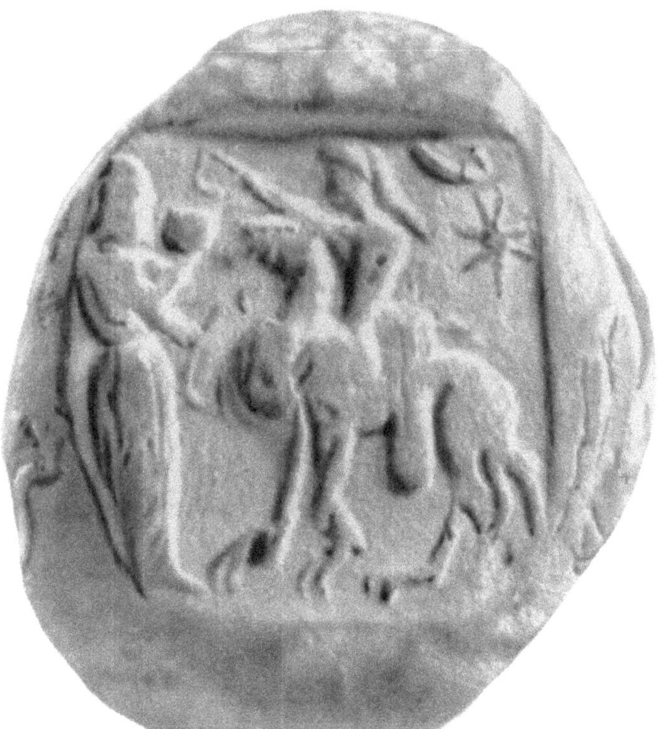

167. A god mounted on a dragon, seal impression from Erkurgan (Abdullaev, Rtveladze and Shishkina 1991: no. 289).

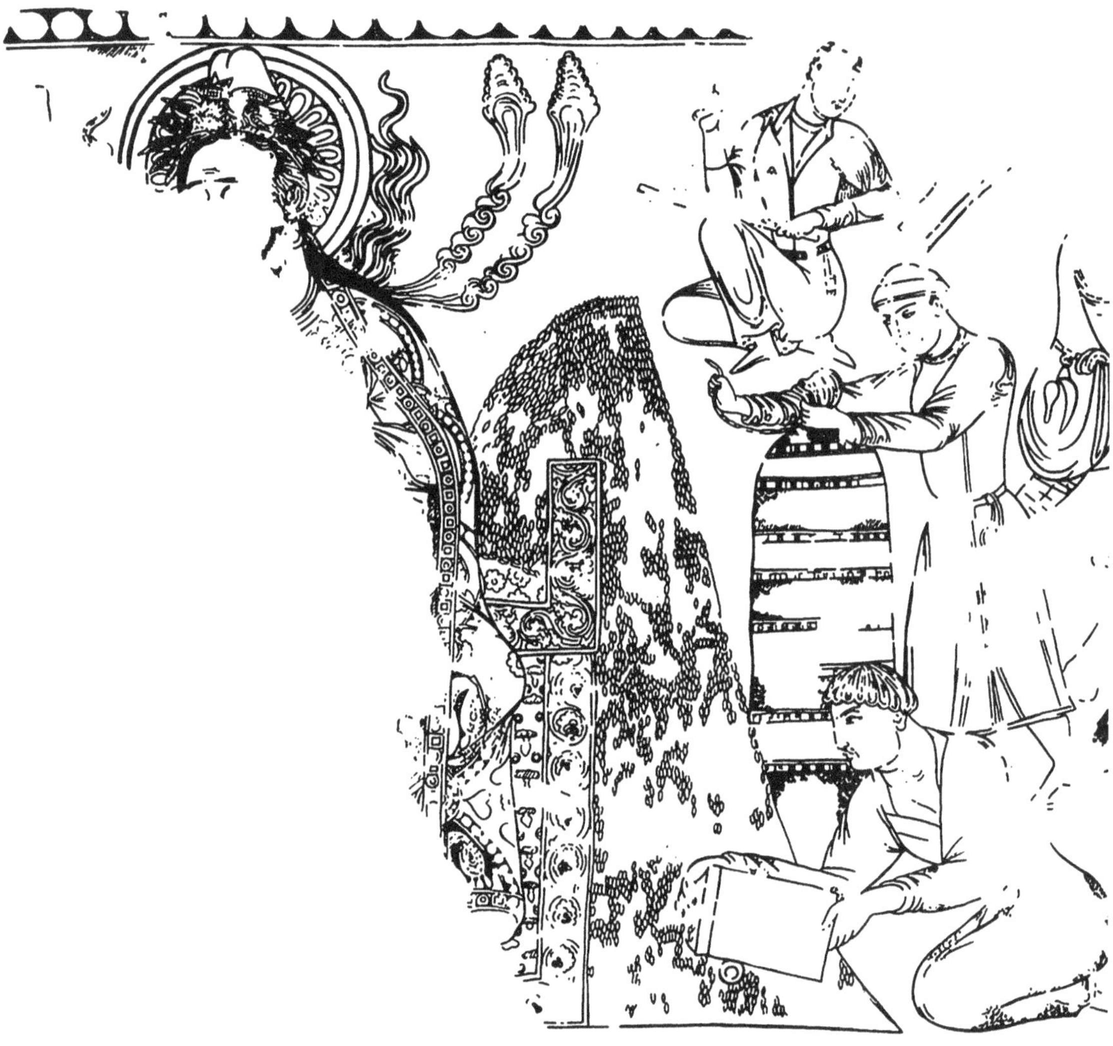

168. The “Grain God”, Panjikent XXV/28, northern wall (Frantz Grenet).

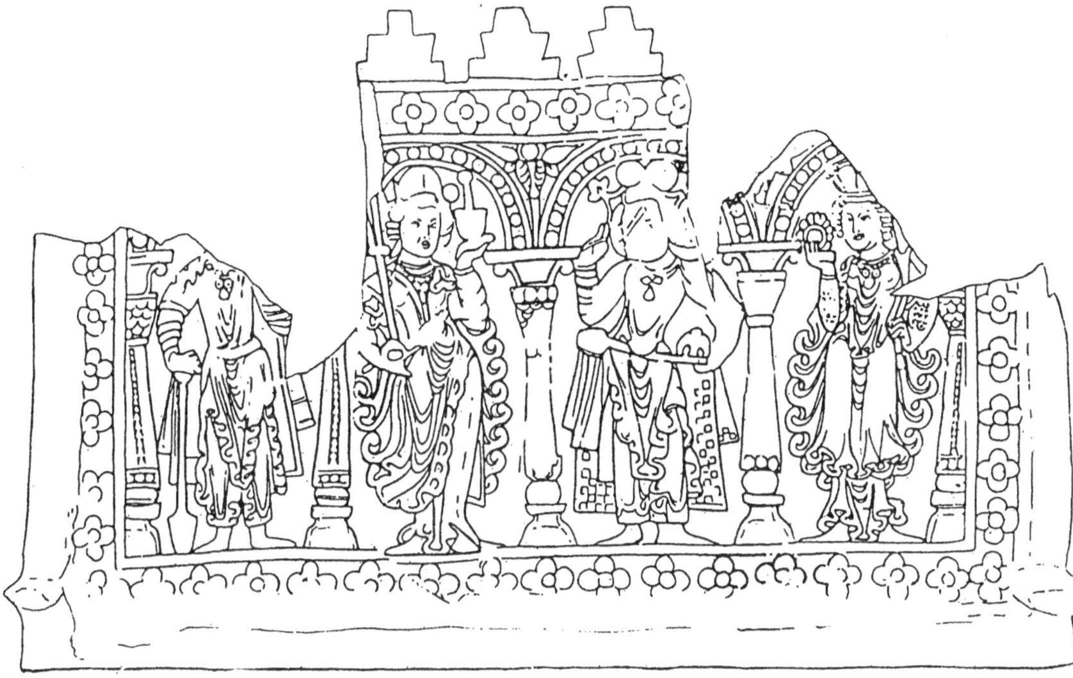

169. The ossuaries from Biyanajman and Miankal, Iš-1 (long side) (Frantz Grenet).

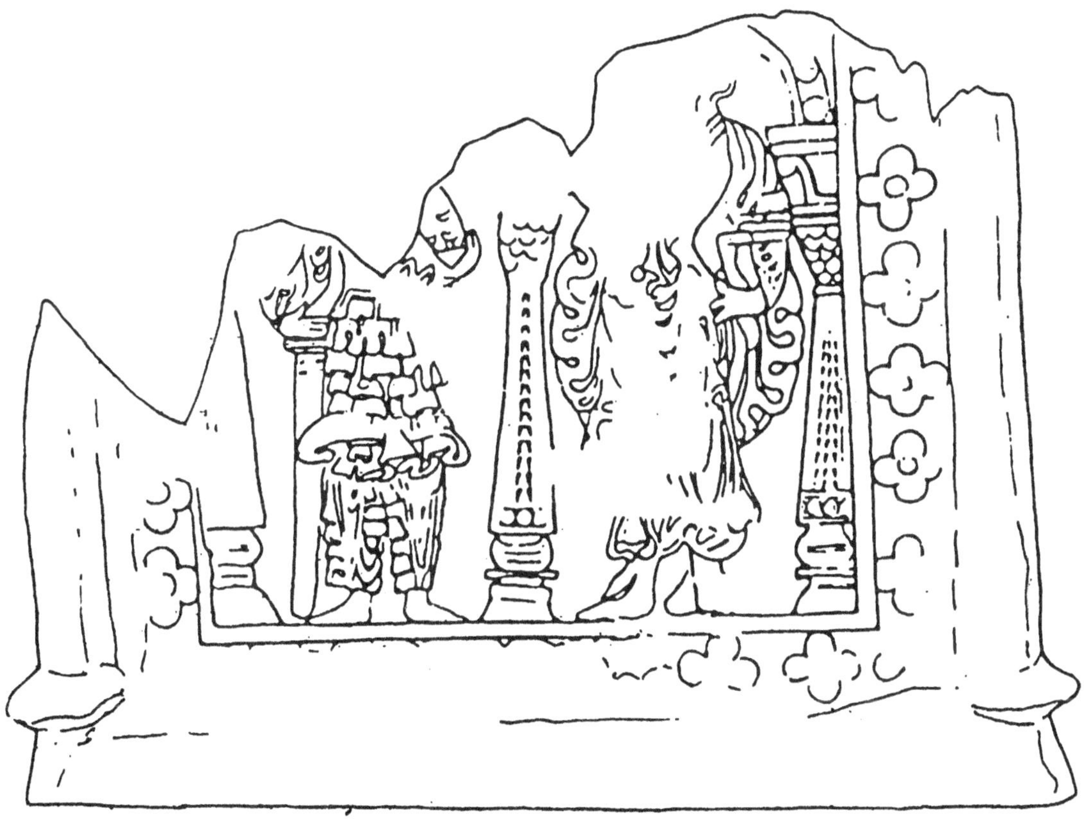

170. The ossuaries from Biyanajman and Miankal, Iš-1 (short side) (Frantz Grenet).

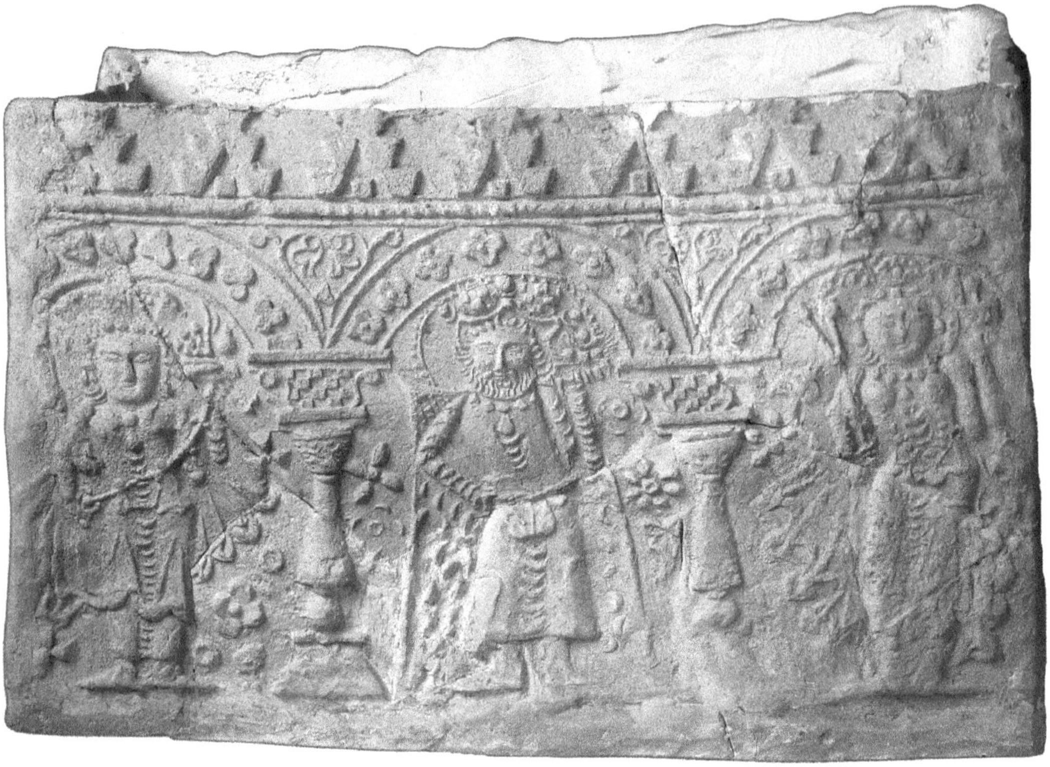

171. The ossuaries from Biyanajman and Miankal, Iš-2 (Frantz Grenet).

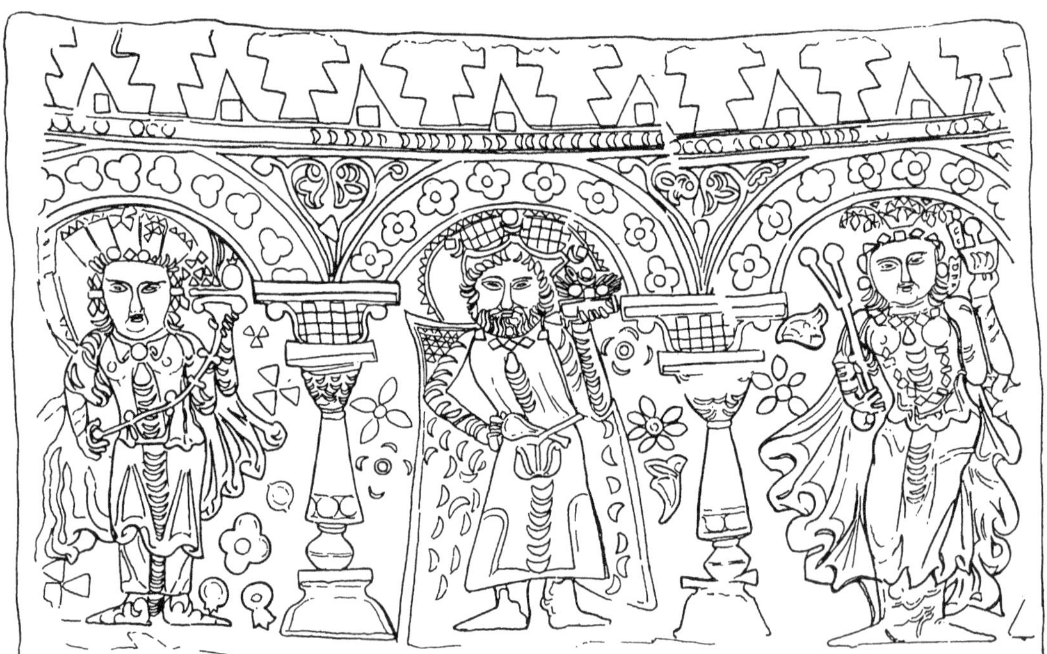

172. The ossuaries from Biyanajman and Miankal, Iš-2, drawing (Frantz Grenet).

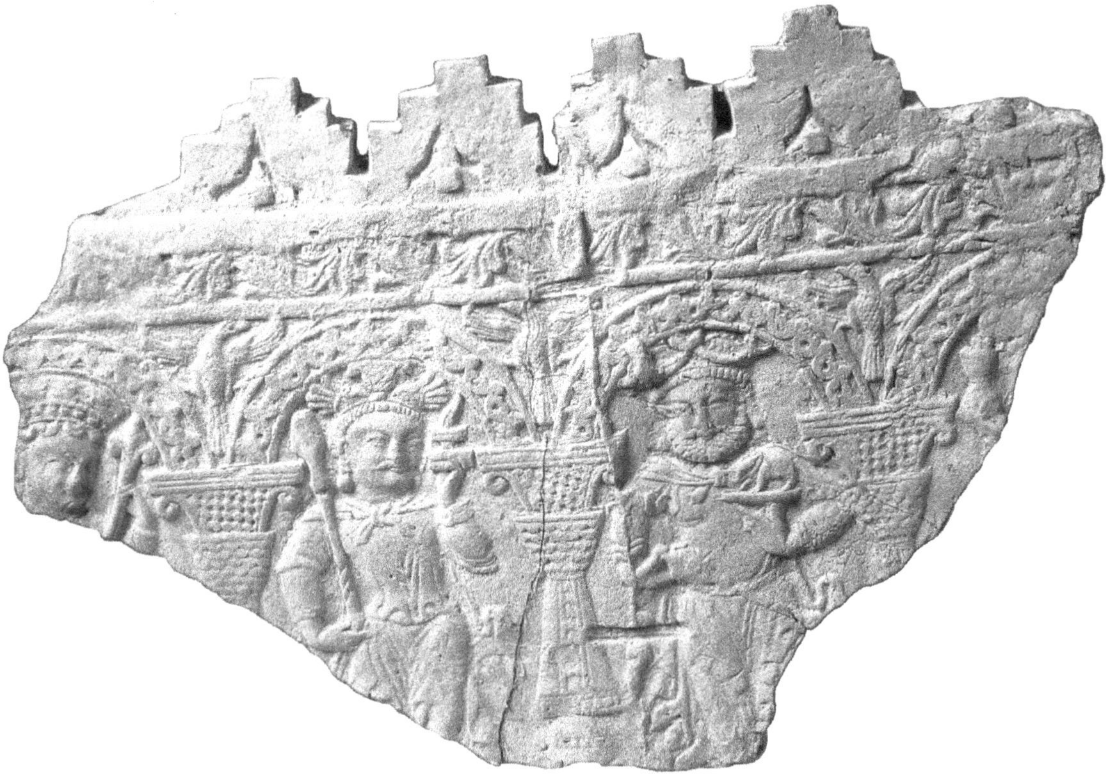

173. The ossuaries from Biyanajman and Miankal, Dt (Frantz Grenet).

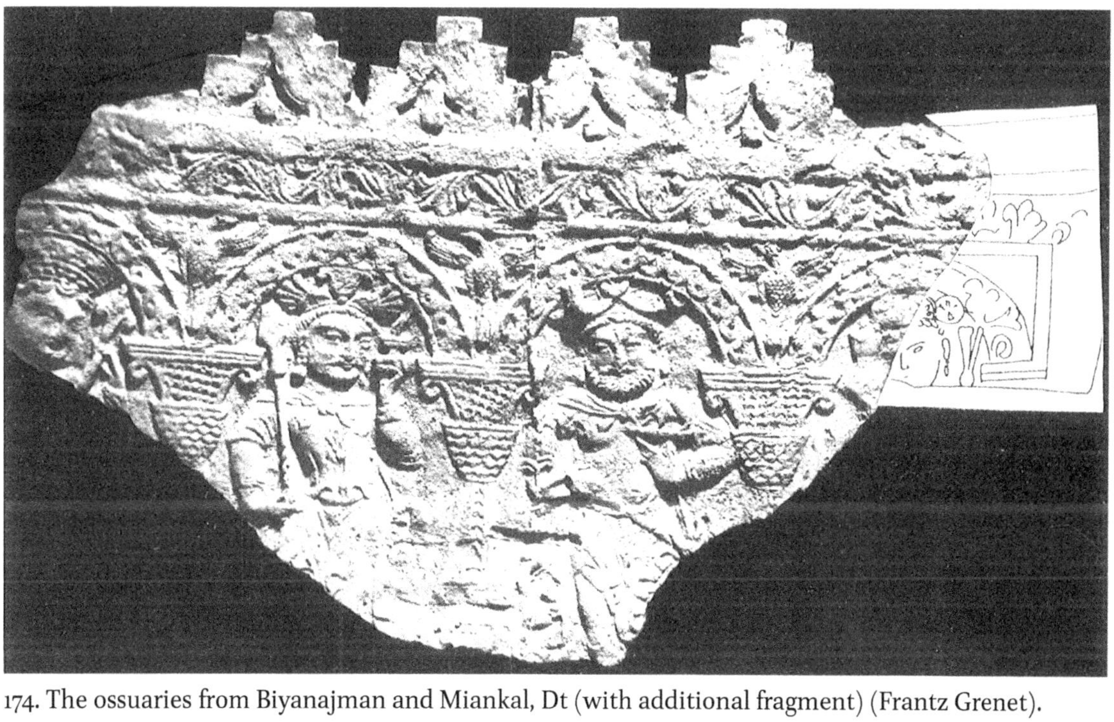

174. The ossuaries from Biyanajman and Miankal, Dt (with additional fragment) (Frantz Grenet).

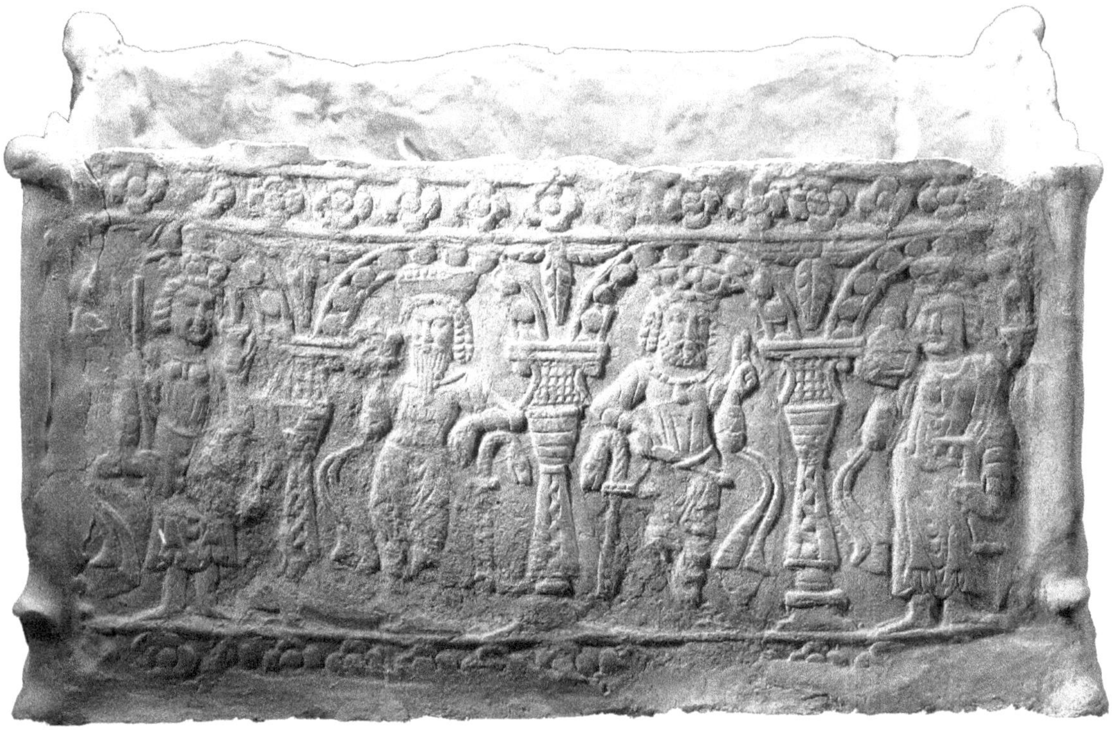

175. The ossuaries from Biyanajman and Miankal, Bn-1 (Frantz Grenet).

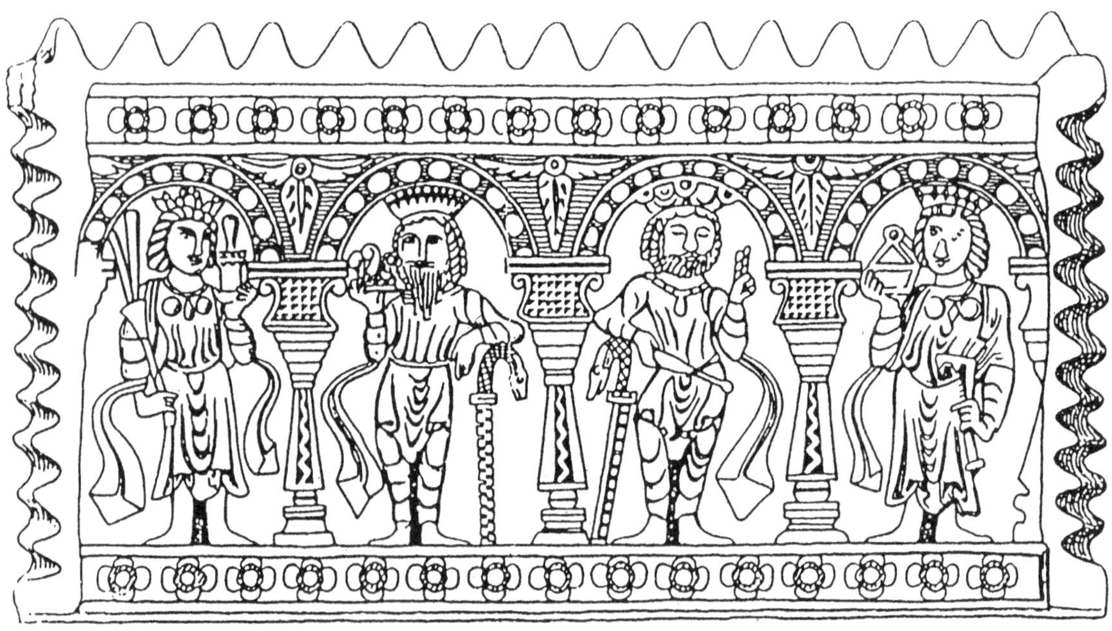

176. The ossuaries from Biyanajman and Miankal, Bn-1, drawing (Frantz Grenet).

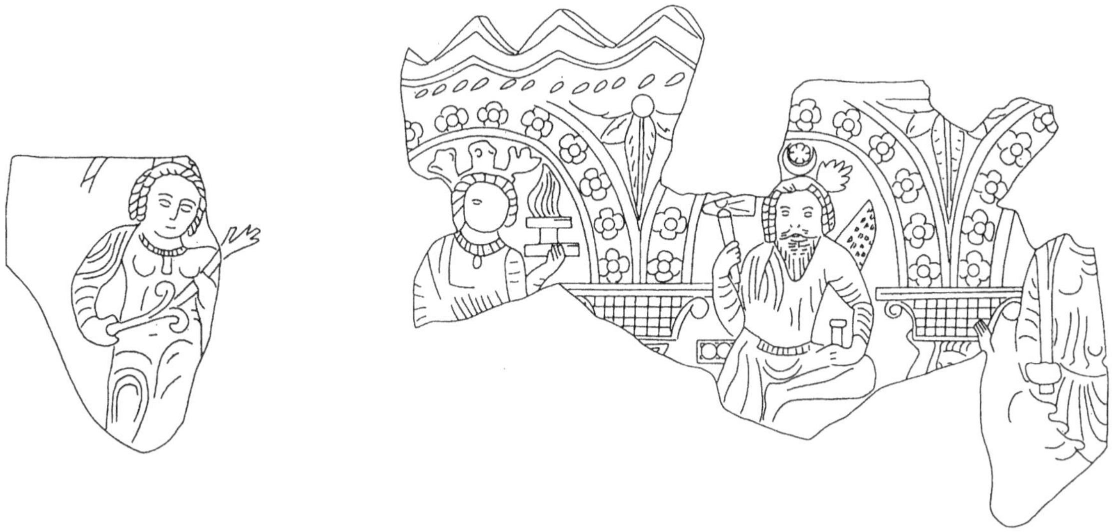

177. The ossuaries from Biyanajman and Miankal, Bn-2 (Frantz Grenet).

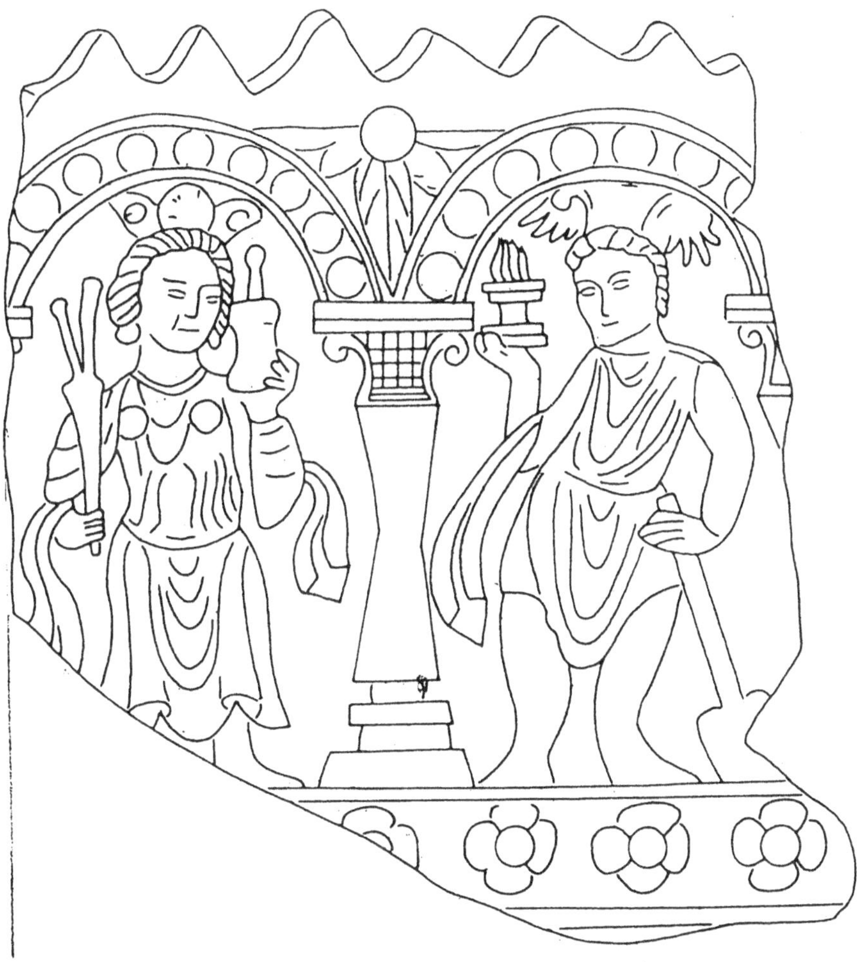

178. The ossuaries from Biyanajman and Miankal, Bn-4 (Frantz Grenet).

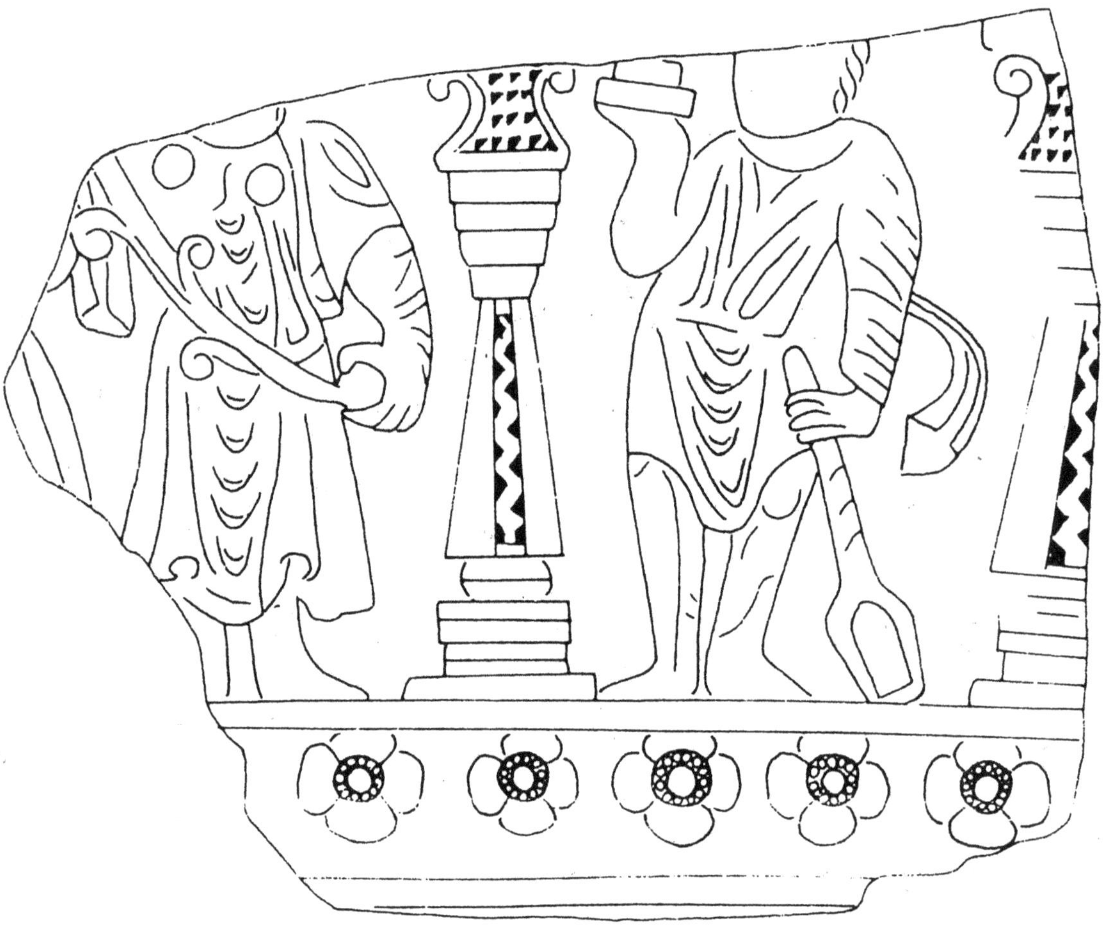

179. The ossuaries from Biyanajman and Miankal, Bn-5 (Frantz Grenet).

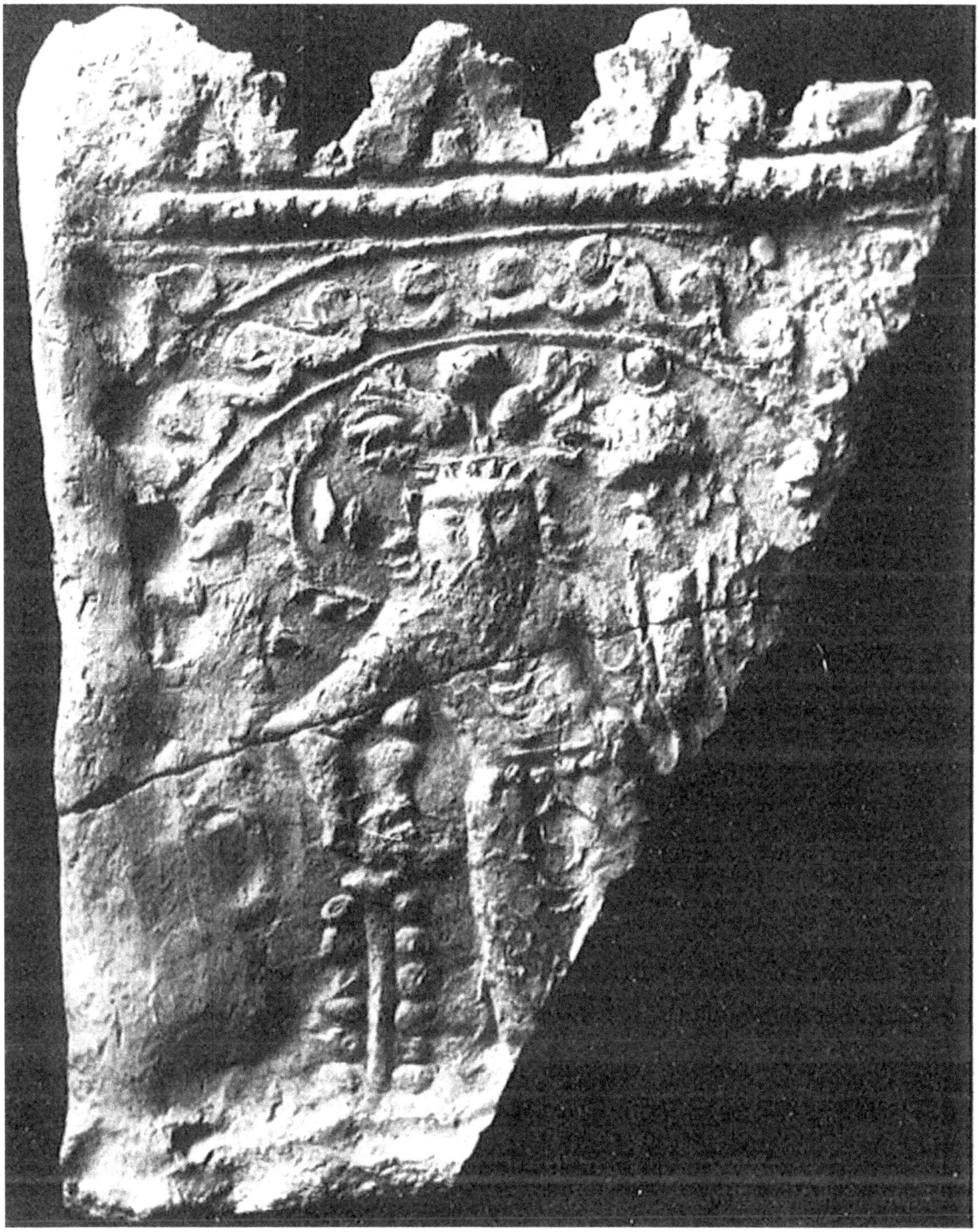

180. The ossuaries from Biyanajman and Miankal, Iš-70 (Frantz Grenet).

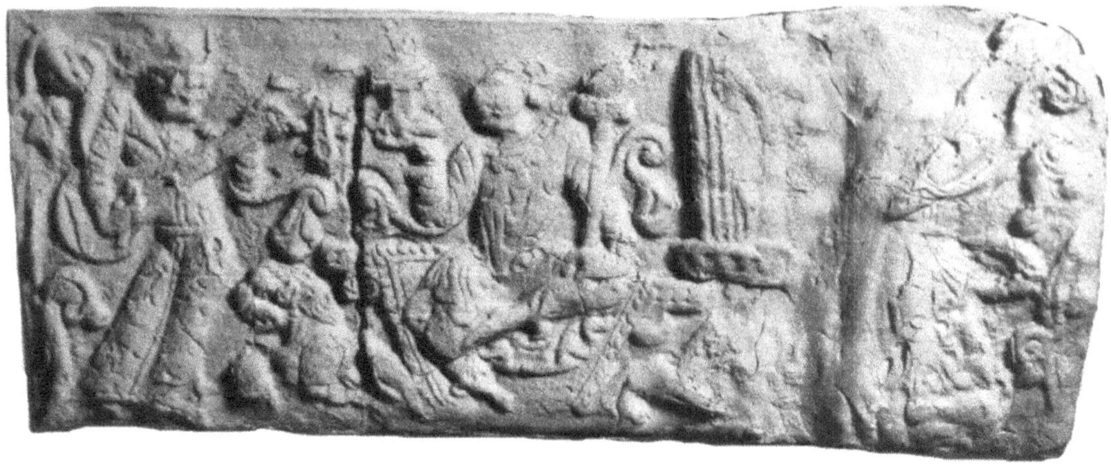

181. The ossuary from Xantepa (Frantz Grenet).

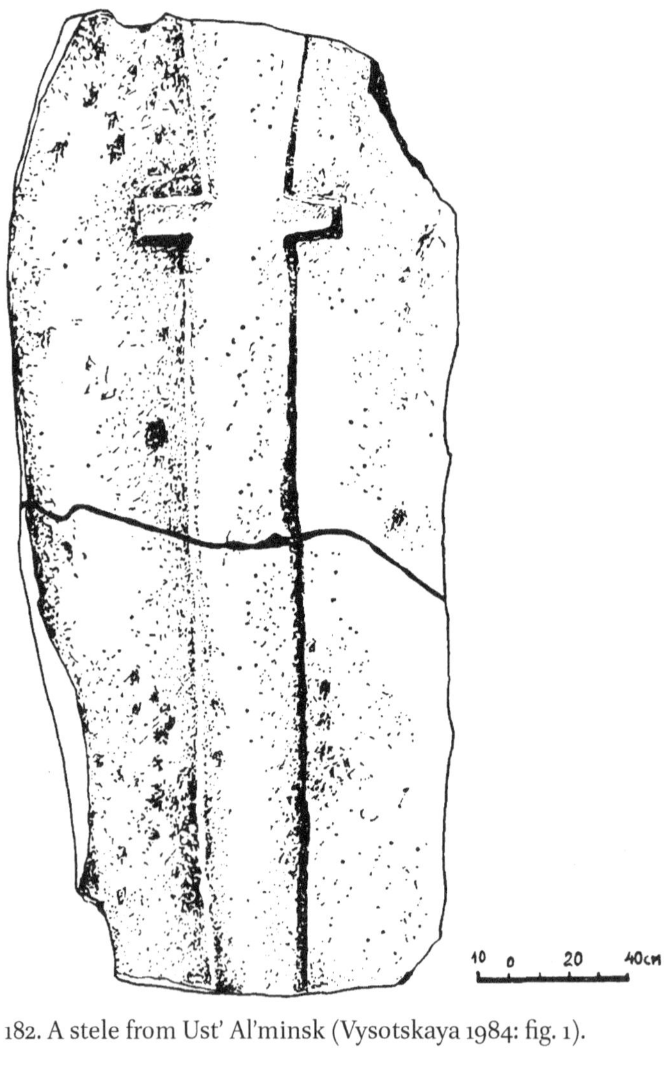

182. A stele from Ust' Al'minsk (Vysotskaya 1984: fig. 1).

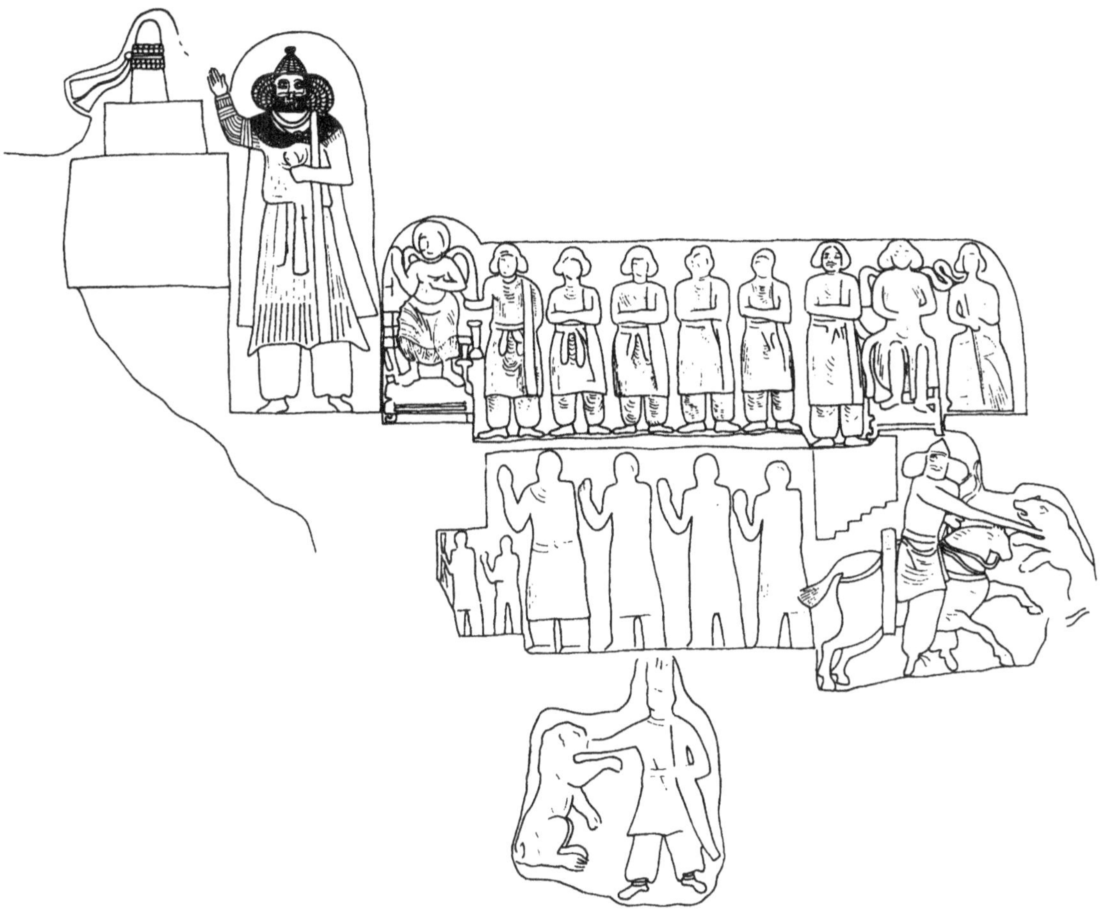

183. Tang-i Sarvak II relief, north-northwestern face (drawing E. Smekens © BAMI).

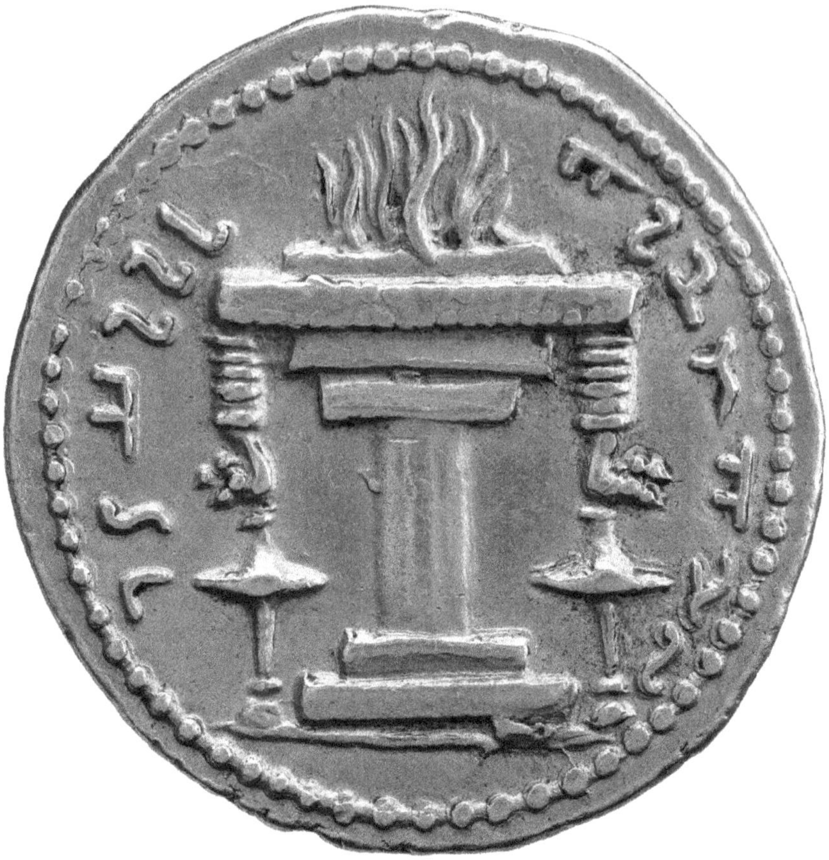

184. Fire-altar on a coin of Ardašīr I (© Trustees of the British Museum).

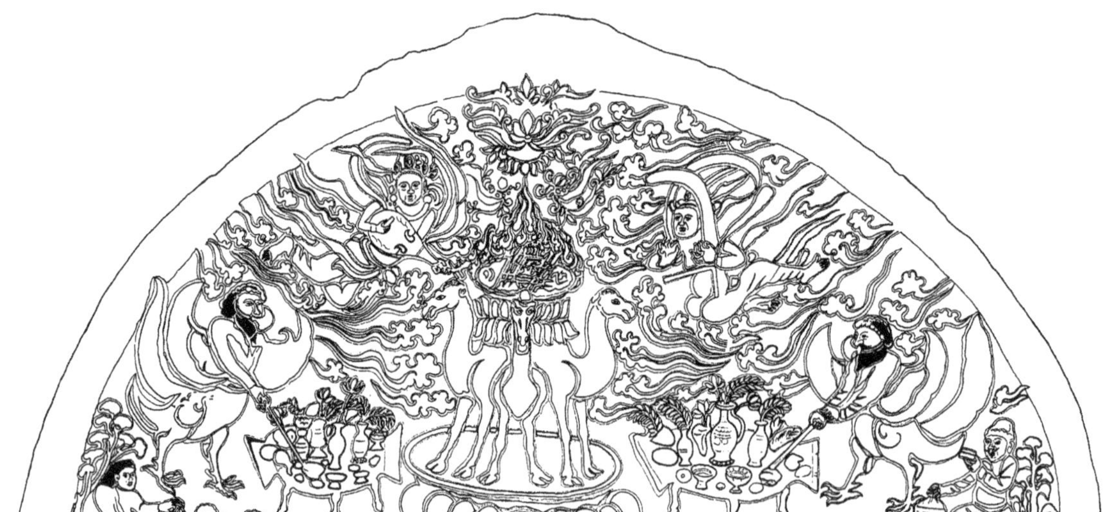

185. A ritual scene carved on the tympanum of the entrance door of the Sino-Sogdian tomb of An Jia (Frantz Grenet).

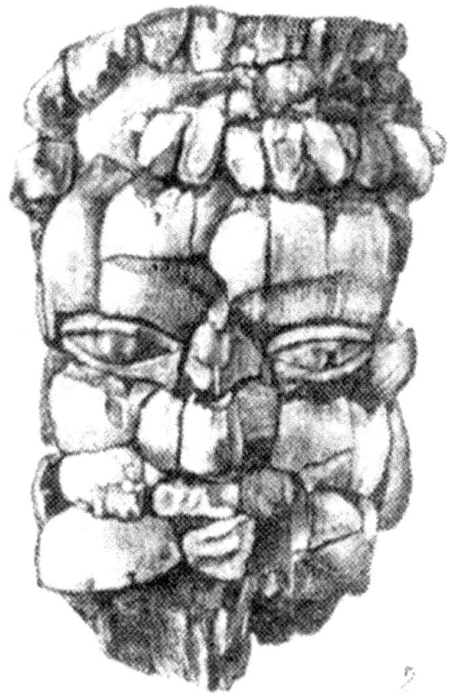

186. Wooden head no. 1, Chilhujra (Pulatov 1975: fig. 47).

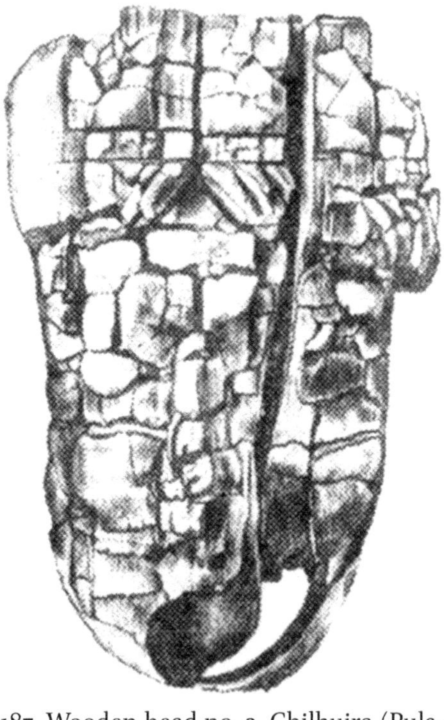

187. Wooden head no. 2, Chilhujra (Pulatov 1975: fig. 48).

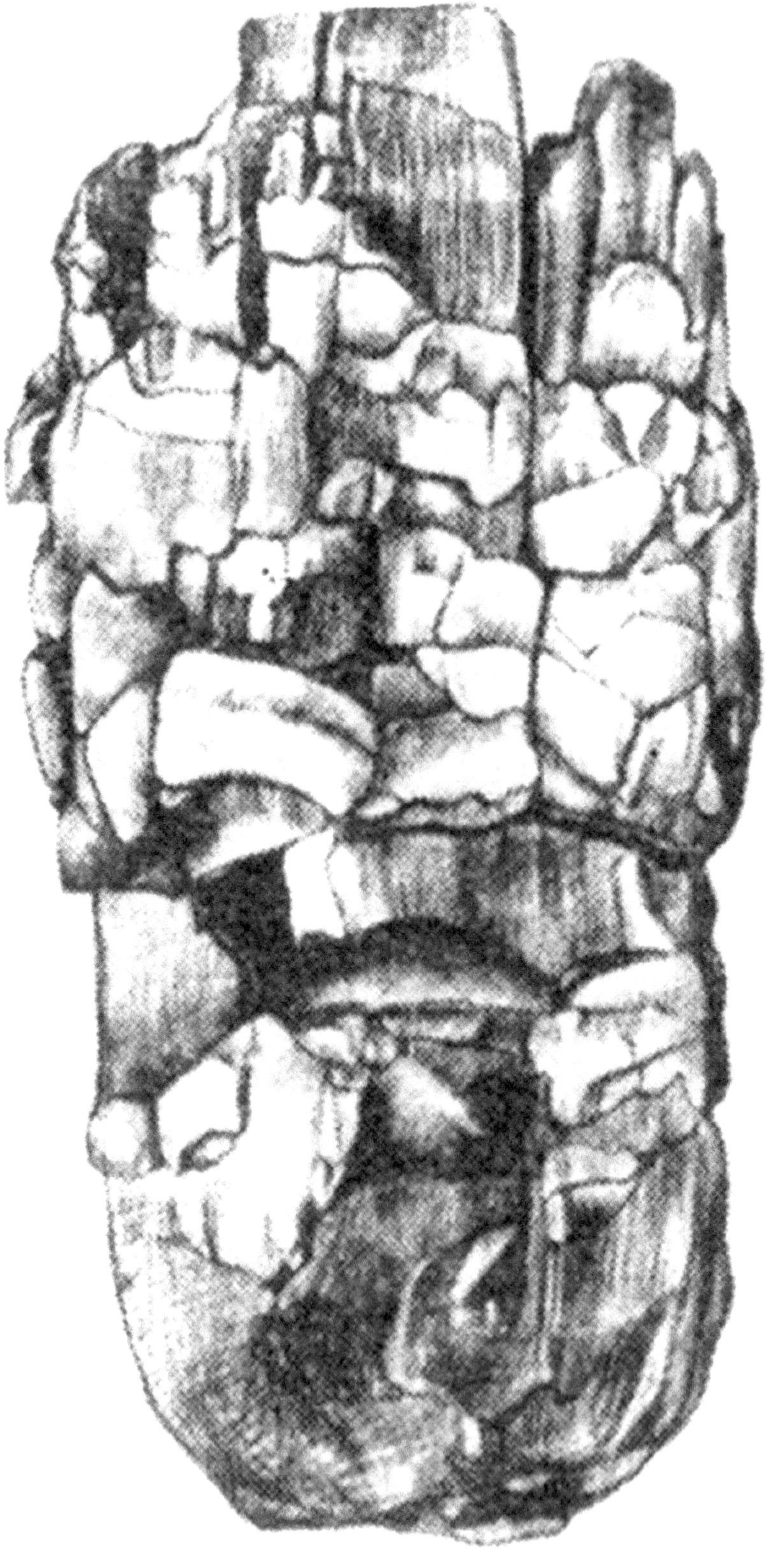

188. Wooden head no. 3, Chilhujra (Pulatov 1975: fig. 49).

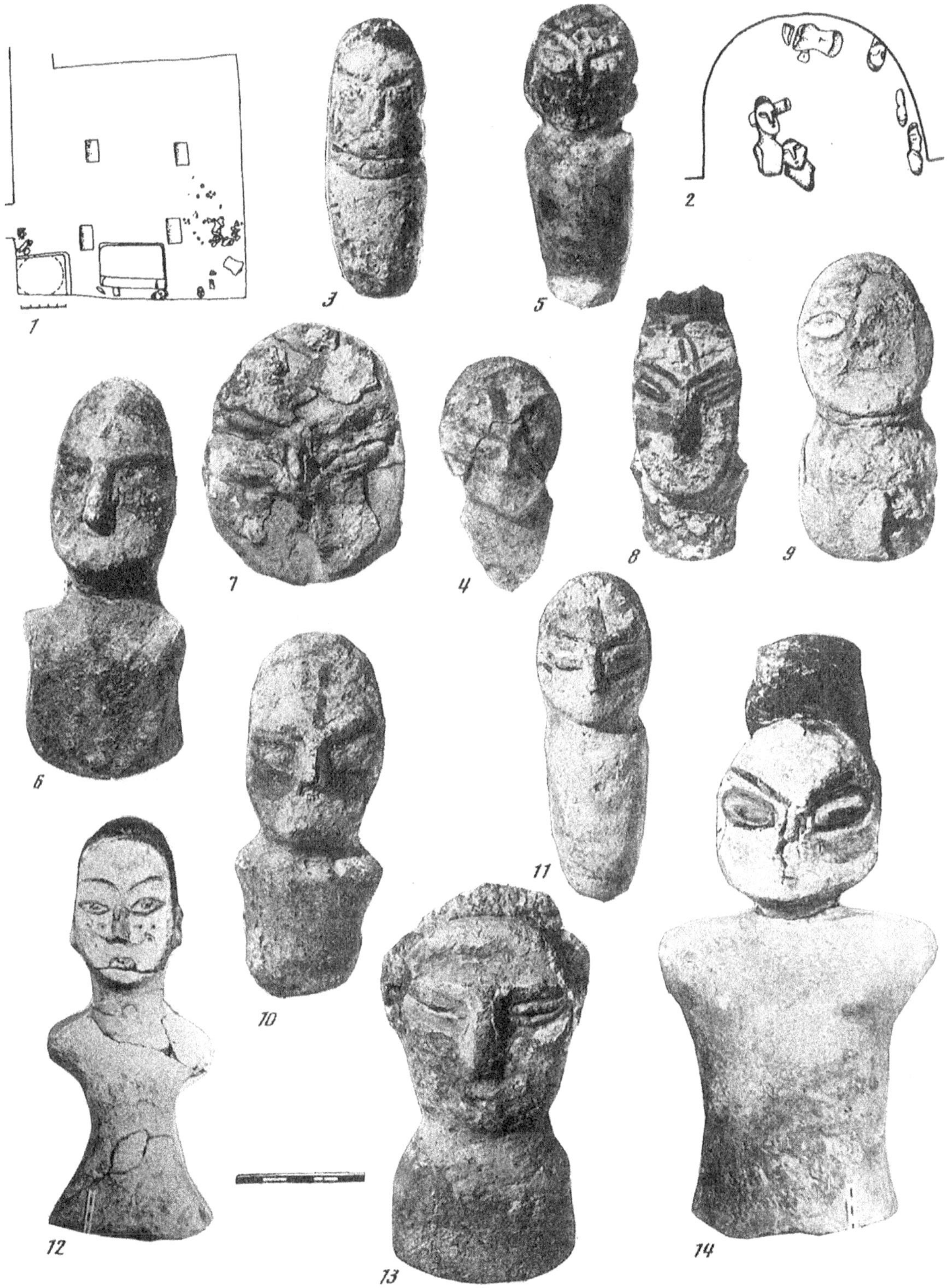

189. Idols from Kayragach (Brykina 1999: fig. 73).

COLOR PLATES

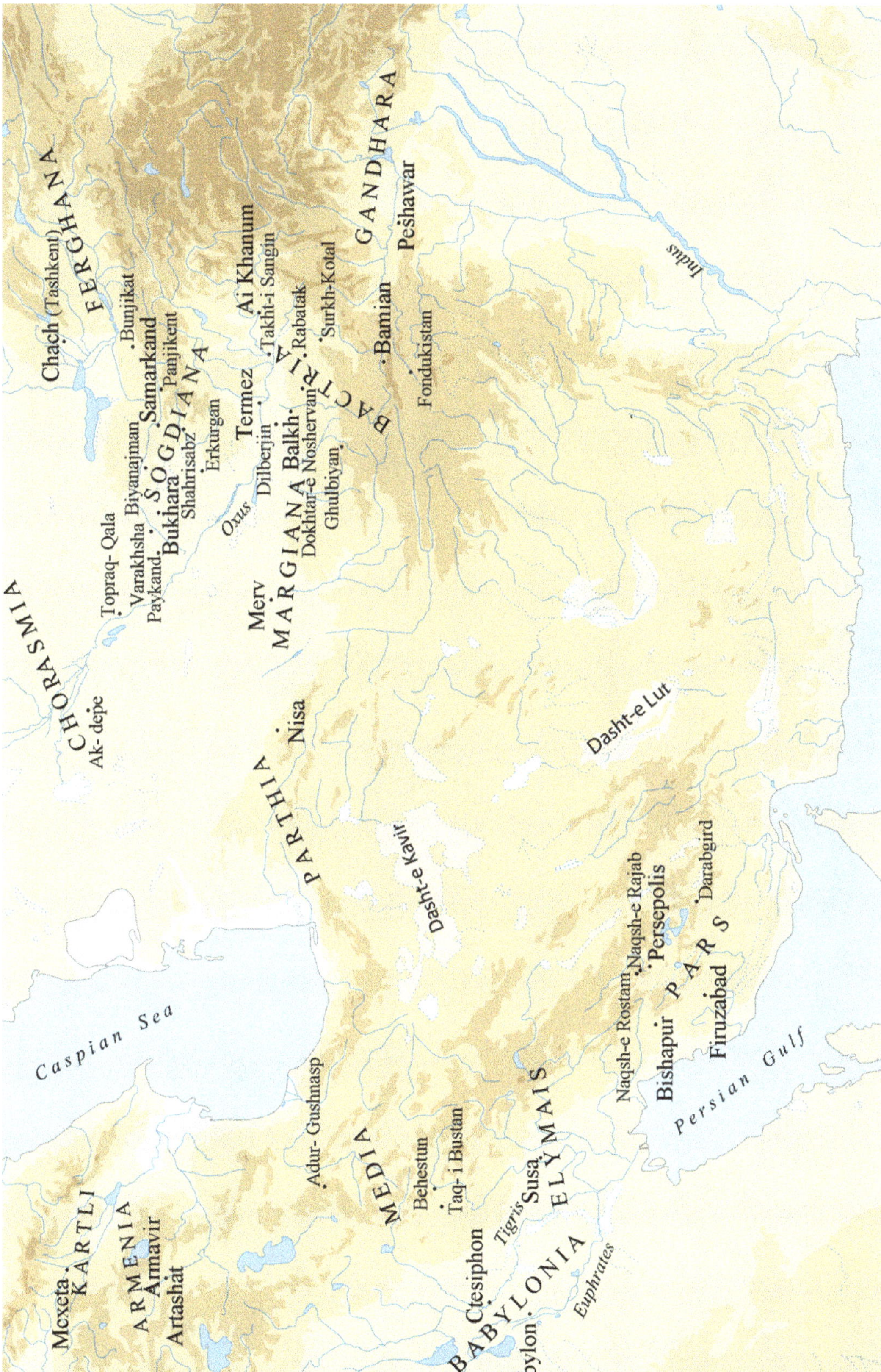

1. Map of the sedentary Iranian world (François Ory).

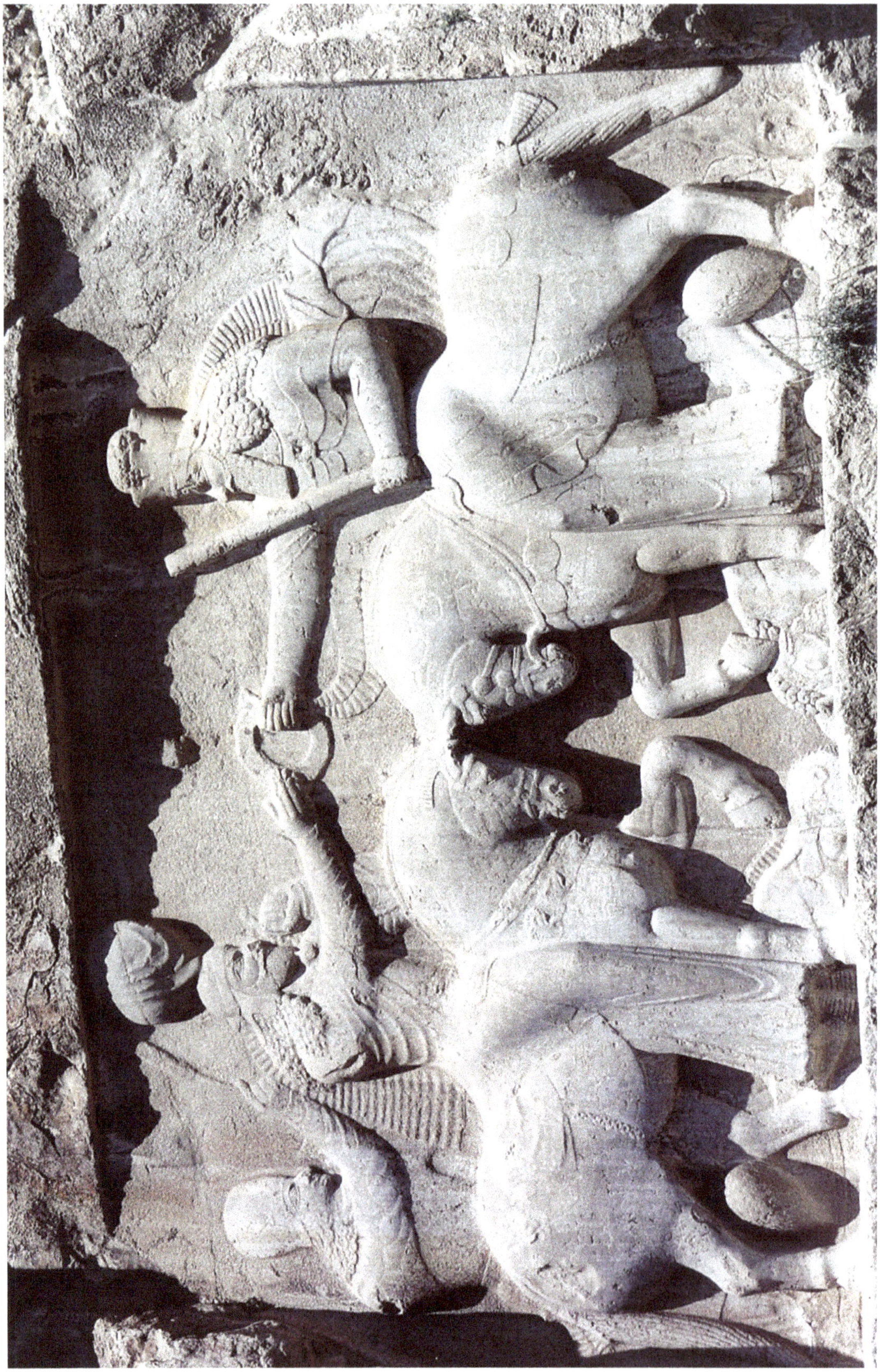

2. Investiture relief of Ardašīr I at Naqš-e Rostam (Photo Ginolerhino 2002).

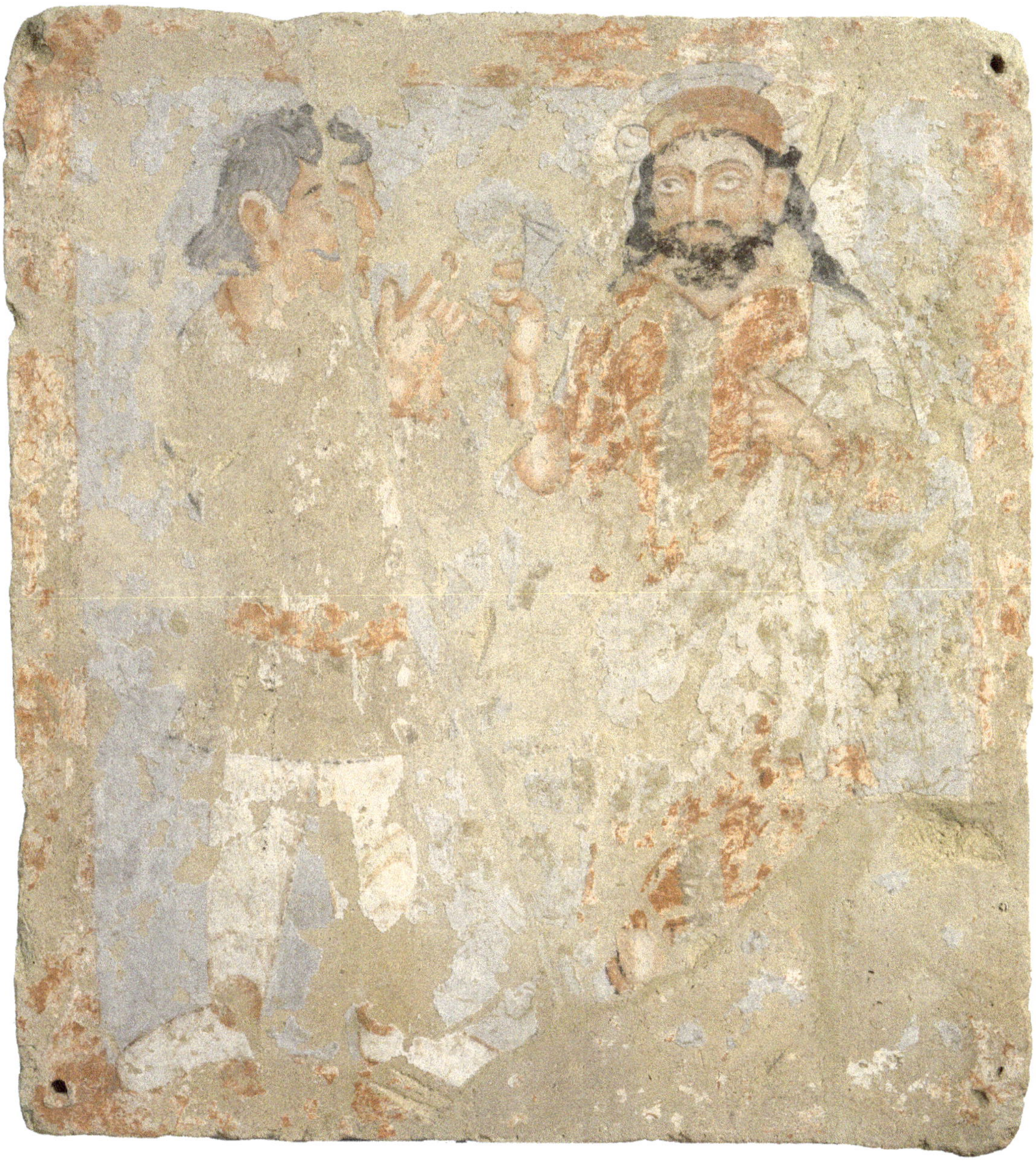

3. Terracotta panel from Afghanistan depicting a Zeus-like deity (© The Metropolitan Museum of Art).

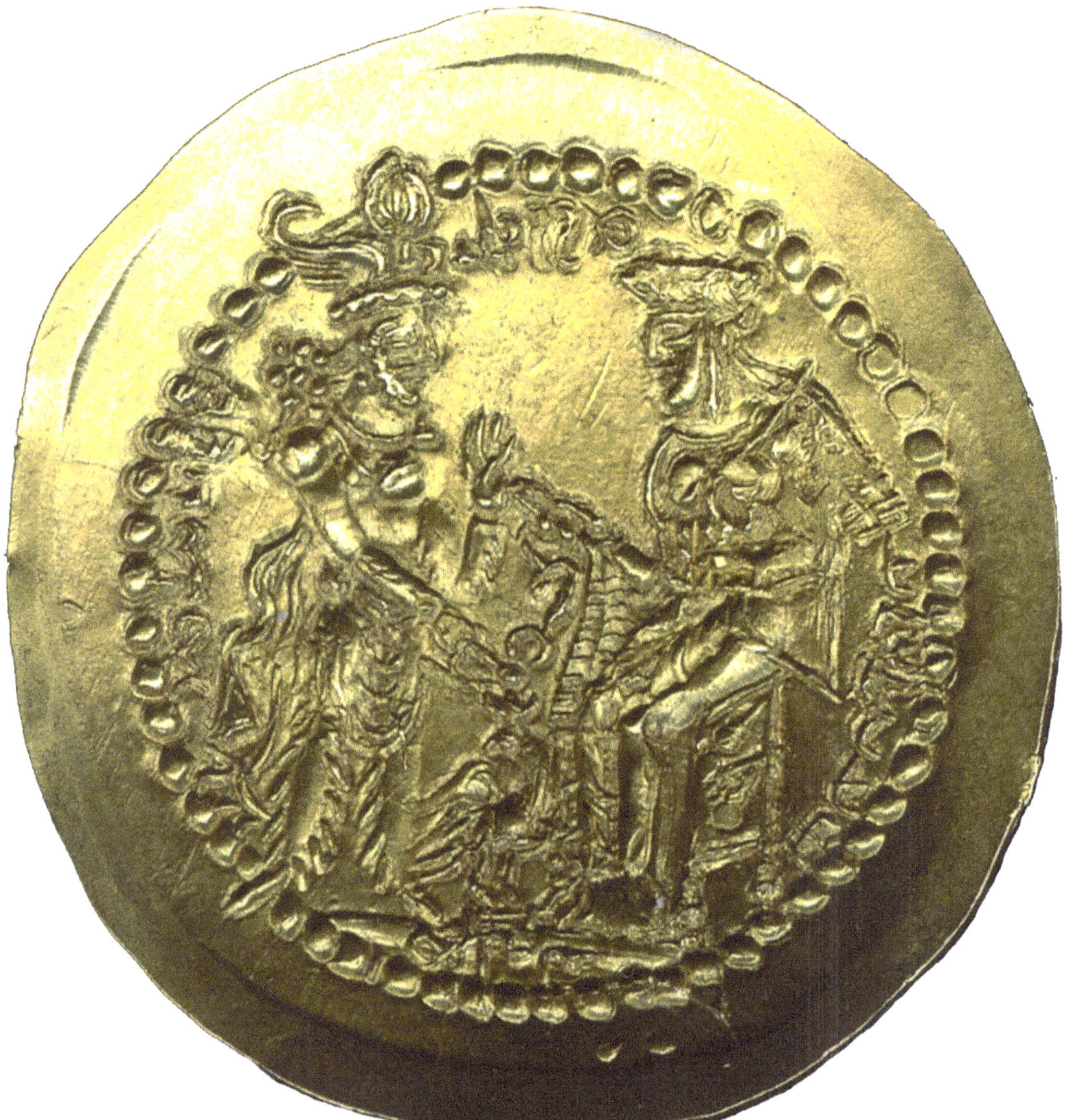

4. Anāhitā on a coin of Kushano-Sasanian King Ōhrmazd I (© Trustees of the British Museum).

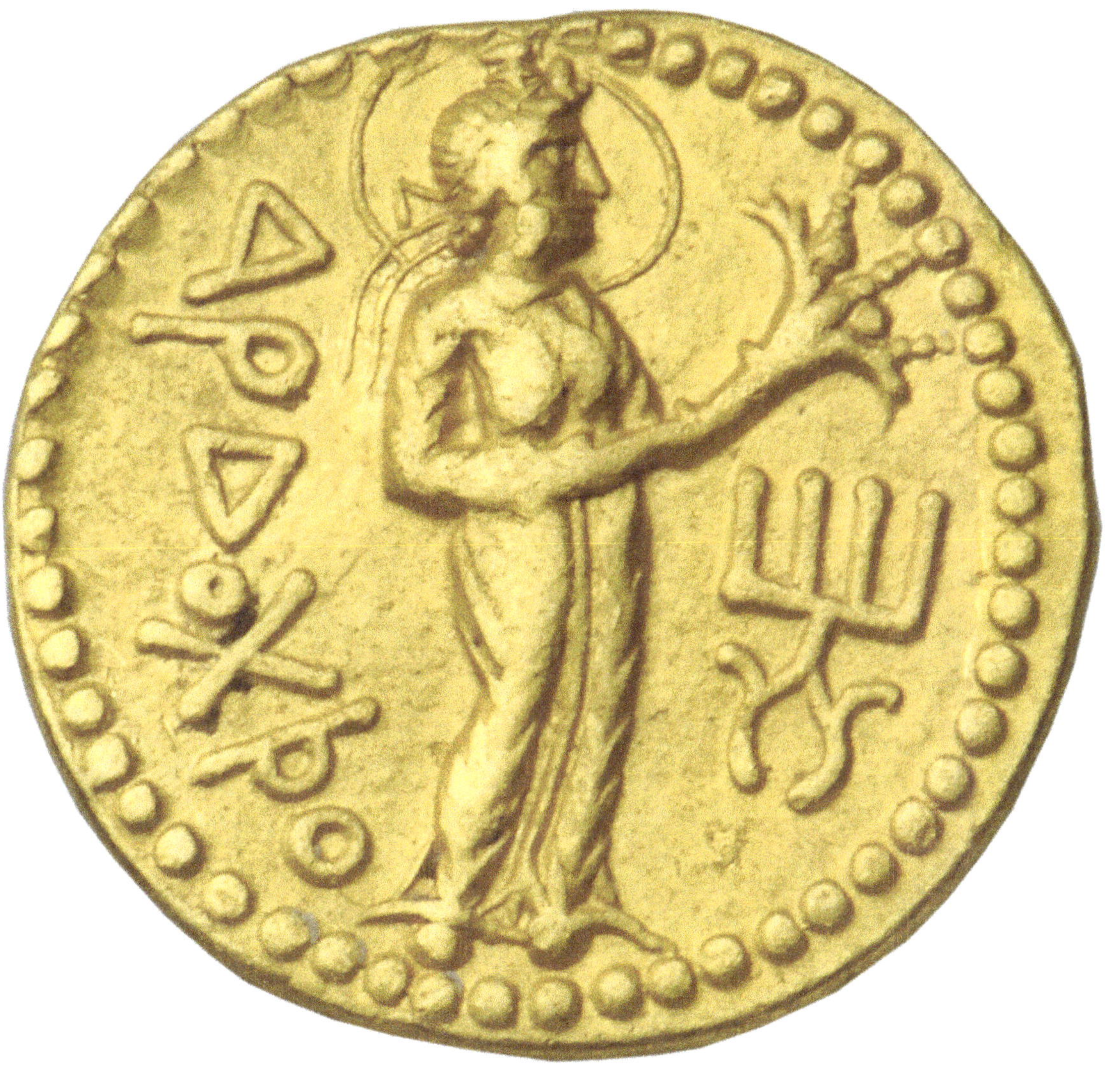

5. Standing Ardoxšo on a Kushan coin (Osmund Bopearachchi).

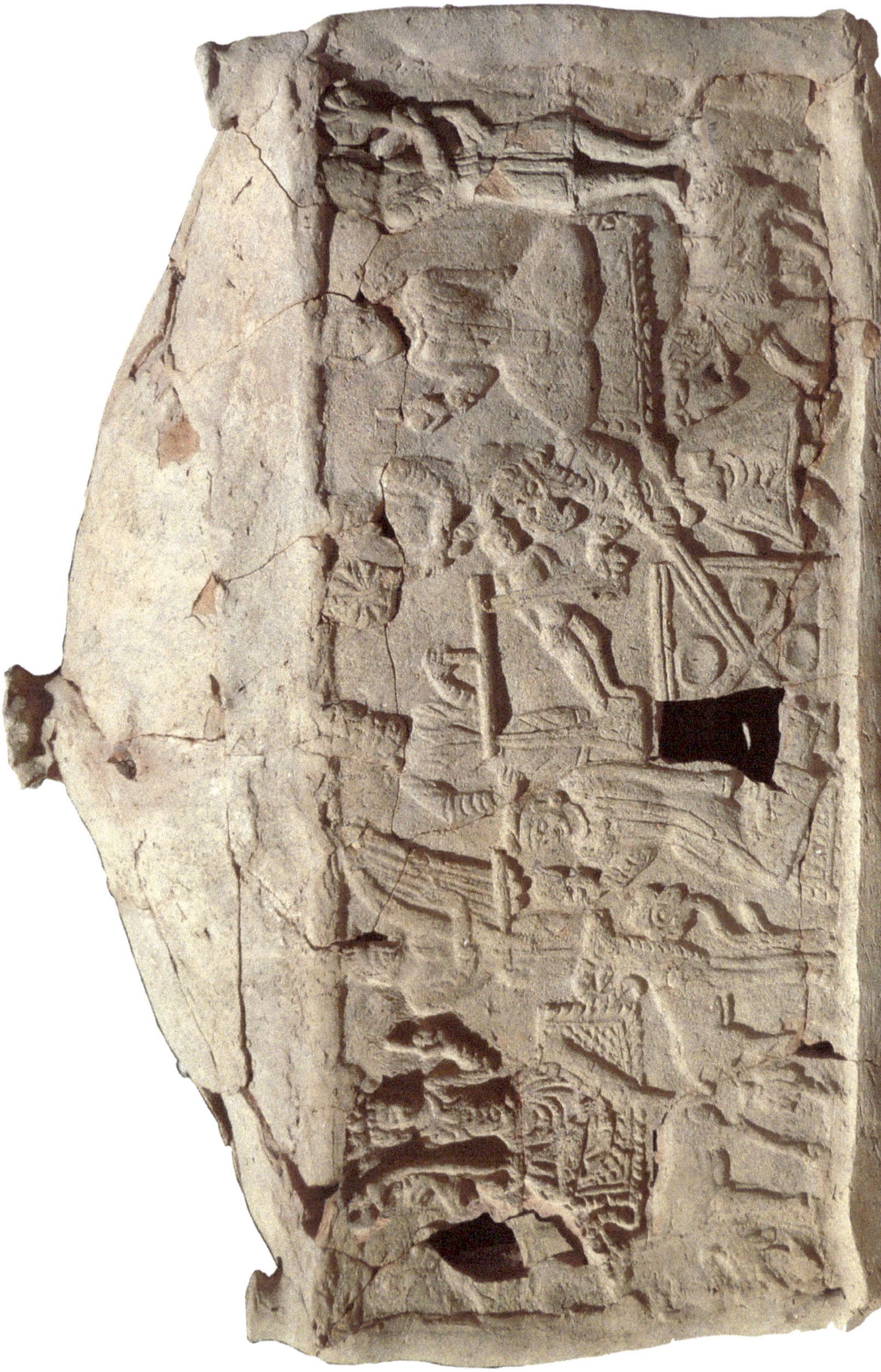

6. Ossuary from Yumalaktepa (Frantz Grenet).

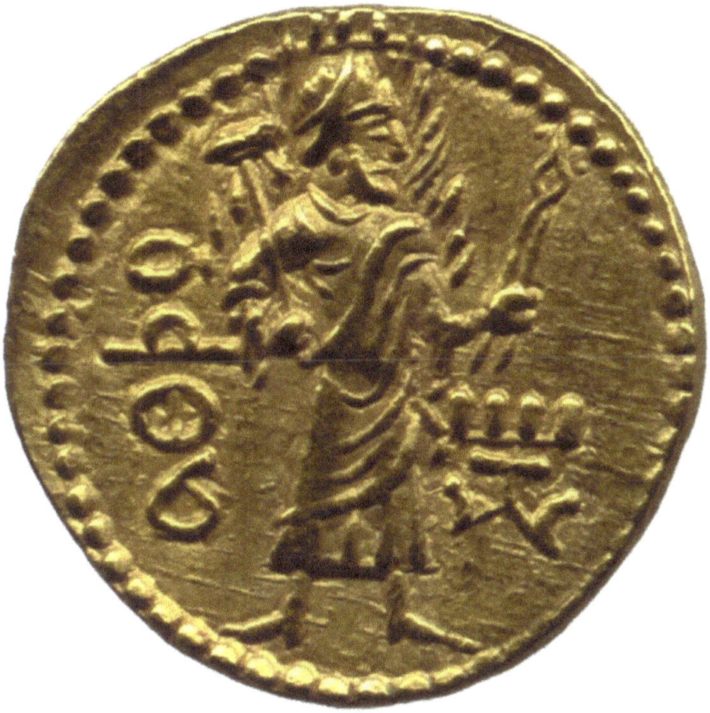

7. Athšo on a Kushan coin, type 2 (© Trustees of the British Museum).

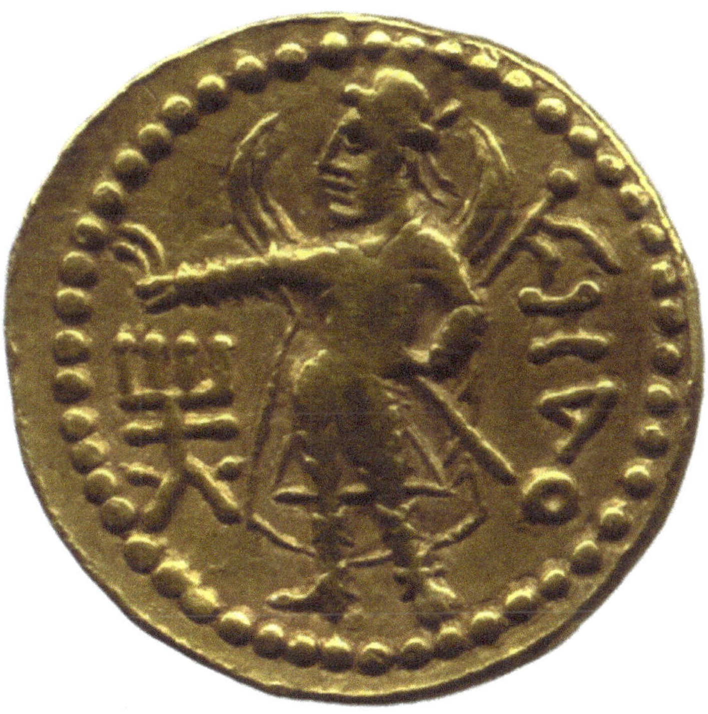

8. Mao on a Kushan coin, Göbl type 1 (© Trustees of the British Museum).

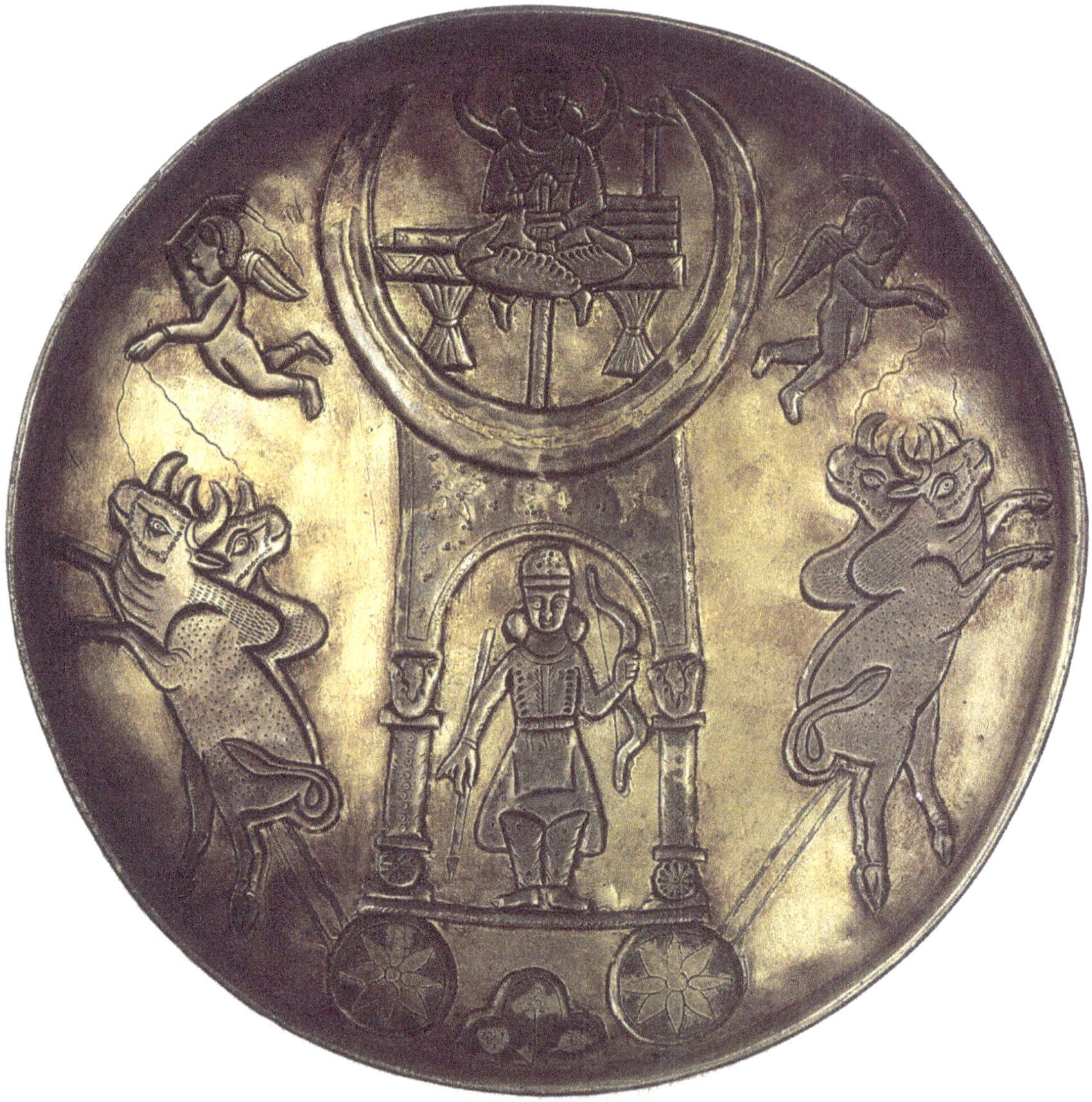

9. The “Klimova plate” (Trever and Lukonin 1987: fig. 29).

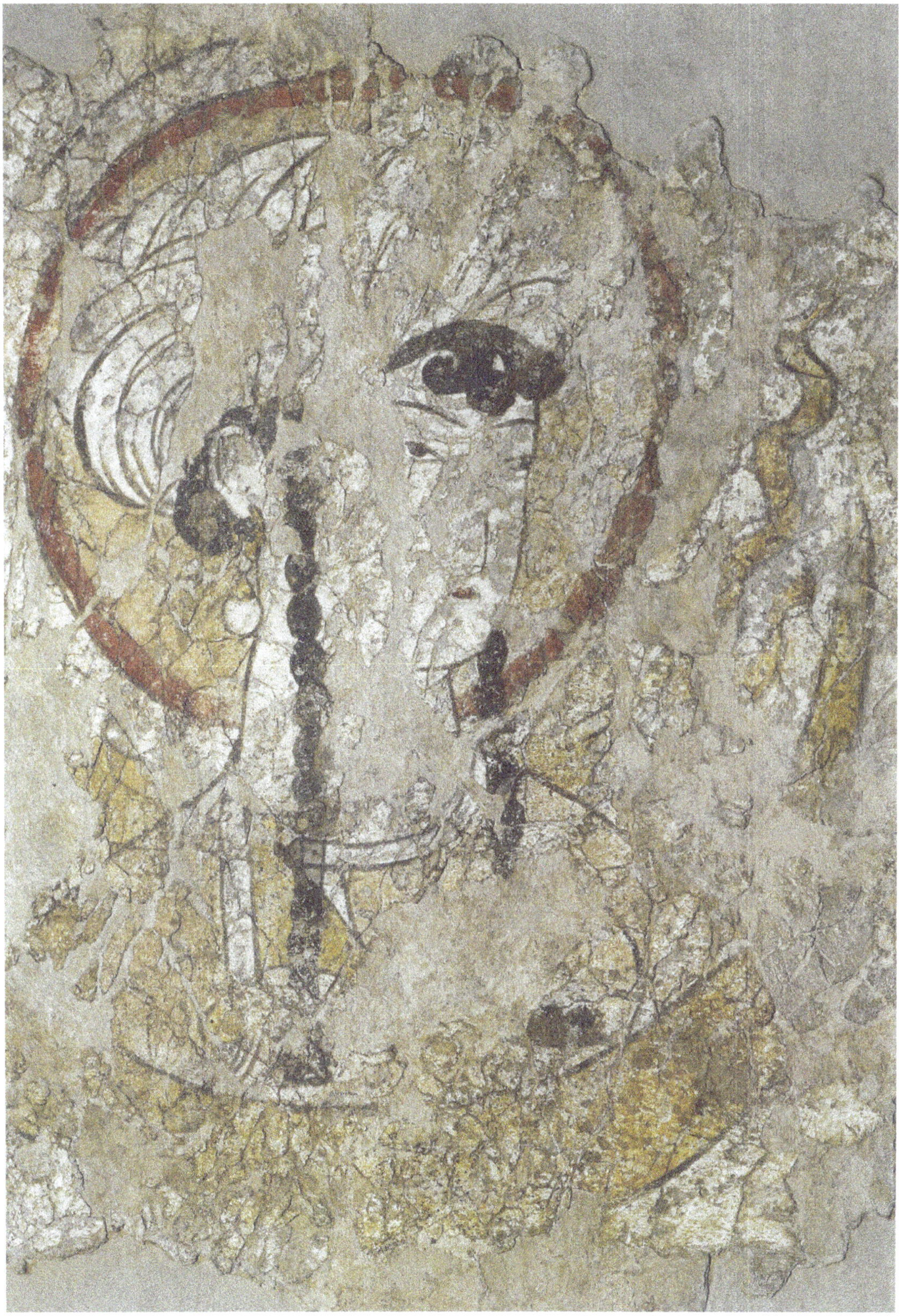

10. The personification of the moon, Panjikent (Marshak 2009: 6).

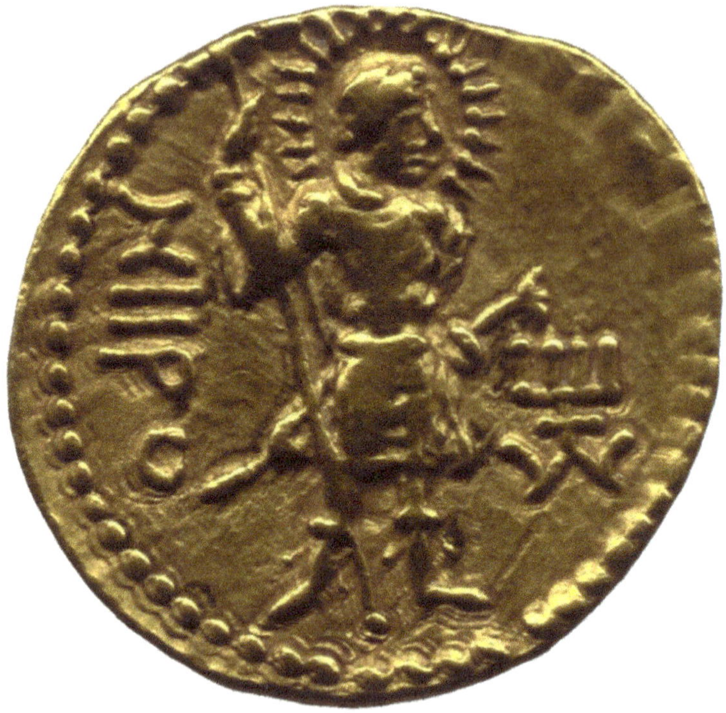

11. Miiro on a Kushan coin, type 9 (© Trustees of the British Museum).

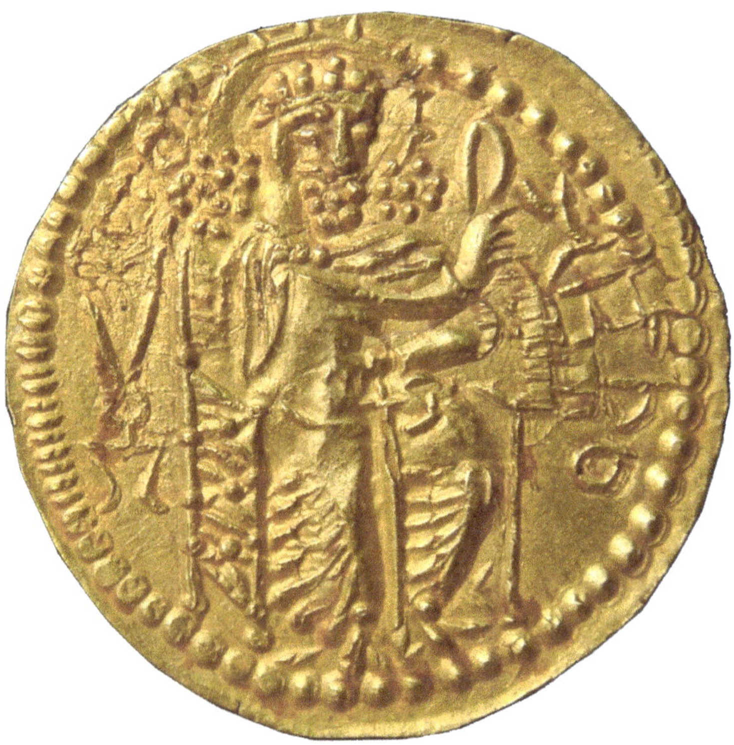

12. Mithra on a coin of the Kushano-Sasanian king Ardašīr I (© Trustees of the British Museum).

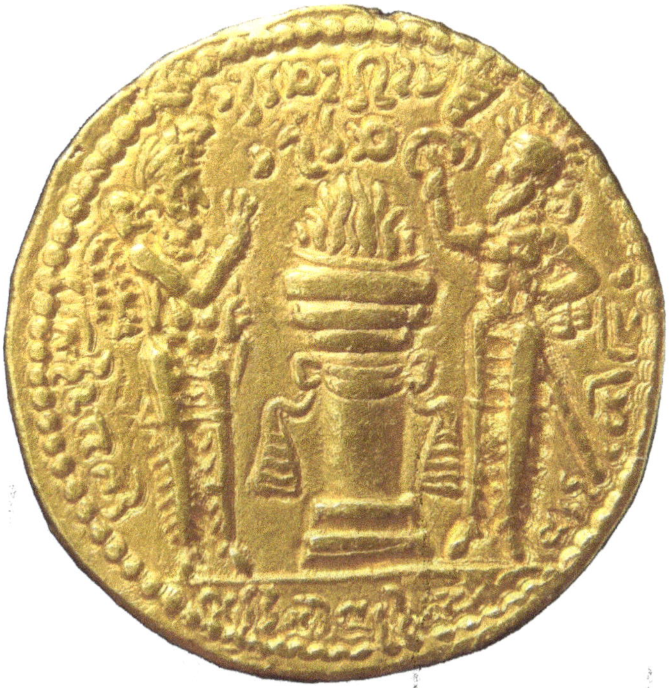

13. Mithra on a coin of the Kushano-Sasanian king Ōhrmazd I minted in Merv (© Trustees of the British Museum).

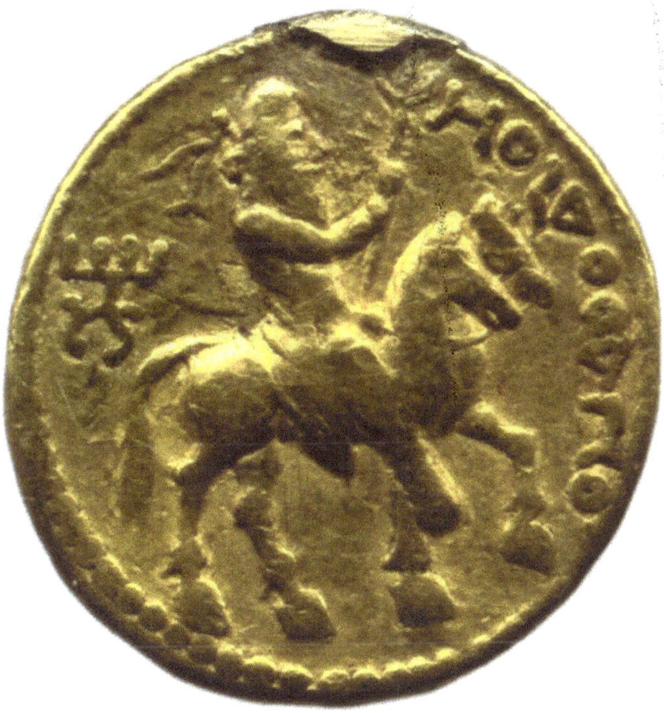

14. Mozdooano on a Kushan coin (© Trustees of the British Museum).

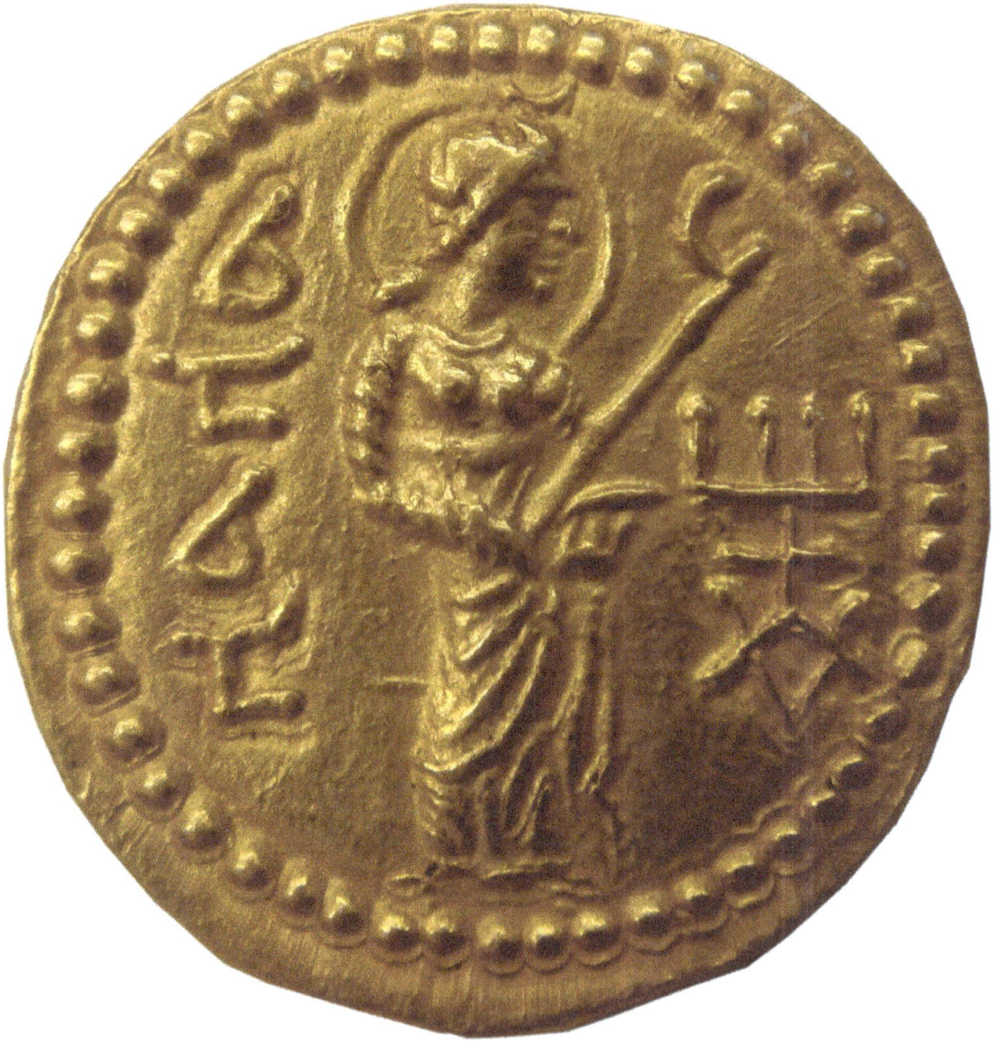

15. Nana on a Kushan coin, standing and holding a staff (© Trustees of the British Museum).

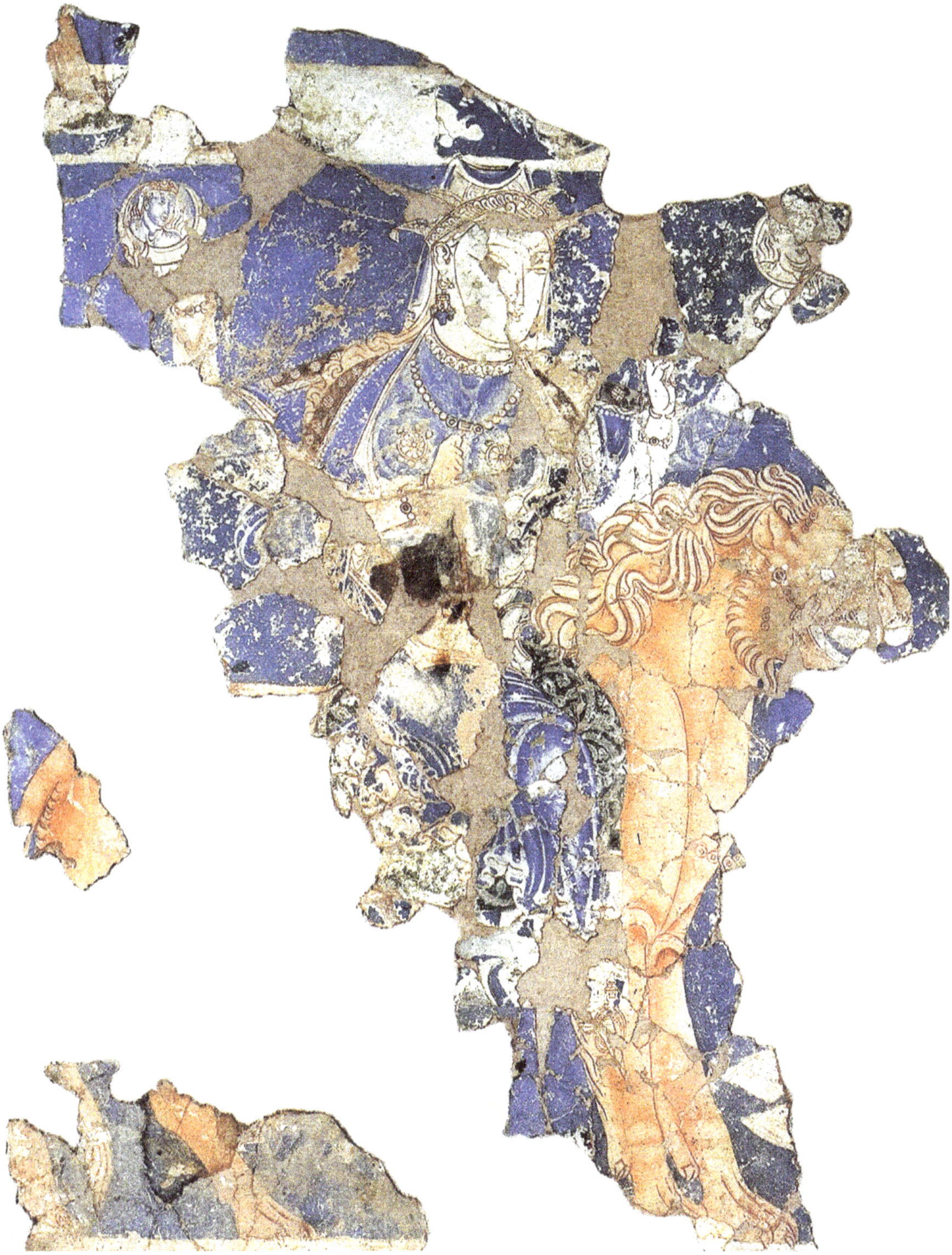

16. Nana on a lion, Bunjikat (Sokolovskiy 2009: fig. 71).

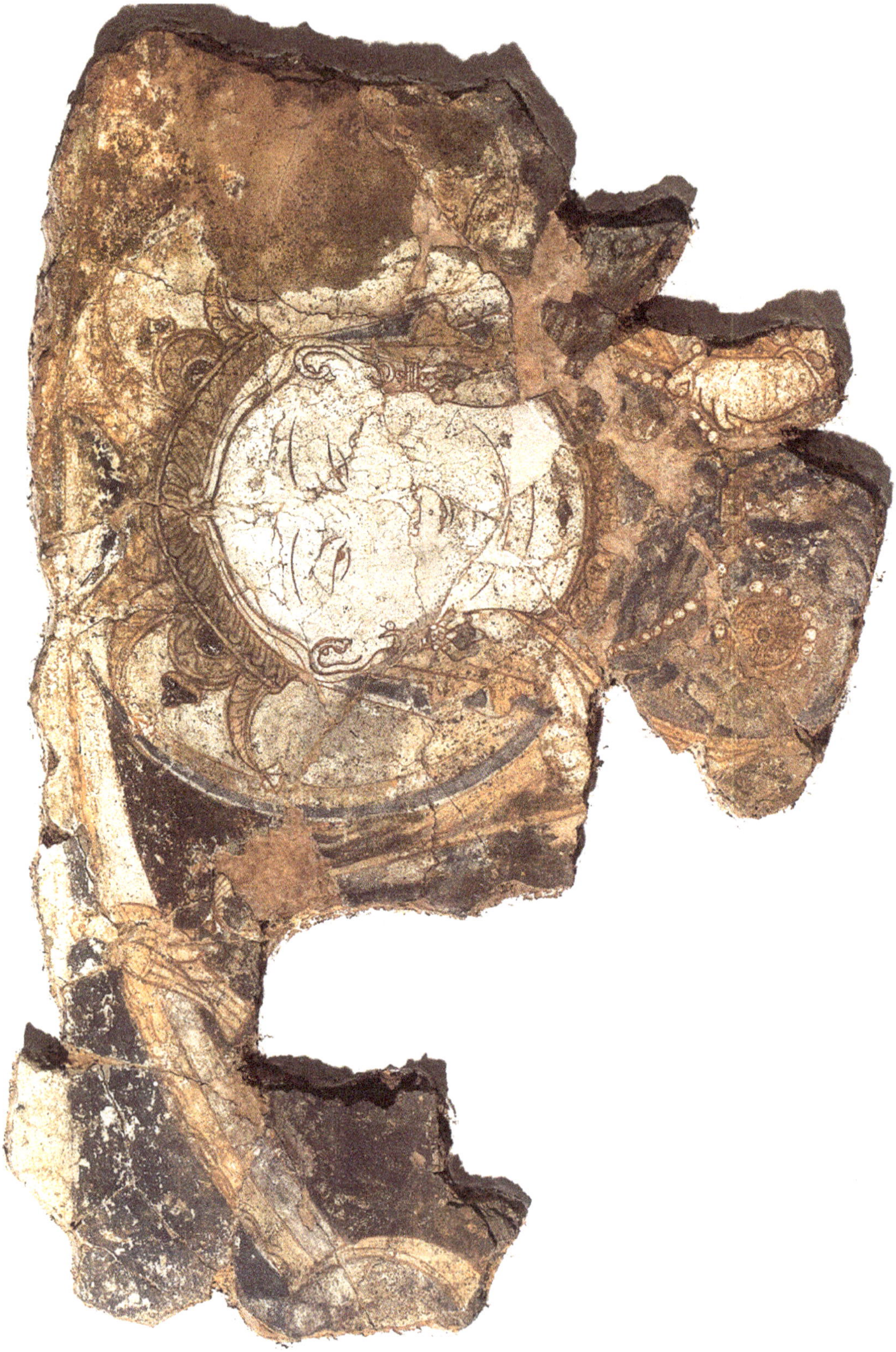

17. Nana depicted *en face*, the eastern wall of the "Small hall" (right side), Bunjikat (Sokolovskiy 2009: fig. 92).

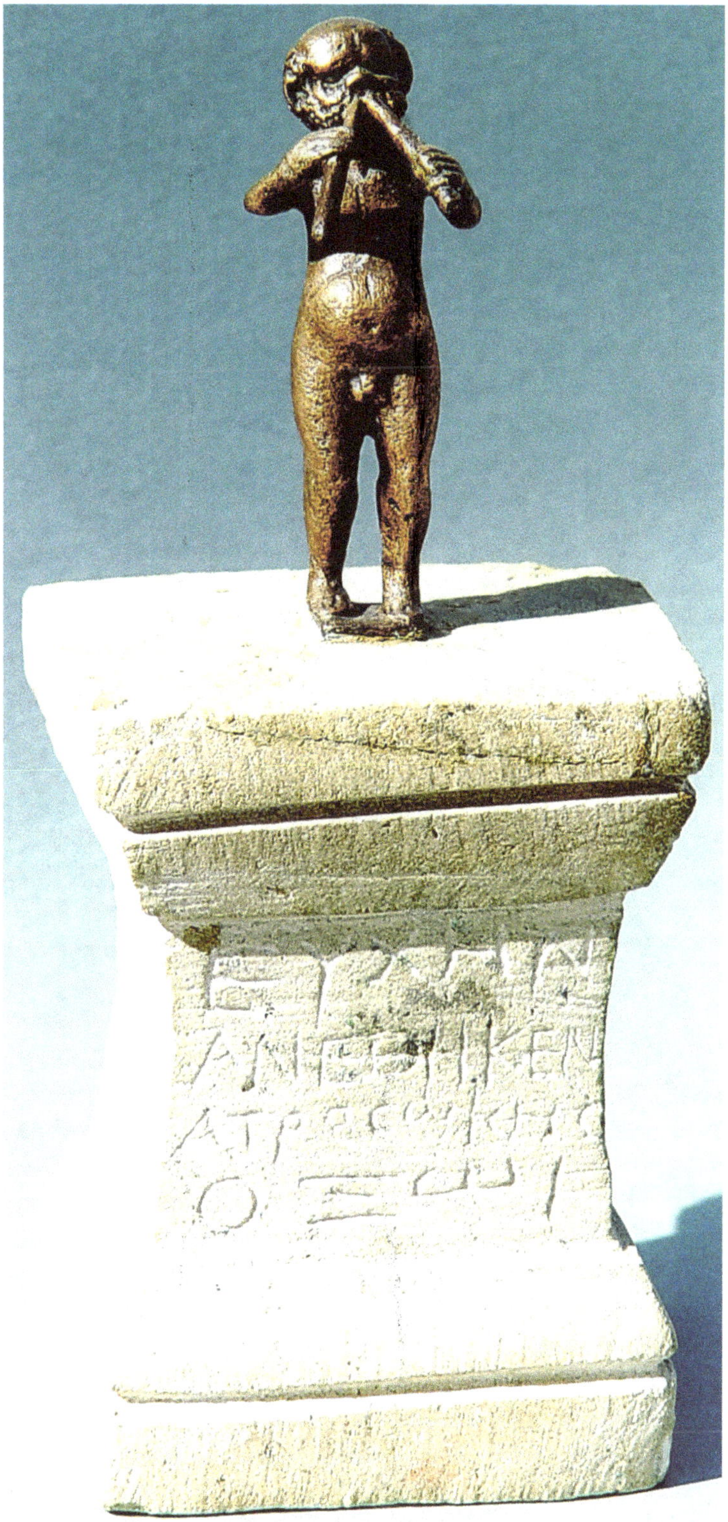

18. A statuette of Marsyas from the Oxus Temple (DAI Eurasien-Abteilung, Gunvor Lindström).

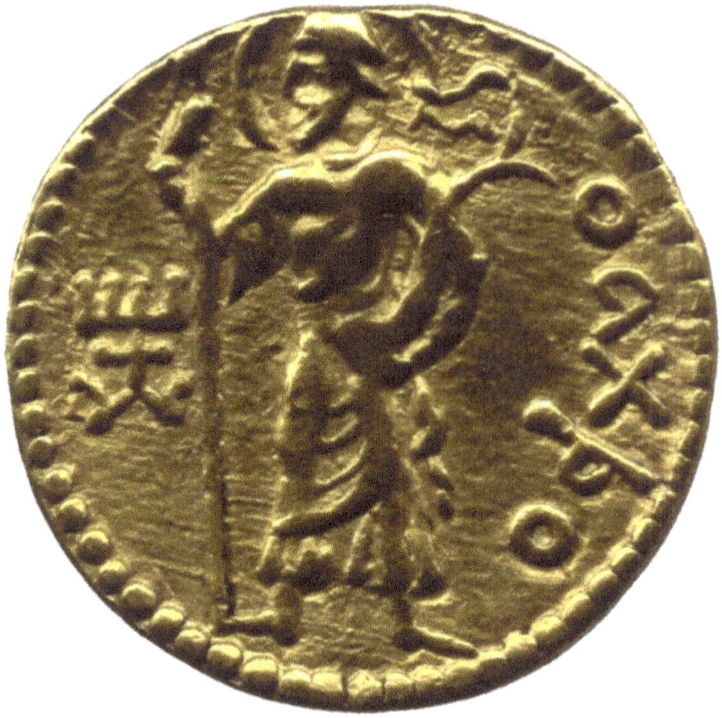

19. Oaxšo on a coin of Huvishka (© Trustees of the British Museum).

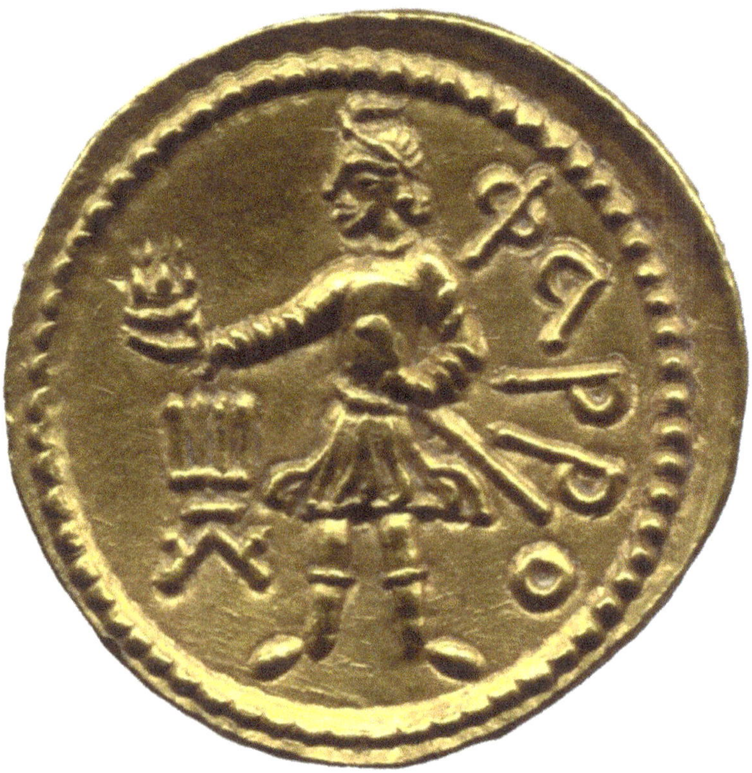

20. Pharro on a Kushan coin, type 5 (© Trustees of the British Museum).

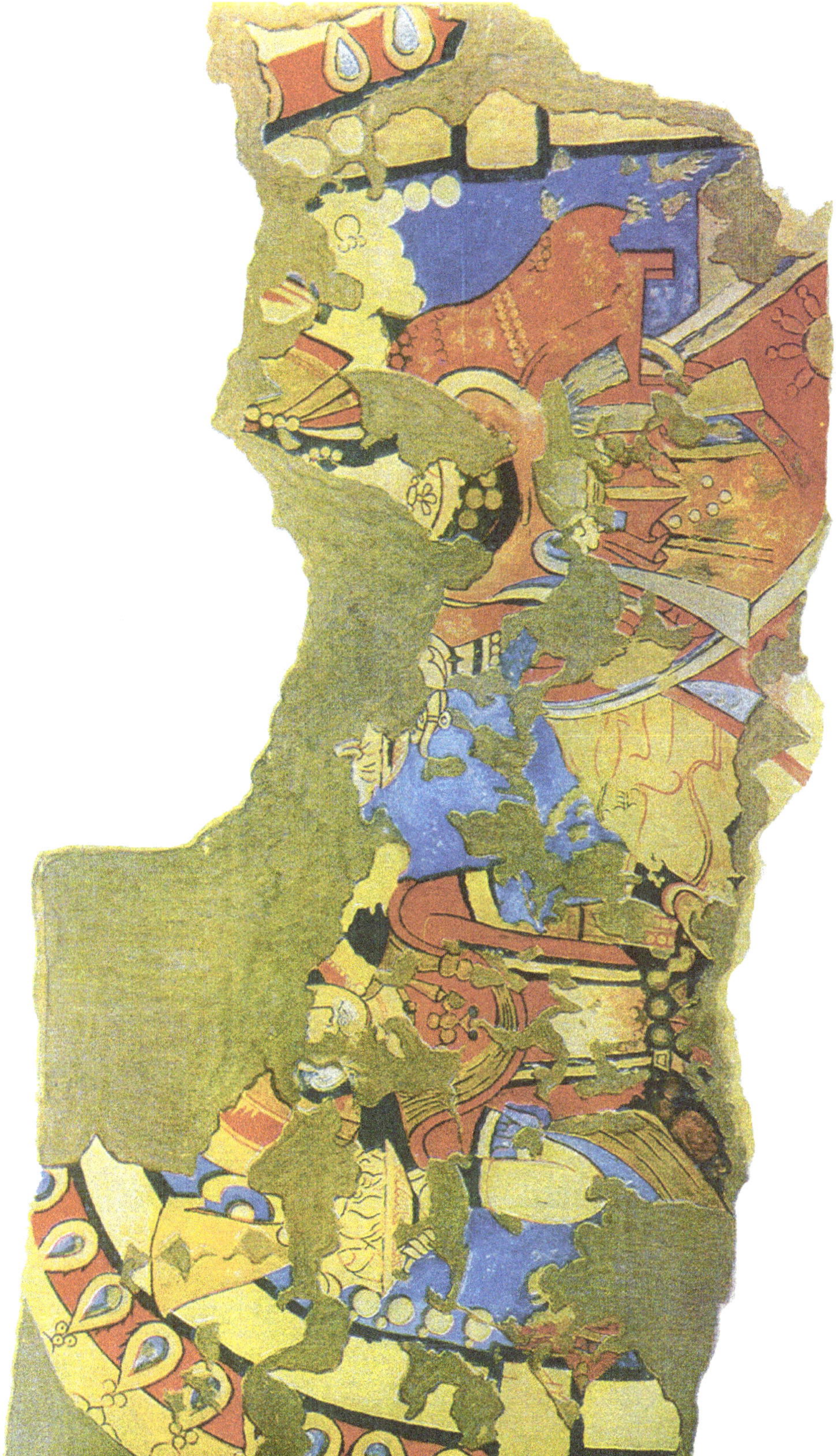

21. Enthroned divine couple, Afrosiab IX (Al'baum 1975: pl. II).

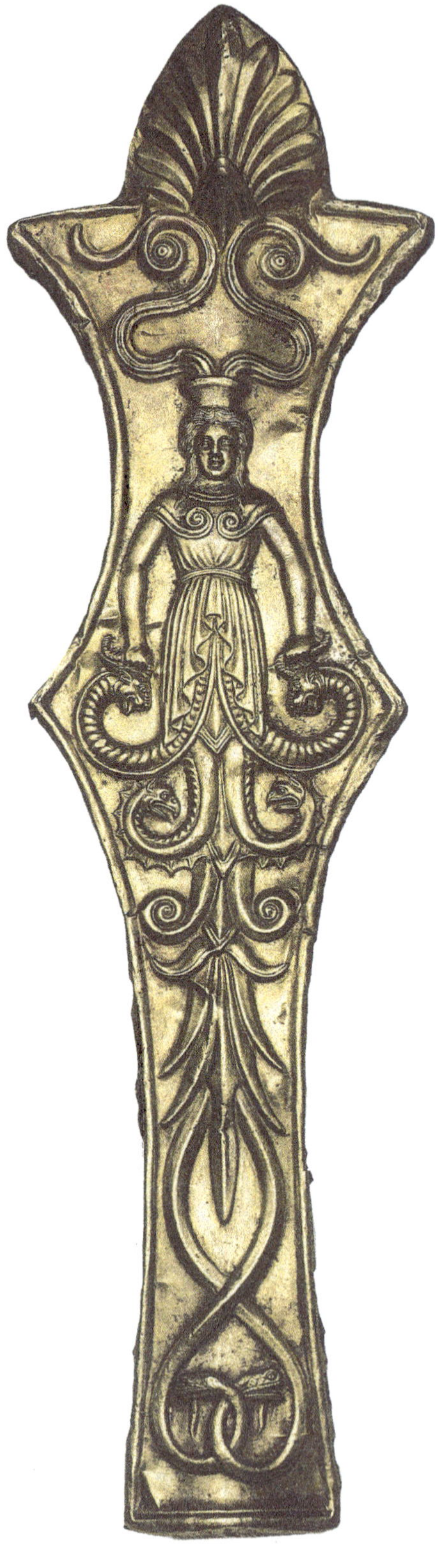

22. Anguipede goddess, Tzymbalova Mogila (Korol'kova 2006: fig. 5).

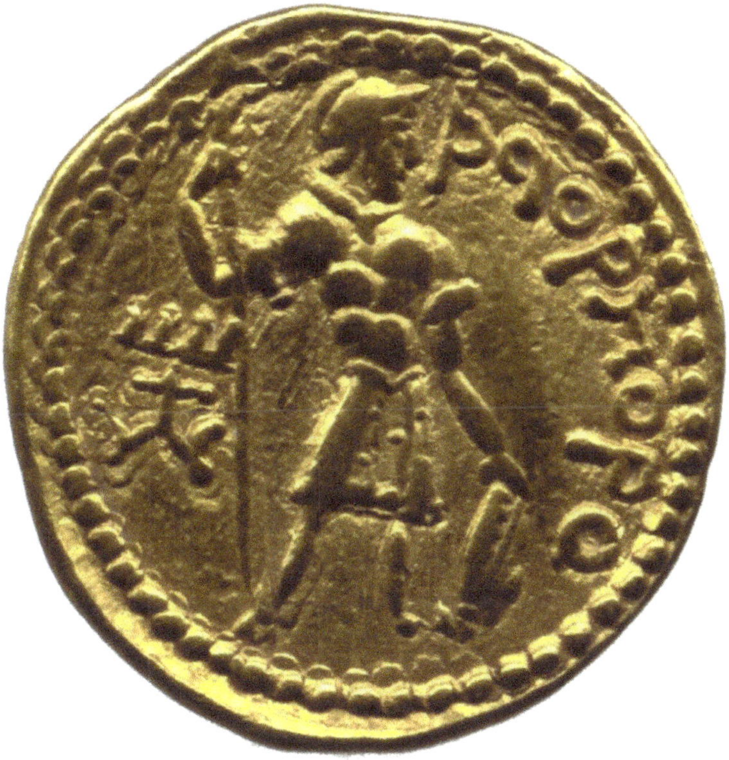

23. Šaoreoro on a Kushan coin, type 1 (© Trustees of the British Museum).

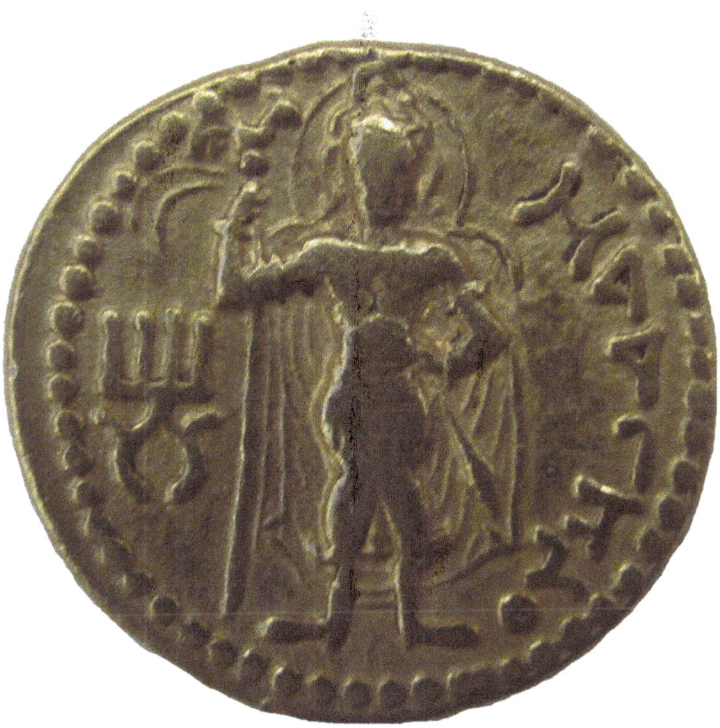

24. Maaseno on a Kushan coin (Osmund Bopearachchi).

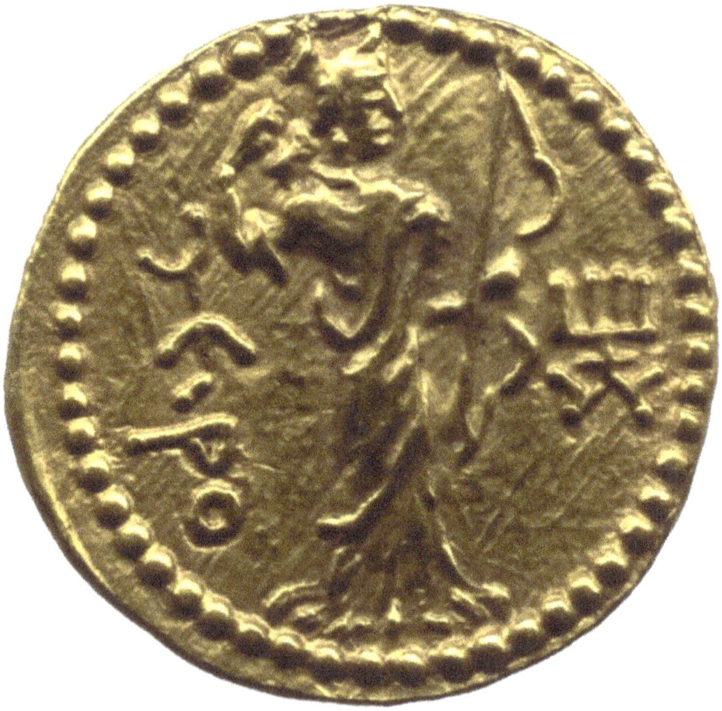

25. Teiro on a Kushan coin (© Trustees of the British Museum).

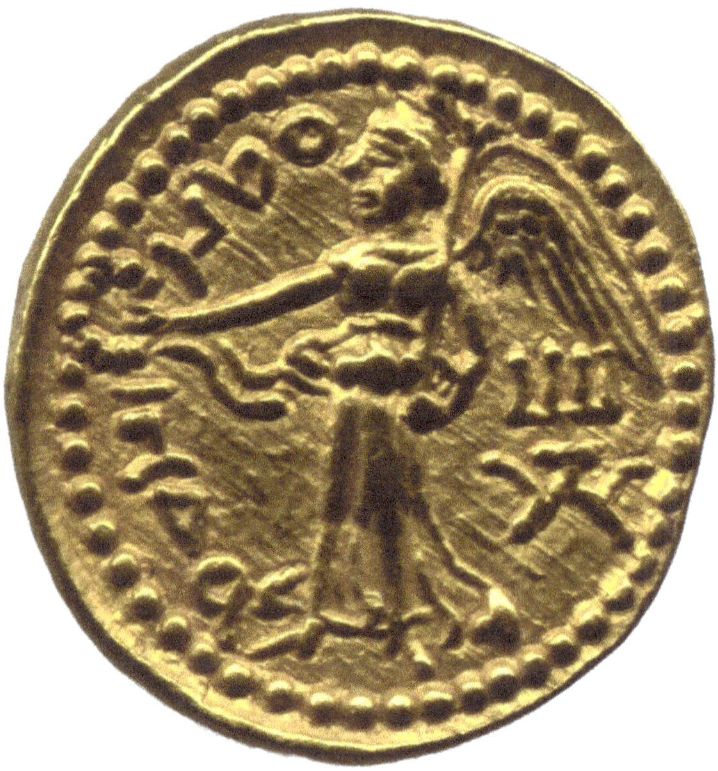

26. Oanindo on a Kushan coin (© Trustees of the British Museum).

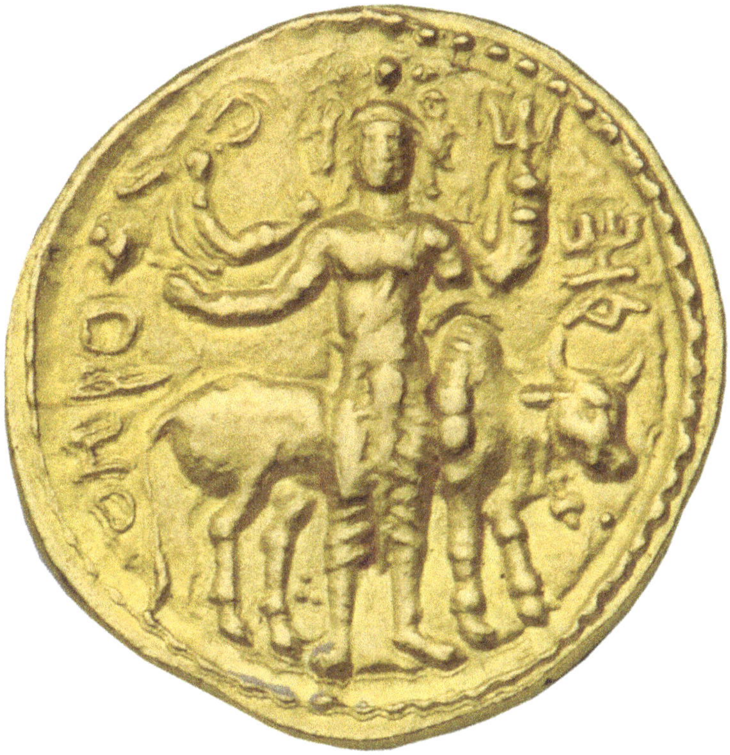

27. Oešo on a Kushan coin, type 4 (Osmund Bopearachchi).

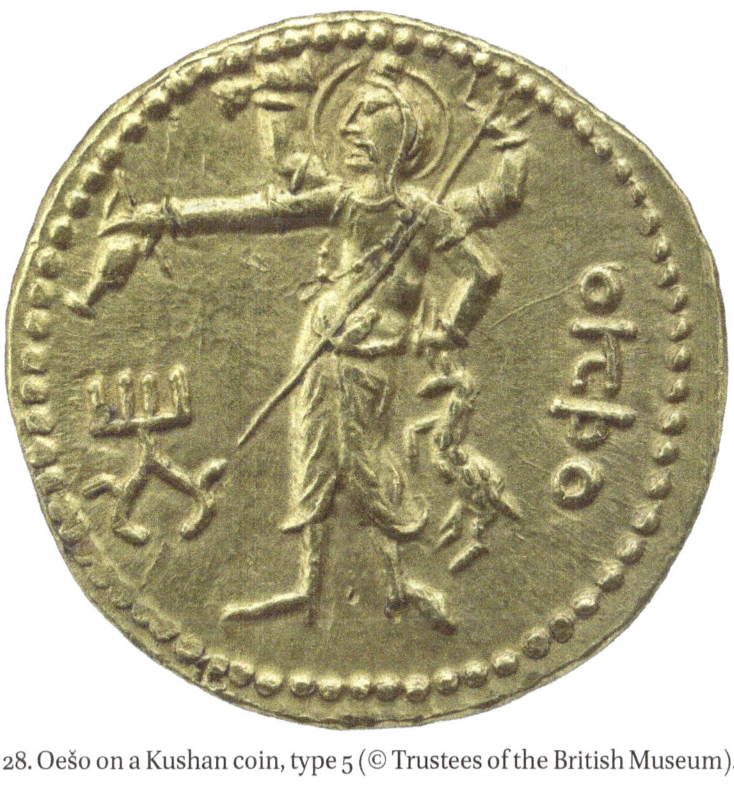

28. Oešo on a Kushan coin, type 5 (© Trustees of the British Museum).

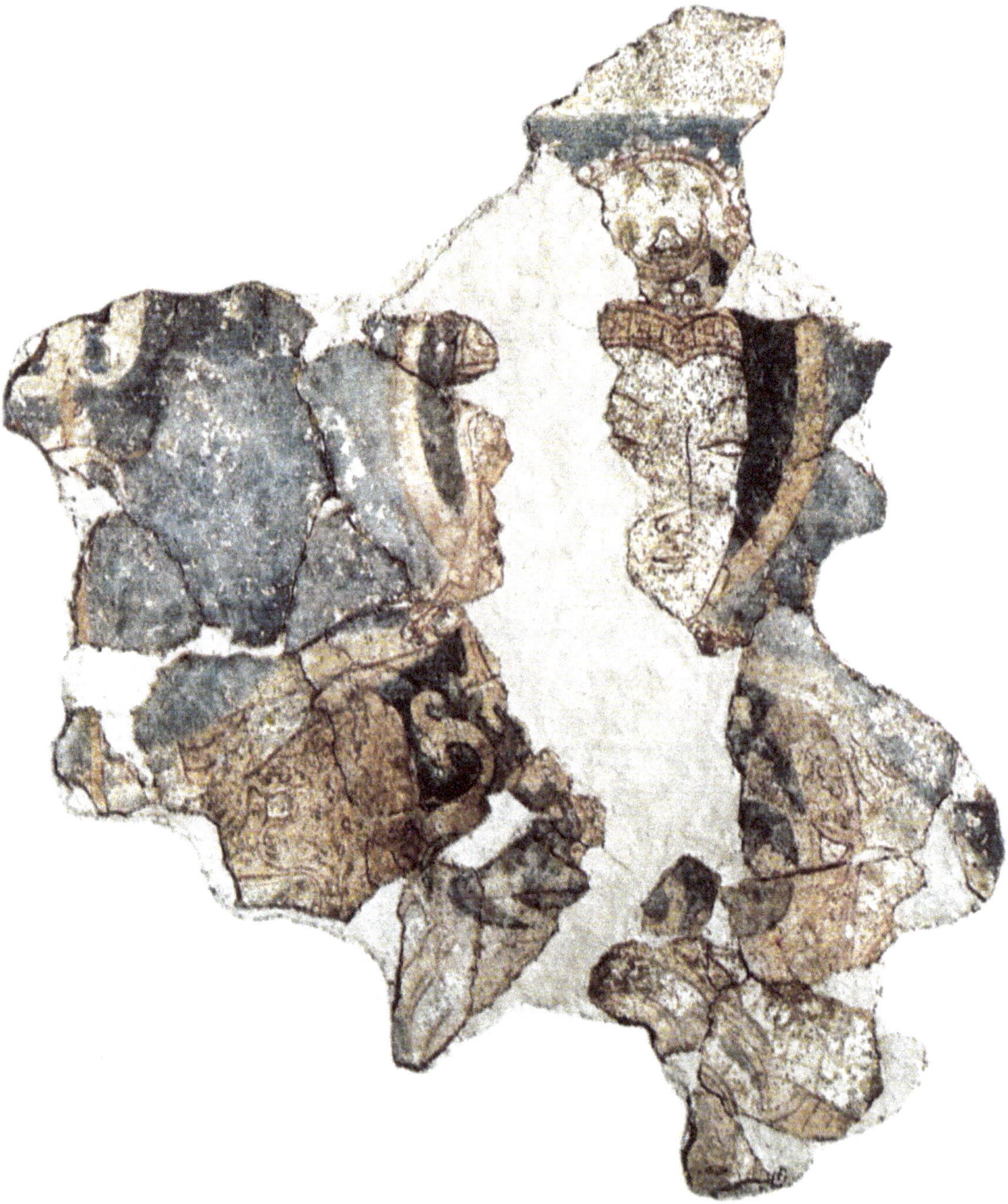

29. Wēšparkar, upper register of the eastern wall of the "Small hall", Bunjikat (Sokolovsky 2009: Fig. 93).

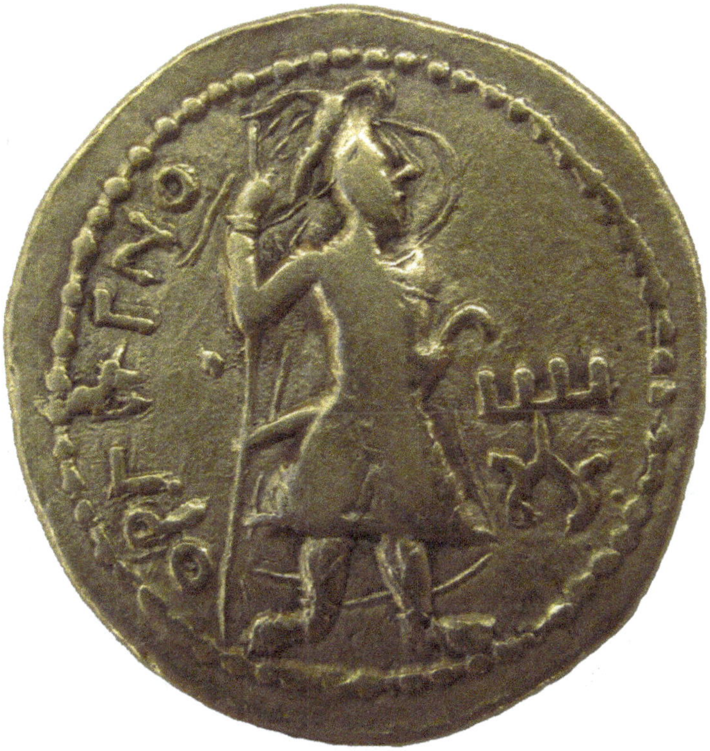

30. Orlagno on a Kushan coin (Osmund Bopearachchi).

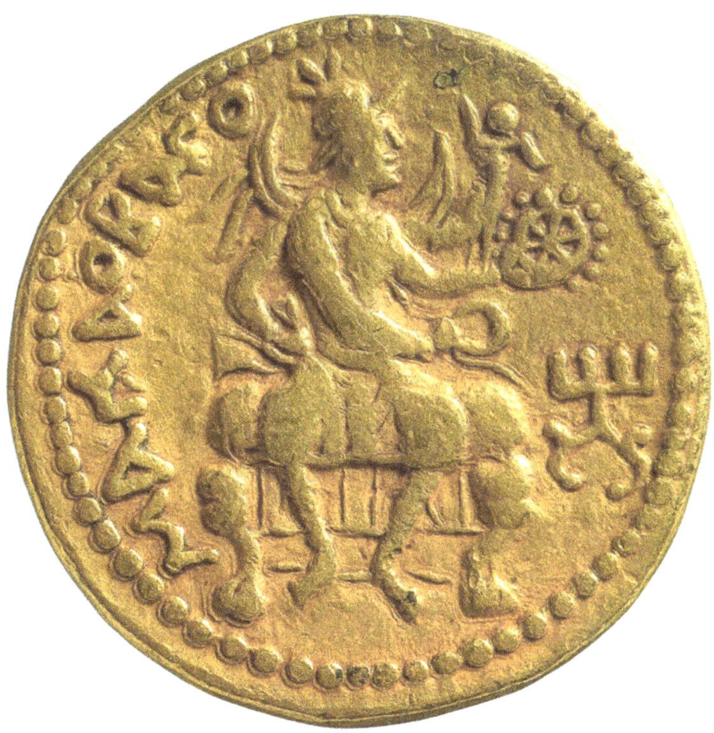

31. Manaobago on a Kushan coin (Frantz Grenet).

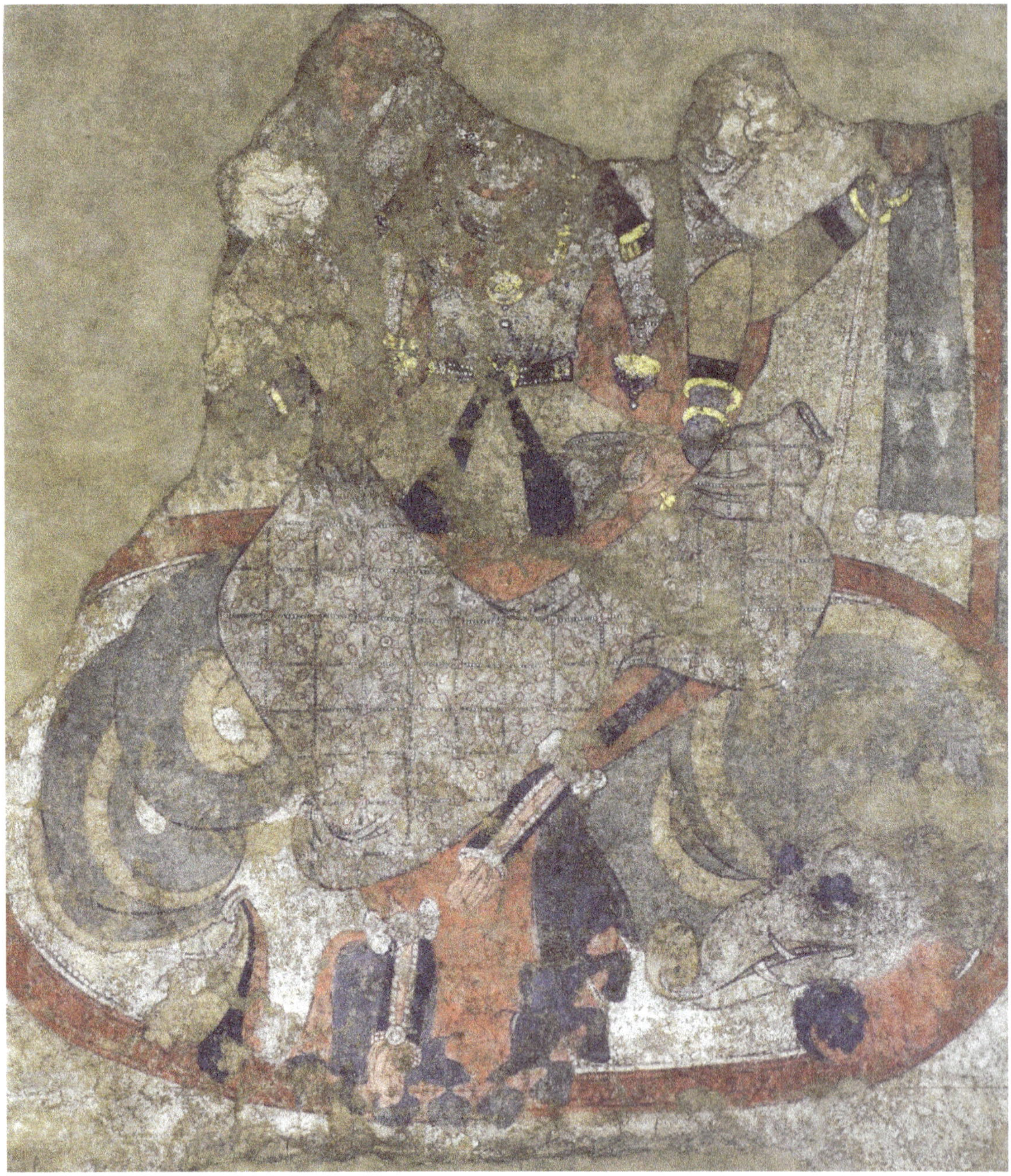

32. A four-armed goddess on a dragon, Panjikent Temple II/5–6 (Marshak 2009: 17).

www.ingramcontent.com/pod-product-compliance
Lightning Source LLC
Chambersburg PA
CBHW080715200926
51611CB00007B/67
* 9 7 8 9 0 0 4 3 6 2 3 4 5 *